Pharmacology: An Introduction

fifth edition

Henry Hitner, Ph.D.

Professor,
Department of Biomedical Sciences
Philadelphia College of Osteopathic Medicine
Philadelphia, Pennsylvania

Barbara Nagle, Ph.D.

Director of Program Planning
Medical and Pharmacy Education Director
III Associates
Bryn Mawr, Pennsylvania

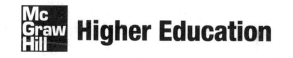 **Higher Education**

Boston   Burr Ridge, IL   Dubuque, IA   Madison, WI   New York   San Francisco   St. Louis
Bangkok   Bogotá   Caracas   Kuala Lumpur   Lisbon   London   Madrid   Mexico City
Milan   Montreal   New Delhi   Santiago   Seoul   Singapore   Sydney   Taipei   Toronto

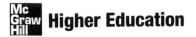

Higher Education

PHARMACOLOGY: AN INTRODUCTION, FIFTH EDITION

Published by McGraw-Hill, a business unit of The McGraw-Hill Companies, Inc., 1221 Avenue of the Americas, New York, NY 10020. Copyright © 2005, 1999, 1994, 1987 by The McGraw-Hill Companies, Inc. All rights reserved. Copyright © 1980 by the Bobbs-Merrill Company. All rights reserved. No part of this publication may be reproduced or distributed in any form or by any means, or stored in a database or retrieval system, without the prior written consent of The McGraw-Hill Companies, Inc., including, but not limited to, in any network or other electronic storage or transmission, or broadcast for distance learning.

Some ancillaries, including electronic and print components, may not be available to customers outside the United States.

♻ This book is printed on recycled, acid-free paper containing 10% postconsumer waste.

4 5 6 7 8 9 0 QPD/QPD 0 9 8 7

ISBN–13: 978–0–07–312275–5
ISBN–10: 0–07–312275–0

Publisher: *David T. Culverwell*
Senior Sponsoring Editor: *Roxan Kinsey*
Developmental Editor: *Patricia Forrest*
Senior Project Manager: *Sheila M. Frank*
Production Supervisor: *Kara Kudronowicz*
Senior Designer: *David W. Hash*
Cover/Interior Designer: *Rokusek Design*
(USE) Cover Images: *©Photodisc Vol. 59*
Compositor: *Carlisle Communications, Ltd.*
Typeface: *9.5/13 Stone Serif*
Printer: *Quebecor World Dubuque, IA*

Library of Congress Cataloging-in-Publication Data

Hitner, Henry.
    Pharmocology: An Introduction / Henry Hitner, Barbara T. Nagle — 5th ed.
        p.   cm.
    Includes bibliographical references and index.
    ISBN 0–07–312275–0
    1. Pharmacology.   I. Nagle, Barbara T.   II. Title

RM300.H57   2005
615.5'8--dc22
                                                    2004040168
                                                            CIP

WARNING NOTICE: The clinical procedures, medicines, dosages, and other matters described in this publication are based upon research of current literature and consultation with knowledgeable persons in the field. The procedures and matters described in this text reflect currently accepted clinical practice. However, this information cannot and should not be relied upon as necessarily applicable to a given individual's case. Accordingly, each person must be separately diagnosed to discern the patient's unique circumstances. Likewise, the manufacturer's package insert for current drug product information should be consulted before administering any drug. Publisher disclaims all liability for any inaccuracies, omissions, misuse, or misunderstanding of the information contained in this publication. Publisher cautions that this publication is not intended as a substitute for the professional judgment of trained medical personnel.

www.mhhe.com

BRIEF CONTENTS

chapter 1   PHARMACOLOGY: AN INTRODUCTION   2

chapter 2   BIOLOGICAL FACTORS AFFECTING THE ACTION OF DRUGS   14

chapter 3   GERIATRIC PHARMACOLOGY   30

chapter 4   MATH REVIEW AND DOSAGE CALCULATIONS   39

chapter 5   AUTONOMIC NERVOUS SYSTEM   51

chapter 6   DRUGS AFFECTING THE SYMPATHETIC NERVOUS SYSTEM   57

chapter 7   DRUGS AFFECTING THE PARASYMPATHETIC NERVOUS SYSTEM   70

chapter 8   DRUGS AFFECTING THE AUTONOMIC GANGLIA   82

chapter 9   SKELETAL MUSCLE RELAXANTS   87

chapter 10   LOCAL ANESTHETICS   98

chapter 11   INTRODUCTION TO THE CENTRAL NERVOUS SYSTEM   111

chapter 12   SEDATIVE-HYPNOTIC DRUGS AND ALCOHOL   118

chapter 13   ANTIPSYCHOTIC AND ANTIANXIETY DRUGS   131

chapter 14   ANTIDEPRESSANTS, PSYCHOMOTOR STIMULANTS, AND LITHIUM   143

chapter 15   PSYCHOTOMIMETIC DRUGS OF ABUSE   154

chapter 16   ANTIEPILEPTIC DRUGS   166

chapter 17   ANTIPARKINSON DRUGS   175

chapter 18   GENERAL ANESTHETICS   183

chapter 19   OPIOID (NARCOTIC) ANALGESICS   193

chapter 20   ANALGESICS NONOPIOID, ANTIINFLAMMATORY, AND ANTIGOUT DRUGS   211

chapter 21   CARDIAC PHYSIOLOGY AND PATHOLOGY   232

chapter 22   CARDIAC GLYCOSIDES AND THE TREATMENT OF CONGESTIVE HEART FAILURE   238

chapter 23   ANTIARRHYTHMIC DRUGS   245

chapter 24   ANTIANGINAL DRUGS   256

chapter 25   DIURETICS   265

chapter 26   ANTIHYPERTENSIVE DRUGS   279

chapter 27   ANTICOAGULANTS AND COAGULANTS   288

chapter 28   NUTRITION AND THERAPY   305

chapter 29   HYPOLIPIDEMIC DRUGS   321

chapter 30   ANTIANEMICS   332

chapter 31   ANTIALLERGIC AND ANTIHISTAMINIC DRUGS   346

chapter 32   BRONCHODILATOR DRUGS AND THE TREATMENT OF ASTHMA   358

chapter 33   THERAPY OF GASTROINTESTINAL DISORDERS: GERD, ULCERS, AND VOMITING   370

chapter 34   AGENTS THAT AFFECT INTESTINAL MOTILITY   397

chapter 35   INTRODUCTION TO THE ENDOCRINE SYSTEM   408

chapter 36   ADRENAL STEROIDS   415

chapter 37   GONADAL HORMONES AND THE ORAL CONTRACEPTIVES   427

chapter 38   DRUGS AFFECTING THE THYROID AND PARATHYROID GLANDS AND BONE DEGENERATION   450

chapter 39   PANCREATIC HORMONES AND ANTIDIABETIC DRUGS   464

chapter 40   POSTERIOR PITUITARY HORMONES AND DRUGS AFFECTING UTERINE MUSCLE   484

chapter 41   ANTIBACTERIAL AGENTS   494

chapter 42   ANTIFUNGAL AND ANTIVIRAL (AIDS) DRUGS   511

chapter 43   ANTIPROTOZOAL AND ANTHELMINTIC DRUGS   542

chapter 44   ANTISEPTICS AND DISINFECTANTS   556

chapter 45   ANTINEOPLASTIC AGENTS   566

chapter 46   IMMUNOPHARMACOLOGY   576

TABLE OF CONTENTS

part I

GENERAL CONCEPTS   1

chapter 1

PHARMACOLOGY: AN INTRODUCTION   2

Drug Sources   3
Terminology Related to Drug Effects   4
Basic Concepts in Pharmacology   5
Drug Safety   7
Drug Nomenclature   8
Chapter Review   10

chapter 2

BIOLOGICAL FACTORS AFFECTING THE ACTION OF DRUGS   14

Drug Forms   15
Routes of Administration   17
Drug Absorption   17
Drug Distribution   19
Drug Metabolism   20
Drug Excretion   20
Half-Life   21
Blood Drug Levels   21
Bioavailablility   21
Factors of Individual Variation   22
Pediatric Drug Considerations   23
Drug Interactions   25
Terminology Associated With Chronic Drug Use and Abuse   25
Chapter Review   27

chapter 3

GERIATRIC PHARMACOLOGY   30

Drug Use in the Elderly   31
Effects of Age on Drug Response   33
Drug Compliance in the Elderly   34
Chapter Review   36

chapter 4

MATH REVIEW AND DOSAGE CALCULATIONS   39

Fractions, Decimals, and Percents   40
Dosage Calculations   42
Systems of Measurement   42
Monitoring IV Infusion Rates   46
Chapter Review   48

part II

PHARMACOLOGY OF THE PERIPHERAL NERVOUS SYSTEM   50

chapter 5

AUTONOMIC NERVOUS SYSTEM   51

Nervous System Organization   52
Physiology and Pharmacology   52
Parasympathetic and Sympathetic Divisions   52
Chapter Review   55

chapter 6

DRUGS AFFECTING THE SYMPATHETIC NERVOUS SYSTEM   57

Adrenergic Nerve Endings   58
Norepinephrine Versus Epinephrine   58
Adrenergic Receptors   58
Alpha-Adrenergic Drugs   60
Beta-Adrenergic Drugs   60
Dopamine   62
Alpha-Adrenergic Blocking Drugs   62
Beta-Adrenergic Blocking Drugs   63
Adrenergic Neuronal Blocking Drugs   65
Chapter Review   67

chapter 7

DRUGS AFFECTING THE PARASYMPATHETIC NERVOUS SYSTEM   70

Parasympathetic System   71
Cholinergic Drugs   73
Anticholinergic Drugs   76
Chapter Review   79

chapter 8

DRUGS AFFECTING THE AUTONOMIC GANGLIA   82

Ganglionic Drugs   83
Chapter Review   85

chapter 9

SKELETAL MUSCLE RELAXANTS   87

Clinical Indications   88
Peripherally Acting Skeletal Muscle
   Relaxants   88
Direct-Acting Skeletal Muscle Relaxants   91
Centrally Acting Skeletal Muscle
   Relaxants   92
Chapter Review   95

chapter 10

LOCAL ANESTHETICS   98

Mechanisms of Action   99
Pharmacology   99
Routes of Administration   100
Adverse Effects   102
Clinical Applications   103
Chapter Review   106

part III

PHARMACOLOGY OF THE CENTRAL NERVOUS SYSTEM   109

chapter 11

INTRODUCTION TO THE CENTRAL NERVOUS SYSTEM   111

Parts of the Brain   112
Functional Components   114
Chapter Review   116

chapter 12

SEDATIVE-HYPNOTIC DRUGS AND ALCOHOL   118

Sleep Cycle   119
Barbiturate Sedatives and Hypnotics   120
Benzodiazepines   123
Miscellaneous Nonbarbiturates   124
Alcohol   125
Chapter Review   128

chapter 13

ANTIPSYCHOTIC AND ANTIANXIETY DRUGS   131

Types of Mental Illness   132
Antipsychotic Drugs   132
Antianxiety Drugs   136
Chapter Review   140

chapter 14

ANTIDEPRESSANTS, PSYCHOMOTOR STIMULANTS, AND LITHIUM   143

Types of Depression   144
Drugs Used to Treat Depression   144
Chapter Review   151

chapter 15

PSYCHOTOMIMETIC DRUGS OF ABUSE   154

LSD-Type Hallucinogens   155
Psychomotor Stimulants   157
Miscellaneous Psychotomimetic Drugs   160
Chapter Review   163

chapter 16

ANTIEPILEPTIC DRUGS   166

Types of Epilepsy   167
Drugs Used to Control Epilepsy   168
Drugs Used in the Treatment of Absence
   Seizures   170
Treatment of Status Epilepticus   171
Use of Antiepileptic Drugs
   During Pregnancy   171
Antiepileptic Drug Interactions   171
Chapter Review   172

chapter 17

ANTIPARKINSON DRUGS   175

Neurotransmitters Affecting the
  Basal Ganglia   176
Drug Therapy   176
Chapter Review   181

chapter 18

GENERAL ANESTHETICS   183

General Anesthesia   184
Use of General Anesthetics   186
Chapter Review   191

chapter 19

OPIOID (NARCOTIC) ANALGESICS   193

Pain   195
Opioid Analgesics   196
Site and Mechanism of Action   199
Pharmacological Effects   199
Absorption and Metabolism   203
Adverse Effects   203
Acute Opioid Poisoning   204
Opioid Antagonists   204
Special Considerations   205
Drug Interactions   206
Chapter Review   208

chapter 20

ANALGESICS NONOPIOD, ANTIINFLAMMATORY, AND ANTIGOUT DRUGS   211

Inflammation Antiinflammatory Drugs   212
Nonopioid Analgesics   213
Salicylates   217
Acetaminophen   220
Drugs Useful in Treating Gout   222
Drug Interactions   224
Chapter Review   227

part IV

PHARMACOLOGY OF THE HEART   231

chapter 21

CARDIAC PHYSIOLOGY AND PATHOLOGY   232

Cardiac Function   233
Main Diseases of the Heart   234
Chapter Review   236

chapter 22

CARDIAC GLYCOSIDES AND THE TREATMENT OF CONGESTIVE HEART FAILURE   238

Cardiac Glycosides   239
Diuretic Therapy of CHF   241
Chapter Review   243

chapter 23

ANTIARRHYTHMIC DRUGS   245

Types of Arrhythmias   246
Class 1 Antiarrhythmic Drugs   248
Class 2 Antiarrhythmic Drugs   251
Class 3 Antiarrhythmic Drugs   252
Class 4 Antiarrhythmic Drugs   252
Other Antiarrhythmic Drugs   253
Special Considerations   253
Chapter Review   254

chapter 24

ANTIANGINAL DRUGS   256

Nitrites and Nitrates   257
Beta-Adrenergic Blocking Drugs   259
Calcium Antagonists   259
Clinical Indications for Antianginal
  Drugs   260
Chapter Review   261

part V

PHARMACOLOGY OF THE VASCULAR AND RENAL SYSTEMS 263

chapter 25

DIURETICS 265

Renal Physiology 266
Conditions Associated With Renal
Dysfunction 268
Osmotic Diuretics 269
Carbonic Anhydrase Inhibitors 270
Thiazide and Thiazide-Like Diuretics 271
Organic Acid Diuretics 273
Potassium-Sparing Diuretics 273
Miscellaneous Diuretics 274
Special Considerations 274
Drug Interactions and Incompatibilities 275
Overdose 276
Chapter Review 277

chapter 26

ANTIHYPERTENSIVE DRUGS 279

Physiological Factors Controlling
Blood Pressure 280
Antihypertensive Therapy 281
Chapter Review 286

chapter 27

ANTICOAGULANTS AND COAGULANTS 000

Coagulation 288
Anticoagulant Mechanism of Action 289
Monitoring Coagulation 296
Thrombolytic Enzymes 299
Coagulants/Hemostatics 300
Chapter Review 302

chapter 28

NUTRITION AND THERAPY 305

Nutrients 306
Vitamins 309
Fat-Soluble Vitamins 309
Water-Soluble Vitamins 312
Body Water 314

Minerals 314
Chapter Review 318

chapter 29

HYPOLIPIDEMIC DRUGS 321

Liver Metabolism and Lipoproteins 322
Monitoring Blood Lipid Levels 323
Bile Acid Sequestrants 324
HMG-CoA Reductase Inhibitors 325
Miscellaneous Hypolipidemics 326
Clinical Indications 327
Contraindications 327
Drug Interactions 327
Chapter Review 330

chapter 30

ANTIANEMICS 332

Causes of Anemia 333
Iron Deficiency Anemia 334
Cyanocobalamin Deficiency 336
Folic Acid Deficiency 338
Erythropoetin 340
Chapter Review 342

part VI

DRUGS THAT AFFECT THE RESPIRATORY SYSTEM 345

chapter 31

ANTIALLERGIC AND ANTIHISTAMINIC DRUGS 346

Action of Histamine 347
Antiallergic Agents 348
Antihistaminic Agents 350
Chapter Review 356

chapter 32

BRONCHODILATOR DRUGS AND THE TREATMENT OF ASTHMA 358

Respiratory Diseases 359
Role of the Autonomic Nervous System 360
Bronchodilator Drugs 361

Antiinflammatory Drugs   363
Antiallergic Agents   364
Mucolytics   364
Expectorants   364
Chapter Review   365

part VII

PHARMACOLOGY OF THE GI TRACT   369

chapter 33

THERAPY OF GASTROINTESTINAL DISORDERS: GERD, ULCERS, AND VOMITING   370

Digestion and Ulcer Production   371
Management of Ulcers   373
Management of Gastroesophageal Reflux
   Disease (GERD)   373
Antisecretory Drugs   376
Antacids   384
Sucralfate   386
Management of Emesis   387
Chapter Review   393

chapter 34

AGENTS THAT AFFECT INTESTINAL MOTILITY   397

Bowel Function   398
Antidiarrheals   398
Laxatives and Cathartics   401
Chapter Review   405

part VIII

PHARMACOLOGY OF THE ENDOCRINE SYSTEM   407

chapter 35

INTRODUCTION TO THE ENDOCRINE SYSTEM   408

Endocrine System   409
Uses of Hormones   409
Chapter Review   413

chapter 36

ADRENAL STEROIDS   415

Glucocorticoids   416
Mineralocorticoids   420
Special Considerations   421
Drug Interactions   423
Chapter Review   425

chapter 37

GONADAL HORMONES AND THE ORAL CONTRACEPTIVES   427

Female Sex Hormones   428
Male Sex Hormones (Androgens)   441
Impotence   444
Chapter Review   447

chapter 38

DRUGS AFFECTING THE THYROID AND PARATHYROID GLANDS AND BONE DEGENERATION   450

Thyroid Function, Pharmacology,
   and Disorders   451
Parathyroid Hormones   456
Chapter Review   461

chapter 39

PANCREATIC HORMONES AND ANTIDIABETIC DRUGS   464

Pancreatic Endocrine Function   465
Diabetes Mellitus   465
Treatment of Diabetes   466
Chapter Review   481

chapter 40

POSTERIOR PITUITARY HORMONES AND DRUGS AFFECTING UTERINE MUSCLE   484

Diabetes Insipidus   485
Drugs Affecting Uterine Muscle   486
Tocolytics   487
Chapter Review   489

part IX

PHARMACOLOGY OF INFECTIOUS DISEASES 493

chapter 41

ANTIBACTERIAL AGENTS 494

Morphology of Bacteria 495
Chemotherapy 496
Penicillins 497
Cephalosporins 499
Aminoglycosides 501
Tetracyclines 502
Sulfonamides 503
Macrolide Antibiotics 504
Fluroquinolone Antimicrobials 505
Miscellaneous Antimicrobial Drugs 505
Drugs Used to Treat Tuberculosis 506
Chemoprophylaxis 507
Chapter Review 508

chapter 42

ANTIFUNGAL AND ANTIVIRAL (AIDS) DRUGS 511

Antifungal Drugs 512
Viral Diseases and Antiviral Drugs 519
Antiviral Drugs 524
Drug Interactions 532
Chapter Review 538

chapter 43

ANTIPROTOZOAL AND ANTHELMINTIC DRUGS 542

Protozoal Infections 543
Malaria 543
Dysentery 547
Other Protozoal Infections 548
Anthelmintic Drugs 549
Chapter Review 553

chapter 44

ANTISEPTICS AND DISINFECTANTS 556

Mechanism of Action 557
Chapter Review 563

part X

ANTINEOPLASTICS AND DRUGS AFFECTING THE IMMUNE SYSTEM 565

chapter 45

ANTINEOPLASTIC AGENTS 566

Types of Cancer 567
Alkylating Drugs 568
Antimetabolites 569
Miscellaneous Antineoplastic Drugs 570
Chapter Review 573

chapter 46

IMMUNOPHARMACOLOGY 576

Immune System 577
Immunosuppressive Drugs 578
Immunostimulant Drugs 581
Chapter Review 582

PREFACE

Pharmacology is a science that deals with the study of drugs. The last half of the twentieth century has witnessed a revolution in pharmacology, an explosion of knowledge that has given rise to many new areas of research. Consequently, the number of drugs has significantly increased. Pharmacology is an ever-changing, growing body of information that continually demands greater amounts of time and education from those in the health professions.

Personnel in the allied health and nursing professions spend much of their working time in direct contact with patients – observing, treating, and administering to the countless requirements and demands that constitute effective and responsible patient care. Therefore, it is important that students in health professions acquire a sound basic understanding of pharmacology as it relates to their particular needs.

Pharmacology: An Introduction is designed for a variety of allied health programs requiring an understanding of pharmacology. It attempts to present a basic rationale for understanding current drug therapy. The drug information and chapter features are designed to be applicable and adaptable to many different educational programs.

In most allied health curricula, pharmacology appears after the basic courses in anatomy and physiology. This textbook presents drugs according to their therapeutic applications. In each section, pertinent physiology and related diseases are reviewed before the pharmacology of the drugs is discussed. This approach by body system serves to provide the necessary background information and to refresh the student's memory of previously learned material through which the therapeutic action of the drugs can be clearly understood.

The fifth edition of *Pharmacology: An Introduction* has been completely updated. Emphasis is placed on current drug therapy. The discussion of each drug classification concentrates on the mechanisms of action, main therapeutic effects, clinical indications, adverse reactions, and drug interactions. Pertinent information on absorption, metabolism, excretion, and other special considerations are also included when appropriate.

Pertinent features of *Pharmacology: An Introduction* include chapters on Geriatric Pharmacology, Nutrition and Vitamins, and a new section on pediatric pharmacology. Also an information diagram for therapeutic drug classes called Drug Class at a Glance is included. This diagram appears in the beginning of each drug chapter and summarizes the over-the-counter and prescription status, FDA pregnancy categories, and main clinical indications for the drugs contained within that chapter. In addition, sections entitled Patient Administration and Monitoring appear in each of the drug chapters. This section summarizes important patient information and patient instructions. A new open and visual design enhances these features and aids in student retention of important concepts.

Drug dosages are included in many of the tables. In addition, both generic and examples of drug trade names are given. The trade name will always appear in italic type within parentheses. It must be emphasized that trade names are subject to constant additions and deletions as companies begin or cease production of a given drug product.

The chapter reviews at the end of each chapter provide immediate reinforcement of terminology and pharmacological concepts important for acquiring knowledge. The clinically relevant on-the-job questions allow students more opportunity to practice critical thinking skills. Another feature is the addition of Internet activities to many of the chapters. This feature provides websites, directions, and suggestions that can be used to access additional information on diseases and the drugs used to treat them.

The Instructor's Manual provides the instructor with materials to help organize lessons and classroom interaction. The manual includes teaching strategies, answers to chapter review questions, and chapter tests.

Students should realize that completion of an introductory pharmacology course is only the beginning step in understanding this complex subject. The information gained in pharmacology must be correlated with other courses and with clinical experience in order to provide responsible patient care.

REVIEWERS

A sincere thanks to our reviewers who helped shape the direction of this book.

Judith K. Ehninger, RN, BS, CMA
Lehigh Carbon Community College

Jannie R. Adams, Ph.D., RN, BSN-MSA-HSA
Clayton College & State University

Dorothy S. Hall, RN, MSN, CST
Ivy Tech State College

Phyllis C. Caviness, RN, BSN, MED
Richmond Community College
Hamlet, NC

Edward J. Barbieri, Ph.D.
National Medical Services

Todd Kudronowicz
Wal-Mart Pharmacy

Jerry Young
El Centro-Dallas

Joan Matsukawa
University of Hawaii
Kapi'olani Community College

April Schroer
San Antonio, TX

Cheri Smith, BS
El Paso Community College

Jim Palmer, Ph.D.
Director Pharmacy Technician Program
Walters State Community College

Cindy B. Johnson, R. Ph, MSW
Arapalwe Community College
Littleton, CO

Tony Ford
Portsmouth, VA

Richelle Laipply
University of Akron
Akron, OH

Suzanne Bitters
CHI Institute
Southampton, PA

Jack L. Jansen, BSN
Medical Department Chair
Las Vegas College
Las Vegas, NV

Candy Dailey, RN, CMA
Nicolet Area Technical College
Rhinelander, WI

Crystal Celeste Contreras-Hinojosa, C. Ph. T.
South Texas Vo-Tech
McAllen, TX

Margaret Lentz, RN, BSN, CMA
Western Wisconsin Technical College
LaCrosse, WI 54601

Barbara E. Kennedy, RN C.Ph.T.
Blair College
Colorado Springs, CO

Teresa S. Frazier, MS, RN
Northeast Technology Center
Afton, KS & Pryar, OK

Sandra Schuler
Montgomery College

Mary Marks, MSN, RN-BC
Mitchell Community College
Mooresville, NC

Connie Price, RN
Center for Technical Studies
Plymouth Meeting, PA

Dr. John A. Ridlon, Ph.D.
Corinthian Colleges
San Antonio, TX

Michael Wolchonok, M.D.
Bay State College
Boston, MA

Sajona Weaver
Sinclair Community College
Dayton, OH

Claudia L. Johnson, MSN, RNC, APN
Polytech Adult Education
Woodside, DE

James Lear
National Institute of Technology
Houston, TX

Chris Crigger, CPht
Pharmacy Technician Instructor
San Antonio College

part

1

GENERAL CONCEPTS

Chapter 1

Pharmacology: An Introduction

Drug Sources
Terminology Related to Drug
   Effects
Basic Concepts in Pharmacology
Drug Safety
Drug Nomenclature

Chapter 2

Biological Factors Affecting the Action of Drugs

Drug Forms
Routes of Administration
Drug Absorption
Drug Distribution
Drug Metabolism
Drug Excretion
Half-Life
Blood Drug Levels
Bioavailability

Factors of Individual Variation
Pediatric Drug Considerations
Drug Interactions
Terminology Associated With
   Chronic Drug Use and Abuse

Chapter 3

Geriatric Pharmacology

Drug Use in the Elderly
Effects of Age on Drug Response
Drug Compliance in the Elderly

Chapter 4

Math Review and Dosage Calculations

Fractions, Decimals, and Percents
Dosage Calculations
Systems of Measurement
Monitoring IV Infusion Rates

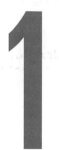

PHARMACOLOGY: AN INTRODUCTION

CHAPTER FOCUS

This chapter provides an introduction to basic pharmacology. It also describes the properties of drugs, their sources, how drugs produce effects, and drug nomenclature.

CHAPTER OBJECTIVES

After studying this chapter, you should be able to

- define pharmacology and its major subdivisions.

- describe what a drug is and explain the differences between a therapeutic effect, side effect, and toxic effect.

- identify a drug receptor and trace how agonists and antagonists interact with receptors.

- explain the relationship between drug dosage and drug response, and the relationship between drug response and time.

- explain drug safety and therapeutic index.

- describe three names by which drugs are known.

- list two common drug reference books.

Key Terms

adverse effect: general term for undesirable and potentially harmful drug effect.

agonist: drug that binds to its receptor and produces a drug action.

antagonist: drug that binds to its receptor and prevents other drugs or substances from producing an effect.

chemical name: name that defines the chemical composition of a drug.

contraindications: situations or conditions when a certain drug should not be administered.

controlled substance: drug that has the potential for abuse and thus is regulated by law.

dose: exact amount of a drug that is administered in order to produce a specific effect.

drug: chemical substance that produces a change in body function.

drug indications: intended or indicated uses for any drug.

ED50:   effective dose 50, or dose that will produce an effect that is half of the maximal response.

generic name: nonproprietary, or common, name of a drug.

LD50:   lethal dose 50, or dose that will kill 50 percent of the animals tested.

mechanism of action: explanation of how a drug produces its effects.

nonprescription, over-the-counter (OTC) drug: drug that can be purchased without the services of a physician.

pharmacology: study of drugs.

potency: measure of the strength, or concentration, of a drug required to produce a specific effect.

prescription drug: drug for which dispensing requires a written or phone order that can only be issued by or under the direction of a licensed physician.

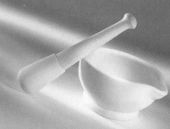

受体
receptor: specific location on a cell membrane or within the cell where a drug attaches to produce its effect.

side effect: drug effect other than the therapeutic effect that is usually undesirable but not harmful.

site of action: location within the body where a drug exerts its therapeutic effect, often a type of specific receptor.

[saraputic]
therapeutic effect: desired drug effect to alleviate some condition or symptom of disease.

therapeutic index (TI): ratio of the LD50 to the ED50.

toxic effect: undesirable drug effect that implies drug poisoning; can be very harmful or life-threatening.

trade name: patented proprietary name of drug sold by a specific drug manufacturer.

INTRODUCTION

Pharmacology is the study of drugs. A drug can be any substance that, when administered to living organisms, produces a change in function. Thus, substances such as water, metals (iron), or insecticides can be classified as drugs. However, the term *drug* commonly means any medication that is used for treating disease.

Pharmacology refers to a very broad area of study. It can be broken down into several topics, each one a major subject area of study. Table 1:1 lists some of these areas. Throughout this book, tables organize information so that the pharmacology of each drug class can be easily understood.

DRUG SOURCES

A logical question to ask about pharmacology is "Where do drugs come from?" There are several sources of drugs. In the early days of medicine, most drugs were obtained from plant or animal sources. Plants and living organisms contain active substances that can be isolated, purified, and formulated into effective drug preparations. Examples of drugs derived from plants that are still widely used today include the analgesics [an·no·gesic] morphine and codeine, which were obtained from the poppy plant (*Papver somniferum*); the heart drug digitalis, which was obtained from the purple foxglove (*Digitalis purpurea*); and the antimalarial drug quinine, which was obtained

a drug used to reduce pain.

	Major Areas of Pharmacology
TABLE 1:1	

AREA	DESCRIPTION
Pharmacodynamics	Study of the action of drugs on living tissue
Pharmacokinetics	Study of the processes of drug absorption, distribution, metabolism, and excretion
Pharmacotherapeutics	Study of the use of drugs in treating disease
Pharmacy	Science of preparing and dispensing medicines
Posology	Study of the amount of drug that is required to produce therapeutic effects
Toxicology	Study of the harmful effects of drugs on living tissue

from the bark of the cinchona tree. Recently, a new anticancer drug, paclitaxel, was isolated from the yew tree. The search for new plant drugs is still very active. It is also interesting that many of the drugs of abuse such as cocaine, marijuana, mescaline, heroin, and others are derived from plants. Most of these drugs were used for hundreds of years by many different cultures in their religious and ritual ceremonies. Drugs obtained from living organisms include hormones such as insulin (from the pig) and growth hormone from pituitary glands. In addition, antibiotics such as cephalosporins and aminoglycosides have been derived from bacteria. The early history of pharmacology is filled with many interesting stories of discovery and medical experimentation. Textbooks devoted to the history of medicine and pharmacology are the best sources for additional information. Despite the many examples of drugs obtained from plants and living organisms, the main source of new drugs today is from chemical synthesis. Also, many of the drugs that once were obtained from plants and animals are now chemically synthesized in pharmaceutical laboratories.

TERMINOLOGY RELATED TO DRUG EFFECTS

Another basic question that should be answered is "What actually is a **drug?**" Every pure drug is a chemical compound with a specific chemical structure. Because of its structure, a drug has certain properties that are usually divided into chemical properties and biological properties. The properties of any drug determine what effects will be produced when the drug is administered. An important fact to remember is that, structurally, the human body is composed mostly of cells, even though these cells are highly organized into tissues, organs, and systems. Consequently, drugs produce effects by influencing the function of cells.

Pharmacologists know that all drugs produce more than one effect. Every drug produces its intended effect, or **therapeutic effect,** along with other effects. The therapeutic use(s) of any drug is referred to as the **drug indication,** meaning indications for use. The term **contraindication** refers to the situation or circumstance when a particular drug should *not* be used. Some drug effects, other than therapeutic effects, are described as undesirable. Undesired

drug effects are categorized as side effects, adverse effects, and toxic effects.

Side Effects

Many **side effects** are more of a nuisance than they are harmful. The dry mouth and sedation caused by some antihistamine drugs is an example. In many cases drug side effects must be tolerated in order to benefit from the therapeutic actions of the drug.

Adverse Effects

Adverse effects are also undesired effects, but these are effects that may be harmful (persistent diarrhea, vomiting, or central nervous system [CNS] disturbances such as confusion) or that with prolonged treatment may cause conditions that affect the function of vital organs such as the liver or kidney. Reduction of dosage or switching to an alternative drug will often avoid or minimize these harmful consequences.

Toxic Effects

Toxic effects, or toxicity, implies drug poisoning, the consequences of which can be extremely harmful and may be life-threatening. In these situations, the drug must be stopped and supportive treatment and the administration of antidotes may be required.

The term most frequently used to describe the undesirable effects of drugs is *adverse effects*. However, you should be familiar with the other terms because they are used and, if used correctly, describe the nature and potential severity of undesired drug effects.

Most drugs will cause all three types of undesired effects, depending on the dose administered. At low doses, side effects are common and often expected. At higher doses, additional adverse effects may appear. At very high doses, toxic effects may occur that can be fatal. Consequently, the undesired effects produced by most drugs are often a function of dosage, which is why a well-known physician from the Middle Ages, Paracelsus (1493–1541), made the famous statement "only the dose separates a drug from a poison"—and we could add, "a therapeutic effect from a toxic effect." Allied health personnel spend the majority of their time in patient contact. Therefore, they have an important responsibility to observe the undesired effects of drugs, to recognize the side effects that are often expected, and to identify and report the adverse and toxic effects that are potentially harmful and that often require medical attention.

BASIC CONCEPTS IN PHARMACOLOGY

As in any subject, fundamental principles and concepts form the basis upon which additional information can be added. Pharmacology is no exception, and the following basic concepts apply to any drug.

Site of Action

The **site of action** of a drug is the location within the body where the drug exerts its therapeutic effect. The site of action of some drugs is not known; however, the site of action for most drugs has been determined. For example, the site of action of aspirin to reduce fever is in an area of the brain known as the hypothalamus. Within the hypothalamus the temperature-regulating center controls and maintains body temperature. Aspirin alters the activity of the hypothalamus so that body temperature is reduced. Throughout this book, when the site of drug action is known or suspected, it will be presented.

Mechanism of Action

Mechanism of action explains how a drug produces its effects. For example, local anesthetic agents produce a loss of pain sensation by interrupting nerve conduction in sensory nerves. In order for nerve impulses to be conducted, sodium ions must pass through the nerve membrane. Local anesthetic agents attach to the nerve membrane and prevent the passage of sodium ions. Consequently, sensory nerve impulses for pain are not conducted to the pain centers in the brain. Knowledge of the mechanism of action of drugs is essential to understanding why drugs produce the effects that they do.

Receptor Site

Drug action is usually thought to begin after a drug has attached itself to some cell membrane. For a few drugs and for some normal body substances, there seems to be a specific location on certain cells. This area is referred to as the **receptor** site. The attachment, or binding, of a drug to its receptors begins a series of cell changes referred to as the drug action.

When a specific receptor site for a drug is known, that receptor site becomes the site of action for that particular drug. Morphine, an analgesic drug, is an example of a drug thought to bind to specific receptors. The receptors for morphine are located in the brain and are known as the morphine, or opioid, receptors. When morphine binds to its receptors, it produces cell changes that reduce the perception of pain. There are many different pharmacological receptors, and they will be described in the appropriate chapters.

Agonists and Antagonists

Drugs that bind to specific receptors and produce a drug action are called **agonists.** Morphine is an example of an agonist. Drugs that bind to specific receptors but do not produce any drug action are called **antagonists.**

Antagonists are also known as blocking drugs. Usually, antagonists bind to the receptors and prevent other drugs or body substances from producing an effect. Naloxone, a morphine antagonist, is administered to prevent, or antagonize, the effects of morphine in cases of morphine overdose. There are many examples in pharmacology where drug antagonists are used to prevent other substances from exerting an effect.

When both agonist and antagonist drugs are administered together, they compete with each other for the same receptor site. This effect is known as competitive antagonism. The amount of drug action produced depends on which drug (agonist or antagonist) occupies the greatest number of receptors. The actions of a drug agonist and antagonist are illustrated in Figure 1:1.

FIGURE 1:1 Competitive Antagonism at Work

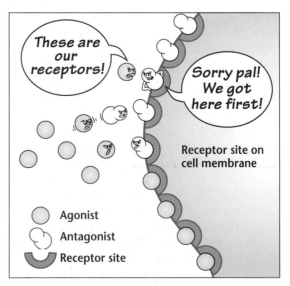

Dose-Response Curve

A fundamental principle of pharmacology is that the response to any drug depends on the amount of drug given. This principle is known as the dose-response relationship. A **dose** is the exact amount of a drug that is administered in order to produce a specific effect. The effect is referred to as the response. When the relationship between the dose and the response is plotted as a graph, it is referred to as a dose-response curve.

Figure 1:2 illustrates the appearance of a typical dose-response curve for two similar drugs. The main feature of the dose-response relationship is that a drug response is proportional to the dose. As the dose increases, so does the magnitude of the response. Eventually, a maximal response is usually attained (100 percent response); further increases in dose do not produce any greater effect. This point on the graph is known as the ceiling effect. The ceiling effect reflects the limit of some drug classes to produce a particular effect. Above a certain dosage no further increase in effect is observed. Doses above those needed to produce the ceiling effect usually cause other undesired, often toxic, drug effects. Drugs within a drug class that are more potent than other drugs in the same class will produce the ceiling effect at a lower dosage, but they will not "raise the ceiling." Drugs that continue to cause an increased effect as long as the dose is increased do not have a ceiling effect.

A graded dose-response curve can be used to evaluate drug response among different drugs. In a graded dose-response curve, the increases in drug dosage are plotted against the increases in drug response. For example, dose-response curves are used to compare the potency of similar drugs. **Potency** is a measure of the strength, or concentration, of a drug required to produce a specific effect. The dose that will produce an effect that is half of the maximal response is referred to as the effective dose 50, or **ED50.**

The ED50 can be used to compare the potency of drugs that produce the same response. In Figure 1:2, the ED50 of drug A is 10 mg while the ED50 of drug B is 20 mg. Therefore, drug A is twice as potent as drug B. Twice the concentration of drug B is needed to produce the same response as drug A.

Quantal (referred to as all-or-none) dose-response curves are used to show the percentage of a human or animal population that responds to a specific drug dosage. This information is important for determining the dosages that are recommended for various treatments. Quantal dose-response curves require an understanding of mathematical statistics that is beyond the scope of this textbook.

Time-Response Curve

The relationship of the drug response and time (duration of action) is known as the time-response relationship. Duration of action is the length of time that a drug continues to produce its effect. Most drugs produce effects over a relatively constant period of time. When the relationship between time and response is plotted on a graph, it is known as a time-response curve. Figure 1:3 illustrates the appearance of a typical time-response curve. In this example, the drug response

FIGURE 1:2 A Typical Dose-Response Curve

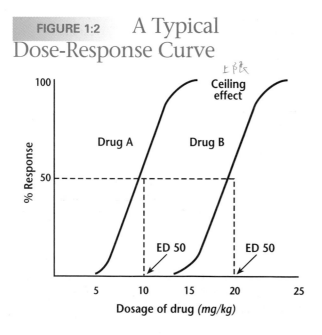

FIGURE 1:3 A Typical Time-Response Curve

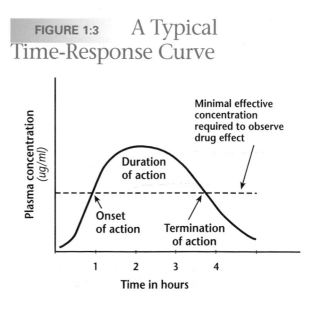

being measured is the plasma concentration of the drug. After drug administration, a certain amount of time is required before a drug will produce an observable effect.

The time from drug administration to the first observable effect is known as the onset of action. The drug response will continue as long as there is an effective concentration of the drug at the site of action. As the drug is metabolized and excreted, the response gradually decreases because the drug level is decreasing. Eventually, the response will no longer be observed. Time-response curves are used for predicting the frequency with which a drug must be administered in order to maintain an effective drug response.

DRUG SAFETY

The federal Food and Drug Administration (FDA) has established guidelines that govern the approval and use of all drugs. Every drug must fulfill two major requirements before it can be approved for use in humans: efficacy (proof of effectiveness) and safety. The drug must be effective in the disease state for which it has been approved. Approved drugs must satisfy specific safety criteria as determined by extensive animal testing and controlled human testing. As discussed previously, the dose separates therapeutic effects from toxic effects.

NOTE TO THE HEALTH CARE PROFESSIONAL

All drugs will act as poisons if taken in excess. Only the dose separates a therapeutic effect from a toxic effect. The goal of drug therapy is to select a dose that is in the therapeutic range and avoid doses that produce toxicity. This task is not easy because many factors influence the amount of drug that reaches its site of action. These factors—such as route of administration, absorption, and drug metabolism—will be discussed in Chapter 2, Biological Factors Affecting the Action of Drugs.

Drug safety receives much attention today. It is a constant source of concern and debate because the public is more aware of the dangers of drugs. In order to receive approval for use in humans, a drug must undergo several years of animal testing and evaluation. Several animal species must be used in order to evaluate the effectiveness and toxicity of a drug. One of the first tests that is performed is the lethal dose 50, or **LD50**. The LD50 is the dose that will kill 50 percent of the animals tested. The results of the LD50 and other tests are used to predict the safety of a drug.

Therapeutic Index

The **therapeutic index (TI)** is a ratio of the LD50 to the ED50 of a drug. It gives an estimate of the relative safety of a drug. The equation is expressed as:

$$TI = LD50/ED50 = 1000 \text{ mg}/100 \text{ mg} = 10$$

In this example, the therapeutic index is 10. This index indicates that ten times as much drug is needed to produce a lethal effect in 50 percent of the animals as is needed to produce the therapeutic effect in 50 percent of the animals. The therapeutic index is used only in animal studies to establish dosage levels for other testing procedures. The goal of drug therapy is to achieve therapeutic effects in all individuals without producing any harmful effects.

Adverse Effects

All drugs produce adverse and toxic effects if taken in excess. Most adverse effects are dose dependent, which means the higher the dose, the greater the chances for producing an adverse effect. Certain tissues are more frequently affected than others. Oral drugs often cause nausea, vomiting, and diarrhea because of gastrointestinal (GI) irritation. The liver, kidneys, brain, and cardiovascular system may be adversely affected because these organs are exposed to the highest concentrations of the drug. Drugs that produce birth defects, such as thalidomide, are known as teratogens. Drugs that promote the growth of cancerous tumors are called carcinogens.

A few adverse effects are not dose dependent. These effects, such as drug idiosyncrasy and drug allergy, are determined by individual variation. Although all human beings are basically similar, there may be minor variations in certain enzymes or other body proteins. These variations may produce changes in drug metabolism that lead to unusual responses to a particular drug. An individual reaction to a drug with an unusual or unexpected response is known as an idiosyncrasy.

Drug allergy occurs when an individual becomes sensitized to a particular drug and produces antibodies against the drug (antigens). Subsequent administration of the drug leads to an antigen-antibody reaction. Antigen-antibody reactions involving drugs usually cause the release of histamine from cells known as mast cells. Histamine produces the characteristic symptoms of allergy, which include rashes, hives, itching, nasal secretion, hypotension, and bronchoconstriction.

In serious allergic reactions, the symptoms may be so severe that death may occur. The term *anaphylaxis* is used to describe these serious allergic reactions.

DRUG NOMENCLATURE

All drugs are chemicals, and many have long **chemical names.** As a result, all drugs are given a shorter name, known as the nonproprietary name, which is usually a contraction of the chemical name. The nonproprietary name is more commonly referred to as the **generic name.**

When the drug is marketed by a pharmaceutical company, it is given a third name, known as the proprietary name, or **trade name.** Since several different pharmaceutical companies may market the same generic drug, there may be several different trade names for any one drug. Figure 1:4 gives three names of a commonly prescribed drug.

Drugs are also divided into prescription and nonprescription drugs. **Prescription drugs** require a written or phone order (the prescription), which can only be issued by or under the direction of a licensed physician, dentist, or veterinarian. The prescription is a legal document that contains instructions for the

pharmacist, who is licensed to dispense prescription medications. **Nonprescription drugs,** usually referred to as **"over-the-counter" (OTC) drugs** (such as aspirin, antacids, cold remedies), can be purchased anywhere and do not require the services of a physician or pharmacist.

Drug References

Medical libraries, hospital libraries, and educational institutions that provide medical education generally stock one or more drug reference books that provide drug information.

The United States Pharmacopeia/National Formulary (USP/NF) is the official drug list recognized by the U.S. government. It provides information concerning the physical and chemical properties of drugs. The *USP/NF* is revised every 5 years and is used primarily by drug manufacturers to ensure drug production according to official government standards.

The Physicians' Desk Reference (PDR®) is the reference most widely used by physicians, pharmacists, and nurses for information relating to the use of drugs in the practice of medicine. It is updated yearly and provides information on indications for use, dosage and administration, contraindications, and adverse reactions. You should learn how to look up drugs in the *PDR®*.

Drug Facts and Comparisons (F&C) is a loose-leaf index and drug information service subscribed to by most medical libraries. Drug information and new drug additions are updated monthly. This index provides the most current drug information on a regular basis.

The United States Pharmacopeial Convention, Inc. publishes a series of volumes under the general title of United States Pharmacopeia Dispensing Information (USP DI) that are updated yearly. Volume I—*Drug Information for the Health Care Professional*—provides in-depth information about prescription and over-the-counter medications, and nutritional supplements. Volume II—*Advice for the Patient*—provides drug information for the patient.

Drug Information—American Hospital Formulary Service—provides detailed drug information. Drugs are organized according to therapeutic use and classification. It is updated yearly.

Chapter Openers

In the chapters that deal with therapeutic drugs, a diagram will appear on the chapter heading page. The purpose of the diagram is to provide

FIGURE 1:4 Drug Nomenclature

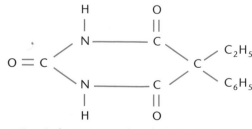

Chemical name: 5,5,-Phenylethylbarbituric acid
Nonproprietary name: Phenobarbital
Proprietary name: Solfoton
   (Trade name)

important information in a quick visual reference about the drugs included in that chapter. The information displayed informs the reader whether the drugs are available over-the-counter (OTC), by prescription, or a combination of both. In addition, it identifies which FDA Pregnancy Category (see Chapter 2) has been designated for the use of these drugs during pregnancy. Finally, the general clinical indications for the chapter drugs are presented. In the event individual drugs differ from the main representative drugs, the exceptions will be identified on the diagram.

Controlled Substances Act

The Federal Comprehensive Drug Abuse Prevention and Control Act of 1970 is designed to regulate the dispensing of certain drugs that have the potential for abuse. These **controlled substances** are assigned to one of five schedules, depending on their medical usefulness and potential for abuse. Table 1:2 describes the schedules and provides examples of some controlled substances.

TABLE 1:2

Drug Schedules Defined in the Federal Comprehensive Drug Abuse Prevention and Control Act

SCHEDULE	DEFINITION	CONTROLLED DRUGS
Schedule I	Drugs with high abuse potential and no accepted medical use	Heroin, hallucinogens, marijuana; these drugs are not to be prescribed
Schedule II	Drugs with high abuse potential and accepted medical use	Narcotics (morphine and pure codeine), cocaine, amphetamines, short-acting barbiturates; no refills without a new written prescription from the physician
Schedule III	Drugs with moderate abuse potential and accepted medical use	Moderate- and intermediate-acting barbiturates, glutethimide, preparations containing codeine plus another drug; prescription required, may be refilled five times in 6 months when authorized by the physician
Schedule IV	Drugs with low abuse potential and accepted medical use	Phenobarbital, chloral hydrate, antianxiety drugs (*Librium*, *Valium*); prescription required, may be refilled five times in 6 months when authorized by the physician
Schedule V	Drugs with limited abuse potential and accepted medical use	Narcotic drugs used in limited quantities for antitussive and antidiarrheal purposes; drugs can be sold only by a registered pharmacist; buyer must be 18 years old and show identification

* Narcotics 麻醉藥 / 鎮靜劑

* codeine (用鴉片制成の止痛鎮咳藥)

* barbiturate 巴比妥酸鹽

* glutethimide - kind of phenobabital

* antitussive [anti·恵sive] 止咳藥

Chapter Review

Understanding Terminology

Match the definition in the left column with the appropriate term in the right column.

_e_ **1.** The study of the amount of drug that is required to produce therapeutic effects.

_g_ **2.** The study of the harmful effects of drugs on living tissue.

_a_ **3.** The study of the action of drugs on living tissue.

_c_ **4.** The study of drugs.

_f_ **5.** The science of preparing and dispensing medicines.

_b_ **6.** The study of the processes of drug absorption, distribution, metabolism, and excretion.

_d_ **7.** The study of the use of drugs in treating disease.

a. pharmacodynamics

b. pharmacokinetics

c. pharmacology

d. pharmacotherapeutics

e. posology

f. pharmacy

g. toxicology

Answer the following questions.

8. Define a drug. _____

_____

9. Differentiate between therapeutic effect, side effect, and toxic effect. _____

_____

_____

10. What is the difference between site of action and mechanism of action?_____

_____

_____

11. What is the relationship between ED50, LD50, and therapeutic index? _____

_____

_____

12. Explain the difference between a prescription drug, OTC drug, and a controlled substance. _____

_____

_____

13. Explain the difference between idiosyncrasy and drug allergy. _____

_____

_____

14. Write a short paragraph describing the terms *receptor site, binding, drug action, agonist, antagonist,* and *competitive antagonism.* _____

_____

_____

Acquiring Knowledge

Answer the following questions.

1. Examine a copy of the *Physicians' Desk Reference (PDR®)*. In the beginning of the book are different colored pages. Briefly describe the information found in the white, pink, and blue pages. How might the information in the glossy gray pages be helpful? _____

_____

_____

2. Look up the popular decongestant pseudoephedrine in the pink pages of the *PDR*®. What is your conclusion based on the available trade names? _____

_____

3. What is a dose-response curve and what information is given by a dose-response curve?_____

_____

4. What is the importance of a time-response curve? How often would you estimate that a drug should be administered per day if the drug is eliminated in 4 hours? In 24 hours? _____

_____

5. It is interesting that a drug can produce a therapeutic effect and an undesired side effect in one situation, and that the same side effect may be considered a therapeutic effect in another situation. Explain this phenomenon using the drug promethazine (*Phenergan*) as an example.____

_____

6. Obtain a copy of *Drug Facts and Comparisons* (F&C) from your school or library. It is divided into many sections. There are five sections that are frequently used. Examine each section and briefly explain how it might be useful in your field.

   a. Table of Contents _____

   _____

   b. Color Locator _____

   _____

   c. Color Locator Index _____

   _____

   d. Chapters; broken down by sections on drug classifications _____

   _____

   _____

   e. Index _____

   _____

7. Using the *F&C,* read the introduction, including the information on how to use the product listing. Answer the following questions.

   a. Where would you find the distribution status of a product? _____

   _____

   b. Where would you find the prescribing information? _____

   _____

   c. Explain what *cost index* is, how to use this, and how this information may be useful to you in your field._____

   _____

8. If you needed to find information on a specific product, would it be easier and faster to look in the appropriate chapter or use the index at the back of the book? _____

_____

_____

Applying Knowledge—On the Job

Use your critical-thinking skills to answer the following questions.

1. Obtain a copy of the *PDR®* from your school, nursing unit, or clinic and use it to do some sleuthing. Find the drugs that solve the following "medical mysteries."

   a. Dan is currently taking the drugs *Mephyton, Biaxin,* and *Entex LA* for his chronic celiac disease and acute sinusitis. He was just prescribed *Coumadin* for thrombosis, and it had no therapeutic effect. Dan's doctor suspects it's a case of drug antagonism. Which drug is Dan taking that is antagonistic with *Coumadin*? _____

   _____

   _____

   b. Mary's grandfather just came home from the doctor with a prescription for *Vaseretic* and he has already forgotten why he is supposed to take it. Explain what this drug is, its indications, and the most common adverse effects. _____

   _____

   _____

   c. Bill's young wife was just prescribed *Vibra-Tabs* for a respiratory infection. Bill asks you what this drug is and is it safe for his wife to take, since she may be pregnant. Is it safe? _____

   _____

   _____

2. Assume that your employer has asked you to help screen patients for potential prescription drug problems. Look up the following frequently prescribed prescription drugs in the *PDR®* and fill in the information requested in the spaces provided.

   a. *Indocin:* What would tip you off that a patient was showing adverse effects to the drug? _____

   _____

   b. *Bicillin:* Describe symptoms of a patient who is allergic to this drug. _____

   _____

   c. *Depakote:* For whom is this drug contraindicated? _____

   _____

Use the F&C to answer the following questions.

3. **a.** A patient calls you and states that he has found a single loose tablet on the carpet. He needs you to identify it for him. He describes it as a small blue tablet with a heart cut out of the middle. There is writing on the tablet, but it is too small to read. What is this medication? __

   _____

   _____

   b. A patient calls with a minor problem. While traveling, she got her medications mixed together. She needs to take her *Cordarone* tablet but isn't sure which one it is. Could you please describe it to her? _____

   _____

4. **a.** A physician wants to know what glucose elevating products are available and whether they require a prescription. Look under the hormone section and find these products. List the available products, strengths, forms, and status. _____

   _____

   _____

   b. A physician wants to know the available forms and strength of *Imitrex*. Using the index, look up the medication and list the available forms, strengths, and package sizes. _____

   _____

   _____

5. Sarah Roberts has liver damage due to a past history of alcohol abuse. She is also taking carbamazepine 400 mg TID. Can she safely take acetaminophen for her chronic headaches? ____

_____

_____

Internet Connection

There are a number of Internet websites that provide drug information. One of these is **Rx List** (http://www.rxlist.com). Rx List has information and drug monographs on the top 200 drugs, based on prescriptions filled, in the United States. When you reach the website, click on the heading _Top 200_. What is the top drug for 2003? Click on this drug heading and explore the information presented. Notice the number of different trade names under which this drug is sold. Select another drug with which you may be familiar and survey the information. This website can be useful throughout your course when you need additional drug information.

Another pertinent website belongs to the **Food and Drug Administration** (http://www.fda.gov). Listed are topics on foods, cosmetics, animal and human drugs, and tobacco. Click on some of these headings to familiarize yourself with the FDA.

Additional Reading

Liang, B. C. 2002. The drug development process I: Drug discovery and initial development. _Hospital Physician_ 38(1):18.

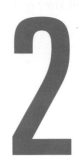

chapter

2

BIOLOGICAL FACTORS AFFECTING THE ACTION OF DRUGS

CHAPTER FOCUS

This chapter provides a description of the basic principles of pharmacokinetics, or the study of what happens to a drug after it is administered. It also describes how different dosage forms, individual variations, drug interactions, and drug dependency affect drug response.

CHAPTER OBJECTIVES

After studying this chapter, you should be able to

- list different forms of drug products and the routes by which they are administered.
- explain the processes of pharmacokinetics.
- identify how half-life, blood drug level, and bioavailability relate to drug response.
- list several factors of individual variation that can alter drug response.
- understand the drug factors that relate to pediatric drug administration.
- define the different types of drug interaction.
- explain the basic terminology of chronic drug administration and drug dependence.

Key Terms

bioavailability: percentage of the drug dosage that is absorbed.

drug absorption: entrance of a drug into the bloodstream from its site of administration.

drug addiction: condition of drug abuse and drug dependence that is characterized by compulsive drug behavior.

drug dependence: condition of reliance on the use of a particular drug, characterized as physical and/or psychological dependence.

drug distribution: passage of a drug from the blood to the tissues and organs of the body.

drug microsomal metabolizing system (DMMS): group of enzymes located primarily in the liver that function to metabolize (biotransformation) drugs.

drug tolerance: decreased drug effect occuring after repeated drug administration.

enzyme induction: increase in the amount of drug-metabolizing enzymes after repeated administration of certain drugs.

enzyme inhibition: inhibition of drug-metabolizing enzymes by certain drugs.

first-pass metabolism: drug metabolism that occurs following oral absorption from the GI tract.

half-life: time required for the body to rid itself of half of the drug dosage that was absorbed (percent bioavailability).

individual variation: difference in the effects of drugs and drug dosages from one person to another.

intramuscular (IM) injection: route of drug administration; drug is injected into gluteal or deltoid muscles.

intravenous (IV) injection: route of drug administration; drug is injected directly into a vein.

loading dose: initial drug dose administered to rapidly achieve therapeutic drug concentrations.

maintenance dose: dose administered to maintain drug blood levels in the therapeutic range.

14

oral administration: route of drug administration by way of the mouth through swallowing.

parenteral administration: route of drug administration that does not involve the gastrointestinal (GI) tract.

INTRODUCTION

The familiar saying "No two people are exactly alike" applies well to the effects produced by drugs. An identical drug and dose may produce an intense response in one individual and no observable effect in another. The major reason for these differences is **individual variation.** Individual variation occurs as a result of several factors, any of which can influence the pharmacological response to drugs. There are also factors that determine how fast a drug reaches its site of action (receptors), how long it remains there, and how long the body takes to eliminate the drug. These important pharmacological considerations are understood by examining the biological factors that affect drug action.

One of the factors that affects drug action is the route of drug administration. The route determines the rate of drug absorption. **Drug absorption** refers to the entrance of a drug into the bloodstream, where it is distributed **(drug distribution)** to the various tissues of the body. The intensity and the duration of drug action depend on primarily the rate of drug metabolism and drug excretion. Figure 2:1 on page 16 shows the interrelationship of these processes.

Individual variation is caused by a number of physical and psychological factors, including differences in age, sex, weight, genetic variation, emotional state, patient expectations (placebo effect), and the presence of other disease conditions (pathology) or other drugs. The remainder of this chapter will describe what happens to a drug between its administration and its elimination from the body. The interplay among the various biological factors determines the actual drug response.

DRUG FORMS

Drugs are prepared in various forms for administration. The physical and chemical properties of a drug usually determine which form will be most effective. In addition to the drug, most drug products contain other ingredients that facilitate the administration and absorption of the drug. Drug preparations should always be taken exactly as prescribed. Some of the more common drug forms and preparations follow.

Aqueous Preparations

Syrups are commonly used aqueous preparations. A syrup is a solution of water and sugar to which a drug is added. Addition of

flavoring agents eliminates the bitter taste of many drugs.

Alcoholic Preparations

Elixirs, spirits, tinctures, and fluid extracts are drugs dissolved in various concentrations of alcohol, usually in the range of 5 to 20 percent.

Solid and Semisolid Preparations

The solid type of preparation is most common. A number of different kinds for different purposes are available.

Powders

Powders are drugs or drug extracts that are dried and ground into fine particles.

Movement of a Drug in the Body

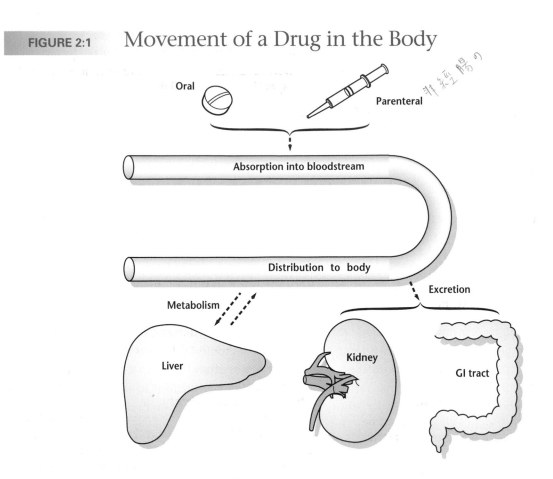

Tablets

Tablets are drug powders that have been compressed into a convenient form for swallowing. They usually disintegrate in the stomach more rapidly than most other solid preparations.

Troches and Lozenges

These flattened tablets are allowed to dissolve in the mouth. They are commonly used for colds and sore throats.

Capsules 膠囊

Gelatin capsules are used to administer drug powders or liquids. Gelatin capsules dissolve in the stomach, thereby releasing the drug.

Delayed-Release Products

These are usually tablets or capsules that are treated with special coatings so that various portions of the drug will dissolve at different rates. Delayed-release products usually contain the equivalent of two or three single-dose units. They are designed to produce drug effects over an extended time.

Enteric-Coated Products

Some drugs are very irritating to the stomach. Also, the gastric juices of the stomach can

inactivate certain drugs. In these cases, the drug tablet or capsule is coated with an acid-resistant substance that will dissolve only in the less acidic portions of the intestines. Enteric-coated products should be taken on an empty stomach with water, either 1 hour before or 2 hours after meals.

Suppositories 塞藥

These are drugs mixed with a substance (cacao butter) that will melt at body temperature. Suppositories are intended for insertion into the rectum, urethra, or vagina.

Ointments 藥膏

Ointments or salves are soft, oily substances (petrolatum or lanolin) containing a drug that is applied to the skin, or in the case of ophthalmic ointments, to the eye.

Transdermal Products

Transdermal products are administered through a bandage or patch system. The drug is released from the bandage or patch and is then absorbed through the skin into the systemic circulation. This method provides a continuous source of the drug over 24 hours or more. Nitroglycerin, estrogen, and clonidine are drugs available in this form.

ROUTES OF ADMINISTRATION

Oral Administration

The most common routes of drug administration are oral (PO) and parenteral. **Parenteral administration** is any route that does not involve the GI tract, including inhalation, hypodermic injection, and topical application. The **oral administration** route is the safest and the most convenient method. Oral administration usually requires 30 to 60 minutes before significant absorption from the GI tract occurs; therefore, the onset of drug action is delayed.

Although some drugs are irritating to the stomach and may cause nausea, heartburn, and vomiting, administration of such drugs with sufficient amounts of water or with meals minimizes gastric irritation. However, food also delays drug absorption and therefore delays the onset of drug action.

Besides convenience, another advantage of oral administration is that drugs given orally can be removed (within the first few hours) by gastric lavage or induced vomiting. This procedure is often employed in drug overdose (sleeping pills) or accidental poisoning.

Parenteral Administration

The most common routes of parenteral administration include intramuscular (IM) injection, intravenous (IV) injection, inhalation, and topical application. **IM injections** are usually delivered into the gluteal or deltoid muscles. Extreme caution should be observed with gluteal injections to avoid injury to the sciatic nerve. The onset of action with IM administration is relatively short, usually within several minutes. **Intravenous (IV) injection** is usually restricted to use in the hospital. IV injection offers the fastest means of drug absorption because the drug is delivered directly into the circulation; therefore, the onset of drug action is almost immediate. However, there is some degree of risk because the drug cannot be withdrawn once it has been injected. Dosage miscalculations resulting in overdose can produce serious, even fatal, consequences. Inhalation involves administration of drug through the nose or mouth and into the lungs during respiratory inspiration. This route is especially useful for the local administration of drugs into the respiratory tract. Topical application of creams and ointments is used for local effects in the skin and in certain conditions

for systemic effects, as with nitroglycerin ointment for the treatment of angina pectoris.

Several other routes of administration are used in specific situations. The most commonly used routes are listed in Table 2:1 with examples of their indications for use. Other routes will be presented in the appropriate chapters.

DRUG ABSORPTION

Drug absorption refers to the entrance of a drug into the bloodstream. In order for absorption to occur, the drug must be dissolved in body fluids. With the exception of IV or intraarterial administration, drugs must pass through membranes of the GI lining and blood vessels before they gain access to the blood. Cell membranes are composed of lipids and proteins, which form a semipermeable barrier.

Cells have special transport mechanisms that allow various substances (including drugs) to pass through the cell membrane. These mechanisms include filtration, passive transport, and active transport. Most drugs pass through membranes by passive transport. An important principle in passive transport is that the concentration of drug on each side of the membrane differs. In passive transport, drug molecules pass from an area of high concentration to an area of low concentration (law of diffusion).

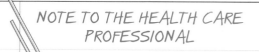

NOTE TO THE HEALTH CARE PROFESSIONAL

It is very important for nurses and other health personnel to always follow the physician's orders and the established guidelines for the administration of drugs. One practical approach to drug administration is referred to as "the five rights." This approach advocates that the person dispensing the drug make a mental checklist that emphasizes giving the *right patient* the *right drug* in the *right dose* by the *right route* at the *right time*.

In addition, a sixth right has been suggested—the *right attitude* on the part of the person administering the drug. This aspect is important for generating a positive attitude in the patient toward therapy and contributes to a positive placebo response on the part of patients.

TABLE 2:1 Routes of Drug Administration

ROUTE	APPROXIMATE ONSET OF ACTION	INDICATIONS	EXAMPLES
Oral (PO)	30 to 60 minutes	Whenever possible, the safest and most convenient route	Most medications—aspirin, sedatives, hypnotics, antibiotics
Sublingual	Several minutes	When rapid effects are needed	Nitroglycerin in angina pectoris
Buccal	Several minutes	Convenient dosage form for certain drugs	Androgenic drugs
Rectal	15 to 30 minutes	When patient cannot take oral medications and parenteral is not indicated, also for local effects	Analgesics, laxatives
Transdermal	30 to 60 minutes	Convenient dosage form that provides continuous absorption and systemic effects over many hours	Nitroglycerin, estrogen 硝酸甘油 此途径性3敦素
Subcutaneous (SC)	Several minutes	For drugs that are inactivated by the GI tract	Insulin
Intramuscular (IM)	Several minutes	For drugs that have poor oral absorption, when high blood levels are required, and when rapid effects are desired	Narcotic analgesics, antibiotics
Intravenous (IV)	Within 1 minute	In emergency situations, where immediate effects are required, also when medications are administered by infusion	IV fluids (dextrose), nutrient supplementation, antibiotics
Intraarterial	Within 1 minute	For local effects within an internal organ	Cancer drugs
Intrathecal	Several minutes	For local effects within the spinal cord	Spinal anesthesia with lidocaine
Inhalation	Within 1 minute	For local effects within the respiratory tract	Antiasthmatic medications such as epinephrine
Topical	Within 1 hour	For local effects on the skin, eye, or ear	Creams and ointments
Vaginal	15 to 30 minutes	For local effects	Creams, foams, and suppositories

For example, following oral administration, there is a large amount of drug in the GI tract and no drug in the blood. Consequently, the drug molecules have a natural tendency to diffuse from the GI tract into the blood. The speed or rate of drug absorption also depends on the chemical properties of the drug and the site of administration. The properties of the drug that most determine absorption are lipid (fat) solubility of the drug and the degree of drug ionization.

Lipid Solubility

Cell membranes are composed of a significant amount of lipid material. In general, the more lipid-soluble a drug is, the faster it will pass through a lipid substance like the cell membrane.

With the exception of general anesthetics (highly lipid soluble), most drugs are primarily water soluble and only partially lipid soluble. Many water-soluble drugs are weak acids or bases that can form charged particles or ions (ionization) when dissolved in body fluids. The absorption of water-soluble drugs is mainly influenced by the degree of drug ionization.

Drug Ionization

Most drugs exist in two forms, ionized and unionized. Like electrolytes (Na^+ and Cl^-), ionized drugs are charged molecules because their atomic structure has lost or gained electrons. The molecules then become either positively or negatively charged. In general, ionized drug molecules do not readily cross cell membranes. The un-ionized (uncharged) form of the drug is required in order for absorption to occur.

The first generalization is that acid drugs (aspirin) are mostly un-ionized when they are in an acidic fluid (gastric juice). Consequently, drug absorption is favored. Conversely, acid drugs are mostly ionized when they are in an alkaline fluid; therefore, absorption is not favored and occurs at a slower rate and to a lesser extent.

The second generalization is that basic drugs (streptomycin, morphine) are mostly un-ionized when they are in an alkaline fluid (lower GI tract after rectal administration). Conversely, these drugs are mostly ionized when they are dissolved in an acidic fluid like the upper GI tract. This is the reason why morphine is usually administered parenterally. In the stomach (pH 1 to 3) and upper intestinal tract (pH 5 to 6), basic drugs like morphine are absorbed more slowly and to a lesser extent than acidic drugs because they are primarily in an ionized form.

The acid and base nature of drugs may be useful in treating drug toxicity (overdose). Drugs are generally excreted by the kidneys in an ionized form. To increase drug excretion, the pH of the urine can be altered. For example, to increase the renal excretion of an acid drug (aspirin), the urine is alkalinized (pH > 7). In an alkaline urine, acidic drugs are mostly ionized and more rapidly excreted. In the same manner basic drugs are more rapidly excreted by acidifying the urine (pH < 7).

Drug Formulation

Drugs must be in solution before being absorbed. Tablets and capsules require time for the dissolution to occur. For this reason, liquid medications are generally absorbed faster than the solid forms. Drug particles can be formulated into different sizes, such as crystals, micronized particles, or ultramicronized particles. The smaller the size of the drug particle, the faster the rate of dissolution and absorption.

DRUG DISTRIBUTION

After a drug gains access to the blood, it is distributed to the various tissues and organs of the body. Several factors determine how much drug reaches any one organ or area of the body. The main factors are plasma protein binding, blood flow, and the presence of specific tissue barriers.

Plasma Protein Binding

Several different proteins (albumin and globulins) are in the plasma and form a circulating protein pool. These plasma proteins help regulate osmotic pressure (oncotic pressure) in the blood and transport many hormones and vitamins. In addition, many drugs are attracted to the plasma proteins, especially albumin. The result is that some drug molecules are bound to plasma proteins while some drug molecules are unbound (free in the circulation). Only the unbound or free drug molecules can exert a pharmacological effect. The ratio of the bound to unbound drug molecules varies with the drug used. Some drugs are highly bound (99 percent), while other drugs are not bound to any significant degree.

Occasionally, there is competition between drugs or other plasma substances for the same plasma protein binding site. In this situation, one drug may displace another. The result is that the concentration of free drug of one of the drugs increases, and this concentration can lead to increased pharmacological and adverse effects similar to overdosage.

Blood Flow

The various organs of the body receive different amounts of blood. Organs such as the liver, kidneys, and brain have the largest blood supply. Consequently, these organs are usually exposed to the largest amount of drug. Some tissues, such as adipose tissue, receive a relatively poor blood supply and, as a result, do not accumulate large amounts of drug. However, highly lipid-soluble drugs can enter adipose tissue easily where they can accumulate and remain for an extended period of time.

Blood-Brain Barrier

In the case of the brain, an additional consideration is the blood-brain barrier. This barrier is an additional lipid barrier that protects the brain by restricting the passage of electrolytes and other water-soluble substances. Since the brain is composed of a large amount of lipid (nerve membranes and myelin), lipid-soluble drugs pass readily into the brain. As a general rule, then, a drug must have a certain degree of lipid solubility if it is to penetrate this barrier and gain access to the brain.

DRUG METABOLISM

Whenever a drug or other foreign substance is taken into the body, the body attempts to eliminate it. This usually involves excretion by one of the normal excretory routes (renal, intestinal, or respiratory). Some drugs can be excreted in the same chemical form in which they were administered. Other drugs, however, must be chemically altered before they can be excreted by the kidneys. Drug metabolism, also referred to as biotransformation, is the chemical alteration of drugs and foreign compounds in the body.

The liver is the main organ involved in drug metabolism. Within the cells of the liver are a group of enzymes that specifically function to metabolize foreign (drug) substances. These enzymes are referred to as the **drug microsomal metabolizing system (DMMS).** The main function of this system is to take lipid-soluble drugs and chemically alter them so that they become water-soluble compounds. Water-soluble compounds can be excreted by the kidneys. Lipid-soluble compounds are repeatedly reabsorbed into the blood. Although most drugs are inactivated by metabolism, a few are initially converted into pharmacologically active metabolites.

An interesting phenomenon occurs with some drugs, especially the barbiturates and other sedative-hypnotic drugs. When these drugs are taken repeatedly, they stimulate the drug microsomal metabolizing system. By stimulating this system, the drugs actually increase the amount of enzymes in the system; this process is referred to as **enzyme induction.** With an increase in the amount of enzymes, there is a faster rate of drug metabolism. Consequently, the duration of drug action is decreased for all drugs metabolized by the microsomal enzymes. In addition, other drugs can inhibit the drug microsomal-metabolizing enzymes to cause **enzyme inhibition.** This action slows the metabolism of all other drugs metabolized by these enzymes. This will increase the duration and intensity of the drugs inhibited. Enzyme induction and enzyme inhibition are common causes of adverse drug interactions.

After oral administration, all drugs are absorbed into the portal circulation, which transports the drugs to the liver before they are distributed throughout the body. Some drugs are metabolized significantly as they pass through the liver this first time. This effect is referred to as **first-pass metabolism.** It can significantly reduce the amount of active drug that reaches the general circulation.

DRUG EXCRETION

The common pathways of drug excretion are renal (urine), GI (feces), and respiratory (exhaled gases). Although the liver is the most important organ for drug metabolism, the kidneys are the most important organs for drug excretion.

Renal Excretion

After the blood is filtered through the glomerulus of the kidneys, most of the filtered substances are eventually reabsorbed into the blood. The exceptions to this are the urinary waste products and anything else that is in a nonabsorbable form. In order for drug excretion to occur, the drug or drug metabolite must be water soluble and preferably in an ionized form. As mentioned, acid drugs are mostly ionized in alkaline urine and basic drugs are mostly ionized in an acid urine. In the case of barbiturate or aspirin overdose (acid drugs), alkalinization of the urine with sodium bicarbonate will hasten elimination of either drug in the urine.

GI Excretion

After oral administration, a certain portion of drug (unabsorbed) passes through the GI tract and is excreted in the feces. The amount varies with the particular drug used.

In addition, there is another pathway involving the intestinal tract, the enterohepatic pathway. Certain drugs (fat-soluble drugs) can enter the intestines by way of the biliary tract. After the drug is released into the intestines (in the bile), it may be absorbed into the blood again. This is referred to as the enterohepatic cycle. The duration of action of a few drugs is greatly prolonged because of this repeated cycling of the drug (liver → bile → intestines → blood → liver).

Respiratory Excretion

The respiratory system does not usually play a significant role in drug excretion. However, some drugs are metabolized to products that can be exchanged from the blood into the respiratory tract. General anesthetic gases are not totally metabolized. These drugs are excreted primarily by the lungs.

Miscellaneous

Some drugs and drug metabolites can also be detected in sweat, saliva, and milk (lactation). Infants can be exposed to significant amounts of certain drugs after nursing (see the Drug Exposure During Infant Nursing section).

HALF-LIFE

The **half-life** of a drug is the time required for the blood or plasma concentration of the drug to fall to half of its original level. It is important in determining the frequency of drug administration. The major factors that determine half-life are the rates of drug metabolism and excretion. The half-life of any drug is relatively constant if the individual has normal rates of drug metabolism and excretion. It can be prolonged when liver or kidney disease is present. In these situations, the dose or the frequency of administration can be reduced.

BLOOD DRUG LEVELS

The intensity of drug effect is mainly determined by the concentration of drug in the blood or plasma. The amount of drug in the plasma is determined by an interplay of all of the pharmacokinetic processes (absorption, distribution, metabolism, and excretion). These processes occur together. As a drug is absorbed and distributed, the liver and kidneys begin the processes of metabolism and excretion. The plasma level of the drug is constantly changing, as illustrated in Figure 1:3 on page 6. In the beginning, absorption and distribution predominate and the plasma level increases. Later, drug metabolism and excretion predominate and the plasma level decreases.

Drug monitoring, the periodic measurement of blood drug levels, is performed to ensure that the level of drug in the blood is within the therapeutic range. Drug levels below the therapeutic range will not produce the desired drug effect, while levels

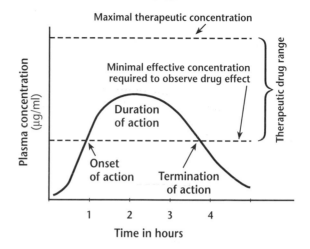

FIGURE 2:2 Illustration of Therapeutic Drug Range

above the therapeutic range cause increased side effects and toxicity. This concept is illustrated in Figure 2:2.

There are some drugs that require several dosages or several days or weeks to reach the desired drug effect. In some clinical situations it may be necessary to reach therapeutic drug levels as rapidly as possible. In these cases, a loading dose may be administered. A **loading dose** is usually an initial higher dose of drug, often administered IV, to rapidly attain the therapeutic drug level and drug effects. Loading doses are usually followed by **maintenance doses** that are smaller and calculated to maintain the drug level within the therapeutic range.

BIOAVAILABILITY

Bioavailability is the percentage of the dose of a drug that is actually absorbed into the bloodstream. Differences in drug formulation, route of administration, and factors that affect GI absorption can influence bioavailability. A particular drug may be manufactured by many different drug companies and sold under different trade names. In these situations, the amount of drug may be the same in each product but the product may be different because of particle size, binders, fillers, and tablet coating. These differences may alter bioavailability. There have been examples of this in the past. Now, however, the Food and Drug Administration (FDA) regulates and requires bioavailability testing.

FACTORS OF INDIVIDUAL VARIATION

Many factors affect individual variation. These factors include age, weight, sex, genetic variation, emotional state, placebo effect, the presence of disease, and patient compliance.

Age

The effects of drugs in different age groups is of particular importance. Infants, children, and the elderly are generally more sensitive to the actions of drugs than are younger adults. Drug considerations during pregnancy on fetal development, during the infant nursing period, and in infants and children are discussed in the section Pediatric Drug Considerations. Drug considerations for the elderly are presented in Chapter 3, Geriatric Pharmacology.

Weight

Most adult dosages are calculated for the average adult weight, 150 pounds between the ages of 16 and 65. Obviously, all adults are not 150 pounds. In small individuals (100 pounds), the dose may have to be reduced. In larger individuals (200 to 300 pounds), the dose may have to be increased. However, this approach does not always hold true, since many other factors are involved.

Sex and Percent Body Fat

Females possess a higher percentage of body fat and a lower percentage of body water than do males of equal weight. Consequently, females may experience a greater drug effect than do males because the drug is dissolved in a smaller volume of body fluid. Lipid-soluble drugs are more widely distributed and may produce longer durations of action than in males. This same concept also applies to the differences in body fat composition between members of the same sex.

Genetic Variation

Individuals tend to inherit the proteins and enzyme patterns of their parents. There is significant genetic variation in some of the drug-metabolizing enzymes, so individual differences can occur. If the difference affects the rate of drug metabolism, there may be a difference in the effects produced by the drug. An enzyme may be missing, in which case drug metabolism is extremely slow. A slowed metabolic rate may result in increased and prolonged drug effects that can lead to serious consequences. Examples of genetic variation will be discussed in specific chapters.

Emotional State

Differences in drug effects can be caused by the emotional state of the individual. For example, an individual who is excited or extremely anxious may require a larger dose of hypnotic or tranquilizer than an individual who is not emotionally stimulated but who still has difficulty sleeping.

Placebo Effect

Patients come to physicians and hospitals with varying expectations. It has been observed that if patients have a positive attitude and think that the drug or treatment will help, chances are the patients claim an improvement whether there actually is one or not.

In some studies, patients have been unknowingly given sugar pills or placebos instead of an actual drug. A large percentage of these patients claim an improved condition even though they received no real drug. Likewise, patients with hostile or negative attitudes, who feel that nothing will help their condition, usually say that they feel no difference or even worse after a specific treatment or medication. The influence of one's mind on the course of treatment is referred to as the placebo effect. This phenomenon can be used by the medical and nursing staff to enhance the positive attitude of patients. Thus, the patients stand a better chance of responding successfully to therapy.

Presence of Disease

The presence of other diseases that are debilitating or that decrease the function of some vital organ usually makes an individual more susceptible to the effects and adverse reactions of drug therapy. As mentioned, the liver and kidneys are especially important, since these two organs are exposed to the highest drug levels. For this reason, liver and kidney function are often adversely affected by drugs. Patients with hepatic or renal disease suffer a greater incidence of adverse drug effects because they are unable to eliminate the drug and its metabolites effectively. Consequently, plasma drug levels are much higher in these patients due to accumulation of the drug in the plasma.

Patient Compliance

Drug compliance refers to taking a drug exactly as prescribed. If dosages are forgotten or skipped, the drug effects will be reduced or absent. This is referred to as noncompliance. Noncompliance is often a problem in geriatric patients who may have memory difficulties and who are easily confused by complicated dosing schedules, especially when several different drugs are involved. Particular care and sufficient patient instructions and training must be given to ensure that all patients understand dosing instructions.

PEDIATRIC DRUG CONSIDERATIONS

Fetal Period during Pregnancy

Before birth the developing fetus will be exposed to most drugs taken during pregnancy. The placenta is not a drug barrier, and drug absorption and distribution to the fetus follow the same principles as with other maternal organs (passive diffusion based on lipid solubility and ionization). Although there are relatively few drugs that have been proven to be teratogenic (cause birth defects), it is recommended that drug exposure during pregnancy should be avoided if possible. This is especially true during the first trimester when organogenesis, the formation of body organs, is occurring. Drugs that are teratogens may cause spontaneous abortion, growth retardation, birth defects, or carcinogenesis (development of cancer). The Food and Drug Administration has established guidelines, the FDA Pregnancy Categories (see Table 2:2), that classify drugs based on fetal risk. Table 2:3 lists some drugs that have been associated with teratogenicity in humans.

Drug Exposure during Infant Nursing

Drugs administered to nursing mothers appear in breast milk to varying degrees. Unfortunately there is a lack of controlled studies and reliable information in this area. The major concern is that the drug concentration in the milk will be high enough to produce undesired or harmful effects in the infant. Generally, the recommendation is to avoid unnecessary drug administration. Usually the infant experiences the same pharmacological effects as in the mother. For example, laxatives may cause infant diarrhea, while sedatives and hypnotics will cause drowsiness and lethargy. Other drugs such as anticancer agents or drugs with increased toxicities are contraindicated unless the benefit to the mother clearly outweighs the risk to the infant. Table 2:4 lists some of the drugs that appear in breast milk.

Pediatric Considerations

There are a number of pharmacokinetic and pharmacodynamic differences between pediatric and adult patients. Neonates (0 to 1 month), infants (1 to 12 months), and children of increasing age are not simply "small adults." There are a number of factors that must be considered that generally require reduction in dosage beyond the obvious difference in body weight. These

---

| **TABLE 2:2** | **Description of FDA Pregnancy Categories** |

CATEGORY	DESCRIPTION
Pregnancy Category A	Drug studies in pregnant women have not yet demonstrated risk to the fetus.
Pregnancy Category B	Drug studies have not been performed in pregnant women; animal studies have not demonstrated fetal risk.
Pregnancy Category C	Drug studies have not been performed in pregnant women or in animals, or animal studies have revealed some teratogenic potential but the risk to the fetus is unknown.
Pregnancy Category D	Drug studies have revealed adverse risk to the fetus. The benefit-to-risk ratio of the drug must be established before use during pregnancy.
Pregnancy Category X	Drug studies have revealed teratogenic effects in women and/or animals. Fetal risk clearly outweighs benefit. Drug is contraindicated in pregnancy.
Pregnancy Category NR	Drug has not yet been rated by FDA.

TABLE 2:3   Examples of Drugs With Demonstrated Teratogenic Risk in Humans

DRUG	TERATOGENIC EFFECT
androgens (male hormone)	Masculinization of female fetus
carbamazepine	Craniofacial and fingernail deformities
diethylstilbestrol	Vaginal tumors and genital malformations in offspring
estrogen (female hormone)	Feminization of male fetus
lithium	Cardiac defects
phenytoin	Craniofacial and limb deformities, growth retardation
retinoic acid	Craniofacial, cardiac, and *CNS defects
thalidomide	Phocomelia (limb deformities)
warfarin	Facial, cartilage, and CNS defects

Abbreviations: *CNS, central nervous system.

TABLE 2:4   Examples of Drugs That Cross Into Breast Milk Following Maternal Use

DRUG CLASS	EXAMPLES
Antibiotics	ampicillin, erythromycin, penicillin, streptomycin, sulfa drugs, tetracyclines
Antiepileptic agents	phenytoin, primidone
Antithyroid agents	thiouracil
CNS stimulants	nicotine
Laxatives	cascara, danthron
Narcotic analgesics	codeine, heroin, methadone, morphine
Nonnarcotic antiinflammatory agents	phenylbutazone
Sedative-hypnotic agents	barbiturates, chloral hydrate
Tranquilizers (antipsychotic agents)	chlorpromazine, lithium

differences tend to decrease with advancing age, especially after the first year of life.

Drug Administration and Absorption

Neonates and infants have a small skeletal muscle mass. In addition, limited physical activity results in a lower blood flow to muscle. Therefore, absorption after IM injections is slower and more variable. There is also increase risk of muscle and nerve damage with IM injections. In serious situations the IV route is more reliable and generally preferred. The skin of neonates and infants is thinner and topically applied drugs are more rapidly and completely absorbed into the systemic circulation. With regard to oral administration, the gastric pH of premature babies and neonates is less acidic. This could result in decreased bioavailability and lower blood levels of orally administered drugs that are acidic in nature.

Drug Distribution

Pediatric patients possess a higher percentage of body water and a lower percentage of body fat. These differences decrease the distribution of lipid-soluble drugs to body tissues and organs. This tends to cause higher drug blood levels. Water-soluble drug distribution is increased (greater peripheral drug distribution), which tends to lower drug blood levels. These effects are all in comparison to the adult effects. While pediatric patients have higher percentages of water, they are more easily dehydrated by vomiting and diarrhea. The resulting reduction of body fluids will increase drug concentrations and drug effects.

Plasma protein levels are also lower, especially in neonates. This results in lower plasma protein binding of drugs and, therefore, greater amounts of unbound or "free" drug. Since only the unbound drug exerts an effect, there will be a greater intensity of drug effect.

Drug Metabolism and Excretion

There is a reduced capacity for drug metabolism and drug excretion during the first several years of life. Consequently, drug elimination occurs more slowly and the duration of drug action is prolonged. The decreases in drug metabolism and excretion are most evident in the neonate and infant. After the first year, drug metabolism and excretion gradually become proportional to those of the adult.

Dosage Adjustment

Dosage calculations in pediatrics are based mainly on age, body surface area, and body weight. The rules and formulas used for these calculations are presented in Chapter 4, Math Review and Dosage Calculations.

DRUG INTERACTIONS

Drug interaction refers to the effects that occur when the actions of one drug are affected by another drug. There are many different types of drug interactions. Some drugs interfere with each other during GI absorption and therefore should not be administered at the same time. Other drugs may interfere with plasma protein binding, drug metabolism, or drug excretion. Throughout this book, the common drug interactions will be given. Table 2:5 explains the general terms that are associated with drug interactions.

TERMINOLOGY ASSOCIATED WITH CHRONIC DRUG USE AND ABUSE

The chronic use of certain drugs results in a number of physiologic and pharmacologic changes in drug response. Drug tolerance and drug dependence are two important phenomena involved in chronic drug use.

Tolerance

Drug tolerance is defined as a decreased drug effect that occurs after repeated administration. In order to attain the previous drug effect, the dosage must be increased. This is a common occurrence

TABLE 2:5	Terminology of Common Drug Interactions
TERM	**EXPLANATION**
Incompatibility	Usually refers to physical alterations of drugs that occur before administration when different drugs are mixed in the same syringe or other container
Additive effects	When the combined effect of two drugs, each producing the same biological response by the same mechanism of action, is equal to the sum of their individual effects
Summation	When the combined effect of two drugs, each producing the same biological response but by a different mechanism of action, is equal to the sum of their individual effects
Synergism	When the combined effect of two drugs is greater than the sum of their individual effects
Antagonism	When the combined effect of two drugs is less than the sum of their individual effects

in individuals who abuse drugs such as cocaine, barbiturates, morphine, and heroin. There is also the phenomenon of cross-tolerance, which is the tolerance that exists between drugs of the same class. Tolerance is caused by changes or adaptations that occur in response to repeated drug exposure. The main types of tolerance are referred to as metabolic tolerance and pharmacodynamic tolerance. Metabolic tolerance is caused by enzyme induction—the drug increases the drug-metabolizing enzymes (DMMS) and the dose must be increased in order to attain the same previous effect. Pharmacodynamic tolerance is caused by the ability of some drugs to decrease the number of drug receptors. This usually takes several weeks or months and is referred to as "down-regulation." With the reduction in drug receptors there is a reduction in intensity of drug effect.

Drug Dependence

Drug dependence is a condition wherein reliance on the administration of a particular drug becomes extremely important to the well-being of an individual. Drug dependence is usually characterized as psychological and/or physical. When the drug is used repeatedly for nonmedical purposes, the term *drug abuse* is implied. Any activity that is repeated and that provides pleasure involves a psychological component of behavior. The smoking of tobacco, for example, is an activity associated with psychological dependence. Deprivation of smoking causes some unpleasant feelings, but does not result in serious medical consequences. All drugs that are abused have varying degrees of psychological dependence associated with them. Many abused drugs also produce physical dependence when taken for prolonged periods of time and usually at increasing dosages. Deprivation of these drugs leads to a physical withdrawal syndrome that is very unpleasant, characterized by measurable changes in many bodily functions, and that may cause serious medical consequences. The withdrawal reactions from alcohol, barbiturates, and opiate drugs are examples of this type of reaction. When drug dependence is particularly severe and compulsive drug behavior dominates all other activities, the term **drug addiction** is used. Information concerning tolerance and dependence of specific drug classes can be found in Chapters 12 (Sedative-Hypnotic Drugs and Alcohol), 13 (Antipsychotic and Antianxiety Drugs), 15 (Psychotomimetic Drugs of Abuse), and 19 (Opoid [Narcotic] Analgesics).

Chapter Review

Understanding Terminology

Match the description in the left column with the appropriate term in the right column.

___ **1.** When the combined effect of two drugs, each producing the same biological response by the same mechanism of action, is equal to the sum of their individual effects.

___ **2.** When the combined effect of two drugs, each producing the same biological response but by a different mechanism of action, is equal to the sum of their individual effects.

___ **3.** When the combined effect of two drugs is greater than the sum of their individual effects.

___ **4.** When the combined effect of two drugs is less than the sum of their individual effects.

___ **5.** Usually refers to physical alterations of drugs that occur before administration when different drugs are mixed in the same syringe or other container.

___ **6.** Decreased drug effects after chronic administration.

a. additive effects

b. antagonism

c. incompatibility

d. summation

e. synergism

f. tolerance

Answer the following questions in the spaces provided.

7. Differentiate between the following terms: *parenteral administration, oral administration, intramuscular injection,* and *intravenous injection.* _____
_____
_____

8. What is the main disadvantage to the IV method of drug administration? _____
_____
_____

9. By what method of cell transport are most drugs absorbed? What are the main requirements for drug absorption? _____
_____

10. Explain why alkalinization of the urine increases the rate of excretion of drugs such as aspirin or phenobarbital. _____
_____

11. Briefly describe the main factors that determine drug distribution. _____
_____
_____

12. What is the major requirement for a drug if it is to gain access to the brain? _____
_____
_____

13. What is the drug microsomal-metabolizing system, and what is its main function? _____
_____
_____

14. List the major pathways of drug excretion. _____
_____

15. Why is the plasma drug concentration important? What are the main factors that determine plasma concentration? _____

_____

16. List the factors that can contribute to individual variation in drug response. _____

_____

_____

Acquiring Knowledge

Answer the following questions in the spaces provided.

1. A single IV injection of 100 mg of a drug with a half-life of 4 hours is administered to a young adult. Approximately how many hours will it take to totally eliminate this dosage from the body?

_____

_____

2. A drug has a bioavailability of 70 percent after oral administration. How many milligrams of drug will be absorbed following a dosage of 200 mg? What would be the expected effect on bioavailability if a large meal was ingested just before administration? _____

_____

_____

3. Your grandmother has just been prescribed a very lipid-soluble drug. Would you expect her dosage to be larger or smaller than that for a younger adult? Explain. _____

_____

_____

4. Rifampin is a drug that causes enzyme induction. Would you have to increase or decrease the dosage of another drug taken concurrently if it required drug metabolism for elimination? What change in dosage would a very water-soluble drug require? _____

_____

_____

5. Individuals who become dependent on drugs such as alcohol or narcotics require a steady supply of drug for administration or they will experience unpleasant and potentially harmful effects. Individuals with diabetes require insulin injections on a daily basis or they will experience potentially harmful effects. Are the individuals taking insulin dependent on the drug? Is there a difference between the dependence on insulin versus alcohol? Explain._____

_____

_____

Applying Knowledge—On the Job

Use your critical thinking skills to answer the following questions in the spaces provided.

1. Assume that your new job in a neighborhood health clinic is to identify individual patient factors that might affect the bioavailability of drugs prescribed for the patients. Following are descriptions of five of the clinic's patients whom you dealt with this morning. For each patient, identify one factor that could affect drug bioavailability and explain how drug dosage could be changed to compensate for it.

   a. Jonathan is a 35-year-old male with a medical history of stomach complaints but no evidence of ulcer. When Jonathan visited the clinic this morning he weighed in at 324 pounds. He presented with upper respiratory symptoms attributable to allergy and was prescribed a decongestant and an antihistamine.

   Factor _____

   Dosage change _____

   _____

b. Lisa is a 25-year-old female weighing 103 pounds. She is in good health. At her clinic visit this morning, she complained of muscle pain caused by moving furniture into her new apartment. She was prescribed a muscle relaxant and a pain reliever.

Factor _____

Dosage change _____

c. Al is a 50-year-old male alcoholic weighing 150 pounds. His history reveals long-term alcohol abuse. Liver function tests run last month showed some enzyme abnormalities. Al's visit to the clinic this morning was for a sinus infection. He was prescribed an antibiotic and a decongestant.

Factor _____

Dosage change _____

d. Janet is a 49-year-old weighing 130 pounds. Her visit to the clinic this morning was for insomnia, which she has suffered since her husband's death 2 weeks ago. It was clear from her behavior at the clinic today that she's emotionally distraught. She was prescribed a mild sedative.

Factor _____

Dosage change _____

e. Jessie is a 5-year-old girl weighing 43 pounds. She presented at the clinic this morning with an upper respiratory virus and strep throat. She was prescribed an antibiotic for the strep throat and pediatric ibuprofen for fever and discomfort.

Factor _____

Dosage change _____

2. Assume that you have volunteered to work a nonprescription drug hotline. Your job is to give people who call assistance with over-the-counter drugs. How would you react—and why—to the following anonymous callers?

a. Caller A is worried about taking too much aspirin. She didn't realize until after she took the capsules that they were double the dose of the product she usually takes. She wants to know if there's something she might have on hand at home that she could take to counter the effects of the extra aspirin in her system. _____

b. Caller B wants to know if it's all right to take a laxative while she is breast-feeding her baby.

_____

_____

Additional Reading

Blodget, J. B. 1995. Managing injection reactions. *Nursing* 25(9):46.

Cohen, M. R., and Cohen, H. G. 1996. Medication errors: Following a game plan for continued improvement. *Nursing* 26(11):34.

Hadaway, L. C. 2002. I. V. infiltration: Not just a peripheral problem. *Nursing* 2002 32(8):36.

Hadaway, L. C. 2001. How to safeguard delivery of high alert I.V. drugs. *Nursing* 2001 31(2):36.

Hussar, D. A. 1995. Helping your patient follow his drug regimen. *Nursing* 25(10):62.

Konich McMahan, J. 1996. Full speed ahead with caution: Rushing intravenous drugs. *Nursing* 26(6):26.

Laskowski Jones, L., and Solati, D. S. 2001. Responding to pediatric trauma. *Nursing* 2001 31(9):36.

Mayer, G. G., and Rushton, N. 2002. Writing easy-to-read teaching aids. *Nursing* 2002 32(3):48.

McLean, J. 1990. The placebo effect: Magic pills. *Nursing Times* 86(28):28.

Smetzer, J. 2001. Take 10 giant steps to medication safety. *Nursing* 2001 31(11):49.

Wichowski, H. C., and Kubsch, S. 1995. Improving your patients compliance. *Nursing* 25(1):66.

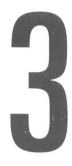

GERIATRIC PHARMACOLOGY

This chapter describes the effects of aging on drug response. It explains the pharmacokinetic and pharmacodynamic alterations that occur with age. In addition, it discusses how age-related drug changes are affected by other factors that increase with age such as nutritional status, disease, and the number of drugs that are often prescribed in the elderly population to maintain health and prolong life in the age of modern medicine.

CHAPTER OBJECTIVES

After studying this chapter you should be able to

- describe the main physiological changes that occur with aging.

- list several factors that affect the absorption and distribution of drugs in the elderly.

- list several factors that affect the metabolism and excretion of drugs in the elderly.

- understand the effects of nutrition and age-related diseases on drug response.

- explain the problems associated with drug compliance in the elderly.

Key Terms

creatinine: a metabolite of muscle metabolism that is excreted in the urine in proportion to renal function.

creatinine clearance: a measure of renal creatinine excretion that is used to evaluate renal function.

drug compliance: following drug prescription directions exactly as written.

enterohepatic cycling: the process of elimination and reabsorption through the liver, biliary ducts, and intestinal tract.

geriatrics: medical specialty that deals with individuals over 65 years of age.

mixed-function oxidase system: drug microsomal metabolizing enzymes that decrease with age and slow the rate of drug metabolism.

polypharmacy: the situation in patients whose treatment involves multiple drug prescriptions.

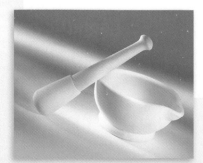

The process of aging begins slowly in the young adult and proceeds at varying individual rates throughout life. The effects of genetics, nutrition, exercise, injury, disease, environment, and many other factors affect the rate of aging. Regardless of the factors that can influence the aging process, there are predictable changes that occur in every individual with the passing of time. This chapter will focus on the age-related changes that influence drug response. The term **geriatric** refers to individuals over 65 years of age. Geriatric medicine, the medical treatment of the elderly, has developed into a medical specialty.

DRUG USE IN THE ELDERLY

The number of older individuals in the population is increasing and will continue to increase in the future. The dramatic increase in life expectancy over the past few decades has been a significant factor in the growth of this population. The progress of medical technology, including the discovery and development of many new and more effective drugs, has played an important role in improving the health and quality of life, in addition to increasing the number of years a person can live. The cost and social impact of new and often expensive treatments have also raised a number of moral and ethical issues concerning the prolongation of life at any cost.

Compared to other age groups, the geriatric population accounts for the highest percentage of drug prescriptions per year. Drug use increases with increasing age and the number of drugs consumed in the geriatric population averages between three and four drugs per individual. Both the nature and frequency of adverse drug reactions increase with age. It is not uncommon for elderly patients with multiple diseases, such as hypertension, arthritis, chronic obstructive pulmonary disease, and heart failure to have prescriptions for ten or more drugs. The number of possible adverse reactions and drug-drug interactions with this number of drugs is almost beyond calculation.

Physiological Effects of Aging on Pharmacokinetic Processes

Aging is a continuous process that begins when life is conceived. However, most healthy individuals do not begin, or will not admit to, feeling the effects of age until the third or fourth decade. It has been estimated that after 25 or 30 years of age, the cardiac output, the amount of blood pumped by the heart per minute, decreases by approximately 1 percent per year. This means that by the age of 65, the liver and kidneys, for example, are receiving significantly less blood per minute than they did 40 years ago. This, in particular, can have important consequences for drug action and the ability of the body to eliminate drugs. In addition, the size of most body organs decreases with age and, therefore, there are fewer cells to carry out organ functions. Each of the pharmacokinetic processes: drug absorption, drug distribution, drug metabolism, and drug excretion are affected to some degree by the aging process.

Drug Absorption

With age there is a decrease in blood flow to the intestinal tract, reduced intestinal absorptive surface area, a decrease in gastric acid secretion, and a decrease in intestinal motility. These changes tend to slow the rate of drug absorption and the onset of drug action. In addition, the peak drug blood level (highest drug concentration attained after administration) may be lower than it would be in a younger adult. While the peak drug level may be lower, the total amount of drug absorbed is usually not significantly affected. Consequently, the main effect of aging is to slow drug absorption and delay the onset of drug action.

Drug Distribution

There are significant alterations in body composition that occur with age. The percentage of lean body mass (muscle) and the percentage of total body water decrease. If one thinks of the body as a big beaker filled with 35 liters (l) of fluid and a drug dose dumped into the beaker, there will be a certain concentration of drug per liter. As the percentage of water decreases, the same dose will produce a higher concentration of drug in the beaker. The same thing occurs in the body. As one becomes older, the same dosage of drug given to a younger adult will produce a higher drug concentration in the elderly.

The percentage of body fat (adipose tissue) increases with age. This causes lipid-soluble drugs to be more widely distributed to the body organs that have a high fat content, such as adipose tissue and muscle (modest fat content, but large mass), and away from the liver and kidneys. Since the liver and kidneys are responsible for drug metabolism and excretion, any diversion from them will slow elimination of drug from the body. The drug will then have a longer half-life and duration of action.

Water-soluble drugs will have less body fluid in which to dissolve and are less widely distributed out to the organs with high fat content. This produces higher plasma drug levels and greater pharmacological effects when compared to the same dosage of drug administered to a younger adult.

The concentration of plasma proteins, mainly albumin, decreases with age. Since most drugs are bound to some extent to plasma proteins and it is only the concentration of "free drug" that produces the pharmacological effect, any decrease in plasma proteins and plasma protein drug binding will increase the amount of free drug (unbound) and, therefore, the intensity of drug effect.

In summary, the overall effect of aging on drug distribution is to generally make any adult drug dosage produce greater pharmacological effects in the elderly if the drug is given in the same dosage. Drugs that are affected by the changes in drug distribution with age usually require a reduction in dosage.

Drug Metabolism

In general, the rate of drug metabolism decreases with age, although there is much variability. The age-related decreases in liver blood flow and production of some drug microsomal metabolizing enzymes reduce the rate of drug metabolism. The enzymes that are most affected appear to be the enzymes that oxidize drugs, referred to as the **mixed-function oxidase system.** The pharmacological effects of drugs requiring oxidation, the benzodiazepines (diazepam, *Valium*) for example, are usually prolonged. In addition, drugs that undergo first-pass metabolism are not as extensively metabolized during the first pass through the liver. This allows a greater amount of drug to be absorbed,

an example of increased bioavailability. Other factors such as smoking, alcohol consumption, and the administration of certain drugs, all of which may cause microsomal enzyme induction, will increase the rate of drug metabolism. Consequently, it is difficult to accurately predict the effects of aging on specific drug metabolism, but the expected effect is a reduction in the rate of metabolism and an increase in the duration of drug action.

Drug Excretion

Drugs are eliminated from the body mainly by renal excretion and gastrointestinal elimination. Some drugs and drug metabolites pass from the liver through the biliary tract and into the intestinal tract for elimination. There are also drugs that can be reabsorbed back into the blood after following this pathway. This is referred to as **enterohepatic cycling.** Enterohepatic cycling can increase the drug half-life and the duration of drug action.

The reduction of renal blood flow with age has a significant effect on the renal elimination of drugs. Renal excretion is probably the most important pharmacokinetic process that is affected by age. Almost all measures of renal function, such as glomerular filtration rate and creatinine clearance, are significantly reduced with age. The duration of drug action, plasma drug concentration, and pharmacological effects will all be increased for drugs that are eliminated primarily by renal excretion. Drugs that are primarily excreted by the urinary tract usually require dosage reduction. The reduction in dosage is usually based on the urinary excretion of **creatinine.** Creatinine is a product of muscle metabolism that is excreted by the kidneys in proportion to glomerular filtration rate. The lab test to evaluate the ability of the kidneys to excrete creatinine is known as **creatinine clearance.** The test involves measuring the concentration of creatinine in the blood and using a mathematical formula (not shown) to determine the creatinine clearance rate. This value is then compared to the expected normal value found in healthy younger adults. Dosage adjustments can then be calculated based on the level of individual renal function. The plasma concentration of creatinine increases with age and renal disease, and reflects the effects of age and disease to decreased renal function. Table 3:1 summarizes the major effects and consequences of aging on the pharmacokinetic processes.

TABLE 3:1   Age-Related Changes in Pharmacokinetic Processes

PHARMACOKINETIC PROCESS	AGE-RELATED CHANGE
Drug absorption	Decreased intestinal blood flow, surface area, and motility delay drug absorption and slow onset of drug action.
Drug distribution	Decreased body water, lean body mass, and plasma proteins along with increased fat content increase plasma drug concentrations and pharmacologic effects.
Drug metabolism	Decreased liver blood flow, liver organ size, and enzyme concentrations decrease the rate of drug metabolism and increase the duration and intensity of drug action.
Drug excretion	Age-related decreases in renal function and blood flow slow the rate of drug excretion, and increase the duration and intensity of drug action.

EFFECTS OF AGE ON DRUG RESPONSE

The effects of age on drug response are difficult to evaluate. Most of the information comes from observations that a specific drug or drug class appears to either produce increased or decreased pharmacological effects in geriatric patients when compared to the effects produced in younger adults. Increased pharmacological effects are more common and usually observed as an increase in adverse or toxic effects. The changes in drug sensitivity may be caused by a number of factors: general state of health, nutritional status, presence of chronic disease, and alteration in the pharmacodynamic response to specific drugs.

Nutritional Status

Nutrition is extremely important to the state of health. Many of the elderly live alone or in unfamiliar surroundings such as nursing homes. The desire, ability, and affordability to prepare well-balanced meals are often lacking. An adequate diet is important in relation to liver function and the ability to metabolize drugs. Lack of adequate protein intake lowers the concentration of plasma proteins, especially albumin, necessary for plasma protein drug binding. Protein intake is also important for synthesis of drug-metabolizing enzymes. Protein deficiencies may increase the concentrations of "free drug" (unbound) and reduce the rate of drug metabolism, both of which can increase the duration and intensity of drug action.

General health and the ability of the body to maintain homeostatic mechanisms such as regulation of body temperature, blood pressure, cardiac output, and many other physiological processes are dependent in part on proper nutrition. Nutritional deficiencies also increase susceptibility to infection, disease, and the adverse effects of drug treatment.

Presence of Disease

The major chronic diseases of aging—hypertension, coronary artery disease, diabetes, cancer, and many others—all have effects that reduce vital organ function, especially of the heart, liver, and kidneys. Reduction of organ function decreases the ability of these organs to metabolize and eliminate drugs. Consequently, the actions and adverse effects of most drugs is increased. The consequences of disease on drug action increase as the number of diseases in any one individual increase. Table 3:2 lists the main effect of some of the more common disease-drug interactions.

Alteration of Pharmacodynamic Response

It is very difficult to evaluate changes in drug response that are not related to changes in the pharmacokinetic processes. While there may be some decreases in the number of drug receptors or drug receptor sensitivity with age, there are very few examples that have been well documented. One example that is often mentioned is a decrease in sensitivity of the elderly to beta-adrenergic drugs. It appears that actually more of a drug, such as isoproterenol, is required to increase the heart

Common Disease-Drug Interactions in the Elderly

DISEASE	DRUGS	CONSEQUENCE
Congestive heart failure	Cardiac depressants: beta-blockers, some calcium blockers (verapamil, diltiazam)	Excessive cardiac depression, hypotension, cardiac arrest
Diabetes mellitis	Thiazide and loop diuretics, beta-blockers	Alteration of blood glucose
Hypertension	Nonsteroidal antiinflammatory drugs	Interfere with antihypertensive actions of diuretics and *ACE inhibitors
Hypokalemia	Thiazide and loop diuretics, cardiac glycosides (digoxin)	Increase loss of potassium and may cause cardiac arrhythmias
Mental depression	**CNS depressants, propranolol, antihypertensives causing CNS depression (clonidine)	Increase mental depression, precipitate depressive episodes
Prostatic hypertrophy	Anticholinergic drugs	Increase difficulty of urination, urinary retention
Renal disease	Nonsteroidal antiinflammatory drugs, aminoglycosides, amphotericin B	Decrease renal function, may cause renal failure
Respiratory diseases, bronchitis, emphysema	Nonselective beta-blockers	Bronchoconstriction, respiratory distress

Abbreviations: *ACE, **angiotensin-converting enzyme**; **CNS, central nervous system.

rate of elderly individuals. However, in most cases the elderly are more sensitive to the actions of drugs and experience greater pharmacological effects and higher incidences of adverse effects.

The elderly are often more sensitive to drugs that depress the central nervous system. Sedatives, hypnotics, antianxiety agents, antipsychotic, and antidepressant drugs often cause excessive pharmacological and adverse effects in the elderly. This is often in the form of mental confusion, disorientation, and other neurological disturbances. Some of the antipsychotic, antidepressant, and antihistamine drugs possess anticholinergic activity (Chapter 7). Excessive anticholinergic effects frequently cause urinary retention, constipation, and a variety of neurological disturbances. There are many examples of drugs that require special consideration when prescribed for the elderly. Additional geriatric considerations with specific drugs will be presented in the appropriate chapters.

DRUG COMPLIANCE IN THE ELDERLY

Drug Compliance is extremely important in the elderly. The elderly are frequently confused by their dosing regimens. They often have difficulty understanding and remembering what the drug is and exactly why it was prescribed. The confusion is increased in those who already have problems with memory, who live alone, and in those who are not provided with sufficient time for instruction and training on the proper procedures for drug administration. The confusion increases in direct proportion to the number of different drugs and administration devices with which the individual is confronted. The term **polypharmacy** is used to describe the situation that involves multiple drug prescriptions. Forgetting to take the drug or not remembering whether or not the drug was already taken is the cause of many missed doses. The presence of unpleasant drug side effects also encourages noncompliance. Since physicians are often too busy to take the time to instruct patients, this is one of the important functions of allied health personnel. Time and patience are of extreme importance in these instructions. The attitude and demeanor of the person providing drug prescribing instructions are sometimes the key ingredients to successful drug compliance.

Another important consideration for compliance is the dosage form; for example, liquid, capsule, or tablet. Many elderly patients have difficulty swallowing large capsules. In addition, they often cannot get the lid off the drug container. There are easy-to-open lids for the elderly, available upon request. The elderly often have trouble reading the small print on drug labels or identifying the different drugs. Sometimes describing the different drugs (the small white one, the large green one, etc.) may help them know which drugs to take at the proper times. Organizing a schedule of specific times for drug dosing, such as before a specific meal or just before bedtime, is also important for establishing a routine that is less likely to be forgotten.

Chapter Review

Understanding Terminology

Match the appropriate answer, a or b, with the numbered statement in relationship to drug use in the elderly.

a. Increased duration and/or intensity of drug action

b. Decreased duration and/or intensity of drug action

___ **1.** Cirrhosis of the liver

___ **2.** Drug noncompliance

___ **3.** An increase in creatinine levels in the blood

___ **4.** Drugs that cause microsomal enzyme induction

___ **5.** Renal disease

___ **6.** Malnutrition

___ **7.** Drugs that increase liver blood flow

___ **8.** Enterohepatic cycling of drugs

___ **9.** Decrease in plasma proteins

___ **10.** Lipid-soluble drugs

Acquiring Knowledge

Answer the following questions in the space provided.

11. Describe three changes in body composition that occur with aging. _____

_____

12. What are the major age-related changes that occur in the liver? _____

_____

13. Briefly explain the importance of creatinine in relation to renal function. _____

_____

14. Describe three factors of drug compliance that are relative to geriatric patients. _____

_____

15. What are adverse effects of excessive anticholinergic drug action in the elderly? _____

_____

16. Explain how lower concentrations of plasma proteins can increase drug response. _____

_____

Applying Knowledge—On the Job

Use your critical thinking skills to answer the following questions in the space provided.

1. Mr. Green is 75 years old and in the doctor's office for his first checkup after being prescribed digoxin (*Lanoxin*) once daily and chlorothiazide (*Diuril*) two times a day (BID) for congestive heart failure. He still has some signs of heart failure and has admitted that he sometimes forgets to take his pills. He also has trouble reading the labels and isn't sure which pill he is supposed to take again at night.

   a. Can you give some instructions that might help Mr. Green become more compliant? _____

   _____

   _____

   b. Two weeks later Mr. Green returns for another office visit. His pulse rate is irregular and he says he feels weak and that he might pass out. What is most likely occurring with the patient? Is this a drug effect? A drug-drug interaction? You may have to look these drugs up in the *Physicians' Desk Reference (PDR®)*. _____

   _____

2. Mrs. Jones is 68 years old and has a history of diabetes and hypertension for which she takes medication. Over the years the diabetes seems to be decreasing her kidney function, and lately her urine samples show the presence of protein. She has recently experienced episodes of dizziness and her blood pressure recording during her checkup today was quite low. Could Mrs. Jones's blood pressure medication dosage be too high? What might be occurring here that may need some adjustment? _____

   _____

3. Mr. Smith has a cancer tumor that has become resistant to chemotherapy. He has experienced dramatic weight loss and his appetite is poor. Medications for his heart condition that were well tolerated in the past have now begun to cause toxicity. List the factors that may be responsible for this recent increase in drug toxicity. _____

   _____

4. Explain how the development of congestive heart failure could lead to a decrease in the rate of drug metabolism and drug excretion. _____

   _____

Use the *PDR®* or *F&C* to answer the following questions.

5. A 74-year-old male is currently taking hydrochlorothiazide, digoxin, isosorbide, and warfarin on a daily basis. He also takes nitroglycerin PRN. The doctor has just prescribed erythromycin for an upper respiratory infection. While you are talking to the patient, he remembers that his cardiologist has recently prescribed Norpace CR 150 mg BID. Is this contraindicated? Should the physician be notified? What action would you expect to follow and why? _____

   _____

6. A 70-year-old male has been diagnosed with Parkinson's disease. The physician has decided to start him on Lodosyn. Does this patient's age have a factor on the dosing of this medication? ___

   _____

7. A 63-year-old female diabetic patient with a history of excellent control with a consistent dose of insulin has recently suffered several hypoglycemic episodes. The only other medication she is taking is OTC ibuprofen 200 mg QID for her arthritis. All tests come back within normal range with the exception of her blood glucose level, which is low. Her physician has advised her to check her blood glucose level BID and explained how to adjust her dose accordingly. What other factors may be involved? _____

   _____

Internet Connection

Two Internet websites that focus on the aging process are the **National Institute of Aging** (http://www.nih.gov/nia) and the **National Council on Aging** (http://www.ncoa.org). After reaching the website for the National Institute of Aging, click on *What's New*. Listed are a variety of topics related to aging; explore some of these to observe the type of information available. Click on *Health Information* and select the heading for *Alzheimer's disease*. Click on the following headings in succession to get a better understanding of the disease: *Alzheimer's Disease Publications: Publications Online, Alzheimer's disease: Unraveling the Mystery.*

Organize a short presentation on Alzheimer's disease and present it to your class. This will provide some background information when the drugs used to treat Alzheimer's disease are discussed in Chapter 7.

Additional Reading

Carlson, J. E. 1996. Perils of polypharmacy: 10 steps to prudent prescribing. *Geriatrics* 51(7):26.

Cohen, G. D. 2002. The psychiatric consultant: Advising older adults who are contemplating retirement. *Geriatrics* 57(8):37.

Hall, G. R. 1996. Acute confusion in the elderly: What to do when the clouds roll in. *Nursing* 26(7):32.

Marin, D. B., Sewell, M. C., and Schlechter, A. 2002. Alzheimer's disease. *Geriatrics* 57(2):36.

Miller, C. A. 2002. Helping older adults reduce the cost of the drugs they need. *Geriatrics Nursing* 23(4):230.

Neugroschle, J. 2002. Agitation. *Geriatrics* 57(4):33.

Sable, J. A., Dunn, L. B., and Zisook, S. 2002. Late-life depression. *Geriatrics* 57(2):18.

Smith, M. K., and Sullivan, J. M. 1997. Nurses' and patients' perceptions of most important caring behaviors in a long-term care setting. *Geriatric Nursing* 18(2):70.

Worfolk, J. B. 1997. Keep frail elders warm. *Geriatric Nursing* 18(1):7.

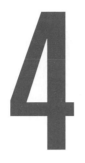

MATH REVIEW AND DOSAGE CALCULATIONS

Key Terms

decimal: another way to write a fraction when the denominator is 10, 100, 1000, and so on.

denominator: bottom number of a fraction; shows the number of parts in a whole.

fraction: part of a whole.

improper fraction: fraction that has a value equal to or greater than 1.

mixed number: number written with both a whole number and a fraction.

numerator: top number of a fraction; shows the part.

percent: decimal fraction with a denominator of 100.

proper fraction: fraction that has a value less than 1.

proportion: a mathematical equation that expresses the equality between two ratios.

ratio: the relationship of one number to another expressed by whole numbers (1:5) or as a fraction ($\frac{1}{5}$).

solute: substance dissolved in a solvent; usually present in a lesser amount.

solution: homogeneous mixture of two or more substances.

solvent: liquid portion of a solution that is capable of dissolving another substance.

CHAPTER FOCUS

This chapter reviews basic mathematical operations required for drug calculation. It also provides examples that clearly show how to set up and solve different types of dosage problems necessary for proper drug administration.

CHAPTER OBJECTIVES

After studying this chapter, you should be able to

- solve basic arithmetical problems involving fractions, decimals, and percents.
- perform conversions from one metric unit of measure to another.
- set up ratio and proportion equations and solve for the unknown term.
- solve drug problems involving solutions and solid dosage forms.
- solve problems involving pediatric dosing.

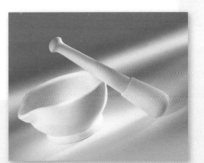

INTRODUCTION

Because the intensity of drug response is directly related to dosage (dose-response relationship), administration of the proper drug dosage is essential to the practice of medicine. Drugs whose names look alike or sound alike (for example, *Demerol*/dicumarol, *Isordil*/isuprel) can cause improper drug selection. Mistakes in dosage calculation can cause insufficient drug response or excessive and potentially harmful drug effects. Consequently, it is essential for anyone responsible for administering medication to understand the proper procedures for dosage calculation.

FRACTIONS, DECIMALS, AND PERCENTS

A brief review of fractions, decimals, and percents is presented to refresh the memory for the basic arithmetical procedures used in dosage calculation.

Fractions

When something is divided into equal parts, one of the parts is referred to as a **fraction** (part of the whole). A fraction is composed of two numbers, a numerator and a denominator. The **numerator** is the top number of a fraction. It indicates how many parts are being referred to. The **denominator** is the bottom number of a fraction. It indicates how many parts something has been divided into (see Figure 4:1).

Proper Fractions

Fractions whose values are less than 1 (the numerator is smaller than the denominator) are called **proper fractions.** The following are examples of proper fractions:

$$\frac{1}{4} \quad \frac{2}{3} \quad \frac{7}{8} \quad \frac{9}{10}$$

Improper Fractions

Fractions whose values are equal to or greater than 1 (the numerator is equal to or greater than the denominator) are called **improper fractions.** The following fractions are improper:

$$\frac{5}{5} \quad \frac{7}{5} \quad \frac{11}{6} \quad \frac{15}{8}$$

An improper fraction can be written as a **mixed number,** which is a whole number plus the fractional remainder. This is calculated by dividing the denominator of the improper fraction into the numerator and placing any remainder over the original denominator. If there is no remainder, the improper fractions have been changed to mixed numbers:

$$\frac{5}{5} = 1 \quad \frac{7}{5} = 1\frac{2}{5}$$

$$\frac{11}{6} = 1\frac{5}{6} \quad \frac{24}{8} = 3$$

The terms of a fraction can be changed without changing its value. Multiplying or dividing the numerator and the denominator of a fraction by the same number does not change the value of the fraction, as shown in the following examples:

$$\frac{2 \div 2}{4 \div 2} = \frac{1}{2} \quad \frac{2 \times 3}{4 \times 3} = \frac{6}{12}$$

Fractions are generally written in their reduced, or lowest, terms. For example:

$$\frac{6}{12} \text{ reduces to } \frac{1}{2}$$

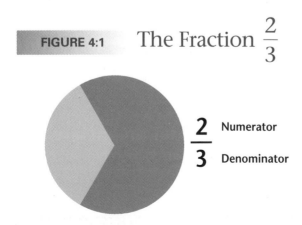

FIGURE 4:1 The Fraction $\dfrac{2}{3}$

$\dfrac{2}{3}$ $\mathbf{2}$ Numerator $\mathbf{3}$ Denominator

The fraction $\frac{2}{3}$ represents two of three equal-sized pieces of a whole.

Reducing Fractions to Their Lowest Terms

Reduce a fraction to its lowest terms by dividing the numerator and denominator by the largest number that will divide into both of them evenly. For example:

$$\frac{15}{20} \div \frac{5}{5} = \frac{3}{4} \qquad \frac{35}{49} \div \frac{7}{7} = \frac{5}{7}$$

Multiplying Fractions

Multiply fractions by multiplying the numerators together and the denominators together and reducing to lowest terms. For example:

$$\frac{2}{3} \times \frac{3}{4} = \frac{6}{12} = \frac{1}{2}$$

If the fractions involve large numbers, reduce the numbers by dividing any numerator and any denominator by the same number. Repeat this cancellation process as often as possible. For example:

$$\overset{1}{\underset{2}{\cancel{\frac{9}{18}}}} \times \overset{1}{\underset{2}{\cancel{\frac{27}{54}}}} = \frac{1}{4}$$

$$\overset{1}{\underset{1}{\cancel{\frac{4}{6}}}} \times \overset{\overset{1}{2}}{\underset{\underset{2}{4}}{\cancel{\frac{12}{16}}}} = \frac{1}{2}$$

To multiply a whole number by a fraction, place the whole number over a denominator of 1, then multiply numerators and denominators. For example:

$$10 \times \frac{1}{2} = \frac{10}{1} \times \frac{1}{2} = \frac{10}{2} = 5$$

Dividing Fractions

Dividing one fraction by another is similar to multiplying fractions. However, first you must invert the divisor before multiplying the numerators together and the denominators together. For example:

$$\frac{2}{3} \div \frac{3}{4}$$

$$\frac{2}{3} \times \frac{4}{3} = \frac{8}{9}$$

If the divisor is a whole number, place it over 1, invert it, and then multiply as before. For example:

$$\frac{3}{4} \div 4 = \frac{3}{4} \div \frac{4}{1} = \frac{3}{4} \times \frac{1}{4} = \frac{3}{16}$$

Decimals

Any whole number may be divided into tenths (0.1), hundredths (0.01), thousandths (0.001), and so on. These divisions of a number by orders of 10 (10, 100, 10,000, etc.) are known as decimal fractions, or **decimals.** Decimals are another way of expressing fractions. For example:

$$\frac{1}{10} = 0.1 \qquad \frac{1}{100} = 0.01 \qquad \frac{1}{1000} = 0.001$$

To change a fraction to a decimal, simply divide the numerator by the denominator. Note that you may need to add zeros after the decimal point in the dividend. For example:

$$\frac{1}{4} = 4\overline{)1.00}^{\,0.25} = 0.25$$

To change a decimal to a fraction, place the decimal number over the order of 10 (10, 100, 1000, etc.) that corresponds to the last place of the decimal and reduce to lowest terms. For example:

$$0.5 = \frac{5}{10} = \frac{1}{2} \qquad 0.25 = \frac{25}{100} = \frac{1}{4}$$
$$\text{tenths} \qquad\qquad\qquad \text{hundredths}$$

$$0.005 = \frac{5}{1000} = \frac{1}{200}$$
$$\text{thousandths}$$

Multiplying Decimals

Multiplying decimals is similar to multiplying whole numbers except for the placement of the decimal point. After multiplying the two decimal numbers, add the total number of decimal places (places to the right of each decimal point) and count off the total number of decimal places in the answer (product). Count from right to left, and put the decimal point in front of the last number you count. For example:

```
      1.25    (2 decimal places)
    ×0.25     (2 decimal places)
     ────
      625
     250
    ──────
    0.3125    (4 decimal places)
```

When an answer has fewer numbers than total decimal places, add zeros as placeholders to make up the difference.

$$\begin{array}{r} 0.5 \quad \text{(1 decimal place)} \\ \times\, 0.1 \quad \text{(1 decimal place)} \\ \hline 0.05 \quad \text{(2 decimal places)} \end{array}$$

Dividing Decimals

When dividing decimals, move the decimal place in the divisor to the far right and then move the decimal place in the number being divided by the same number of places. For example:

$$25 \div 0.05 = 0.05\overline{)25.000}^{\,500.0}$$
$$\text{(2 places)} \qquad \text{(2 places)}$$

$$0.010 \div 0.5 = .5\overline{)0.010}^{\,0.02}$$
$$\text{(1 place)} \qquad \text{(1 place)}$$

Percents

Percent means per hundred. So, **percents** are decimal fractions with denominators of 100. See the following examples:

$$10\% = \frac{10}{100} = 0.10$$

$$25\% = \frac{25}{100} = \frac{1}{4} = 0.25$$

Multiplying Percents

Change the percent to a decimal (in hundredths) and multiply. For example:

15 percent of 75

$$\begin{array}{r} 75 \\ \times\, 0.15 \\ \hline 375 \\ 75 \\ \hline 11.25 \end{array} \quad \begin{array}{l} \text{(2 decimal} \\ \text{places)} \\ \\ \\ \text{(2 decimal places)} \end{array}$$

0.2 percent of 50

$$\begin{array}{r} 50 \\ \times\, 0.002 \\ \hline 0.100 \end{array} \quad \begin{array}{l} \text{(3 decimal places)} \\ \\ \text{(3 decimal places)} \end{array}$$

DOSAGE CALCULATIONS

Health professionals today are very fortunate because pharmaceutical manufacturers prepare and market most drugs in convenient dosage forms. The metric system has essentially replaced the apothecaries' system, so mathematical conversions are rarely necessary. Also, the concept of unit dose packaging eliminates much of the time that was previously required for drug calculation and preparation. However, in certain situations, drug calculations are still required. These situations primarily involve the preparation of a drug dosage from a stock solution, vial, scored tablet, or calculation of dosage based on body weight or other body measurement.

Basic Calculations

Ratio is the relationship of one number to another expressed by whole numbers (1:5) or as a fraction $\frac{1}{5}$. The lowest form of the ratio is determined by dividing the smaller number into the larger number. In this example, the ratio would be 5:1.

Proportion is a mathematical equation that expresses the equality between two ratios.

EXAMPLE 25:5 = 50:10
The first (25) and last terms (10) are called the extremes. The second (5) and third terms (50) are called the means. The product (multiplication) of the extremes must equal the product of the means.

$$\begin{array}{c} \text{means} \\ \downarrow \quad \searrow \end{array}$$
EXAMPLE $\quad 25{:}5 = 50{:}10$
$$\begin{array}{c} \nwarrow \qquad \nearrow \\ \text{extremes} \end{array}$$
$$25 \times 10 = 5 \times 50$$
$$250 = 250$$

When one of the numbers in the proportion is not known, the proportion equation can be solved for the unknown (referred to as X).

EXAMPLE There are 10 milligrams (mg) of drug per milliliter (ml) of solution. How many milliliters must be administered in order to provide 65 mg of drug?

10 mg:1 ml (what you know) = 65 mg:X ml (what you need to know)

$$10X = 65$$
$$X = 6.5 \text{ ml}$$

Remember, the smaller known ratio is put to the left of the equal sign and the unknown ratio is put to the right of the equal sign. Solve for X by multiplying the means and the extremes.

SYSTEMS OF MEASUREMENT

Metric System

The metric system is the preferred system for scientific measurement. The units of measure for the metric system are meter (length), gram (weight), and liter (volume). A convenient feature of the metric system is that measurements are in decimal progression, so that 10 units of one size equal 1 unit of the next-higher size.

The names of the metric system are formed by joining Greek and Latin prefixes with the terms *meter, gram,* and *liter:*

milli—$\frac{1}{1000}$ (0.001)   deka—10

centi—$\frac{1}{100}$ (0.01)   hecto—100

deci—$\frac{1}{10}$ (0.1)   kilo—1000

Apothecaries' System

The apothecaries' system is an older system of measurement that is rarely used today. The basic unit of measurement is the grain (gr). Only a few conversion values are included to show the relationship to the metric system.

Household System

The household system is a less accurate system of measurement. It is mainly used in the home where dosages can be expressed in terms of common household measurements: teaspoon (tsp), tablespoon (tbsp), and liquid ounces (oz).

Conversion Tables

Weights

1 kilogram (kg) = 1000 grams (g)

1 gram (g) = 1000 milligrams (mg)

1 milligram (mg) = 1000 micrograms (μg)

1.5 grains (gr, apothecaries' system) = 100 mg

1 grain (gr, apothecaries' system) = 60.0 mg

$\frac{1}{2}$ grain (gr, apothecaries' system) = 30.0 mg

Volumes

1 liter (l) = 1000 milliliters (ml), 1000 cubic centimeters (cc), or approximately 1 quart

500 ml = approximately 1 pint

250 ml = approximately 8 fluid ounces = 1 cup

30.0 ml = approximately 1 fluid ounce

1.0 ml = 1.0 cc (cubic centimeters)

Approximate Household Measures

60 drops (gtt) = 1 teaspoon (tsp)

1 teaspoonful (tsp) = approximately 5.0 ml

1 tablespoonful (tbsp) = approximately 15.0 ml

2 tablespoons (tbsp) = approximately 1 fluid ounce (oz)

1 measuring cup = approximately 8 fluid ounces (oz)

Conversions

It is frequently necessary to make conversions of solution concentrations from liters (l) to milliliters (ml) and drug weights from grams (g) to milligrams (mg) or micrograms (μg). Knowledge of metric system equivalents is essential to performing these simple conversions. Conversion problems can be set up as a proportion and solved for X.

EXAMPLE Convert 1.5 liters (l) to ml.

$$1 \text{ l}:1000 \text{ ml} = 1.5 \text{ l}:X$$
$$1 X = 1500 \text{ ml}$$
$$X = 1500 \text{ ml}$$

Alternate setup of proportion equation as a fraction:

EXAMPLE Convert 1.5 liters to ml.

$$\frac{1 \text{ l}}{1000 \text{ ml}} = \frac{1.5 \text{ l}}{X \text{ ml}}$$
$$X = 1000 \times 1.5$$
$$X = 1500 \text{ ml}$$

EXAMPLE Convert 750 ml to liters (l).

$$\frac{1000 \text{ ml}}{1 \text{ l}} = \frac{750 \text{ ml}}{X \text{ l}}$$
$$1000 X = 750$$
$$X = \frac{750}{1000}$$
$$X = 0.75 \text{ l}$$

EXAMPLE Convert 0.25 g to milligrams (mg).

$$\frac{1 \text{ g}}{1000 \text{ mg}} = \frac{0.25 \text{ g}}{X \text{ mg}}$$
$$X = 1000 \times 0.25$$
$$X = 250 \text{ mg}$$

EXAMPLE Convert 350 mg to grams (g).

$$\frac{1000 \text{ mg}}{1 \text{ g}} = \frac{350 \text{ mg}}{X \text{ g}}$$

$$1000 X = 350$$

$$X = \frac{350}{1000}$$

$$X = 0.35 \text{ g}$$

Sometimes it is necessary to convert from one system of measurement to another.

EXAMPLE Convert 500 ml to ounces (oz).

$$\frac{250 \text{ ml}}{8 \text{ oz}} = \frac{500 \text{ ml}}{X \text{ oz}}$$

$$250 X = 500 \times 8$$

$$250 X = 4000$$

$$X = 16 \text{ oz}$$

PRACTICE PROBLEMS

Convert the following:

1. 500 mg = _____ g
2. 0.45 g = _____ mg
3. 0.03 l = _____ ml
4. 4 tbsp = _____ ml
5. 60 ml = _____ oz

Solve the following conversions by setting up a proportion equation:

6. 6 teaspoons (tsp) to tablespoons (tbsp)
7. 1.5 pints to ml
8. 5 grains (gr) to mg
9. 500 micrograms (μg) to mg
10. 2500 grams (g) to kg

Solutions

A **solution** is a homogeneous mixture of two or more substances. The liquid portion of the solution is known as the **solvent** and the substance dissolved within the solvent is the **solute.** Solutions are commonly expressed as percentages. There are three types of percentage solutions:

Weight in Weight (W/W)

Weight in weight solutions contain a given weight of drug (or other solute) in a definite weight of solvent so that the final solution is 100 parts by weight.

EXAMPLE A 10 percent (W/W) solution of sodium chloride would contain 10 g of sodium chloride in 90 g of water.

Weight in Volume (W/V)

Weight in volume solutions contain a given weight of solute (drugs, salts) in enough solvent so that the final solution contains 100 parts by volume.

EXAMPLE A 10 percent (W/V) solution of sodium chloride would contain 10 g of sodium chloride in enough water to make 100 ml of final solution.

Volume in Volume (V/V)

Volume in volume solutions contain a definite volume of solute added to enough water so that the final solution would be 100 parts by volume.

EXAMPLE A 10 percent (V/V) solution of sodium chloride would contain 10 ml of sodium chloride (100 percent solution) in enough water to make 100 ml of final solution.

Calculating Dosages

The proportion equation is useful for calculating dosages. Whenever three of the terms of a proportion are known, the unknown term can be determined if the equation is properly constructed.

EXAMPLE Morphine sulfate injection for intravenous use is available in a concentration of 8 mg/ml of solution. Calculate the number of ml required to administer a dosage of 20 mg of morphine sulfate.

$$\frac{8 \text{ mg}}{1 \text{ ml}} = \frac{20 \text{ mg}}{X \text{ ml}}$$
$$8X = 20$$
$$X = 2.5 \text{ ml}$$

EXAMPLE There is a drug order for 50 mg of secobarbital (elixir). The stock bottle contains 22 mg of secobarbital in 5 ml of solution. How many milliliters should the patient receive?

$$\frac{22 \text{ mg}}{5 \text{ ml}} = \frac{50 \text{ mg}}{X \text{ ml}}$$
$$22X = 50 \times 5$$
$$22X = 250$$
$$X = 11.3636, \text{ or } 11.4 \text{ ml}$$

EXAMPLE There is a drug order for 75 mg of meperidine (*Demerol*) to be administered intramuscularly (IM). *Demerol* is supplied in a 5 percent solution (W/V). A 5 percent solution (W/V) would be 5 g of *Demerol* in 100 cc or 50 mg/1 ml as it is written on the vial label. How many ml of *Demerol* should be administered to the patient?

$$\frac{50 \text{ mg}}{1 \text{ ml}} = \frac{75 \text{ mg}}{X \text{ ml}}$$
$$50X - 75$$
$$X = \frac{75}{50}$$
$$X = 1.5 \text{ ml}$$

EXAMPLE Insulin is usually administered in a syringe that corresponds to the concentration of the stock solution (40 units per ml U-40 and a U-40 syringe; 100 units per ml U-100 and a U-100 syringe). If an insulin syringe is not available, a tuberculin syringe may be used. However, the unit dosage must be converted to ml using the proportion method. What would be the dose in milliliters for an order of 20 units of insulin when only U-100 insulin is available?

$$\frac{100 \text{ units}}{1 \text{ ml}} = \frac{20 \text{ units}}{X \text{ ml}}$$

$$100X = 20$$
$$X = \frac{20}{100}$$
$$X = 0.2 \text{ ml}$$

EXAMPLE There is a drug order for 60 mg of drug. The drug is available in 20-mg tablets. How many tablets are required? The problem requires setting up a fraction based on the formula:

$$\frac{\text{desired dosage}}{\text{available dosage}} = \frac{\overset{3}{60 \text{ mg}}}{\underset{1}{20 \text{ mg}} \ (1 \text{ tablet})} = 3 \text{ tablets}$$

A variation on this problem could be that 10 mg of a drug are desired:

$$\frac{\text{desired dosage}}{\text{available dosage}} = \frac{\overset{1}{10 \text{ mg}}}{\underset{2}{20 \text{ mg}} \ (1 \text{ tablet})} = \frac{1}{2} \text{ tablet}$$

(tablet must be scored for breakage)

EXAMPLE An injection of 1000 units of tetanus antitoxin is ordered. The tetanus antitoxin is available in an ampul labeled 1500 units/ml. How many milliliters should be injected?

$$\frac{\text{desired dosage}}{\text{available dosage}} = \frac{\overset{2}{1000 \text{ units}}}{\underset{3}{1500 \text{ units}} \ (\text{per milliliter})}$$

$$= \frac{2}{3} \text{ ml} = 3\overline{\smash{)}2.00}^{\ 0.66 \text{ ml}}$$

Pediatric Dosage Calculations

Dosage calculations in pediatrics are based on age, body surface area (BSA), and body weight. Following are the formulas used for these calculations. The BSA formula is the formula most commonly used.

Young's rule:

$$\frac{\text{age of child}}{\text{age of child}} + 12 \times \text{adult dose} = \text{child's dose}$$

Clark's rule:

$$\frac{\text{weight of child}}{150 \text{ lb}} \times \text{adult dose} = \text{child's dose}$$

Fried's rule:

$$\frac{\text{age in months}}{150} \times \frac{\text{average}}{\text{adult dose}} = \text{child's dose}$$

Body surface area (BSA) rule:

$$\frac{\text{body surface area of child (square meters)}}{1.7} \times \text{adult dose} = \text{child's dose}$$

EXAMPLE   Katie has just turned 3 years old and weighs 30 pounds. Her mother wants to know how much cough syrup to give Katie. The directions have worn off the bottle and she can only make out the dosage for adults—2 teaspoons every 4 hours. How much should Katie receive?

Young's rule: $\frac{3}{3}+12 \times 10$ ml = Katie's dose

$$\frac{1}{5} \times 10 \text{ ml} = 2 \text{ ml}$$

Clark's rule: $\frac{30}{150} \times 10$ ml $\quad$ = Katie's dose

$$\frac{1}{5} \times 10 \text{ ml} = 2 \text{ ml}$$

Fried's rule: $\frac{36}{150} \times 10$ ml = Katie's dose

$$0.24 \times 10 \text{ ml} = 2.4 \text{ ml}$$

Dosage Calculations Based on Body Weight

Drug dosages are sometimes administered on a body weight basis, for example, in mg/kg. This may require conversion of pounds to kilograms (1 kg = 2.2 lbs). The dose/kg is then multiplied by the number of kilograms.

EXAMPLE   There is a drug order for the antibiotic amikacin 7.5mg/kg administered intravenously (IV) for a patient weighing 110 pounds. Amikacin is available as 100 mg per 2-ml vial. How many milligrams of drug are required and in what volume?

Step 1: Convert pounds to kilograms.
110 lbs divided by 2.2 lb/kg = 50 kg

Step 2: Determine how many mg of drug are required.
7.5 mg/kg × 50 kg = 375 mg

Step 3: Determine how many ml of stock solution contains 375 mg, using the

proportion equation method.

100 mg:2 ml = 375 mg:X ml

100 X = (375) (2) or 750

X = 750/100 = 7.5 ml of vial solution ($3\frac{3}{4}$ vials)

EXAMPLE   If the patient in the previous problem was an infant weighing 20 lbs with a body surface area of 0.44 square meters, what would be the dose according to the BSA rule?

BSA rule: BSA of child (square meters)/1.7 × adult dose

$\frac{0.44}{1.7} \times 375$ mg

= 0.258 × 375 = 96.75 mg or 97 mg

Since vials contain $\frac{100 \text{ mg}}{2 \text{ ml}}$, calculate volume

$\frac{100 \text{ mg}}{2 \text{ ml}} = \frac{97 \text{ mg}}{X \text{ ml}}$

100 X = (2) (97) or 194

X = 1.94 ml of vial solution

EXAMPLE   A loading dose of digoxin capsules (*Lanoxicaps*), 10 μg/kg, has been ordered for a patient weighing 154 pounds. *Lanoxicaps* are available as 50-, 100-, and 200-μg capsules. How many capsules should be administered?

Step 1: Convert pounds to kilograms.
154 lbs divided by 2.2 lb/kg = 70 kg

Step 2: Determine how many micrograms are required.
70 kg × 10 μg/kg = 700 μg or 0.7 mg

Step 3: Determine how many capsules are required.
0.2 mg:capsule = 0.7 mg:X
0.2 X = 0.7
X = 3.5 capsules (3 capsules of 200 μg and 1 capsule of 100 μg)

MONITORING IV INFUSION RATES

Hospitalized patients often receive drug administration by slow IV infusion. Drugs are added to various sterile IV solutions such as sodium chloride injection, United States Pharmacopeia (USP) or dextrose (5%) injection,

USP. Drug concentrations and solutions are prepared by the hospital pharmacy. The IV drug infusion solutions must be prepared under aseptic conditions, the drugs and solutions mixed must be chemically compatible, and often the infusion solution must be adjusted to a specific pH value. Preparation of these solutions should always follow established hospital procedures and be reviewed by a pharmacist.

After establishment of an open IV line, the drug solution is administered according to a specific infusion rate, in drops per minute. Usually there are 15 drops/ml of solution, but this number can vary with the viscosity of different solutions. Since allied health personnel are sometimes called upon to monitor IV infusion rates, the following example is presented to illustrate the principles involved.

Formula for adjusting IV infusion rate:

$$\frac{\text{ml of IV solution} \times \text{number of drops/ml}}{\text{hours of administration} \times 60 \text{ minutes}} = \text{drops per minute}$$

EXAMPLE   An IV infusion of furosemide (*Lasix*) 2 mg/min for 4 hours was ordered for a patient with severe edema. The hospital pharmacy prepared the infusion solution by adding 480 mg (2 mg/min × 60 × 4) in 500 ml of sodium chloride injection, USP. How many drops per minute should be administered?

$$\frac{500 \text{ ml} \times 15 \text{ drops/ml}}{4 \text{ hours} \times 60 \text{ minutes}} = \frac{7500}{240} = 31.25 \text{ drops/min}$$

Regulate the IV flow by counting the drops (to nearest whole number) for 15 seconds and multiplying by 4 (for 1 min). Adjust the IV tube clamp until the correct rate is attained.

Chapter Review

Understanding Terminology

Match the term in the left column with the appropriate set of examples to the right. Use each set of examples only once.

___ **1.** Mixed numbers

___ **2.** Decimals

___ **3.** Proper fractions

___ **4.** Denominator

___ **5.** Fractions

___ **6.** Numerator

___ **7.** Improper fractions

a. $\dfrac{8}{16}, \dfrac{13}{27}, \dfrac{3}{4}$

b. $\dfrac{15}{12}, \dfrac{4}{3}, \dfrac{39}{18}$

c. $1\dfrac{1}{2}, 15\dfrac{4}{5}, 5\dfrac{17}{18}$

d. 1.5, 0.75, 12.3333

e. the 3 in $\dfrac{3}{4}$

f. the 4 in $\dfrac{3}{4}$

g. $\dfrac{1}{2}, \dfrac{7}{10}, \dfrac{5}{12}$

Answer the following question in the spaces provided.

8. Define *solution, solute,* and *solvent.* _____

_____

_____

Acquiring Knowledge

Answer the following questions and solve the following problems in the spaces provided.

1. Convert 0.125 g to milligrams. _____
2. Convert 1200 ml to liters. _____
3. Two teaspoons of cough syrup equals how many milliliters? _____
4. One-quarter grain equals how many milligrams? _____
5. Four fluid ounces equals how many milliliters? _____
6. There is a drug order for 2.5 mg of glipizide (*Glucotrol*). Scored tablets are available in 5- and 10-mg strengths. Calculate the dosage. Why is the drug being given? (Refer to the *PDR*®.) _____

_____

_____

7. After several days, the dosage of glipizide for the patient in Problem 6 has been increased to 7.5 mg. Calculate the dosage. _____
8. There is an order for 75 mg of *Demerol Hydrochloride* syrup (USP). The syrup contains 50 mg of *Demerol Hydrochloride* per 5 ml. Calculate the dosage. What is the generic name of this drug? (Refer to the *PDR*®.) _____

_____

_____

9. Several hours later, the patient in Problem 8 complained of severe pain. The order was changed to 100 mg administered by intramuscular (IM) injection. *Demerol Hydrochloride* is supplied as a solution in vials labeled 50 mg/ml. Calculate the parenteral dosage. _____

10. A drug vial for parenteral injection is labeled "1 ml contains 50 mg." Calculate the amount required to administer a 30-mg dose. _____

Applying Knowledge—On the Job

Use your critical thinking skills to answer the following questions in the spaces provided.

1. Assume that you're spending your summer as an intern in a university hospital pharmacy. One of your duties is to prepare desired dosages from available dosages to arrive at the correct weight or number of units of drug for each order the pharmacist fills. Show the calculations for the correct amount of drug for each of the following orders that were filled on your first day of work.

    a. The first order called for 90 mg of drug. The drug is available in 30-mg tablets. How many tablets are required? _____

    b. The second order called for 2000 units of tetanus antitoxin. The tetanus antitoxin is available in an ampul of 1500 units/ml. How many milliliters should be injected? _____

    c. The third order called for 70 mg of secobarbital. The stock bottle contains 22 mg of secobarbital in 5 ml of solution. How many milliliters should the patient receive? _____

2. Bert just finished his training as a pharmacist assistant and started working in a nursing home dispensary last week. One of his job duties is to calculate the number of milliliters of drug-for-drug orders given in milligrams. Show how you would deal with the following patient orders if you had Bert's job.

    a. There's a drug order for 100 mg of *Demerol* to be administered IM. The label on the stock bottle of *Demerol* says it's in a 5 percent solution, or 50 mg per ml. _____

    b. There's an order for a diabetic patient of 30 units of insulin. The stock bottle is labelled U-100, or 100 units per ml. _____

3. There is a drug order for diazepam (*Valium*), 0.5 mg/kg, administered orally. The patient weighs 110 pounds. *Valium* is available in 2-, 5-, and 10-mg tablets. How many milligrams and what combination of tablets will you administer? _____

4. Ampicillin (*Omnipen*) oral suspension is available as 125 mg/5 ml. There is a drug order for 500 mg four times a day (QID). How many milliliters will you administer with each dose? How often will you administer the dose? _____

5. The usual oral dose of ampicillin is 500 mg. How much should a 15-month-old baby receive according to Fried's rule? How much should a 50-pound child receive according to Clark's rule?

PHARMACOLOGY OF THE PERIPHERAL NERVOUS SYSTEM

Chapter 5

Autonomic Nervous System

Nervous System Organization
Physiology and Pharmacology
Parasympathetic and Sympathetic
   Divisions

Chapter 6

Drugs Affecting the Sympathetic Nervous System

Adrenergic Nerve Endings
Norepinephrine Versus Epinephrine
Adrenergic Receptors
Alpha-Adrenergic Drugs
Beta-Adrenergic Drugs
Dopamine
Alpha-Adrenergic Blocking Drugs
Beta-Adrenergic Blocking Drugs
Adrenergic Neuronal Blocking
   Drugs

Chapter 7

Drugs Affecting the Parasympathetic Nervous System

Parasympathetic System
Cholinergic Drugs
Anticholinergic Drugs

Chapter 8

Drugs Affecting the Autonomic Ganglia

Ganglionic Drugs

Chapter 9

Skeletal Muscle Relaxants

Clinical Indications
Peripherally Acting Skeletal Muscle
   Relaxants
Direct-Acting Skeletal Muscle
   Relaxants
Centrally Acting Skeletal Muscle
   Relaxants

Chapter 10

Local Anesthetics

Mechanisms of Action
Pharmacology
Routes of Administration
Adverse Effects
Clinincal Applications

Autonomic Nervous System

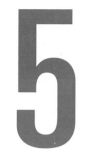
Key Terms

acetylcholine (ACH): neurotransmitter of parasympathetic (cholinergic) nerves; stimulates the cholinergic receptor.

adrenergic receptor: receptor located on internal organs that responds to norepinephrine.

afferent nerve: transmits sensory information to the brain and spinal cord (central nervous system).

autonomic nervous system (ANS): system of nerves that innervate smooth and cardiac muscle (involuntary) of the internal organs and glands.

cholinergic receptor: receptor located on internal organs that responds to acetylcholine.

efferent nerve: carries the appropriate motor response from the brain and spinal cord.

epinephrine: hormone from adrenal medulla that stimulates adrenergic receptors, especially during stress.

fight or flight reaction: response of the body to intense stress; caused by activation of the sympathetic division of the ANS.

homeostasis: normal state of balance among the body's internal organs.

neurotransmitter: substance that stimulates internal organs to produce characteristic changes associated with sympathetic and parasympathetic divisions.

norepinephrine (NE): neurotransmitter of sympathetic (adrenergic) nerves that stimulates the adrenergic receptors.

parasympathetic: refers to nerves of the ANS that originate in the brain and sacral portion of the spinal cord; they are active when the body is at rest or trying to restore body energy and function.

sympathetic: refers to nerves of the ANS that originate from the thoracolumbar portion of the spinal cord; they are active when the body is under stress or when it is exerting energy.

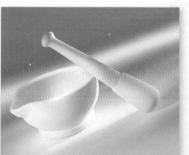

CHAPTER FOCUS

This chapter describes the basic organization of the autonomic nervous system (ANS) and how it functions to maintain homeostasis as the body experiences stress. It also explains the role of the sympathetic and parasympathetic divisions of the ANS and how the nerves of these systems regulate the activities of the individual body organs.

CHAPTER OBJECTIVES

After studying this chapter, you should be able to

- describe the two divisions of the ANS and explain how they differ.

- explain how sympathetic and parasympathetic nerves interact with each other to regulate organ function (maintain homeostasis).

- describe the fight or flight reaction and explain how it affects the activities of the different organs.

- list four effects caused by parasympathetic stimulation.

- list two autonomic neurotransmitters and explain the role of each in the function of the ANS.

NERVOUS SYSTEM ORGANIZATION

The nervous system is an elaborate system that functions at both conscious (under control of the will, or voluntary) and unconscious (not under control of the will, or involuntary) levels.

Central Nervous System (CNS)

The central nervous system (CNS), consists of the brain and spinal cord. The CNS receives and interprets sensory information (via peripheral **afferent nerves**) and then initiates appropriate motor responses (via peripheral **efferent nerves**).

Peripheral Nervous System (PNS)

The peripheral nervous system is composed of 12 pairs of cranial nerves and 31 pairs of spinal nerves. It is separated into two divisions based on the type of muscle to which these nerves travel (innervate).

Somatic Division

The somatic nerves are the branches of the cranial and spinal motor nerves that innervate skeletal muscle (voluntary). These nerves are under conscious, or voluntary, control of the cerebral cortex.

Visceral Division (Autonomic Nervous System)

The visceral nerves are the branches of the cranial and spinal motor nerves that innervate cardiac and smooth muscle (involuntary). The visceral nerves, which are not under conscious control, are regulated by the hypothalamus and the medulla oblongata. The visceral nerves are commonly referred to as the **autonomic nervous system (ANS).**

PHYSIOLOGY AND PHARMACOLOGY

It is important to emphasize that understanding the physiology and pharmacology of the ANS can be challenging to beginning students. However, understanding the ANS is essential to understanding the actions of many drugs.

The ANS is composed of the nerves that innervate (or travel to) smooth and cardiac muscle. These two types of muscle are found in the walls of the internal organs and possess a special property, autorhythmicity, which allows them to initiate their own contractions. This process can be demonstrated by removing the heart or a piece of intestine from a frog, placing the organ in oxygenated Ringer's solution, and observing the contractions that occur without any stimulation.

If the internal organs can initiate their own contractions, why is the autonomic nervous system needed? The answer is the key to the purpose of the ANS: the ANS functions to regulate the rate at which these organs work, either increasing or decreasing their activity. In this way, **homeostasis,** the normal balance among the body's internal organs, can be maintained.

Whether the activity of the organ increases or decreases depends upon body activity. But the question arises, "How can an autonomic nerve going to any visceral organ both increase *and* decrease the activity of the organ?" The answer is that it cannot. Two different types of autonomic nerves, sympathetic and parasympathetic, innervate most internal organs.

PARASYMPATHETIC AND SYMPATHETIC DIVISIONS

The ANS has two subdivisions: the parasympathetic and sympathetic divisions. The nerves of the **parasympathetic** division (also known as the craniosacral division) originate from the brain (cranial nerves 3, 7, 9, and 10) and spinal cord (sacral nerves S2 to S4). The nerves of the **sympathetic** division (known as the thoracolumbar division) originate from the thoracic and lumbar spinal nerves (T1 to L3). Figure 5:1 shows how some of these nerves are linked to organs and glands.

As a result, most of the major body organs and glands receive a nerve from each division. There are exceptions; for example, most blood vessels do not receive parasympathetic innervation. In this situation, blood pressure is controlled by either increasing sympathetic activity or decreasing (inhibiting) sympathetic activity. However, the general plan is that one division is responsible for increasing the activity of a particular organ, while the other division decreases the activity of that organ. Unfortunately, one division does not *always* increase activity and the other division *always* decrease activity in each of the organs. How is the effect of each division predicted? The answer is that sympathetic stimulation produces

FIGURE 5:1 The Origin and Distribution of the Autonomic Nervous System Divisions

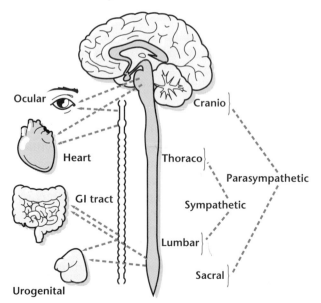

Each organ receives two nerves: one from either the cranio (eye, heart) or sacral (GI, urogenital) portion of the parasympathetic division, and one from either the thoraco (eye, heart) or lumbar (GI, urogenital) portion of the sympathetic division. Sympathetic nerves are shown originating from their ganglia along the spinal cord.

changes in the body that are similar to changes observed during frightening or emergency situations. These changes are collectively referred to as **fight or flight reaction.**

During the fight or flight reaction, the sympathetic division increases the activity of certain organs to allow a greater expenditure of energy for both physical and mental exertion. At the same time, there is a decrease in the activity of the remaining organs, whose functions are not required for the fight or flight reaction.

The parasympathetic division is more active during periods of rest and restoration of body energy stores. The parasympathetic nerves regulate body functions such as digestion and elimination of waste products (urination, defecation).

Normally, we do not experience situations in which we need the fight or flight reaction to enable us to fight or run. However, the daily stresses, anxieties, and illnesses we do experience are sufficient to activate the sympathetic system to produce changes that are similar to the fight or flight reaction. When the sympathetic division is stimulated, all sympathetic nerves are activated at the same time. Therefore, the whole body is stimulated. With the parasympathetic division, only selected nerves can be stimulated, and the stimulation can be confined to a particular body system, for example, contraction of the urinary bladder during urination. The overall effects of sympathetic and parasympathetic stimulation are summarized in Table 5:1.

Usually in a beginning discussion of the ANS, only the peripheral motor (efferent) nerves are discussed. Peripheral autonomic nerves are the branches of the cranial and spinal nerves that travel to the cardiac muscle and smooth muscle of the internal organs. A typical peripheral nerve is composed of many neurons traveling together to the same destination. In an autonomic nerve, two groups of neurons are linked together by synapses as the nerve travels from the spinal cord to the internal organ. In the peripheral nervous system, a collection of synapses is referred to as a ganglion.

In the ANS, neurons that emerge from the spinal cord form the preganglionic nerve. Neurons that travel from the ganglion to the internal organ form the postganglionic nerve. The ganglion is the collection of synapses between the preganglionic and postganglionic nerve fibers, as illustrated in Figure 5:2.

The main pharmacological difference between the sympathetic nerves and the parasympathetic nerves is the **neurotransmitter** released from the postganglionic nerve ending. The

TABLE 5:1   Effects of Sympathetic and Parasympathetic Stimulation

AREA	SYMPATHETIC EFFECT	PARASYMPATHETIC EFFECT
Adrenal medulla	Release of epinephrine	—
Arteries	Vasoconstriction (*exceptions are the coronary arteries and arteries to skeletal muscle, which are dilated*)	Most arteries are not supplied by parasympathetic nerves
Heart	Increases rate	Decreases rate
	Increases contractility	Decreases contractility
Intestines, GI motility, and secretions	Decreased	Increased
Postganglionic neurotransmitter	Norepinephrine released	acetylcholine released
Pupil of the eye	Dilation (mydriasis)	Constriction (miosis)
Respiratory passages, lower	Bronchodilation	Bronchoconstriction
Urinary bladder	Relaxation	Contraction
Urinary sphincter	Contraction	Relaxation

FIGURE 5:2   A Diagrammatic Representation of a Typical Sympathetic and Parasympathetic Efferent Nerve

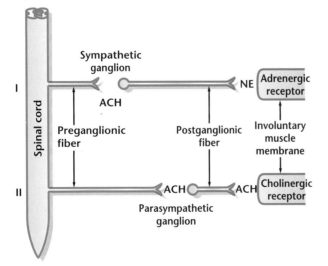

I. Sympathetic pre-, and postganglionic fibers from the thoracolumbar division.
II. Parasympathetic pre-, postganglionic fibers from the sacral division (ACH = acetylcholine; NE = norepinephrine).

neurotransmitter stimulates the internal organs and produces the characteristic changes that are associated with each division of the ANS as listed in Table 5:1.

In the parasympathetic nervous system, the neurotransmitter released at the ganglia and the postganglionic nerve endings is **acetylcholine (ACH).** In sympathetic nerves, the neurotransmitter released at the ganglia is ACH, but at the postganglionic nerve endings, it is **norepinephrine (NE).** Nerves that release acetylcholine are referred to as cholinergic, while nerves that release norepinephrine are referred to as adrenergic. The cardiac and smooth muscle membrane sites where these neurotransmitters act are known as the **cholinergic receptors** (ACH) and the **adrenergic receptors** (NE) as shown in Figure 5:2.

In summary, the effects of parasympathetic stimulation are produced by the release of acetylcholine, which bind to the cholinergic receptors. The effects of sympathetic stimulation are produced by the release of norepinephrine from adrenergic nerve endings and also by **epinephrine** released from the adrenal medulla. Both norepinephrine and epinephrine bind to and stimulate adrenergic receptors.

Chapter Review

Understanding Terminology

Answer the following questions.

1. What is the difference between an afferent nerve and an efferent nerve?_____
_____

2. Differentiate between adrenergic receptors and cholinergic receptors. _____
_____

3. What is the meaning of homeostasis? _____
_____

4. What terminology is applied to nerves that release acetylcholine? _____
_____

5. What terminology is applied to nerves that release norepinephrine? _____
_____

Acquiring Knowledge

Answer the following questions.

1. What are the two main divisions of the autonomic nervous system? _____
_____

2. What is the main function of each division? _____
_____

3. From what areas of the CNS does each division originate? _____
_____

4. What is the significance of "dual autonomic innervation" to most internal organs? _____
_____

5. What property of smooth and cardiac muscle allows them to initiate their own contractions? ___
_____

6. Describe what is meant by the fight or flight reaction. What conditions activate this reaction?___
_____

7. During what body activities is the parasympathetic division active? _____

8. Think of an emergency situation requiring immediate and intense physical exertion. List as many body organs as you can and predict the desired level of activity (increased or decreased). Which neurotransmitter would produce this effect? Do your predictions correctly correspond to the fight or flight reaction? _____
_____

Applying Knowledge—On the Job

Use your critical thinking skills to answer the following questions in the spaces provided.

1. Use the *PDR*® product category index to look up drugs that mimic (parasympathomimetics) and drugs that inhibit (parasympatholytics) cholinergic activity. List one or two drugs from each category, the main drug effect, and clinical indications. Do your findings correspond to the expected effects of cholinergic stimulation and inhibition? _____
_____
_____

2. Use the *PDR*® product category index to find drugs that mimic (sympathomimetics) and drugs that inhibit (sympatholytics) adrenergic activity. List one or two drugs, the main drug effect, and clinical indications. Do your findings correspond to the expected effects of adrenergic stimulation and inhibition? _____

_____

_____

_____

_____

Use *F&C* to answer the following questions.

3. Using the index, look up *acetylcholine*. Answer the following questions.
   a. What is the listed indication? _____

   _____

   b. What is the expected onset and duration of action? _____

   _____

   c. What is the concentration or strength(s) that this is available in? _____

   _____

4. Using the index, look up *Yocon* and *Yohimex*. Answer the following questions.
   a. What is the generic name for these products? _____

   _____

   b. What are the contraindications? _____

   _____

   c. Are there any drug interactions listed? _____

   _____

5. Using the index, look up *Regitine*. Answer the following questions.
   a. What are the listed indications? _____

   _____

   b. What are the listed precautions? _____

   _____

   _____

Additional Reading

Changeux, J-P. 1993 Chemical signalling in the brain. *Scientific American* 269:58.

Finocchiaro, D. N., and Herzfeld, S. T. 1990. Understanding autonomic dysreflexia. *American Journal of Nursing* 90 (9):56.

Schatz, I. J. 1997. Autonomic failure and orthostatic hypotension. *Hospital Practice* 32 (5):15.

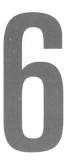
DRUGS AFFECTING THE SYMPATHETIC NERVOUS SYSTEM

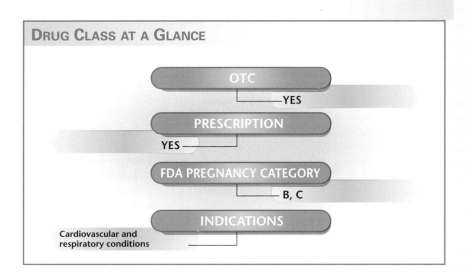

DRUG CLASS AT A GLANCE

OTC
— YES

PRESCRIPTION
YES —

FDA PREGNANCY CATEGORY
— B, C

INDICATIONS
Cardiovascular and
respiratory conditions

Key Terms

adrenergic neuronal blocker: drug that acts at the neuronal endings to reduce the formation or release of NE.

alpha-adrenergic blocker: drug that blocks the alpha effects of NE and EPI.

alpha-adrenergic receptor: receptor located on smooth muscle that mediates contraction.

beta-adrenergic receptor: receptor located either on the heart (beta-1) or smooth muscle (beta-2). Beta-1 stimulation increases heart function, while beta-2 stimulation relaxes smooth muscle.

catecholamine: refers to norepinephrine, epinephrine, and other sympathomimetic compounds that possess the catechol structure.

false transmitter: drug-induced substance in nerve endings that reduces neuronal activity.

nonselective beta-adrenergic blocker: drug that blocks the beta effects of EPI.

selective beta-1 adrenergic blocker: drug that blocks only beta-1 receptors.

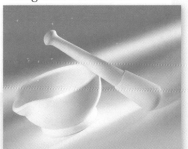

CHAPTER FOCUS

This chapter describes the pharmacology of drugs that affect the sympathetic nervous system. It also explains the ways in which adrenergic drugs (agonists) stimulate adrenergic receptors to increase sympathetic activity, while other drugs (antagonists) block adrenergic receptors to reduce sympathetic activity.

CHAPTER OBJECTIVES

After studying this chapter, you should be able to

- explain how the adrenergic nerve endings function both to release and inactivate norepinephrine.
- name three different adrenergic receptors and describe the actions they mediate.
- explain the effects of norepinephrine (NE) and epinephrine (EPI) on alpha and beta receptors.
- name three alpha-adrenergic agonists and describe the main pharmacological effects and uses of each.
- name three beta-adrenergic agonists and describe the main pharmacological effects and uses of each.
- describe the three major types of adrenergic-blocking drugs and the pharmacological effects produced by each type.

selective beta-2 adrenergic drug: drug that stimulates only beta-2 receptors at therapeutic doses.

sympatholytic: "blocking" drug or effect that decreases sympathetic nervous system activity.

sympathomimetic: adrenergic drug or effect that increases sympathetic nervous system activity.

INTRODUCTION

The sympathetic nervous system regulates the activity of the internal organs and glands during physical exertion and other stressful situations. Peripheral sympathetic nerves, known as adrenergic nerves, release the neurotransmitter norepinephrine (NE). Norepinephrine binds to its adrenergic receptors and produces the effects that are associated with sympathetic stimulation (fight or flight) (see Chapter 5).

The adrenal medulla releases the hormone epinephrine (EPI), which also stimulates the adrenergic receptors. EPI (adrenaline) is released from the adrenal medulla in larger amounts during stress and emergency situations. Norepinephrine and epinephrine are chemically similar and are generally referred to as the **catecholamines.**

ADRENERGIC NERVE ENDINGS

It is important to have an understanding of how the adrenergic nerve endings function. The nerve endings are mainly concerned with the formation of NE. Norepinephrine is then stored within granules inside the nerve endings. When the adrenergic nerves are stimulated, NE is released. Norepinephrine then travels to the smooth or cardiac muscle membrane, attaches to adrenergic receptors, and produces the sympathetic response. Most of the NE then passes back into the nerve endings (reuptake). Inside the nerve endings, the NE may be reused or may be destroyed by the

enzyme monoamine oxidase (MAO). These actions are illustrated in Figure 6:1.

NOREPINEPHRINE VERSUS EPINEPHRINE

Although NE and EPI are both adrenergic neurotransmitters, there are some important differences in the effects that each produces. Both NE and EPI stimulate many of the internal organs to increase sympathetic activity. However, EPI causes an inhibition or relaxation of smooth muscle in a few of the organs. For example, the respiratory passageways are relaxed (bronchodilation) by EPI. This effect fits into the fight or flight reaction because more oxygen passes into the lungs when the respiratory tract is dilated. Because of the differences in the responses produced by NE and EPI, two main types of adrenergic receptors are believed to exist.

ADRENERGIC RECEPTORS

The two main adrenergic receptors are known as the alpha- and the beta-adrenergic receptors. Although some organs contain more than one type of receptor, one receptor type usually predominates and determines the overall response of the organ. **Alpha-adrenergic receptors** are found predominantly on smooth muscle

FIGURE 6:1 The Adrenergic Nerve Ending Illustrating the Release, Reuptake, and Metabolism of Norepinephrine (NE)

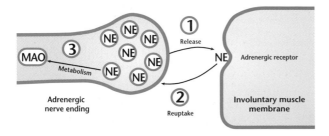

	TABLE 6:1	Effects of Norepinephrine and Epinephrine on Alpha and Beta Receptors		

RECEPTOR	ORGAN	NOREPINEPHRINE EFFECT	EPINEPHRINE EFFECT
Alpha (contraction of smooth muscle)	Most arteries and veins	Vasoconstriction	Vasoconstriction
	Pupils of eye	Dilation	Dilation
Beta-1 (stimulation of cardiac muscle)	Heart	Moderate increase in heart rate, force of contraction, and atrioventricular conduction	Greater increase in heart rate, force of contraction, and atrioventricular conduction
Beta-2 (relaxation of smooth muscle)	Bronchiolar smooth muscle	Norepinephrine does not stimulate beta-2 receptors	Bronchodilation
	Uterus		Relaxation
	Skeletal muscle vessels and coronary artery vessels		Vasodilation

membranes and when stimulated by NE or EPI, they produce contraction; for example, vasoconstriction of most blood vessels.

Beta-adrenergic receptors are found on both cardiac and some smooth muscle membranes. In the heart, the predominant beta receptors are classified as beta-1 receptors, and when stimulated by NE or EPI, they increase heart rate and force of contraction. In smooth muscle, the predominant beta receptors are classified as beta-2 receptors, and when stimulated by EPI, they produce vasodilation (mainly skeletal muscle blood vessels and coronary arteries) and bronchodilation (relaxation of bronchiolar smooth muscle). Norepinephrine does not stimulate beta-2 receptors and this is the main difference between NE and EPI. Note that alpha-receptor stimulation causes smooth muscle contraction at some organ sites while beta-2 receptor stimulation causes smooth muscle relaxation at other organ sites. Table 6:1 summarizes the effects of NE and EPI on the adrenergic receptors of several organs.

Although the classification system for the adrenergic receptors seems confusing, it is useful for classifying drugs. There are two main classes of drugs that affect the sympathetic system. The first, adrenergic drugs **(sympathomimetics),** produces effects that are similar to stimulating or mimicking the sympathetic nervous system. There is an increase in blood pressure, heart rate, and diameter of the respiratory passageways (bronchodilation). These responses are clinically useful in patients suffering from shock, cardiac arrest, or respiratory difficulty.

Drugs, including NE and EPI, that produce contraction of smooth muscle by stimulating the alpha receptors are referred to as alpha-adrenergic drugs. Drugs, including EPI, that both stimulate the heart (stimulate beta-1 receptors) and cause relaxation of smooth muscle (stimulate beta-2 receptors) are referred to as beta-adrenergic drugs. EPI is one of the few substances that stimulates both alpha and beta receptors. There are also a few beta-adrenergic drugs that selectively stimulate only the beta-2 receptors at therapeutic doses. These drugs are referred to as the **selective beta-2 adrenergic drugs** and are used primarily as bronchodilators.

The second main class of drugs that affects the sympathetic nervous system is the adrenergic blocking drugs **(sympatholytics).** These drugs produce effects that would be expected by inhibiting or blocking sympathetic activity. Therefore, a decrease in blood pressure and heart rate usually occurs. Clinically, these effects are beneficial in patients with hypertension, angina pectoris, and certain types of cardiac arrhythmias.

Drugs that block the alpha effects of NE and EPI are known as the **alpha-adrenergic blockers.** Drugs that block the beta effects of EPI (beta-1 and beta-2) are known as the **nonselective beta-adrenergic blockers.** Drugs that block only beta-1 receptors are known as **selective beta-1 adrenergic blockers.** The effect of these alpha- and beta-blockers is to decrease sympathetic activity, especially in the cardiovascular system. The blocking drug competes with NE or EPI for the

TABLE 6:2   Alpha-Adrenergic Drugs

DRUG (TRADE NAME)	MAIN USE	DOSAGE FORMS
ephedrine	Nasal decongestant	Capsule, Parenteral Injection
metaraminol (Aramine)	To increase blood pressure	Parenteral Injection
methoxamine (Vasoxyl)	To increase blood pressure	Parenteral Injection
norepinephrine (Levophed)	To increase blood pressure	Parenteral Injection
phenylephrine (many)	Nasal decongestant	Nasal spray, drops; Tablets, Parenteral injection
pseudoephedrine (many)	Nasal decongestant	Tablets, Caplets, Oral Liquids
tetrahydrozoline (Visine)	Ophthalmic decongestant	Ocular drops
tetrahydrozoline (Tyzine)	Nasal decongestant	Nasal drops

receptor sites. When the drug occupies the receptors, it prevents NE and EPI from producing an effect. Another method to inhibit the sympathetic system is to decrease the formation or the release of NE. Drugs that act at the neuronal endings to reduce the formation or release of NE are known as the **adrenergic neuronal blockers.**

ALPHA-ADRENERGIC DRUGS

Norepinephrine is considered to be the parent or prototype drug for the alpha drug class. The alpha-adrenergic drugs have chemical structures and produce effects that are almost identical to those of NE. The most important clinical effect produced by the alpha-adrenergic drugs is contraction of smooth muscle. This includes vasoconstriction of most blood vessels, contraction of sphincter muscles in the gastrointestinal (inhibits movement of intestinal contents) and urinary (restricts passage of urine) tracts, and dilation of the pupil of the eye (mydriasis).

Clinical Indications

Alpha drugs are used (usually intravenous [IV] infusion) in hypotensive states; for example, after surgery, to increase blood pressure and maintain circulation. Vasoconstriction of blood vessels in mucous membranes of the nasal sinuses produces a decongestant effect. Consequently, some of these drugs are included in over-the-counter (OTC) cold and allergy preparations for relief of nasal congestion. A few of the alpha drugs are also used in ophthalmology to dilate the pupils (mydriatic drugs) and as ocular decongestants. Alpha drugs

that pass the blood-brain barrier—for example, amphetamines—produce a central effect to suppress appetite. These drugs and other appetite suppressants will be discussed in Chapter 33. Table 6:2 lists the alpha drugs and their main uses.

Adverse Effects

The major adverse effects of the alpha-adrenergic drugs are due to excessive vasoconstriction of blood vessels. This may result in hypertension, hypertensive crisis, or heart palpitations. In some patients, this can lead to either hemorrhage (usually cerebral) or to cardiac arrhythmias. Consequently, extreme caution must be observed with hypertensive or cardiac patients. Patients receiving parenteral administration of these drugs should have blood pressure recordings taken at frequent intervals. The most common side effect of decongestant use is irritation of the nasal sinuses or eyes due to excessive dryness caused by the vasoconstrictive decrease in blood flow.

Caution

The IV needle should be checked frequently to make certain that the drug is not infiltrating the skin. Infiltration by alpha drugs causes intense vasoconstriction of skin blood vessels, which can lead to death of skin cells and gangrene.

BETA-ADRENERGIC DRUGS

The beta-adrenergic drugs have a selective action to combine with beta receptors. With the exception of EPI, most beta drugs produce very few alpha effects.

TABLE 6:3　Beta-Adrenergic Drugs

DRUG (TRADE NAME)	CLASSIFICATION	MAIN USE
epinephrine *(Adrenaline)*	Alpha, beta-1, beta-2	Vasopressor, cardiac stimulant, bronchodilator
isoproterenol *(Isuprel)*	Beta-1, beta-2	Cardiac stimulant, bronchodilator
isoetharine *(Bronkometer)*	Beta-2	Bronchodilator
metaproterenol *(Alupent)*	Beta-2	Bronchodilator
terbutaline *(Brethine)*	Beta-2	Bronchodilator
albuterol *(Proventil, Ventolin)*	Beta-2	Bronchodilator
fenoterol *(Berotec)*	Beta-2	Bronchodilator
salmeterol *(Serevent)*	Beta-2	Bronchodilator

Beta Drug Effects

The most important actions of the beta drugs are stimulation of the heart (beta-1) and bronchodilation (beta-2). Isoproterenol is the most potent beta-adrenergic drug that produces both of these effects. This dual action (heart and respiratory passages) is the main disadvantage of isoproterenol in treating bronchoconstriction caused by asthma or allergy. With isoproterenol, there is often overstimulation of the heart along with the bronchodilator effect. For this reason, a search was conducted to discover beta drugs that would selectively stimulate only the beta-2 receptors without causing excessive stimulation of beta-1 receptors in the heart. Several of these selective beta-2 drugs were discovered and are now widely used as bronchodilators. These beta-adrenergic drugs are further discussed in Chapter 32 with the treatment of asthma.

Beta-2 receptors are also found in uterine smooth muscle. Stimulation of beta-2 receptors within the uterus relaxes smooth muscle and inhibits uterine contractions. Table 6:3 lists the various beta drugs and their main clinical uses.

Clinical Indications for Epinephrine

Epinephrine is the drug of choice for the immediate treatment of acute allergic reactions, such as anaphylaxis. Anaphylaxis can be caused by insect stings, drugs, or other allergens in sensitized individuals. There is difficulty in breathing, decreased blood pressure, and other symptoms of shock. In these situations, EPI (stimulates both alpha and beta receptors)

administered by subcutaneous injection is the preferred treatment. The alpha actions of EPI are also used during surgical procedures or in combination with local anesthetics to produce vasoconstriction. The alpha effect decreases blood flow and bleeding, and prolongs the action of local anesthetics at the site of injection. The beta effects of EPI are useful for cardiac stimulation (beta-1) in emergencies (such as cardiac arrest) and for bronchodilation (beta-2) in the treatment of asthma. Both EPI and isoproterenol are available as OTC bronchodilators.

Adverse Effects

The beta drugs may produce central nervous system (CNS) stimulation resulting in restlessness, tremors, or anxiety. The main adverse effect of the older beta drugs (EPI or isoproterenol) is overstimulation of the heart, which may result in palpitations or other cardiac arrhythmias. These drugs are used with extreme caution in patients with existing heart disease. Drugs that produce beta-2 effects dilate the blood vessels of skeletal muscle. This dilation may lower blood pressure but rarely results in hypotension. At higher than therapeutic doses, the selective beta-2 drugs can also stimulate cardiac beta-1 receptors, which may cause overstimulation of the heart. Use of beta-2 drugs to arrest preterm labor can cause a variety of cardiovascular effects and complications. Fetal heart rate and maternal pulse rate and blood pressure should be closely monitored.

DOPAMINE

Dopamine functions as a neurotransmitter in the brain and is also formed as a precursor in the synthesis of NE in peripheral adrenergic nerve endings. When prepared as a drug (*Intropin*) and administered intravenously, dopamine produces several cardiovascular effects that are useful in the treatment of circulatory shock.

At low doses (0.5 to 2.0 μg/kg/minute), dopamine stimulates dopaminergic receptors in renal and mesenteric blood vessels, resulting in vasodilation and increased renal blood flow. At moderate doses (2 to 10 μg/kg/minute), dopamine also stimulates beta-1 receptors, which increase myocardial contractility and increase cardiac output. Increasing cardiac output and renal blood flow are important actions during shock, when blood pressure and cardiac function are drastically reduced. At higher dosages, dopamine stimulates alpha receptors to produce vasoconstriction.

Dopamine is administered by continuous IV infusion, and the effects disappear shortly after the infusion is stopped. Adverse effects from overdosage usually involve excessive stimulation of the heart and increased blood pressure (alpha effect).

Dobutamine (*Dobutrex*) is a drug, similar to dopamine, that possesses greater beta-1 effects to increase myocardial contractility. The main use of dobutamine is in acute heart failure, where it is administered by IV infusion.

 Patient Administration and Monitoring

Check vital signs (heart rate, blood pressure, respiration) frequently during parenteral administration of adrenergic drugs.

Check to ensure that IV lines are properly adjusted and needles have not infiltrated.

Observe for sympathetic signs of drug overdosage: sweating, trembling, chest pain, respiratory difficulty, significant increases in blood pressure.

Instruct patient to report signs of trembling, sweating, chest pain, shortness of breath, heart irregularities, weakness, or feelings of faintness.

ALPHA-ADRENERGIC BLOCKING DRUGS

The alpha-blockers compete with NE for binding to the alpha-adrenergic receptors. If NE binds to the receptors, the characteristic effects of NE are produced. When the alpha-blocker binds to the receptors, it prevents NE from producing sympathetic responses. Consequently, normal sympathetic activity is decreased in organs that have alpha receptors. Since the major alpha organ is the blood vessels, the effect of alpha blockade is vasodilation and lowering of blood pressure.

Clinical Indications

The alpha-blockers are widely used in the treatment of hypertension. The antihypertensive drugs are discussed in Chapter 26. The alpha-blockers are also used in peripheral vascular conditions (poor blood flow to skin and extremities) such as Raynaud's disease. In addition, they may be used to diagnose pheochromocytoma, a tumor of the adrenal medulla, which produces excessive catecholamine levels and causes severe hypertension. The alpha-blockers produce a dramatic reduction in blood pressure in individuals with pheochromocytoma. In benign prostatic hyperplasia there is enlargement of the prostate gland, which interferes with urine flow through the ureter. Alpha-blocking drugs relax the smooth muscle of the ureter, which improves urinary flow. Table 6:4 lists the alpha-blockers and their main uses.

Adverse Effects

Whenever the activity of one division of the autonomic nervous system is blocked (sympathetic), activity in the other division (parasympathetic) appears to increase. After alpha blockade, when sympathetic activity is blocked, the side effects are similar to an increase in parasympathetic activity in the organs that are blocked. You should note this generalization, that blocking one division of the ANS usually produces some effects that are similar to stimulating the other division. Constriction of the pupils (miosis), nasal congestion, and increased GI activity are commonly experienced after alpha blockade. Compensatory reflex tachycardia also occurs if the blood pressure is significantly lowered. In addition, the alpha-blockers interfere with normal cardiovascular reflexes. Consequently, some patients experience orthostatic hypotension and fainting.

TABLE 6:4   Alpha-Adrenergic Blocking Drugs

DRUG (TRADE NAME)	MAIN USE	COMMON DAILY DOSAGE RANGE
doxazosin (*Cardura*)	Treatment of hypertension Treatment of benign prostatic hyperplasia	1–16 mg PO 1–8 mg PO
phentolamine (*Regitine*)	Diagnosis of pheochromocytoma	5 mg IV
prazosin (*Minipress*)	Treatment of hypertension	1–20 mg PO
tamsulosin (*Flomax*)	Treatment of benign prostatic hyperplasia	0.4–0.8 mg PO
terazosin (*Hytrin*)	Treatment of hypertension Treatment benign prostatic hyperplasia	1–5 mg PO 1–10 mg PO
yohimbine (*Aphrodyne*)	Treatment of male impotence	5.4–16.2 mg PO

BETA-ADRENERGIC BLOCKING DRUGS

Beta-blocking drugs bind to beta-adrenergic receptors and antagonize the beta effects of EPI and NE. Patients with hypertension, angina pectoris, and cardiac arrhythmias often have increased sympathetic activity, with excessive amounts of EPI and NE being released. By occupying beta receptors, the beta-blockers prevent EPI and NE from producing beta sympathetic effects. The heart (beta-1) is one of the most important beta organs and the main clinical use of beta-blockers is to decrease the activity of the heart. Blockade of the beta-1 receptors produces a decrease in heart rate, force of contraction, and impulse conduction through the conduction system of the heart. There are no specific therapeutic indications for blocking the beta-2 receptors.

Types of Beta-Blockers

The beta-blockers are divided into the nonselective beta-blockers (block both beta-1 and beta-2 receptors) and the selective beta-1 blockers. At therapeutic doses, the selective beta-blockers block only beta-1 receptors. At higher doses, the selective beta-blockers may also begin to block beta-2 receptors. Propranolol was the first beta-blocker used clinically; it blocks both beta-1 and beta-2 receptors. The other beta-blockers produce similar effects. The major differences among these drugs are the duration of action and the extent of drug metabolism. Table 6:5 lists the beta-blockers that are currently available.

Pharmacologic Effects

The main effects produced by propranolol are a decrease in rate, force of contraction, and conduction velocity of the heart. In addition, there is usually a lowering of blood pressure. Reducing the effort and work of the heart causes a decrease in oxygen consumption. This effect is beneficial in the treatment of various cardiovascular conditions, especially when there is hyperactivity of the sympathetic nervous system.

Propranolol is administered either orally or intravenously. After oral administration, the drug is carried directly to the liver by the portal system. With propranolol, there is significant metabolism on the first passage through the liver (first-pass metabolism), which reduces the amount of drug that eventually reaches the systemic circulation.

Beta-blockers also affect carbohydrate and lipid metabolism. Interference with carbohydrate metabolism is usually insignificant; however, diabetic patients may experience hypoglycemia. Serum lipid levels (triglycerides) may be increased by continuous therapy with these drugs.

Propranolol is the most lipid-soluble beta-blocker and passes into the brain, where it can exert pharmacological effects. These effects include CNS sedation, depression, and decreased central sympathetic activity, which may contribute to the lowering of blood pressure in the treatment of hypertension. Nadolol and atenolol are lipid-insoluble (water-soluble) beta-blockers, which do not pass into the brain and are excreted mostly unmetabolized in the urine.

Clinical Indications

Propranolol is used in the treatment of angina pectoris (Chapter 24), hypertension (Chapter 26),

TABLE 6:5   Beta-Adrenergic Blocking Drugs

DRUG (TRADE NAME)	MAIN USE	COMMON DAILY DOSAGE RANGE
Nonselective Blockers:		
carvedilol (Coreg)	Hypertension Congestive heart failure	12.5–50 mg PO 6.25–100 mg PO
labetalol (Normodyne)	Hypertension	200–800 mg PO
nadolol (Corgard)	Hypertension, angina pectoris	80–240 mg PO
pindolol (Visken)	Hypertension	10–60 mg PO
propranolol (Inderal)	Hypertension, migraine Angina pectoris Arrhythmias Life-threatening arrhythmias Post-myocardial Infarction	80–240 mg PO 80–320 mg PO 40–120 mg PO 1–3 mg IV 180–240 mg PO
timolol (Blocadren)	Hypertension, post-myocardial infarction Glaucoma	20–40 mg PO Topical drops
Selective Beta-1 Blockers:		
acebutolol (Sectral)	Hypertension Ventricular arrhythmias	400–800 mg PO 400–1200 mg PO
atenolol (Tenormin)	Hypertension, angina pectoris	50–100 mg PO
bisoprolol (Zebeta)	Hypertension	5–20 mg PO
esmolol (Brevibloc)	Supraventricular tachycardia	IV infusion (dose variable)
metoprolol (Lopressor)	Hypertension, angina pectoris	100–400 mg PO

and various cardiac arrhythmias (Chapter 23). Other uses include the treatment of glaucoma, where it decreases intraocular pressure; treatment of migraine headaches, where it often reduces the number of migraine attacks; and after myocardial infarctions, where with chronic therapy beta-blockers appear to decrease the incidences of additional myocardial infarctions and sudden cardiac death.

Esmolol is a short-acting drug that is administered intravenously in emergency situations. It has a quick onset of action to lower ventricular heart rate in cases of supraventricular tachycardia.

Adverse Effects

Common side effects of propranolol include nausea, vomiting, and diarrhea. More serious adverse effects occur when heart function is excessively reduced. This reduction usually produces bradycardia and may lead to congestive heart failure or cardiac arrest. In general, propranolol should not be used in patients with asthma or other respiratory conditions. By blocking beta-2 receptor sites, propranolol and other nonselective beta-blockers may cause bronchoconstriction in individuals with asthma or other respiratory conditions. This bronchoconstriction may precipitate a respiratory emergency. The selective beta-1 blockers have less of a tendency to do this. However, at higher than therapeutic doses, they may also begin to block beta-2 receptors and cause bronchoconstriction. Beta-blockers that gain access to the brain may cause drowsiness, mental depression, and other CNS disturbances.

Drug Interactions

The most serious drug interactions involve therapy of beta-blockers with other drugs that decrease cardiovascular function. These include cardiac glycosides, antiarrhythmic drugs, and calcium blockers. These drug interactions usually lower heart rate and cardiac output, which can lead to hypotension and drug-induced congestive heart failure.

Patient Administration and Monitoring

Check vital signs frequently with parenteral drug administration.

Observe patient frequently for signs of cardiac depression (beta-blockers) and hypotension (alpha- and beta-blockers).

Explain to patient the common drug side effects: weakness, fatigue, dizziness, and sedation.

Instruct patient to report slow pulse rate, chest pain, respiratory difficulties, mental confusion, nightmares, or impotency.

Diabetic patients should be warned that beta-blockers may affect insulin and blood glucose levels, and that they should report any changes.

ADRENERGIC NEURONAL BLOCKING DRUGS

The main activity that occurs inside the adrenergic nerve endings is the formation and storage of NE. Norepinephrine is synthesized from amino acids, either phenylalanine or tyrosine. Several drugs interfere with the formation or the storage of NE. Such drugs are called adrenergic neuronal blockers. Figure 6:2 shows the biochemical steps in the synthesis of NE and the specific sites of action of the neuronal blocking drugs.

FIGURE 6:2 Synthesis of Norepinephrine (NE) and the Sites of Action of the Adrenergic Neuronal Blockers

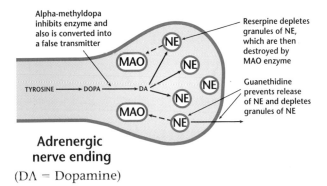

Alpha-methyldopa inhibits enzyme and also is converted into a false transmitter

Reserpine depletes granules of NE, which are then destroyed by MAO enzyme

Guanethidine prevents release of NE and depletes granules of NE

Adrenergic nerve ending

(DA = Dopamine)

Methyldopa (Aldomet)

Methyldopa (alpha-methyldopa) interferes with the synthesis of NE in the nerve endings and greatly reduces the amount of NE that is formed. Consequently, less NE is released, and the activity of the sympathetic system is decreased. There is evidence that the adrenergic nerve endings convert methyldopa into alpha-methylnorepinephrine, which is stored and released by the nerve endings like NE. The term **false transmitter** is used to describe drugs that produce neurotransmitter-like substances, but reduce neuronal activity. The main use of methyldopa is in the treatment of hypertension to lower blood pressure. The most important site of action of methyldopa to reduce blood pressure is in the vasomotor center of the medulla oblongata (central effect). In the medulla, the formation and release of alpha-methylnorepinephrine leads to a decrease in sympathetic activity to vascular smooth muscle, which produces vasodilation and a lowering of blood pressure. The usual oral dose is 250 to 2000 mg/day (divided doses).

During initial treatment with methyldopa, many patients experience drowsiness and/or sedation, but these effects tend to disappear as drug treatment continues. Other side effects include nausea, vomiting, diarrhea, nasal congestion, and bradycardia. In some patients, adverse reaction may cause one or more of the following: drug fever, liver dysfunction, hemolytic anemia, or a lupus-like syndrome resulting in skin eruptions and symptoms of arthritis.

Reserpine

Reserpine is obtained from a plant, *Rauwolfia serpentina*, found mainly in India. The site of action of reserpine is the adrenergic nerve endings. Within the nerve endings, reserpine prevents the storage of NE inside the storage granules. Consequently, the adrenergic nerve endings are depleted of NE. When this occurs, the level of sympathetic activity is greatly reduced.

The most important clinical use of reserpine is in the treatment of hypertension. By reducing sympathetic activity, reserpine produces vasodilation and a lowering of blood pressure. Reserpine is usually administered in combination with a diuretic in the treatment of hypertension.

In addition to its antihypertensive effect, reserpine produces CNS sedation and tranquilization. Before the introduction of the modern antipsychotic drugs, reserpine was widely used to treat psychoses. Today, reserpine is primarily reserved for patients who have not responded to other antipsychotic drugs.

Most of the side effects of reserpine are caused by the decreased sympathetic activity. Side effects are similar to parasympathetic stimulation and include increased salivation, diarrhea, nasal congestion, bradycardia, and excessive hypotension. In the CNS, reserpine may produce excessive sedation, psychic disturbances such as confusion and hallucinations, or mental depression. The mental depression may lead to suicide attempts. At high doses, reserpine may produce symptoms of parkinsonism, which include tremors and muscular rigidity.

Guanethidine *(Ismelin)*

Guanethidine is a potent adrenergic neuronal blocker. There are two main actions that guanethidine exerts on the nerve endings. First, guanethidine prevents the release of NE from the nerve endings, and second, guanethidine depletes the NE storage granules similarly to reserpine. These two effects produce a significant reduction of sympathetic activity.

The main clinical use of guanethidine is to treat severe hypertension; the usual oral dose is 25 to 300 mg/day. The half-life of guanethidine is relatively long. Therefore, the effects of guanethidine continue for up to 10 days after drug treatment is terminated.

The main adverse effects of guanethidine are caused by the decreased sympathetic activity and include diarrhea, nasal congestion, bradycardia, orthostatic hypotension, and impotency in males.

Guanadrel *(Hylorel)*

Guanadrel produces effects similar to those produced by guanethidine. It is used in the treatment of hypertension and generally produces a lower incidence of adverse effects than does guanethidine.

Summary of Sites of Action for Adrenergic Drugs

Figure 6:3 provides a diagramatic summary of typical adrenergic nerve fibers, adrenergic receptors, and representative drugs that act on each receptor site.

FIGURE 6:3 Diagrammatic Summary of Adrenergic Receptor Sites and Sites of Action of Adrenergic Drugs and Adrenergic Blocking Drugs

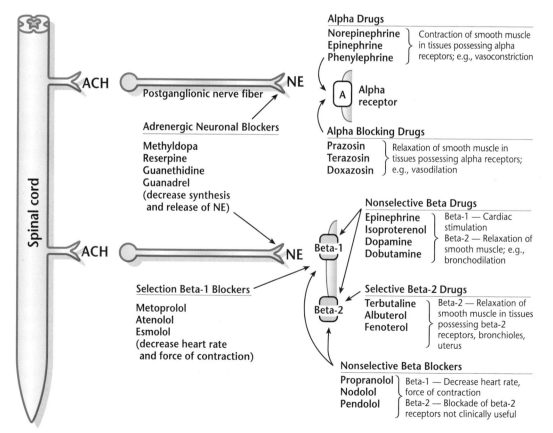

Chapter Review

Understanding Terminology

Match the definition or description in the left column with the appropriate terms in the right column.

_____ 1. Drug that blocks or decreases sympathetic nervous system activity.

_____ 2. Drug that acts at the neuronal endings to reduce the formation or release of NE.

_____ 3. Mediates contraction, located on smooth muscle.

_____ 4. Adrenergic receptor located on either the heart or smooth muscle.

_____ 5. Drug that blocks the beta effects of EPI.

_____ 6. Drug that blocks the alpha effects of NE and EPI.

_____ 7. Norepinephrine and epinephrine.

_____ 8. Adrenergic drug or effect that increases sympathetic nervous system activity.

_____ 9. Hormone released from the adrenal medulla that stimulates the sympathetic nervous system.

a. adrenergic neuronal blocker

b. alpha-blocker

c. alpha receptor

d. beta receptor

e. catecholamine

f. epinephrine

g. nonselective beta-blocker

h. sympatholytic

i. sympathomimetic

Acquiring Knowledge

Answer the following questions in the spaces provided.

1. What is the main function of the sympathetic nervous system? _____
_____

2. List the different types of adrenergic receptors and relate them to specific organ functions. _____
_____

3. What two neurotransmitter substances are associated with the sympathetic nervous system? Describe the effects of each. _____

4. A patient brought into the emergency room is experiencing severe hypotension. Blood pressure reads 90/50. What class of drugs is indicated for treatment? What precautions should be observed when these drugs are administered? What would be the first indication that too much drug has been administered? _____
_____

5. Following cardiac surgery, a patient suddenly experiences a drop in cardiac function and blood pressure. The patient may be developing heart failure. What drugs would most likely be indicated in this situation? What autonomic receptor, in particular, needs to be acted upon? Should it be stimulated or blocked? _____
_____

6. Alpha- and beta-blockers are both indicated for the treatment of hypertension. Explain the difference in the mechanism of action of these two drug classes to lower blood pressure. _____

_____

_____

Applying Knowledge—On the Job

Use your critical thinking skills to answer the following questions in the spaces provided.

1. Following emergency administration of epinephrine subcutaneously (SQ) for an acute asthmatic attack, the physician prescribes terbutalin (Brethine) tablets three times daily. How is this drug classified? What is it supposed to do? What are its advantages over epinephrine in the treatment of chronic asthma? _____

_____

2. One of your coworkers has been taking propranolol (Inderal) regularly for a fast heart rate (tachycardia). Recently she has been complaining of tiredness and a feeling that she might faint. Is this effect drug related and if so, what is occurring? What advice might you give her? _____

_____

_____

3. Assume that your employer, a busy physician, has asked you to help screen patients for potential prescription drug problems. Patient X visited the doctor's office today complaining of "sinus"—sinus congestion, pressure, and headache. The doctor diagnosed an upper respiratory virus and prescribed phenylephrine for the sinus congestion and discomfort. You study Patient X's chart and note that he has a history of hypertension. What should you advise the doctor about the drug she has prescribed for Patient X? _____

_____

4. Betty has asthma and diabetes. She has also developed high blood pressure, for which her doctor just prescribed the drug propranolol. One of your duties as physician's assistant is to make sure patients are not prescribed drugs that are contraindicated because of other health problems. What should you tell the doctor about Betty's prescription for propranolol? _____

_____

_____

5. Linda is a 24-year-old with bronchial asthma that is well-controlled. She is in her 26th week of pregnancy and is experiencing preterm labor. Using the PDR® or F&C, determine whether ritodrine or terbutaline would be indicated to arrest her preterm labor. _____

_____

_____

6. Bill is a 38-year-old with a history of duodenal ulcers. He is currently maintained on cimetadine 800 mg HS. Today he was diagnosed with hypertension and his physician wants to initiate treatment with Lopressor. What dosing considerations should be made, if any? _____

_____

_____

7. Susan is a 26-year-old with a history of migraine headaches. Standard treatment has continuously failed, leaving her to rely on narcotic therapy. Desperate to find a nonnarcotic alternative, she has asked her physician about using DHE-45 injection (dihydroergotamine mesylate). What side effects should she be warned about? _____

_____

_____

Internet Connection

MedicineNet (http://www.medicinenet.com) is a search engine that provides information on many diseases and drugs. After reaching the website, click *Diseases and Treatment* and then highlight the letter "R." Go down the list until you find *Raynaud's Disease,* click on this heading and learn about this condition. What are some of the classes of drugs used to treat this condition? What adrenergic-blocking drugs may be used? What other medications can aggravate this condition?

Another topic at this website under *Diseases and Treatment* at letter "B" is *Bee Stings.* Click on this heading and determine the immediate treatment for a severe allergic reaction. What is the most serious type of reaction called?

Also under *Diseases and Treatment* highlight the letter "B." Go down the list until you find *Benign Prostatic Hyperplasia.* Click on this heading and learn about this condition and its treatment.

Additional Reading

Albertsen, P. C. 1997. Prostate disease in older men 1. Benign hyperplasia. *Hospital Practice* 32 (5):61.

Atenolol for high-risk patients undergoing noncardiac surgery. 1997. *Emergency Medicine* 29 (4):36.

Frishman W. H. 1992. Beta-adrenergic blockers as cardioprotective agents. *American Journal of Cardiology* 70:21.

Oral albuterol for acute cough. 1996. *Emergency Medicine* 28 (10):57.

Schatz, I. J. 1997. Autonomic failure and orthostatic hypotension. *Hospital Practice* 32 (5):15.

Sohl, L. L., and Applefeld, M. M. 1990. A new direction for dobutamine. *Nursing* 20 (10):42.

Urbano, F. L. 2001. Raynaud's phenomenon. *Hospital Physician* 37 (9):27.

Wilde, M. I., Fitton, A., and Sorkin, E. M. 1993. Terazosin. A review of its pharmacodynamic and pharmacokinetic properties, and therapeutic potential in benign prostatic hyperplasia. *Drugs and Aging* 3:258.

7

DRUGS AFFECTING THE PARASYMPATHETIC NERVOUS SYSTEM

CHAPTER FOCUS

This chapter describes the basic pharmacology of drugs that affect the parasympathetic nervous system. It also explains how cholinergic drugs increase parasympathetic activity and anticholinergic drugs decrease it.

CHAPTER OBJECTIVES

After studying this chapter, you should be able to

- describe the neuronal release and inactivation of acetylcholine.

- list the three types of cholinergic receptors and the tissues where they are located.

- explain the effects of acetylcholine on the major internal organs and glands of the body.

- name two direct- and two indirect-acting cholinergic drugs and the effects they produce.

- name three anticholinergic drugs and the main effects they produce on the major body systems.

- list the most frequently observed adverse effects of both cholinergic and anticholinergic drug therapy.

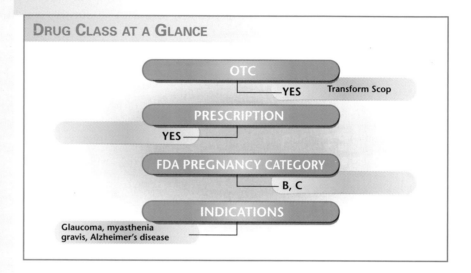

DRUG CLASS AT A GLANCE

OTC — YES — Transform Scop

PRESCRIPTION — YES

FDA PREGNANCY CATEGORY — B, C

INDICATIONS — Glaucoma, myasthenia gravis, Alzheimer's disease

Key Terms

acetylcholinesterase: an enzyme that inactivates acetylcholine.

anticholinergic: refers to drugs or effects that reduce the activity of the parasympathetic nervous system.

cholinergic: refers to the nerves and receptors of the parasympathetic nervous system; also refers to the drugs that stimulate this system.

muscarinic receptor: an older but more specific term for the cholinergic receptor on smooth and cardiac muscle.

nicotinic-muscle (Nm) receptor: cholinergic receptor located at the neuromuscular junction of skeletal muscle.

nicotinic-neural (Nn) receptor: cholinergic receptor located on both sympathetic and parasympathetic ganglia.

parasympatholytic: refers to drugs (anticholinergic) that decrease activity of the parasympathetic nervous system.

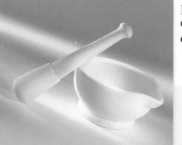

parasympathomimetic: refers to drugs (cholinergic) that mimic stimulation of the parasympathetic nervous system.

INTRODUCTION

The autonomic nervous system regulates the functions of the internal organs and glands. As discussed, the sympathetic division controls activity during physical exertion and stress (fight or flight). The parasympathetic division regulates body functions mainly during rest, digestion, and waste elimination. Parasympathetic stimulation increases the activity of the gastrointestinal (GI) and genitourinary systems and decreases the activity of the cardiovascular system.

PARASYMPATHETIC SYSTEM

The neurotransmitter of the parasympathetic system is acetylcholine (ACH). Nerves that release ACH are called cholinergic nerves; receptors that respond to cholinergic stimulation are called cholinergic receptors. Therefore, other drugs that bind to cholinergic receptors and produce effects similar to those of ACH are referred to as **cholinergic** drugs. Drugs that bind to cholinergic receptors and do not produce any effect (antagonism) are referred to as cholinergic blocking drugs. The cholinergic blocking drugs prevent ACH from acting upon its receptors.

Cholinergic Nerve Endings

Acetylcholine (ACH) is produced and stored within the cholinergic nerve endings. When a nerve is stimulated, ACH is released from its storage granules, travels to the smooth or cardiac muscle membrane, and binds to the cholinergic receptors. The binding of ACH to the receptors initiates the changes that result in parasympathetic stimulation. In the area of the cholinergic receptors is an enzyme, acetylcholinesterase. **Acetylcholinesterase** inactivates ACH only when it is outside a nerve ending and not on the receptor. Inactivation of ACH occurs so quickly that the effects of ACH last for only a few seconds. A cholinergic nerve ending is shown in Figure 7:1.

FIGURE 7:1 Characteristics of the Cholinergic Nerve Ending

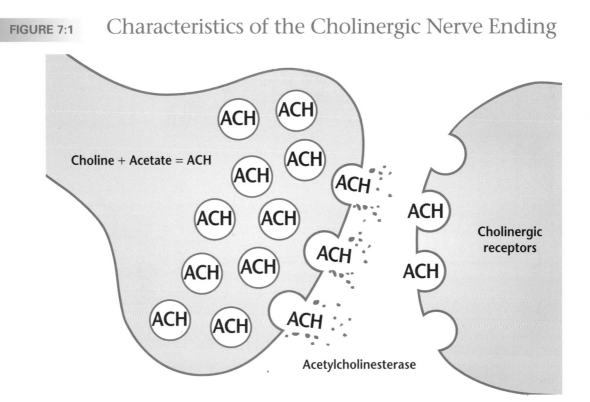

Presynaptic nerve releases acetylcholine (ACH). Postsynaptic membrane contains the cholinergic receptor. Acetylcholinesterase inactivates ACH.

Cholinergic Receptors

Three types of cholinergic receptors are in the peripheral nervous system. Acetylcholine is the neurotransmitter for each receptor site. However, each of the cholinergic receptor types reacts differently to drugs that block the cholinergic receptors. There are three distinct classes of cholinergic blocking drugs, one for each type of receptor. All three types of cholinergic blockers are required clinically to block all of the effects of ACH. Although the terminology used for the cholinergic receptors is confusing to beginning students, learning the terminology is essential for understanding the mechanism of drug action.

Muscarinic Receptors

The cholinergic receptors at the parasympathetic postganglionic nerve endings (as shown in Figure 7:2A) are known as **muscarinic receptors.** The term *muscarinic* is derived from the drug muscarine, which is an alkaloid obtained from a particular type of mushroom. One of the first drugs used to establish the function of the autonomic nervous system (ANS), muscarine produces effects that are similar to those of ACH, but only at these particular receptor sites. Consequently, early pharmacologists referred to these receptors as muscarinic, and the terminology is still in use. Drugs that act like ACH or muscarine at these receptors are referred to as

---

FIGURE 7:2 The Three Cholinergic Sites of Action and Their Specific Receptors

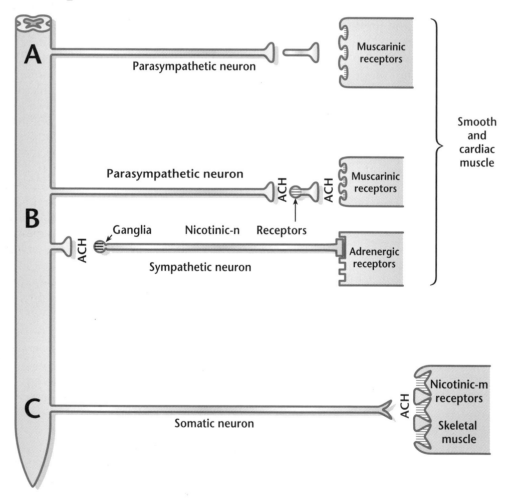

A illustrates a parasympathetic neuron with pre- and postganglionic fibers innervating smooth or cardiac muscle via the muscarinic receptor. **B** illustrates the nicotinic-Nn receptor located on the ganglia of both parasympathetic and sympathetic neurons. **C** illustrates a somatic neuron that innervates skeletal muscle via nicotinic-Nm receptors (ACH = acetylcholine).

cholinergic, or muscarinic, drugs. Drugs that block ACH at the muscarinic receptors are referred to as anticholinergic, or antimuscarinic, drugs. Presently, the terms *cholinergic* and *anticholinergic* are preferred.

Nicotinic-neural (Nn) Receptors

The cholinergic receptors at the ganglionic sites of both sympathetic and parasympathetic nerves (as seen in Figure 7:2B) are known as **nicotinic-neural (Nn) receptors.** Acetylcholine is the neurotransmitter for these receptors. The term *nicotinic* is derived from the drug nicotine, which is an alkaloid obtained from the tobacco plant. Early pharmacologists also used nicotine to study the pharmacology of the ANS, since nicotine stimulates the autonomic ganglia (sympathetic and parasympathetic) in low doses and blocks the autonomic ganglia in high doses. Drugs that act like ACH or low doses of nicotine at these receptors are known as ganglionic stimulants. Drugs that block ACH at these receptors or act like high doses of nicotine are referred to as ganglionic blockers. The ganglionic drugs will be discussed in Chapter 8.

Nicotinic-muscle (Nm) Receptors

The cholinergic receptors at the neuromuscular junction (NMJ) of skeletal muscle (seen in Figure 7:2C) are known as **nicotinic-muscle (Nm) receptors.** Nicotine also stimulates or acts like ACH at the neuromuscular junction. Drugs that block the effects of ACH at the NMJ are neuromuscular blockers or skeletal muscle relaxants. The skeletal muscle relaxant drugs will be discussed in Chapter 9.

CHOLINERGIC DRUGS

Cholinergic drugs mimic the actions of ACH at the muscarinic receptors. Another term with essentially the same meaning is **parasympathomimetic.** Cholinergic drugs are subdivided into two groups: the direct-acting and the indirect-acting drugs. The direct-acting drugs bind to the muscarinic receptors and produce effects similar to those of ACH. The indirect-acting drugs inhibit the enzyme acetylcholinesterase. By inhibiting acetylcholinesterase, these drugs allow ACH to accumulate at each of the cholinergic receptor sites (nicotinic and muscarinic). Consequently, a greater number of receptors become stimulated and the effects of ACH are prolonged.

Direct-Acting Cholinergic Drugs

Direct-acting cholinergic drugs bind to the muscarinic receptors. Acetylcholine is not useful

as a drug because of its extremely short duration of action. Therefore, several derivatives of ACH were synthesized (methacholine and bethanechol) that produce effects like those of ACH, but they are more slowly inactivated by acetylcholinesterase. Consequently, the durations of action of these drugs are considerably longer than is the duration of action for ACH. In all other respects, the derivatives of ACH stimulate the parasympathetic system similarly to ACH.

Pharmacological Effects

The main effects are an increase in GI secretions and motility, an increase in genitourinary activity, bronchoconstriction, miosis, a decrease in blood pressure (vasodilation), and a decrease in heart rate. The cholinergic drugs are listed in Table 7:1.

In addition to the derivatives of ACH, there are a few alkaloids, such as muscarine and pilocarpine, that have parasympathomimetic effects. Muscarine has no clinical importance except in cases of accidental poisoning. Pilocarpine is another alkaloid that acts like ACH and is used only in the form of eyedrops for the treatment of glaucoma.

Clinical Indications

Because of the short duration of ACH and some of its derivatives, the direct-acting cholinergic drugs are rarely used systemically. Bethanechol is the exception; this drug is administered orally to stimulate the urinary and intestinal tracts. Certain drugs (general anesthetics) and conditions, especially in the elderly, cause urinary retention and intestinal stasis. Bethanechol may be administered several times a day to stimulate urination and defecation. The main adverse effects are due to overstimulation of the bladder and intestines resulting in increased urinary frequency and diarrhea.

Cholinergic drugs are used locally during ophthalmic examinations (miotic, to constrict pupil) and in the treatment of glaucoma. In glaucoma there is increased intraocular pressure. Increased intraocular pressure will gradually destroy the retina of the eye and cause blindness. Topical application (eyedrops) of cholinergic drugs produces miosis (pupillary constriction), which promotes better drainage of intraocular fluid from the eye. This lowers pressure and helps prevent retinal damage.

Indirect-Acting Cholinergic Drugs

The indirect-acting drugs are known as the anticholinesterases. These drugs inhibit the

TABLE 7:1   Cholinergic Drugs and Their Major Clinical Uses

DRUG (TRADE NAME)	MAIN USE
Direct Acting:	
acetylcholine *(Miochol-E)*	Miotic in cataract surgery
bethanechol *(Urecholine)*	Nonobstructive urinary retention
carbachol *(Miostat)*	Treatment of glaucoma
pilocarpine *(Pilocar, Ocusert-Pilo)*	Treatment of glaucoma
Indirect Acting:	
ambenonium *(Mytelase)*	Treatment of myasthenia gravis
demacarium *(Humorsol)*	Treatment of glaucoma
edrophonium *(Tensilon)*	Diagnosis of myasthenia gravis, antidote for curare-type drugs
galantamine *(Reminyl)*	Treatment of Alzheimer's disease
neostigmine *(Prostigmin)*	Treatment of myasthenia gravis, antidote for curare-type drugs
physostigmine *(Antilirium, Eserine)*	Antidote to anticholinergic drugs, treatment of glaucoma
pyridostigmine *(Mestinon)*	Treatment of myasthenia gravis, antidote for curare-type drugs
tacrine *(Cognex)*	Treatment of Alzheimer's disease
donepezil *(Aricept)*	Treatment of Alzheimer's disease

enzyme acetylcholinesterase and allow the accumulation of ACH at all cholinergic receptor sites. The anticholinesterase drugs are subdivided into the reversible inhibitors and the irreversible inhibitors of acetylcholinesterase.

Reversible Inhibitors

The reversible inhibitors are used in the diagnosis and treatment of myasthenia gravis, and as antidotes to reverse the effects of drugs that block cholinergic and nicotinic receptors. Myasthenia gravis, which affects the skeletal muscle, is characterized by insufficient acetylcholine activity. Edrophonium has the shortest duration of action, about 30 minutes, and is used intravenously to diagnose myasthenia gravis. The durations of neostigmine (2 to 4 hours), pyridostigmine (3 to 6 hours), and ambenonium (4 to 8 hours) are longer. These drugs are administered orally for the treatment of myasthenia gravis and intravenously to reverse the effects of excessive cholinergic blockade. The previously mentioned drugs are all quarternary amines (charged compounds) that do not cross the blood-brain barrier and produce effects only at peripheral receptor sites.

Physostigmine is not a charged compound and does produce effects in the brain. It is used parenterally to reverse the central nervous system (CNS) effects of excessive anticholinergic blockade and as eyedrops in the treatment of glaucoma.

Irreversible Inhibitors

The irreversible inhibitors of acetylcholinesterase are derivatives of organophosphate compounds widely used as insecticides, pesticides, and as chemical warfare agents. These compounds have extremely long durations of action because they form irreversible bonds with the acetylcholinesterase enzyme. A few of these derivatives—for example, echothiophate (Phospholine)—are used in very small doses as drugs, primarily as eyedrops in the treatment of glaucoma. In larger doses these drugs produce severe toxicity, referred to as cholinergic crisis, that can quickly cause respiratory paralysis and death.

All of the anticholinesterase drugs, reversible and irreversible, produce effects that are similar to those of ACH and parasympathetic stimulation (parasympathomimetic).

Adverse and Toxic Effects of Cholinergic Drugs

The most common adverse effects of these drugs are caused by excessive stimulation of the parasympathetic nervous system. The symptoms include nausea, vomiting, diarrhea, blurred vision, excessive sweating, muscular tremors, bronchoconstriction, bradycardia, and hypotension. In toxic overdosage, muscular paralysis and respiratory depression may cause death. The main antidote is the administration of anticholinergic drugs, such as atropine, which compete with ACH for the muscarinic receptor and reverse the effects of excessive cholinergic stimulation.

Cholinergic Crisis

Cholinergic crisis is the term usually used to describe the effects of excessive drug dosage in patients with myasthenia gravis. At high concentrations ACH causes excessive stimulation of cholinergic (muscarinic) receptors, but blockade (paralysis) of nicotinic receptors. This may result in respiratory paralysis because respiratory muscles are skeletal (voluntary) in nature. In these situations, anticholinesterase drug administration must be stopped until the levels of ACH return to normal. Atropine can be administered to block the effects of excessive muscarinic stimulation.

Farmers who spray their fields with derivatives of the irreversible anticholinesterases (organophosphates) may also experience a cholinergic crisis. Unless protective masks or enclosed tractor cabs are used, the farmer may inhale too much of the insecticide or pesticide and develop signs of cholinergic crisis. With the irreversible drugs, the antidote is atropine to reverse the effects of excessive ACH and also an additional drug, pralidoxime (Protopam). Pralidoxime is a drug that can reactivate the acetylcholinesterase enzyme after it has been inhibited by an irreversible inhibitor. Pralidoxime is most effective immediately after organophosphate exposure. Pralidoxime is also the antidote to organophosphate chemical warfare agents.

Clinical Indications for Anticholinesterase Drugs

The anticholinesterase drugs are more widely used than the direct-acting cholinergic drugs. They are used in the treatment of glaucoma, myasthenia gravis, urinary retention, intestinal paralysis, Alzheimer's disease, and as antidotes to the curare-type skeletal muscle blockers and the anticholinergic drugs.

Patient Administration and Monitoring

Check and observe for signs of cholinergic overdosage, especially after parenteral administration: visual disturbances, salivation, nausea, increased frequency of urination, diarrhea, slow heart rate, respiratory difficulties, seizures (physostigmine).

Explain to patient the common drug side effects: visual disturbances (especially after eyedrops), sweating, increased frequency of urination, and defecation.

Instruct patient to report eye irritation or inflammation, excessive salivation, sweating, urination, and diarrhea, slow pulse rate, muscle weakness, respiratory difficulties.

Topical Use in Glaucoma

Several of these drugs (Table 7:1) are used topically as eyedrops to lower intraocular pressure in glaucoma. By inhibiting the metabolism of ACH, they increase ACH levels in the eye to produce miosis, improved drainage of intraocular fluid, and lower intraocular pressure.

Treatment of Myasthenia Gravis

Myasthenis gravis is a disease of the skeletal muscle endplate where ACH functions to stimulate muscle tone and contraction. The condition is believed to be due to an autoimmune reaction where the body produces antibodies that attack the Nm receptor. The result is loss of skeletal muscle tone and strength. The eyelids droop and as the disease progresses there is difficulty in physical movement. Eventually patients may become bedridden and have difficulty breathing. The longer-acting reversible anticholinesterase drugs, pyridostigmine and ambenonium, are preferred and used orally to increase ACH levels and increase skeletal muscle tone and strength.

Treatment of Urinary Retention and Intestinal Stasis

Urinary retention (also referred to as atony of the bladder), and intestinal stasis or paralysis (also referred to as paralytic ileus) are usually treated with neostigmine. The increased levels of ACH stimulate bladder contraction and intestinal peristalsis.

Treatment of Alzheimer's Disease

Alzheimer's disease is a degenerative brain condition that occurs in some individuals with advanced age. There appears to be a loss of neuronal synapses and, in particular, a reduction of ACH levels in the brain. These changes cause memory loss, dementia, and general deterioration of mental function. Very few drugs have been discovered that are effective in treating this condition. Currently, two centrally acting, reversible anticholinesterase drugs, tacrine *(Cognex)* and donepezil *(Aricept),* are used to increase ACH levels in the brain. Beneficial effects of the drugs are most notable in the early stages of the disease and lessen as the disease progresses. Lecithin *(Phoschol)* is a precursor of ACH and is often administered with the anticholinesterase drugs in an attempt to further increase ACH levels.

Antidotes to Skeletal Muscle Blockers

Skeletal muscle blockers (see Chapter 9) are used in surgery to produce paralysis of skeletal muscles (Nm receptor). At high doses they may cause respiratory paralysis. In these situations, administration of neostigmine will increase ACH levels and antagonize the actions of the skeletal muscle blockers.

Antidotes to Anticholinergic Drug Poisoning

Anticholinergic drugs, such as atropine and scopolamine (see Anticholinergic Drugs section that follows) block the cholinergic receptors (muscarinic) and produce effects similar to decreasing the activity of the parasympathetic system (parasympatholytic). This includes urinary and intestinal inhibition, cardiac stimulation (tachycardia), and central effects in the brain that can cause a variety of stimulant (seizures) and depressant effects (coma). The antidote is usually to administer physostigmine because this drug can pass the blood-brain barrier. The increased levels of ACH produced compete with the anticholinergic drug for the receptor. As the levels of ACH increase, the central effects of excessive anticholinergic blockade are reversed.

ANTICHOLINERGIC DRUGS

The cholinergic blocking drugs that bind to the muscarinic receptors are referred to as the **anticholinergic,** or **parasympatholytic,** drugs. They act by competitive antagonism of ACH. In the presence of anticholinergic drugs, sufficient amounts of ACH are unable to bind to the cholinergic receptors to produce an effect. The oldest anticholinergic drugs, such as atropine and scopolamine, were obtained from the belladonna plant (deadly nightshade) and are commonly referred to as the belladonna alkaloids. Atropine, scopolamine, and the newer synthetic drugs are listed in Table 7:2.

Pharmacological Actions and Clinical Indications

Cardiovascular System

By blocking the effects of ACH, anticholinergic drugs decrease the activity of the vagus nerve (parasympathetic nerve) on the heart. Consequently, there is an increase in heart rate. In patients with excessively slow heart rates (bradycardia), anticholinergic drugs are used to increase heart rate and speed up atrioventricular conduction.

Respiratory System

ACH increases the secretions of the respiratory tract and may cause bronchoconstriction. Anticholinergic drugs are administered preoperatively to inhibit secretions that can interfere with the administration of general anesthetics. In addition, anticholinergic drugs produce bronchodilation and are used in the treatment of asthma (see Chapter 32).

GI System

Anticholinergic drugs reduce salivary and GI secretions. In addition, they decrease the motility of the GI tract and therefore they should not be administered when there is intestinal obstruction. The anticholinergic drugs are used as antispasmodics in GI disorders such as irritable bowel syndrome. In the treatment of peptic ulcers, the anticholinergic drugs, which decrease gastric acid secretion, have been replaced by newer and more effective drugs (see Chapter 33).

Genitourinary System

Anticholinergic drugs inhibit urinary peristalsis and the voiding of urine. These drugs may be

TABLE 7.2

Anticholinergic Drugs and Their Main Uses

DRUG (TRADE NAME)	MAIN USE	COMMON DAILY DOSAGE RANGE
Belladonna Alkaloids:		
atropine	To increase heart rate, preop medication, enuresis, GI and biliary colic, antidote to cholinergic drugs	0.4–0.6 mg PO, IV, IM, SC
	Mydriatic and cycloplegic	Topical eyedrops
hyoscyamine *(Levsin)*	Same as atropine	0.25–1.0 mg PO, IV
scopolamine *(Transderm*-Scop)	Motion sickness	1 patch every 3 days
Semisynthetic Drug:		
homatropine	Mydriatic	Ophthalmic solution
Synthetic Drugs:		
dicyclomine *(Bentyl)*	Treatment of GI disorders such as ulcers, colitis	80–160 mg PO
glycopyrrolate *(Robinul, Robinul Forte)*	Treatment of ulcers	2–6 mg PO
methscopolamine *(Pamine)*	Treatment of GI disorders such as ulcers, colitis	2.5–10 mg PO
oxybutynin *(Ditropan, Ditropan XL)*	Treatment of overactive bladder	5–15 mg PO
propantheline *(Pro-Banthine)*	Treatment of GI disorders such as ulcers, colitis	22.5–60 mg PO
tolterodine (Detrol, Detrol-LA)	Treatment of overactive bladder	2–4 mg PO

used in individuals suffering from enuresis (urinary incontinence) to promote urinary retention and in the treatment of overactive bladder that involves spasm and increased urinary urgency. However, anticholinergic drugs are contraindicated in males with hypertrophy of the prostate gland. These drugs increase urinary retention and further increase the difficulty of urination associated with this condition.

Central Nervous System

Most anticholinergic drugs that gain access to the brain produce a depressant effect, which generally results in drowsiness and sedation. Some over-the-counter preparations contain limited amounts of scopolamine and are used as sleep aids. At higher doses, there can be a mixture of both CNS stimulant and depressant effects. At toxic doses, both atropine and scopolamine may produce excitation, delirium, hallucinations, and a profound CNS depression that can lead to respiratory arrest and death. Anticholinergic actions are useful in the treatment of Parkinson's disease (see Chapter 17) and as antiemetics (see Chapter 33) in the treatment of motion sickness.

Ocular Effects

The anticholinergic drugs produce mydriasis (pupillary dilation) and cycloplegia (loss of accommodation). They are used in ophthalmology to facilitate examination of the retina and lens. Anticholinergic drugs increase intraocular pressure and should *never* be administered to patients with glaucoma. In glaucoma, there is a blockage of the drainage pathway for intraocular fluid. The anticholinergic effect causes pupillary dilation, which in glaucoma increases closure of the drainage pathway. The result can be a sudden increase in intraocular pressure and damage to the eye.

Adverse and Toxic Effects

The most frequently occurring adverse effects of the anticholinergic drugs are caused by excessive blockade of the parasympathetic nervous system. The symptoms include dry mouth, visual disturbances, urinary retention, constipation, flushing (redness) and dryness of the skin, fever (hyperpyrexia), tachycardia, and symptoms of both CNS stimulation and depression. The effects on the skin are due to anticholinergic effects that inhibit the sweating mechanism and that vasodilate certain blood vessels to cause a flushing reaction. In toxic doses, hyperpyrexia and CNS depression can be severe and may be accompanied by depression of the vital centers in the brain. If untreated this may result in respiratory paralysis and death.

The belladonna alkaloids are present in some over-the-counter preparations and in many common plant substances and noneatable plant berries. Poisoning usually occurs in children who have mistakenly eaten the berries. Such children usually develop fever, tachycardia, dryness and flushing of the skin, and mydriasis. Emergency treatment is essential. If sufficient quantities have been ingested, respiratory paralysis, coma, and death may occur within a few hours.

Treatment involves inducing emesis or performing gastric lavage to limit absorption. Activated charcoal and saline cathartics are administered to inactivate the drug and accelerate its elimination. Physostigmine, given intravenously, antagonizes the actions of the anticholinergic drugs and is useful when CNS symptoms such as delirium and coma are present.

Patient Administration and Monitoring

Observe patient for signs of excessive anticholinergic effects, especially after parenteral administration: tachycardia, flushing of skin (redness), decreased urination, CNS stimulation or depression, respiratory difficulties.

Explain to patient the common anticholinergic side effects: dry mouth, blurred vision (pupillary dilation), sedation, or mental confusion.

Instruct patient to report excessive blurred vision, fast pulse rate, difficulty with urination, constipation, mental confusion, or hallucinations.

Geriatric patients are particularly susceptible to anticholinergic effects and should be observed more closely, especially for mental confusion and disorientation.

Anticholinergic drugs are contraindicated in patients with narrow-angle glaucoma, males with prostate hypertrophy, and patients with urinary or intestinal obstruction.

The antidote to anticholinergic overdose is administration of anticholinesterase drugs, especially physostigmine when there are CNS symptoms.

Chapter Review

Understanding Terminology

Match the drug effect or drug use in the left column with the appropriate drug in the right column. Each answer can be used more than once.

___ **1.** Reactivates acetylcholinesterase.

___ **2.** Directly stimulates muscarinic receptor.

___ **3.** Increases ACH levels in the CNS.

___ **4.** Used to reverse CNS anticholinergic toxicity.

___ **5.** Used to treat myasthenia gravis.

___ **6.** Used to prevent motion sickness.

___ **7.** Used before surgery to dry respiratory secretions.

___ **8.** Indicated for treatment of Alzheimer's disease.

___ **9.** Irreversibly inhibits acetylcholinesterase.

___ **10.** Used to treat nonobstructive urinary retention.

a. Bethanechol *(Urecholine)*

b. Ambenonium *(Mytelase)*

c. Scopolamine *(Transdermscope)*

d. Echothiophate *(Phospholine)*

e. Atropine

f. Physostigmine *(Antilirium)*

g. Pralidoxime *(Protopam)*

h. Tacrine *(Cognex)*

11. Differentiate between parasympatholytic and parasympathomimetic. _____
_____
_____

12. Explain the terms *cholinergic* and *anticholinergic*. _____
_____
_____

Acquiring Knowledge

Answer the following questions in the spaces provided.

1. What is the function of the parasympathetic nervous system? _____

2. What is the function of acetylcholinesterase? Where is it found? _____
_____
_____

3. Where are the three different cholinergic receptors located? What class of drug is needed to block each receptor? _____
_____
_____

4. How do the direct-acting and the indirect-acting cholinergic drugs produce their parasympathetic effects? _____
_____

5. List the potential adverse effects of the cholinergic drugs. _____
_____
_____

6. List the potential adverse effects of the anticholinergic drugs. _____
_____
_____

7. Why are the side effects of the anticholinergic drugs similar to the side effects of the sympathetic drugs? _____
_____
_____

Applying Knowledge—On the Job

Use your critical thinking skills to answer the following questions in the spaces provided.

1. As a nurse working for a team of doctors in a busy practice, you are sometimes given the task of screening patients for potential prescription drug problems. Patient X has just been diagnosed as having colitis, for which his doctor has prescribed dicyclomine. You note that in his first visit last year, Patient X mentioned he takes the drug timolol. You decide you'd better check the *PDR*® to see what timolol is used to treat before Patient X starts taking the dicyclomine. What should you report to the doctor? _____
_____
_____

2. Your next-door neighbor knows you are studying pharmacology so she sometimes comes to you when she has questions about health problems. A few minutes ago, she came to your door in a state of panic. She said her 3-year-old had just swallowed some scopolamine tablets, which your neighbor takes for her irritable bowel syndrome. What should you do?_____
_____
_____

3. Your elderly patient who was prescribed an antispasmotic drug for GI hyperactivity is complaining of increased sensitivity to light and notices that she has difficulty urinating. What do you think is happening to this patient? What class of drugs do you think she was most likely prescribed? What drug class would be indicated if her condition worsened and treatment was required? _____
_____
_____

4. Mr. Jones is being treated for myasthenia gravis. During his regular checkup you notice that he is sweating and his heart rate is below normal. You ask him how he's feeling and he says he's had diarrhea for the past few days and that he feels very weak. Can you explain what may be happening to Mr. Jones? Explain why some of his symptoms appear to be due to excessive cholinergic stimulation, yet he has skeletal muscle weakness. _____
_____
_____

5. An elderly woman in a nursing facility is being treated with bethanechol for urinary retention. She is complaining of abdominal discomfort, excessive salivation, and feeling hot and sweaty. Could these symptoms be due to the medication? If so, what do they indicate? _____
_____
_____

6. A 28-year-old male has been diagnosed with irritable bowel syndrome. His health care provider has prescribed dicyclomine 20 mg TID. What side effects should be included in the patient counseling? _____
_____

7. Dan has just been diagnosed with glaucoma for which his physician has prescribed pilocarpine 1 percent—2 gtts OU QID with a return visit in one month. What should Dan be told regarding this medication? _____

_____

_____

Internet Connection

Visit the **MedicineNet** website (http://www.medicinenet.com), under *Diseases and Treatments*, click on letter "E" and look for *Eye, Glaucoma*. Organize a brief presentation that explains the causes, symptoms, detection, and treatments for glaucoma. Under *Diseases and Treatments*, click on the letter "M" and find *Myasthenia Gravis*. Read about the prognosis and treatment of this condition in relation to the drugs presented in this chapter. Also, click on the letter "I" for *Irritable Bowel Syndrome*, "O" for *Overactive Bladder*, and "M" for *Motion Sickness*. Read about the treatments for these conditions.

Additional Reading

Bayer, M. J. and McKay, C. 1997. Reversing the effects of pesticide poisoning Part 1: Insecticides and herbicides. *Emergency Medicine* 29 (4):72.

Bayer, M. J. and McKay, C. 1997. Reversing the effects of pesticide poisoning Part 2: Rodenticides and miscellaneous agents. *Emergency Medicine* 29 (5):78.

Keeping an eye on vision: Primary care of age-related ocular disease. 1997. *Geriatrics* 52 (8):30.

Marin, D. B., Sewell, M. C., and Schlechter, A. 2002. Alzheimer's disease. *Geriactrics* 57 (2):36.

Ramsey, F. 1991. Reversal of neuromuscular blockade. *Current Reviews for Nurse Anesthetists* 514 (7):50.

Seybold, M. E. 1991. Update on myasthenia gravis. *Hospital Medicine* 27 (4):71.

Teplitz, L. 1989. Clinical close-up on atropine. *Nursing* 19 (11):44.

chapter

8

DRUGS AFFECTING THE AUTONOMIC GANGLIA

CHAPTER FOCUS

This chapter describes the drugs that affect autonomic ganglia and examines how ganglionic blocking drugs affect both sympathetic and parasympathetic activity.

CHAPTER OBJECTIVES

After studying this chapter, you should be able to

- describe the pharmacological effects of both ganglionic stimulation and ganglionic blockade.
- list three ganglionic blocking drugs and describe their clinical uses.
- discuss the adverse effects associated with the use of ganglionic blocking drugs.

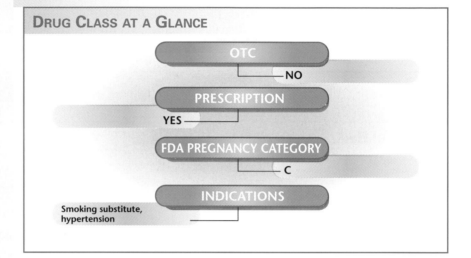

DRUG CLASS AT A GLANCE

OTC — NO

PRESCRIPTION — YES

FDA PREGNANCY CATEGORY — C

INDICATIONS — Smoking substitute, hypertension

Key Terms

ganglionic blocker: drug that blocks the nicotinic-neural receptors and reduces the activity of the autonomic nervous system.

ganglionic stimulant: drug that stimulates the nicotinic-Nn receptors to increase autonomic activity.

nicotine: alkaloid drug in tobacco that stimulates ganglionic receptors.

nicotinic-neural (Nn) receptor: cholinergic receptor at the ganglia.

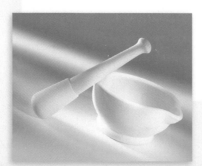

INTRODUCTION

The autonomic ganglia of both sympathetic and parasympathetic nerves are pharmacologically identical. Acetylcholine (ACH) is the neurotransmitter at the ganglionic synapses. Acetylcholinesterase is responsible for inactivation of ACH. Before the discovery of ACH, nicotine was found to stimulate the autonomic ganglia, and so the receptors at the ganglia were known as the **nicotinic-neural (Nn) receptors.** Drugs that stimulate the Nn receptors are called **ganglionic stimulants.** There are no clinical conditions where ganglionic stimulation is of significant clinical value. Therefore, as a drug class, the ganglionic stimulants are of little interest.

Individuals who smoke tobacco inhale **nicotine,** which produces ganglionic stimulation affecting both sympathetic and parasympathetic activity. Theoretically, if both systems are stimulated at the same time, the effects should cancel out. However, sympathetic stimulation appears to predominate in the cardiovascular system while parasympathetic stimulation predominates in the gastrointestinal (GI) tract. Consequently, after smoking, there is usually an increase in heart rate, blood pressure, and GI activity. Nicotine also stimulates the central nervous system (CNS) to produce tremors and, most importantly, the pleasurable effects of smoking.

GANGLIONIC DRUGS

Ganglionic Stimulants

A chewing gum containing nicotine *(Nicorette)* is available for individuals who are trying to stop smoking. The gum releases nicotine that is meant to substitute for the nicotine supplied by smoking. In addition, transdermal skin patches *(Habitrol, Nicoderm)* have recently been introduced that slowly deliver nicotine into the bloodstream. The intention of these products is to prevent any withdrawal reactions caused by quitting the smoking habit. Later, the use of these products can be reduced and then eliminated altogether.

Cautions and Contraindications

Pregnancy

Nicotine and tobacco smoke (contains nicotine) have been shown to be harmful to the fetus. Consequently, tobacco smoking and the use of nicotine substitutes should be avoided during pregnancy.

Adverse Effects

Drugs that block the effects of ACH at the Nn receptors are called **ganglionic blockers.** At toxic doses, ACH and nicotine act like ganglionic blockers and can block both ganglionic and neuromuscular transmission. This blockade can result in respiratory paralysis and death.

The ganglionic blockers that are used clinically compete with ACH for the Nn receptors. These drugs interfere with ganglionic transmission at both the sympathetic and parasympathetic ganglia. Consequently, the effects are a combination of anticholinergic and sympathetic blocking effects. The main disadvantage of the ganglionic blockers is that there is no selectivity. As a result, many side effects are associated with their use. Newer drugs with greater selectivity have been discovered, and these have gradually replaced the ganglionic blockers.

Main Effects of Ganglionic Blockade

Ganglionic blockade decreases the activity of the cardiovascular, gastrointestinal (GI), and genitourinary systems. The major effects are hypotension, bradycardia, decreased intestinal secretions and motility, and reduced urination. In males, impotence may occur. In addition, there are usually varying degrees of mydriasis and cycloplegia.

Pharmacokinetics

The first ganglionic blockers that were discovered (hexamethonium, pentolinium, and trimethaphan) possessed a quaternary ammonium ion. Quaternary ammonium ions are permanently

Drugs Affecting the Autonomic Ganglia   **83**

TABLE 8:1	Drug Interactions with Ganglionic Blocking Drugs	
DRUG CLASS	**RESULT**
Adrenergic drugs	Antagonism of antiadrenergic effect of ganglionic blockade, especially on cardiovascular system
Adrenergic blocking drugs	Additive antiadrenergic effect to produce hypotension and possible cardiovascular collapse
Cholinergic drugs	Antagonism of anticholinergic effect of ganglionic blockade, especially on GI and urinary tracts
Anticholinergic drugs	Additive anticholinergic effect
Vasodilator drugs	Additive vasodilating effect to produce hypotension and possible cardiovascular collapse

charged molecules and are poorly absorbed from the GI tract. Therefore, parenteral administration (intramuscular [IM] or intravenous [IV]) is usually required. On the other hand, one of the ganglionic blockers, mecamylamine, is not a quaternary ion and is almost completely absorbed after oral administration.

Clinical Indications

The only ganglionic blocker currently available is mecamylamine *(Inversine)*. The main indication for mecamylamine is for the treatment of severe hypertension when other drugs have not been effective. The pharmacologic action of mecamylamine is due to ganglionic blockade of sympathetic ganglia, which causes profound vasodilation. Although mecamylamine is a very potent antihypertensive drug, it produces numerous adverse effects which many patients cannot tolerate. Mecamylamine usually is used in combination with other antihypertensive drugs, this allows reduction of the mecamylamine dosage and the frequency and severity of adverse effects.

Adverse Effects

Almost all of the adverse effects of the ganglionic blockers are caused by excessive blockade of the autonomic ganglia. The result is a combination of anticholinergic and antiadrenergic effects, which usually include decreased GI activity (dry mouth and constipation), visual disturbances (mydriasis and cycloplegia), decreased cardiovascular function (hypotension and decreased cardiac output), and decreased genitourinary function (urinary retention and impotency). The ganglionic blockers are contraindicated in patients with glaucoma because the mydriatic effect increases intraocular pressure.

Drug Interactions

Many drugs act on autonomic receptors, and the possibility of a drug interaction with ganglionic blockers is significant. Table 8:1 lists the potential drug interactions with ganglionic blockers.

Chapter Review

Understanding Terminology

Answer the following questions in the spaces provided.

1. Differentiate between a ganglionic stimulant and a ganglionic blocker. _____

_____

2. What is the name of the cholinergic receptors at the ganglia? _____

Acquiring Knowledge

Answer the following questions in the spaces provided.

1. What neurotransmitter regulates ganglionic transmission? _____

2. List the main effects of ganglionic stimulation. _____

_____

3. List the main effects of ganglionic blockade. _____

_____

4. What are the main therapeutic uses of the ganglionic blocking drugs? _____

_____

5. What is the major advantage of mecamylamine *(Inversine)?* _____

_____

_____

6. List the adverse effects of the ganglionic blocking drugs. _____

_____

_____

7. What other drugs might interact with the ganglionic blockers? _____

_____

_____

Applying Knowledge—On the Job

Use your critical thinking skills to answer the following questions in the spaces provided.

1. Assume that you work in a health maintenance organization (HMO), where you act as patient liaison. Patients are encouraged to talk over problems with you if they feel that the problems have not been resolved by a doctor or if they feel uncomfortable discussing the problems with a doctor. One of the patients wants to talk to you about an "embarrassing problem." He says that ever since he started taking that "strong medicine" for his high blood pressure, he hasn't been able to make love to his wife. He also has a dry mouth, and he's constipated all of the time. What drug is the patient most likely taking? What other drugs might be tried to help control his hypertension without causing the side effects he's experiencing?_____

_____

_____

2. A patient has been brought by ambulance to the emergency room where you work. He's suffering from hypotension, and he's on the verge of cardiovascular collapse. The patient's wife, who accompanied him in the ambulance, says he was fine until he took some new medication for his high blood pressure. She has the bottle with her—the medication is mecamylamine. You ask her if he's taking any other medicine, and she replies that he takes something for his angina but she doesn't remember what it is. What might the other medication be, and why is it producing these effects in this patient? _____

_____

_____

Look up the medication *Habitrol* using the *PDR*® or *F&C*. Answer the following questions.

3. List the symptoms of nicotine withdrawal. _____

_____

_____

4. List the symptoms of nicotine toxicity. _____

_____

_____

5. Once a patient has quit smoking, he or she may be able to reduce the dosage of several medications. List five of those medications. _____

_____

_____

Internet Connection

Open the homepage of your computer browser, YAHOO, NETSCAPE, etc. and click open the headings under the Health/Disease category. In the search space, type in *Smoking Cessation* or *Smoking Addiction* and investigate the available information and programs. Websites (http://www.lungusa.org/tobacco) and (http://www.nlm.nih.gov/medlineplus) are also excellent sites for this information.

Additional Reading

The nicotine patch: A good deal? 1997. *Emergency Medicine* 29 (1):55.

Safety of the nicotine patch in cardiac patients. 1997. *Emergency Medicine* 29 (6):45.

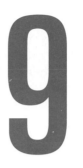

SKELETAL MUSCLE RELAXANTS

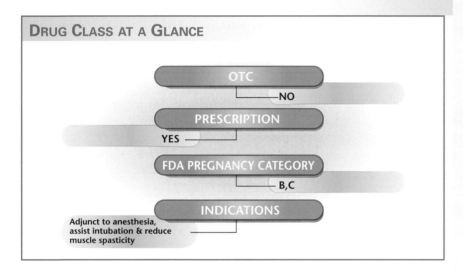

DRUG CLASS AT A GLANCE

- OTC — NO
- PRESCRIPTION — YES
- FDA PREGNANCY CATEGORY — B,C
- INDICATIONS — Adjunct to anesthesia, assist intubation & reduce muscle spasticity

Key Terms

centrally acting skeletal muscle relaxant: drug that inhibits skeletal muscle contraction by blocking conduction within the spinal cord.

depolarizing blocker: produces paralysis by first causing nerve transmission, followed by inhibition of nerve transmission.

fasciculation: twitchings of muscle fiber groups.

hyperthermia: abnormally high body temperature.

incompatibility: undesirable interaction of drugs not suitable for combination or administration together.

malignant hyperthermia: condition in susceptible individuals resulting in a life-threatening elevation in body temperature.

neuromuscular junction (NMJ): space (synapse) between a motor nerve ending and a skeletal muscle membrane that contains acetylcholine (ACH) receptors.

nondepolarizing blocker: produces paralysis by inhibiting nerve transmission.

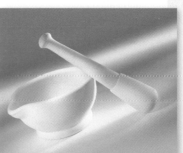

CHAPTER FOCUS

This chapter describes drugs that reduce the contraction of skeletal muscles affecting posture and motor function. It also explains how surgery may be aided by removing the normal tone of skeletal muscles and how spastic muscle disorders are controlled.

CHAPTER OBJECTIVES

After studying this chapter, you should be able to

- describe at least two ways in which skeletal muscles may be relaxed.

- explain why muscle relaxation is necessary during diagnostic and surgical procedures.

- trace how these drugs may alter the ability to control respiration.

- explain how tranquilizers relax skeletal muscles through a different mechanism of action than nondepolarizing blockers.

- identify which drugs are used in the chronic treatment of spastic muscle disorders.

- list three potential adverse effects associated with muscle relaxants.

peripheral skeletal muscle relaxant: drug that inhibits muscle contraction at the neuromuscular junction or within the contractile process.

potentiates: produces an action that is greater than either of the components can produce alone.

vagolytic: inhibition of the vagus nerve to the heart, causing the heart rate to increase (counteraction to vagal tone that causes bradycardia).

vasodilator: substance that relaxes the muscles (sphincters) controlling blood vessels, leading to increased blood flow.

INTRODUCTION

Contraction of skeletal muscles is voluntarily controlled by impulses that originate in the central nervous system (CNS). Impulses from the brain are conducted through the spinal cord to the somatic motor neurons (Figure 9:1). Somatic motor neurons eventually connect with skeletal muscle fibers forming a **neuromuscular junction (NMJ).** The neuronal endings of the somatic motor fibers contain the neurotransmitter acetylcholine (ACH). When ACH is released into the neuromuscular synapses, it combines with cholinergic receptors known as nicotinic-II (NII) receptors. Although these receptors are cholinergic, they are not identical to the muscarinic (parasympathetic) and ganglionic receptors previously discussed in Chapter 5.

Depolarization of the muscle fibers occurs when ACH combines with the NII receptors. Following depolarization, the contractile elements of the muscle fibers (actin and myosin) produce muscle contraction. Muscle relaxation occurs after ACH is hydrolyzed by acetylcholinesterase; this terminates the action of ACH. Skeletal muscle function is essential to life, since respiration depends upon the rhythmic contraction of the diaphragm and chest muscles. In addition, skeletal muscle tone permits coordinated movement of the entire body to maintain posture. This muscle activity occurs continually without our conscious awareness.

CLINICAL INDICATIONS

Many drugs inhibit skeletal muscle contraction by interfering with neuromuscular function. Drugs that inhibit skeletal muscle contraction by blocking conduction within the spinal cord are known as **centrally acting skeletal muscle relaxants** (Figure 9:1, site 1). In contrast, **peripheral skeletal muscle relaxants** inhibit muscle contraction at the NMJ (Figure 9:1, site 2) or within the contractile process (Figure 9:1, site 3). Regardless of the site of action, drugs classified as skeletal muscle relaxants are clinically valuable because they selectively inhibit neuromuscular function. This inhibition then results in skeletal muscle relaxation. Skeletal muscle relaxation is desirable in spastic diseases (multiple sclerosis and cerebral palsy), conditions in which the spinal cord has been damaged (trauma, paraplegia), and injuries in which pain accompanies overexertion of the muscles. In addition, surgical and orthopedic procedures and intubation (for example, bronchoscopy) are often facilitated by the use of skeletal muscle relaxants. Without administering these agents prior to invasive diagnostic procedures, there is a greater possibility for the reacting muscles to tear or become strained.

PERIPHERALLY ACTING SKELETAL MUSCLE RELAXANTS

Mechanism of Action

Neuromuscular blockers inhibit skeletal muscle contraction by interfering with the NII receptors. There are two types of neuromuscular blockers: nondepolarizing (curare, gallamine, and pancuronium) and depolarizing (succinylcholine).

The **nondepolarizing blockers** combine with the NII receptors but do not stimulate the

Innervation of Skeletal Muscle by Somatic Motor Neurons

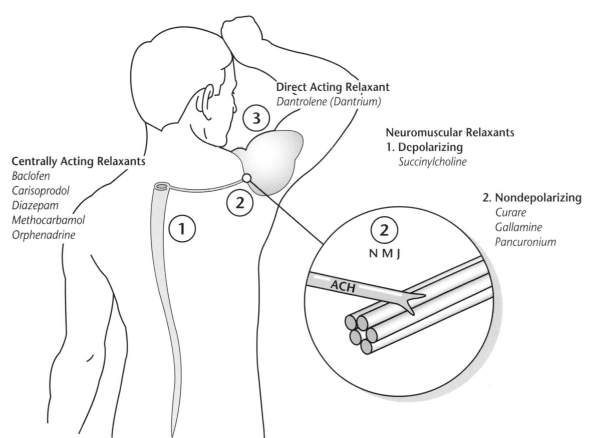

Direct Acting Relaxant
Dantrolene (Dantrium)

Centrally Acting Relaxants
Baclofen
Carisoprodol
Diazepam
Methocarbamol
Orphenadrine

Neuromuscular Relaxants
1. Depolarizing
Succinylcholine

2. Nondepolarizing
Curare
Gallamine
Pancuronium

NMJ

ACH

Site 1: Impulse conduction from the CNS through the spinal cord.
Site 2: Neuromuscular junction (NMJ).
Site 3: Skeletal muscle fibers (ACH = acetylcholine).

receptors. These agents occupy the NII sites so that ACH cannot combine with the receptors and depolarization cannot occur (nondepolarizing, *no* depolarization).

The **depolarizing blockers** inhibit muscle contraction by a two-step process: (1) succinylcholine attaches to the NII receptors and induces depolarization, observed as muscle **fasciculations;** and (2) then succinylcholine alters the NII receptors so that they cannot respond to endogenous ACH stimulation. This phase represents the neuromuscular blockade.

Route of Administration

The nondepolarizing neuromuscular blockers are usually administered intravenously (IV) because they are not well absorbed when taken by mouth. Following a single injection of a nondepolarizing blocker, neuromuscular blockade occurs within 3 to 5 minutes and lasts from 20 to 30 minutes. The muscles of the eyes and face are the first to become relaxed, followed by the limbs, trunk, and diaphragm. Recovery of muscle function occurs as the drug is metabolized and excreted. Curare and pancuronium are metabolized in the liver to some extent, whereas gallamine is excreted unchanged in the urine.

The depolarizing blocker succinylcholine is metabolized so rapidly that it is often administered by intravenous infusion to maintain skeletal muscle relaxation. Succinylcholine is rapidly hydrolyzed by the enzyme plasma cholinesterase, which is present in the blood. Some individuals do not have enough plasma cholinesterase, or because of a genetic abnormality, they produce an abnormal (atypical) enzyme. These people metabolize succinylcholine very slowly, so its duration of action and potential toxicity increase. The IV doses of the peripheral neuromuscular blockers are given in Table 9:1.

TABLE 9:1 — Peripheral Skeletal Muscle Relaxant Doses and Routes of Administration

DRUG (TRADE NAME)	TYPE	ADULT DOSE
atracurium besylate *(Tracrium)*	Nondepolarizing	0.4–0.5 mg/kg IV bolus
cisatricurium besylate *(Nimbex)*	Nondepolarizing	0.15 or 0.2 mg/kg IV
dantrolene *(Dantrium)*	Direct-acting	25 mg PO BID, QID
doxacurium *(Nuromax)*	Nondepolarizing	0.025–0.05 mg/kg IV
gallamine triethiodide *(Flaxedil)*	Nondepolarizing	2.0–2.5 mg/kg IV
mivacurium *(Mivacron)*	Nondepolarizing	0.15 or 0.2 mg/kg IV
pancuronium bromide *(Pavulon)*	Nondepolarizing	0.06–0.1 mg/kg IV
pipecuronium *(Arduan)*	Nondepolarizing	70–85 mcg/kg IV
rapacuronium *(Raplon)*	Nondepolarizing	1.5–2.5 mg/kg IV
roncuronium bromide *(Zemuron)*	Nondepolarizing	0.6–1.2 mg/kg IV
succinylcholine chloride *(Anectine, Quelicin, Sucostrin)*	Depolarizing	0.3–1.1 mg/kg IV, 1–2 mg/ml at 2.5 mg/min continuous IV infusion
tubocurarine (curare)	Nondepolarizing	0.1–0.6 mg/kg IV
vecuronium bromide *(Norcuron)*	Nondepolarizing	0.08–0.10 mg/kg IV

Effects on Cardiopulmonary Systems

Although the primary site of action is the NMJ, neuromuscular blockers also produce cardiovascular changes at therapeutic doses through a different mechanism of action. Curare may cause hypotension because it releases histamine **(vasodilator)** and inhibits sympathetic tone on the blood vessels (ganglionic blockade). In contrast, gallamine may produce tachycardia by blocking the vagal tone on the sino-atrial (SA) node of the heart **(vagolytic).** Gallamine may also increase blood pressure.

Although pancuronium has no effect on the autonomic ganglia or histamine release, it may cause tachycardia by a vagolytic action. Succinylcholine has been reported to produce ventricular arrhythmias and changes in blood pressure, which vary with the amount of drug administered. Since succinylcholine causes potassium leakage from the muscle cells, patients with electrolyte imbalances (burns or trauma) may develop arrhythmias more easily.

All of the blockers except pancuronium cause a release of histamine from mast cells, which leads to the production of bronchospasms and increased bronchial secretions in sensitive patients. Asthmatic patients are especially sensitive to the respiratory complications induced by histamine. Therefore, in asthmatic patients, pancuronium may be preferred to minimize bronchial (respiratory) complications.

Adverse and Toxic Effects

The major toxicity associated with all neuromuscular blockers is paralysis of the respiratory muscles. This is life-threatening because the patient can no longer control breathing, consciously or unconsciously. Skeletal muscle paralysis caused by the nondepolarizing blockers may be reversed by the use of neostigmine or edrophonium. Neostigmine and edrophonium inhibit acetylcholinesterase so that ACH accumulates within the junctions. The ACH displaces the blocker from the NII receptors and, since their receptors are not damaged or changed, initiates depolarization and muscle contraction. An added benefit of neostigmine and edrophonium is their ability to directly stimulate the NII receptors so that skeletal muscle paralysis is reversed.

Succinylcholine overdose presents a special problem because this drug alters the ability of NII receptors to become stimulated. There is no known antidote that reverses the neuromuscular blockade produced by succinylcholine. Administration of the anticholinesterase drugs may worsen the respiratory paralysis. Respiration must be supported artificially until the drug is metabolized and receptor responsiveness returns to normal. Skeletal muscle paralysis may be dangerously prolonged when succinylcholine is used in a patient who has atypical plasma cholinesterase.

Succinylcholine produces an unusual acute toxicity that is probably due to an existing genetic abnormality in 1 out of 20,000 individuals. Occasionally, a normal dose of succinylcholine in combination with an inhalation anesthetic produces a condition known as **malignant hyperthermia.** This condition is associated with a drastic increase in body temperature, acidosis, electrolyte imbalance, and shock. The mechanism by which **hyperthermia** occurs is believed to be related to the anesthetic-induced potentiation of calcium hyperreactivity in susceptible individuals. The hyperactive biochemical reactions progress so quickly that treatment must be started immediately to reduce the risk of death. Treatment of hyperthermia includes reducing body temperature with ice packs and controlling arrhythmias and acidosis with appropriate drugs. Unfortunately, the incidence of fatality in malignant hyperthermia is high. Prevention is primarily directed at obtaining a good family history about other episodes of difficulty during operative procedures. Muscle biopsy and elevated muscle enzyme levels may identify potentially sensitive patients. Such a workup prior to an operation allows the surgical team to avoid the use of sensitizing agents.

Cautions and Drug Interactions

Neuromuscular blocking drugs should be used with extreme caution in patients with impaired neuromuscular function (myasthenia gravis and spinal cord lesions). Any medication that inhibits skeletal muscle function **potentiates** neuromuscular blockers. Antibiotics, antiarrhythmic drugs, and some general anesthetics directly inhibit neuromuscular function, causing skeletal muscle relaxation. Succinylcholine-induced neuromuscular blockade is potentiated by drugs that promote a loss of potassium, such as diuretics and digitalis. In contrast, drugs that stimulate the NII receptors or inhibit acetylcholinesterase antagonize nondepolarizing blockers. Drug interactions associated with skeletal muscle relaxants can

potentiate or eliminate the pharmacologic action of muscle relaxants. Drugs that decrease the effect of any neuromuscular blocker include corticosteroids, carbemazepine, insecticides, acetylcholinesterase inhibitors, and theophylline. Drugs that increase the effect of muscle relaxants include alcohol, antiarrhythmics (lidocaine, procainamide, quinidine), antibiotics (clindamycin, kanamycin, lincomycin, neomycin, pipericilllin, streptomycin, tetracyclines), general anesthetics, narcotic analgesics, tranquilizers, and sedatives. Succinylcholine is potentiated by digitalis and diuretics because these drugs induce a shift in potassium ions that enhances the action of succinylcholine. The only contraindication is the use in patients with a known hypersensitivity to any of these drugs.

The nondepolarizing and depolarizing neuromuscular blockers are prepared as solutions for parenteral administration. Mixing some solutions can result in drug **incompatibility** and should be avoided. Drug incompatibility may result in discoloration of the solution, precipitation of drug, or, most important, alteration of drug potency. Succinylcholine has been reported to be unstable when mixed in alkaline solution (pH > 7.0). Admixture to solutions of barbiturates should be avoided because the combination results in hydrolyzation (breakdown) of succinylcholine.

Clinical Indications

The peripheral neuromuscular blockers are used primarily during surgical procedures to relax abdominal skeletal muscle. These agents are also used during electroconvulsive shock therapy and to reduce muscle spasms produced during tetanus. Because of its short action, succinylcholine may be used to aid intubations for surgical and diagnostic procedures (endoscopy).

Curare can be used as a diagnostic test for myasthenia gravis. Myasthenic patients have impaired neuromuscular function and are five times more sensitive to drug-induced neuromuscular blockade. Administration of curare to a myasthenic patient produces a rapid loss of muscle tone.

DIRECT-ACTING SKELETAL MUSCLE RELAXANTS

Dantrolene is considered a direct-acting peripheral skeletal muscle relaxant because it inhibits the skeletal muscle fiber (Figure 9:1, site 3).

Mechanism of Action

By interfering with biochemical pathways, dantrolene prevents actin and myosin contraction. The skeletal muscle contractile process cannot respond to stimulation, but conduction of impulses through the spinal cord and transmission across the neuromuscular junction are not affected.

Clinical Indications

Dantrolene is used in the treatment of malignant hyperthermia and spastic diseases. Muscle spasms associated with multiple sclerosis, cerebral palsy, and spinal cord injuries may reduce patients' ability to function. Dantrolene, taken orally, allows these individuals to use their residual motor function. In the prevention and treatment of malignant hyperthermia, dantrolene, given intravenously, interferes with the release of calcium in the sensitized muscles, reversing the biochemical crisis.

Adverse Effects

The most frequent adverse effects include dizziness, vomiting, fatigue, and weakness. Dantrolene has a potential for hepatotoxicity. As deaths have occurred due to hepatotoxicity, serum enzymes indicative of changes in liver function, serum glutamic oxaloacetic transaminase (SGOT) and serum glutamic pyruvic transaminase (SGPT), should be monitored frequently during dantrolene therapy. Contraindication to the use of dantrolene includes hepatitis and cirrhosis, as well as other active hepatic diseases. The long-term safety of dantrolene is being evaluated through its continued use. Any drug that decreases muscle strength or depresses the CNS may potentiate the muscle weakness produced by dantrolene. Drugs that increase the effect of dantrolene on skeletal muscle include alcohol, antiarrhythmics (lidocaine, procainamide, quinidine), antibiotics (clindamycin, kanamycin, lincomycin, neomycin, pipericilllin, streptomycin, tetracyclines), general anesthetics, narcotic analgesics, tranquilizers, and sedatives.

CENTRALLY ACTING SKELETAL MUSCLE RELAXANTS

Spastic contraction of skeletal muscles may occur in response to overexertion, trauma, or nervous tension. Usually, the muscles undergoing spasm are limited to the area of trauma (neck, back, or calf). Reflexes within the spinal cord repeatedly stimulate the motor neurons so that localized muscle fibers contract intermittently. This perpetuates a cycle of irritation or inflammation within localized muscle areas.

Mechanism of Action

Drugs that relax skeletal muscle by a central mechanism depress reflex impulse conduction within the spinal cord. This change in conduction reduces the number of impulses available to produce muscle contraction. Centrally acting skeletal muscle relaxants do not alter the function of the NII receptors or the skeletal muscle fibers. Some of these muscle relaxants interfere with select areas of the brain to interupt the spasticity. Although all of the drugs listed in Table 9:2 relieve muscle spasticity, chlordiazepoxide (Librium) and diazepam (Valium) are primarily used as tranquilizers (antianxiety). These agents will be discussed in Chapter 11.

Many people encounter muscle relaxants as outpatient therapy for muscle strain and overexertion during leisure activities; however, two relatively new drugs, baclofen and tizanidine, reduce the spasms which interfere with daily activities in patients with multiple sclerosis. Baclofen (Lioresal) is chemically related to a substance that naturally occurs in the brain (gamma-aminobutyric acid [GABA]). Like other centrally acting muscle relaxants, it inhibits reflexes at the spinal level. Baclofen is primarily used to relieve the symptoms of spasticity (flexor spasms, clonus, muscle rigidity) in patients with multiple sclerosis but may also be of value in patients with spinal cord injury resulting in severe spasticity. Through a different mechanism of action, tizanidine (Zanaflex) reduces spasticity by interacting with alpha-2-adrenergic receptors in the CNS. Neither of these drugs reverses the pathology of multiple sclerosis. Both are adjunct medications that improve the quality of life for many patients with spastic muscle conditions.

Route of Administration and Adverse Effects

The centrally acting skeletal muscle relaxants may be administered orally or parenterally. To some degree, these drugs are metabolized in the liver and excreted in the urine. The most frequently reported adverse effects include blurred vision, dizziness, lethargy, and decreased mental alertness. The intensity of these effects may require patients to avoid driving or

TABLE 9:2   Centrally Acting Skeletal Muscle Relaxants

DRUG (TRADE NAME)	ADULT DOSE
baclofen *(Lioresal)*	10–80 mg PO
carisoprodol *(Rela, Soma)*	350 mg PO TID, QID
chlordiazepoxide* *(Librium)*	2–10 mg PO TID, QID
	2–20 mg IM*, * IV elderly 2–2.5 mg QD, BID
chlorzoxazone *(Parafon Forte DSC)*	250–750 mg PO TID
cyclobenzaprine *(Flexeril)*	10 mg PO TID
diazepam* *(Valium)*	2–10 mg PO TID
	5–10 mg IM**
metaxalone *(Skelaxin)*	800 mg PO TID, QID
methocarbamol *(Robaxin)*	1.0–1.5 g PO QID
orphenadrine citrate *(Norflex)*	100 mg PO BID
	60 mg IV, IM (every 12 hours as needed)**
tizanidine *(Zanaflex)*	4–12 mg PO every 6–8 hours

*These drugs are used primarily as antianxiety agents, rather than skeletal muscle relaxants.
**Should be changed to tablets as soon as the symptoms are relieved.

operating mechanical equipment. With large doses, skeletal muscle tone decreases, resulting in ataxia and hypotension. Tizanidine has the potential to decrease blood pressure because of its action on the sympathetic alpha-2 receptors. This may result in orthostatic hypotension in patients with multiple sclerosis. Prolonged use of diazepam and chlordiazepoxide may lead to dependency. Discontinuation of therapy in patients who have received any of these drugs for long periods (chronically) must be gradual to avoid precipitating withdrawal symptoms. Usually, the dose is decreased over a 4- to 8-week period. Special precautions must be taken when reducing the dose of baclofen during chronic therapy. If an adverse reaction occurs that prompts termination of baclofen therapy, the dose must be reduced gradually. Although not associated with dependence, hallucinations and/or seizures have been reported to occur when the drug was abruptly stopped. Any of the muscle relaxants should be discontinued under medical supervision if a hypersensitivity reaction develops.

Overdose of centrally acting skeletal muscle relaxants will produce symptoms of confusion, somnolence, and depression of vital functions including respiration, heart, and pulse rates. Coma may precede death if the patient does not receive adequate evaluation and treatment in time. There is no specific antidote for overdose associated with centrally acting muscle relaxants. The patient must be monitored for respiratory and cardiovascular activity while a clear airway is maintained and ventilation supported. In the event that hypotension develops, an IV infusion should be available for parenteral fluid therapy. There is a specific benzodiazepine antagonist, flumazenil *(Romazicon)*, which may be of value in the treatment of midazolam overdose. This antagonist has no ability to reverse the depression associated with other centrally acting muscle relaxants.

Drug Interactions
Drugs that depress the CNS (alcohol, sedatives, and tranquilizers) or impair neuromuscular function potentiate the actions and adverse effects of all skeletal muscle relaxants.

Patient Administration and Monitoring

When skeletal muscle relaxants are used in surgical settings, the potential for adverse effects may be minimized through close observation of the patient during recovery. Following diagnostic procedures or intubations under outpatient conditions, or chronic therapy for spastic muscle conditions, there is a greater likelihood that patients may experience adverse effects that could put them at risk for injury. For this reason patients should receive clear instructions about which adverse effects are worthy of physician notification. The centrally acting skeletal muscle relaxants may cause persistent drowsiness that interferes with mental alertness and concentration. For chronic spastic conditions, this effect is usually tolerable so the treatment schedule does not need to be interrupted. It should be noted that dose adjustment does not always mitigate the drowsy effect. Therefore, with short-term therapy of muscle strain, the patient may need to incorporate other solutions to circumvent the difficulties associated with drowsiness.

Patient Instructions

The patient should be asked whether he or she performs tasks that require special equipment or machinery (sewing machines, motor vehicles) or coordination, focus, or physical dexterity (drill press, motor tools, assembly tools). Extra caution is needed, including identifying a coworker, on-site medical personnel, or a relative who is aware of the patient's medication schedule. If necessary, alternate transportation when driving is required may be necessary until treatment is completed.

Alcohol and other CNS depressant drugs should be avoided. This includes over-the-counter (OTC) medications that contain alcohol as a significant active ingredient. These drugs may potentiate poor coordination, drowsiness, and dizziness (postural hypotension).

Skin rash, nasal congestion, persistent fever, or yellowish discoloration of the skin or eyes should be reported to the physician or clinic immediately for further evaluation.

Dantrolene causes photosensitivity so prolonged exposure to sunlight should be avoided.

Baclofen may cause nausea, headache, insomnia, and frequent or painful urination that should be reported to the physician for further evaluation.

Use in Pregnancy

Drugs in this class have been designated Food and Drug Administration (FDA) Pregnancy Category B or C. Safety for use during pregnancy has not been established. It is recommended that no drug should be administered during pregnancy unless it is clearly needed and the potential benefits to the patient outweigh the potential risks to the fetus.

Patients who become pregnant or who expect to become pregnant during therapy should discuss the potential risks of therapy to the fetus with the physician.

Chapter Review

Understanding Terminology

Answer the following questions in the spaces provided.

1. Differentiate between depolarizing blockers and nondepolarizing blockers. _____
_____

2. Explain the difference between peripheral skeletal muscle relaxants and centrally acting skeletal muscle relaxants. _____
_____

3. Use the following terms in a short paragraph: *fasciculation, hyperthermia, vagolytic,* and *vasodilator.* _____
_____

Acquiring Knowledge

Answer the following questions in the spaces provided.

1. What are the physiological events that precede skeletal muscle contraction? _____
_____

2. What is a neuromuscular junction (NMJ)? _____
_____

3. What sites are involved in the production of skeletal muscle relaxation? _____
_____

4. What are the two types of neuromuscular blockers? How do they differ in their mechanism of action? _____
_____

5. Why are neuromuscular blockers administered IV? _____
_____

6. What adverse effects are produced by the neuromuscular blockers as a result of histamine release? _____
_____

7. Describe the major toxicity associated with neuromuscular blockers and the antidote used. _____
_____
_____

8. How does dantrolene differ from neuromuscular blockers? _____
_____

9. What is the mechanism of action of centrally acting skeletal muscle relaxants? _____
_____

10. When are centrally acting skeletal muscle relaxants used? _____
_____

Applying Knowledge—On the Job

Use your critical thinking skills to answer the following questions in the spaces provided.

1. As a health care worker in a busy health maintenance organization (HMO), you work with dozens of patients each day. You've noticed that each of the following three patients who were treated today has been prescribed a drug that could cause problems. For each patient, identify and explain the potential drug problem.

   a. Patient A came to the HMO this morning complaining of muscle pain following a back injury. He was prescribed the muscle relaxant cyclobenzaprine. Patient A is always joking with the nurses about how much he drinks. It's clear that he takes several drinks of whiskey every day. _____

   _____

   b. Patient B came into the HMO last week with strep throat, for which he was prescribed streptomycin. Today, he's complaining of neck and shoulder pain, which he attributes to driving his car for a total of 20 hours over the past 2 days. Patient B was prescribed metaxalone for the muscle pain. _____

   _____

   c. Patient C takes lidocaine for a heart arrhythmia. Yesterday, she injured herself doing calisthenics and spent a sleepless night in pain. Today, she visited the doctor and was prescribed methocarbamol to relax her sore muscles. _____

   _____

   _____

2. Assume that you work in a surgical unit where you coordinate patient medications. For each of the following patients, identify a potential drug problem and how it might be avoided.

   a. Jeri is about to have a type of orthopedic surgery that requires a muscle relaxant for best results. Jeri's medical history indicates that she has asthma but is otherwise in good health.

   _____

   _____

   b. Linda is scheduled for surgery on her back. Her surgeon is planning to give her succinylcholine to relax her muscles during the procedure. As far as the surgeon is aware, Linda is in great health other than the vertebrae that require surgery. Linda has confided in you, however, that she has bulimia, which you know can lead to electrolyte imbalance. ____

   _____

   c. Susan has knee surgery scheduled. A note on her chart indicates that she will be given succinylcholine during the operation to relax the muscles in her leg. Her chart also indicates that she takes digitalis for a heart problem. _____

   _____

   _____

Internet Connection

Web pages that present information on adjuncts to anesthesia, malignant hyperthermia, and the management of malignant hyperthermia discuss the use of skeletal muscle relaxants. This material is designed to be read by medical associates and the general public and therefore is user friendly to access and comprehend. Go on the Internet and select Yahoo (search engine) by entering www.Yahoo.com. You will be presented a list of topics—click on *Health, Medicine, and Drugs*. When the next screen appears do one of the following:

a. Select *Medicine* to access the next menu of medical conditions and diseases. Then select *Anesthesiology* and subsequently, select *Malignant Hyperthermia*. You will have entered the **Malignant Hyperthermia** home page. The Malignant Hyperthermia Associations of America (MHAUS) and Japan maintain the categories of information identified on the home page, including a North American Registry of patients who are malignant hyperthermia susceptible, and a quarterly newsletter, *The Communicator*. This online service provides the most current information on malignant hyperthermia and its management. Conditions that trigger muscle spasticity are described on the home page, with a simple color schematic explaining the action at the neuromuscular junction.

b. Remain on the *Malignant Hyperthermia* web page. Select the category *FAQ* (frequently asked questions). At the next screen, scroll down to the end of the document to review a list of drugs that can be used safely in patients with malignant hyperthermia.

Additional Reading

Anonymous. 1995. New Drugs. Roncuronium (Zemuron): A safer, faster muscle relaxant? *American Journal of Nursing* 95 (3):56.

Biddle, C. 1996. Use and abuse of muscle relaxants. *Current Reviews for Nurse Anesthetists* 15 (16):131.

Gianino, J. 1993. Intrathecal baclofen for spinal spasticity: Implication for nursing practice. *Journal of Neuroscience in Nursing* 2:254:263.

Haslego, S. S. 2002. Malignant hyperthermia: How to spot it early. *RN* 65 (7):31.

Porter, B. 1997. Surgical nursing: A review of intrathecal baclofen in the management of spasticity. *British Journal of Nursing* 6 (5):253.

Ward, L. A. 2001. Spasticity in kids. An intrathecal option. *RN* 64 (1):39.

Waldman, H. J. 1994. Centrally acting skeletal muscle relaxants and associated drugs. *Journal of Pain and Symptom Management* 9 (7):434.

Stump, L. 2000. Rapacuronium bromide. *Journal of Perianesthetic Nursing* 15 (4):258.

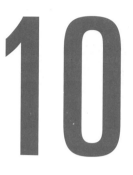

chapter

10

LOCAL ANESTHETICS

CHAPTER FOCUS

This chapter describes the drugs that influence patients' responses to pain and how painful stimuli can be inhibited without affecting consciousness (without depressing higher centers of the brain).

CHAPTER OBJECTIVES

After studying this chapter, you should be able to

- describe how a local anesthetic works (mechanism of action).

- explain how a local anesthetic can reduce pain without affecting the muscles that control posture.

- identify which local anesthetics must be administered by injection.

- describe the adverse effects associated with local anesthetic use.

- identify two local anesthetic drugs that are important in the treatment of cardiac dysfunction because of their action on the heart (antiarrhythmic).

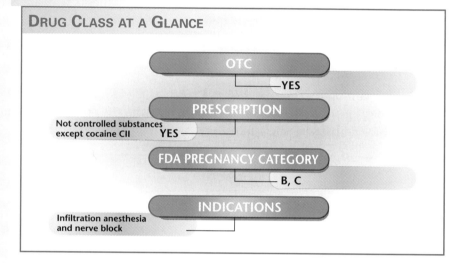

DRUG CLASS AT A GLANCE

OTC
└─ YES

PRESCRIPTION
Not controlled substances
except cocaine CII   YES ─┘

FDA PREGNANCY CATEGORY
└─ B, C

INDICATIONS
Infiltration anesthesia
and nerve block ─┘

Key Terms

amide local anesthetic: anesthetic that has a long duration of action.

cardiac arrhythmia: variation in the normal rhythm (motion) of the heart.

caudal anesthesia: injection of a local anesthetic into the caudal or subcaudal spinal canal.

epidural anesthesia: injection of a local anesthetic into the extradural space.

ester local anesthetic: anesthetic that has a short or moderate duration of action.

general anesthetic: drug that abolishes the response to pain by depressing the central nervous system (CNS) and producing loss of consciousness.

hypersensitivity: exaggerated response such as rash, edema, or anaphylaxis.

infiltration anesthesia: injection of a local anesthetic directly into the tissue.

intradermal anesthesia: injection of a local anesthetic under the skin.

local anesthetic: drug that reduces response to pain by affecting nerve conduction. The action can be limited to an area of the body according to the site of administration.

nerve conduction: transfer of impulses along a nerve by the movement of sodium and potassium ions.

spinal anesthesia: injection of a local anesthetic into the subarachnoid space.

topical application: placing a drug on the surface of the skin or a mucous membrane (for example, mouth, rectum).

vasoconstriction: tightening or contraction of muscles (sphincters) in the blood vessels, which decreases blood flow through the vessels.

vasodilation: relaxation of the muscles (sphincters) controlling blood vessel tone, which increases blood flow through the vessels.

INTRODUCTION

Drugs may be used in many different ways to control pain. **General anesthetics,** to be discussed in Chapter 18, abolish the response to pain by depressing the CNS and producing loss of consciousness. However, it may be desirable to relieve pain without altering the alertness or mental function of the patient. To accomplish this, analgesics (opioid and non-opioid) or local anesthetics may be used. The source and intensity of the pain determine which of these pharmacological agents is most useful to decrease the response to the painful stimuli. **Local anesthetics,** as their name suggests, produce a temporary loss of sensation or feeling in a confined area of the body.

MECHANISM OF ACTION

The most common clinical use of local anesthetics is to abolish painful stimulation prior to surgical, dental (tooth extraction), or obstetric (delivery) procedures. In addition, local anesthetics are ingredients in many over-the-counter (OTC) products for sunburn, insect bites, and hemorrhoids.

Local anesthetics abolish the response to pain because they inhibit sensory nerves that carry painful stimuli to the CNS. In particular, local anesthetics block nerve fiber conduction by acting directly on nerve membranes. Local anesthetics interact with nerve membranes to inhibit sodium ions from crossing the membranes. If sodium ion movement is inhibited, nerves cannot depolarize, and conduction of impulses along the nerves is blocked (Figure 10:1). This blockade of **nerve conduction** is reversible, which means that when the local anesthetic is carried away from the nerve by the circulation, the action of the local anesthetic ends. The local anesthetic is then metabolized.

Sensory nerves carry impulses for pain, touch, warmth, and cold to the brain. The sensory and autonomic nerves are the first fibers to become blocked by local anesthetics because these fibers are relatively small in diameter and unprotected by myelin sheaths. Therefore, local anesthetics can easily penetrate the membranes and inhibit nerve conduction. In contrast, the motor nerves that supply skeletal muscle are the last fibers to be inhibited because motor nerves are large fibers with thick myelin coverings. The importance of this varying degree of nerve depression, presented in Table 10:1, is that pain fibers can be blocked without altering skeletal muscle function (for example, diaphragm, posture). In addition, the pain fibers are the last to recover from local anesthetic blockade.

PHARMACOLOGY

The most commonly used local anesthetics are listed in Table 10:2 on page 101. These agents produce adequate nerve block by inhibiting nerve conduction. They differ in their duration of action, site of metabolism, and potency. There are two classes of local anesthetics: ester local anesthetics and amide local anesthetics.

In general, the **ester local anesthetics** have a short or moderate duration of action because they

FIGURE 10:1 The Action of Local Anesthetics on Nerve Conduction

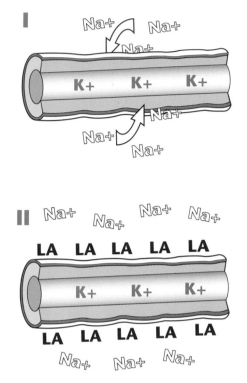

I. Normal conduction along a nerve membrane.
II. Local anesthetics (LA) inhibit nerve conduction by blocking sodium (Na⁺) movement.

are metabolized by enzymes (cholinesterases) that are present in the blood and skin. Examples of ester local anesthetics are benzocaine, cocaine, cyclomethycaine, procaine, and tetracaine. However, tetracaine is the only ester derivative that has a very long duration of action. It is too large a molecule to be rapidly metabolized by the liver.

The **amide local anesthetics** are usually the longer-acting drugs because these agents must be metabolized in the liver. The amide group includes dibucaine, lidocaine, mepivacaine, and procainamide.

ROUTES OF ADMINISTRATION

The duration of action and potency of local anesthetics determine which route of administration to employ. Local anesthetics are administered topically or by injection. Ester anesthetics, particularly those found in OTC preparations, are applied topically to the skin or mucous membranes. **Topical application** of local anesthetics is also known as surface anesthesia. Topical preparations are available as creams, lotions, ointments, sprays, suppositories, eyedrops, and lozenges. The most recent development in topical anesthesia includes combination local anesthetics applied to open and intact skin to reduce pain prior to suturing. The first available combination was TAC (tetracaine, adrenaline, cocaine). This preparation, although extremely effective, is being phased out by combinations that do not contain

TABLE 10:1 Order of Depression of Nerve Fibers by Local Anesthetics

ORDER OF DEPRESSION	TYPE OF NERVE FIBERS
EARLIEST	A. Small-diameter unmyelinated nerves, postganglionic, autonomic sensory → pain → temperature: warmth, cold → itch → tickle
INTERMEDIATE	B. Intermediate-diameter myelinated nerves, preganglionic, autonomic
LAST	C. Large-diameter myelinated nerves somatic motor → skeletal muscle → proprioception sensory (visceral) → sharp pain

TABLE 10:2 — Characteristics of Commonly Employed Local Anesthetics

DRUG (TRADE NAME)	DURATION	ROUTE	PREPARATIONS
Esters:			
benzocaine *(Boil-ease, Dermoplast, Lanacane, Solarcaine)***	0.5–0.75 hr	Topical	5% cream, ointment 2–20% spray
cocaine***	0.25–0.75 hr	Topical	1–4% solution
chloroprocaine *(Nesacaine)*	0.25–0.50 hr	Injection	1–3% solution
procaine *(Novocain)* infiltration	0.25–1.0 hr	Injection	1–2% and 10% solutions
tetracaine *(Pontocaine)*	2–3 hr	Injection	0.2, 0.3, and 1% solutions
(Pontocaine cream/ointment)**	—	Topical	1% cream, 5% ointment
Amides:			
articaine *(Septoaine)*	Varies with dose	Injection	4% solution
bupivacaine *(Marcaine)*	2–4 hr	Injection	0.25–0.75% solution
dibucaine *(Nupercaine)*	3–4 hr	Injection	0.25% solution
*(Nupercainal)***		Topical	0.5% cream, 1% ointment
etidocaine *(Duranest)*	5–10 hr	Injection	1% solution
lidocaine *(Xylocaine, Solarcaine Aloe Extra)*	0.5–1 hr	Injection	2 and 4% solution
lidocaine *(Lidoderm)*	3 hr	Topical	5% lidocaine patch
(Bactine spray, *Unguentine Plus)***		Topical	2% jelly, 2.5 and 5% ointment
mepivacaine *(Carbocaine)*	0.75–1.5 hr	Injection	1 and 2% solutions
ropivicaine *(Naropin)*	2–6 hr	Injection	0.5–2% solution
prilocaine *(Citanest)*	0.5–1.5 hr	Injection	1–4% solutions
Combinations:			
EMLA (lidocaine, prilocaine)	0.5–2 hr	Topical	2.5% of each anesthetic in thick layer
LET (lidocaine, epinephrine, tetracaine)	Not established	Topical	4% lidocaine 0.5% tetracaine 1:2000 epinephrine
Ravocaine (propoxycaine) Novocaine (procaine) and Levophed (norepinephrine)	2–3 hr	Topical	
Septocaine (articaine and Epinephrine)	Varies with dose	Injection	4% articaine 1:100,000 epinephrine
TAC (tetracaine, adrenaline, cocaine)	Not established	Topical	0.5% tetracaine 11.8% cocaine 1:2000 epinephrine
Other:			
Ethyl chloride	Minutes	Topical*	Spray
Fluroethylchloride			
Fluori-methane aerofreeze			
Prez-Pak			

*Decreases surface temperature.   **Over-the-counter preparations.   ***Federally restricted drug, Schedule II.

cocaine. LET (lidocaine, epinephrine, tetracaine) is not available commercially in this combination; it must be compounded as a liquid or gel by the pharmacist. EMLA (a eutectic mixture of local anesthetics) represents a major breakthrough in dermal anesthesia. Lidocaine and prilocaine are combined with a thickener and an emulsifier, applied as a thick layer to intact skin, and covered with clear plastic wrap to promote penetration through the skin. The breakthrough is that this preparation permits much higher concentrations of local anesthetic to be absorbed topically than possible by individual surface preparations. EMLA also can be used to anesthetize skin before intramuscular injections, venipuncture, and procedures such as biopsies.

Injection of local anesthetics may involve several different sites, including under the skin **(intradermal)** and into the spaces around the spinal cord **(spinal, epidural,** or **caudal anesthesia).** The long-acting, potent amide anesthetics are administered primarily by injection.

NOTE TO THE HEALTH CARE PROFESSIONAL

Local anesthetic solutions occasionally contain epinephrine to counteract the vasodilation that occurs. Always read the contents of the bottle before administering a local anesthetic. Local anesthetic preparations that contain epinephrine should not be used for nerve block in the areas of the fingers, toes, ears, nose, or penis. In such areas, epinephrine may produce intense vasoconstriction, leading to ischemia and gangrene. Epinephrine also is contraindicated in conjunction with general anesthetics that increase cardiac excitability (arrhythmogenic).

Infiltration anesthesia is achieved by injecting a local anesthetic directly into the tissue. The extent of anesthesia is determined by the depth of tissue penetrated—that is, the tissue infiltrated. The duration of action following infiltration anesthesia for several injectable local anesthetics is presented in Table 10:2. When these local anesthetics are administered in combination with epinephrine (usually 1:200,000 dilution), the duration of anesthesia may be doubled. For example, prilocaine, mepivacaine, dibucaine, and bupivacaine administered with epinephrine may have their duration of action extended up to 6 hours. The addition of epinephrine retards transport of the local anesthetic away from the site of injection.

ADVERSE EFFECTS

Local anesthetics are administered to produce a pharmacological response in a well-defined area of the body. However, a local anesthetic occasionally is absorbed into the blood from the site of administration and, passing through the circulation, it affects tissues and organs along the way. The most frequent and serious side effects from systemic absorption of a local anesthetic involve the blood vessels, heart, and brain.

Vascular Effects

Cocaine was the first local anesthetic to be discovered. Although it has potent local anesthetic activity, cocaine cannot be used by injection because it produces intense **vasoconstriction.** Cocaine interferes with the sympathetic nervous system and the blood vessels. Today, cocaine is used topically in surgical procedures on the eyes and nasal mucosa because its vasoconstrictor action decreases operative bleeding and improves surgical visualization. Additional information on cocaine is presented in Chapter 15, Psychotomimetic Drugs of Abuse.

All of the other local anesthetics used today produce **vasodilation;** procaine, in particular, produces a marked dilation of blood vessels, which may lead to hypotension. Except for cocaine, toxic levels of the local anesthetics relax vascular smooth muscle and produce significant hypotension. These effects may lead to cardiovascular collapse.

Cardiac Effects

Local anesthetics depress the function of the cardiac conduction system and the myocardium. Usually, these drugs produce a negative chronotropic (bradycardia) and a negative ionotropic response on the heart. In toxic doses, local anesthetics produce **cardiac arrhythmias.** It must be pointed out that in therapeutic (subtoxic) doses, two of the local anesthetics can be administered intravenously to correct certain cardiac arrhythmias. Lidocaine and procainamide are unique drugs because at very low doses they can protect cardiac function, while at toxic doses they inhibit normal cardiac function. The role of lidocaine and procainamide in the therapy of cardiac arrhythmias is discussed further in Chapter 23.

Central Nervous System Effects

All of the local anesthetics can affect the CNS. In large or toxic doses, the local anesthetics can cross the blood-brain barrier and initially stimulate the cerebral cortex. The symptoms of cortical stimulation are nervousness, excitation, tremors, and convulsions. In general, the more potent the anesthetic, the more readily convulsions occur. As the concentration of local anesthetic increases in the brain, all areas of the CNS become depressed. Finally, at toxic levels, local anesthetics produce coma and death due to total depression of the CNS.

Treatment of a local anesthetic overdose when CNS excitation is present includes barbiturates and diazepam *(Valium)*. Once total CNS depression has occurred, the only available treatment is supportive restoration of breathing and blood pressure. In particular, artificial respiration is the essential feature of treatment in the late phase of anesthetic intoxication.

CLINICAL APPLICATIONS

Topical application of local anesthetics relieves pain and itching associated with sunburn, skin abrasions, insect bites, and other allergic reactions, and skin eruptions from chicken pox. Rectal suppositories relieve the pain produced by hemorrhoids. Introduction of a patch containing local anesthetic has use in dental procedures to reduce the pain associated with anesthetic injection and to alleviate painful discomfort following *Herpes zoster* neuralgia. A patch containing 5% lidocaine *(Lidoderm)* is the first FDA-approved medication indicated to relieve the pain of postherpetic neuralgia. Injection of local anesthetics, especially the long-acting amides, is used for surgical, suturing, and obstetrical procedures (epidural, caudal, spinal anesthesia) where the patients remain conscious. Dentistry is one of the most frequent clinical applications of local anesthetics.

Cautions and Contraindications

Local anesthetics may release histamine from mast cells located at the site of injection, producing a rash and local itching typical of a histaminic response of Lewis (see Chapter 31). Occasionally, a patient is hypersensitive to local anesthetics. If a rash or edema occurs, the drug should be stopped immediately. **Hypersensitivity** may develop to ester local anesthetics when they are used frequently. For this reason, topical preparations (creams, ointments, and sprays) should never be used continually for prolonged periods. If hypersensitivity develops and a local anesthetic is required, amide derivatives may be substituted usually without fear of enhancing the allergic response.

Topical application of local anesthetics for sunburn, skin abrasions, and corneal wounds may result in systemic drug levels and toxic responses. When the skin is damaged or opened, local anesthetics can easily reach the blood vessels, and when the pain is intense, patients usually apply local anesthetics several times a day. It is not unusual for a patient to develop hypotension, tremors, and convulsions due to overdose of a local anesthetic.

Special Considerations

When administering a local anesthetic parenterally, monitor cardiovascular and respiratory vital signs after each injection. Restlessness, dizziness, blurred vision, and slurred speech may be early signs of CNS toxicity. Always inject an anesthetic slowly to avoid systemic reactions. Debilitated patients, as well as elderly and pediatric patients, may require reduced doses because these patients are often more susceptible to the actions of local anesthetics. Local anesthetic solutions that contain a vasoconstrictor must be used with extreme caution in patients who have a medical history of hypertension, cerebral vascular insufficiency, heart block, thyrotoxicosis, or diabetes. (Review the effects of sympathomimetic drugs on the cardiovascular and metabolic systems.)

Overdose of topical anesthetics may result in the same life-threatening response as from parentally administered drugs. If convulsions occur, it is an acute emergency. There is no specific antidote. Supportive treatment includes maintaining a clear airway and assisting ventilation with oxygen. If convulsions persist, an ultrashort-acting barbiturate or benzodiazepine may be given parenterally. Intravenous fluids and vasopressors are used when the circulation and organ perfusion are compromised.

Drug Interactions

Local anesthetics are not involved in many drug interactions. However, they may enhance hypotension that occurs with antihypertensive drugs and muscle relaxants. Drugs that directly relax skeletal muscle are enhanced by the use of local anesthetics introduced into the spinal canal. Local anesthetics may increase the release of histamine even when they are being used to relieve an allergic reaction, and this histamine release will only worsen the clinical condition.

Procaine has been shown to inhibit the action of sulfonamide antibiotics. Procaine is metabolized to p-aminobenzoic acid, which competes with the sulfonamide for the bacterial site of action.

Patients who have experienced a hypersensitivity reaction to an ester local anesthetic are more likely to experience a similar reaction if exposed to other ester local anesthetics. Generally, it is advisable to use an amide local anesthetic as an alternative; rarely, cross-sensitivity with lidocaine has been reported.

Sedatives may interact with spinal local anesthetics to potentiate CNS depression. Combination anesthetics that contain epinephrine may produce an increased sympathetic response and sustained hypertension when a patient is taking tricyclic antidepressants or MAO inhibitors.

Patient Administration and Monitoring

Assuming the patient is closely monitored during the procedure, adverse effects may be minimized when local anesthetics are used in operating and emergency rooms. The use of anesthetics in dental procedures as well as available products for self-medication exposes the general population to greater risk of experiencing certain adverse effects. Patients should be instructed about predictable local anesthetic action that could cause problems—namely, loss of sensory perception and motor function.

Patient Instructions

The patient should be advised that loss of sensory perception and motor function may persist for a short time. This means the anesthetized region cannot respond to hot or cold stimuli or to deep scratching. Avoid exposing the skin or mucous membranes (gums) to extreme temperature foods for at least 1 hour or until full pain sensation has returned.

Following topical application to relieve sore throat, the patient should not eat for 1 hour. Since sensation is impaired there is always the danger that the patient may aspirate food particles.

Dental anesthesia will more than likely leave the patient with numbness of the tongue, lip, and/or oral mucosa for up to 1 hour after the procedure. The patient should be alerted to the possible annoying effect of accidentally biting the lips or cheeks during this time. Since pressure perception is impaired, the patient may unconsciously bite extremely hard and find terrific pain and blisters after the anesthetic has subsided. It is advisable that while the tissue is still anesthetized, the patient should not eat or chew gum because of the potential for aspiration to occur.

Notify the Physician

Patients routinely use OTC products containing local anesthetics for a multitude of conditions from sore throat to vaginal and/or rectal itch. While the patient may have ten preparations for use on different body parts, they all probably contain a local anesthetic. Moreover, these are the type of products used by the more sensitive patients such as the elderly and children. The patient should be reminded that any time the skin or mucous membrane is broken, as in sunburn, minor scratches, or irritated mucosa, the local anesthetic may be more well absorbed. Development of mental confusion and changes in pulse or respiration should be reported to the physician for further evaluation.

A small percentage of people are allergic (hypersensitive) to the para-aminobenzoic acid metabolites of procaine and tetracaine. Local swelling, edema, itching, difficulty in breathing, and bronchospasm may indicate hypersensitivity to the anesthetic. If such symptoms occur while using any local anesthetic, the patient should notify the doctor immediately and discontinue the anesthetic.

Use in Pregnancy

Drugs in this class have been designated Food and Drug Administration (FDA) Pregnancy Category B and C. The safety of local anesthetic use in pregnancy has not been established through research in humans, however, the short-term exposure to these drugs during labor and delivery limits the potential risk to the patient and newborn. Adverse effects observed in the newborn, primarily depression of the CNS and cardiovascular tone, quickly reverse once exposure is terminated. The degree of depression is related to the type and amount of local anesthetic administered to the mother.

Chapter Review

Understanding Terminology

Answer the following questions in the spaces provided.

1. Differentiate between local and general anesthetics. _____

_____

2. Explain the difference between vasodilation and vasoconstriction. _____

_____

Match the definition in the left column with the appropriate term in the right column.

____ 3. An exaggerated response (such as rash or edema) to a local anesthetic.

____ 4. Placing a drug on the surface of the skin or a mucous membrane.

____ 5. Injection of a local anesthetic into the subarachnoid space.

____ 6. Injection of a local anesthetic into the extradural space.

____ 7. Injection of a local anesthetic into the caudal or subcaudal canal.

____ 8. Injection of a local anesthetic directly into the tissue.

____ 9. Injection of a local anesthetic under the skin.

a. caudal anesthesia

b. epidural anesthesia

c. hypersensitivity

d. infiltration anesthesia

e. intradermal anesthesia

f. spinal anesthesia

g. topical application

Acquiring Knowledge

Answer the following questions in the spaces provided.

1. Explain how local anesthetics block the response to pain. _____

_____

_____

2. Which nerves are first affected when a local anesthetic is applied? What is the order of depression? _____

_____

_____

3. What are two classes of local anesthetics? How do they differ? _____

_____

_____

4. What body systems are mainly affected by systemic absorption of local anesthetics? _____

_____

5. What are the adverse effects of local anesthetics on the heart? _____

_____

6. What are the adverse effects of local anesthetics on the CNS? _____

_____

7. Compare the effects of cocaine and procaine on blood pressure. _____

_____

8. Why is epinephrine added to some local anesthetic preparations? _____

_____

9. What precautions are associated with the use of local anesthetics and vasoconstrictors? _____
_____
_____

10. What drugs may interact with local anesthetics to produce undesirable effects? _____
_____
_____

Applying Knowledge—On the Job

Use your critical thinking skills to answer the following questions in the spaces provided.

1. Mrs. Brown was rushed to the emergency room by ambulance after her husband found her lying on the kitchen floor having convulsions. She has no previous history of convulsions and appeared to be in good health earlier in the day. You notice that Mrs. Brown has abrasions on her lower right arm, which her husband says she received when she fell to the pavement when bicycling yesterday. He says that she has been self-medicating with an over-the-counter ointment for pain ever since. What do you think caused Mrs. Brown's convulsions?

_____
_____

Use the *PDR®* or *F&C* to answer the following questions.

2. Lidocaine is available in a topical viscous solution preparation. List the strength, peak effect and duration times, and the indications.

_____
_____

3. Bupivacaine is available in the following strengths, 0.25%, 0.5%, and 0.75%. This is commonly used for obstetrical lumbar epidural. One strength is contraindicated for this procedure. Which strength is contraindicated and why?

_____
_____

Use *F&C* to answer the following question.

4. You are reviewing the medication orders for the cataract extraction procedures scheduled for the next day. The anesthetic that will be used is proparacaine (*Opthetic*). What dosing would you expect to find?

_____
_____

Internet Connection

Web pages that present information on local anesthetics include sites directed at parents and health care providers to explain local anesthetic use in dental procedures. These sites also provide links to information, such as gender differences in pain perception, and options for anesthesia. The material is expected to be read by the general public and is therefore user friendly.

Enter www.parentsplace.com. At the search box, enter "local anesthetics or pain management". A list of hyperlinked topics presented include, use of local anesthetics in allergic reactions, dental procedures, and use of local anesthetics during pregnancy. The information at the website is provided by a dentist and clinical practitioner.

The FDA and National Institutes of Health provide up-to-date information through medical and consumer links such as www.healthfinder.gov. This site discusses different formulations of lidocaine and other local anesthetics. Select Health Library, then select prescription drug information, and enter the name of the drug in the search box.

Additional Reading

Edlick, R. F. 1994. Repair of lacerations: Sedation & anesthesia. *Hospital Medicine* 30 (10):39.

Gottschalk, A. 2001. New concepts in acute pain therapy: Preemptive analgesia. *American Family Physician* 63 (10):1979.

Hersch, E. V. 1996. Analgesic efficacy and safety of an intraoral lidocaine patch. *Journal of American Dental Association* 127 (11):1626.

Hussey, V. P. 1997. Perioperative pharmacology: Effectiveness of lidocaine HCl on venipuncture sites. *Association of Operating Room Nurses Journal* 66 (3):472.

Johansson, A. 1996. Nerve blocks with local anesthetics and corticosteroids in chronic pain: A clinical follow-up study. *Journal of Pain and Symptom Management* 11 (3):181–187.

Kundu, S. 2002. Principles of office anesthesia: Part I. Infiltrative anesthesia. *American Family Physician* 66 (1):91.

Kundu, S. 2002. Principles of office anesthesia: Part II. Topical anesthesia. *American Family Physician* 66 (1):99.

Yaster, M. 1994. Local anesthetics in the management of acute pain in infants and children. *Journal of Pediatrics,* Vol. 124, 165.

PHARMACOLOGY OF THE CENTRAL NERVOUS SYSTEM

Chapter 11

Introduction to the Central Nervous System

Parts of the Brain
Functional Components

Chapter 12

Sedative-Hypnotic Drugs and Alcohol

Sleep Cycle
Barbiturate Sedatives and
    Hypnotics
Benzodiazepines
Miscellaneous Nonbarbiturates
Alcohol

Chapter 13

Antipsychotic and Antianxiety Drugs

Types of Mental Illness
Antipsychotic Drugs
Antianxiety Drugs

Chapter 14

Antidepressants, Psychomotor Stimulants, and Lithium

Types of Depression
Drugs Used to Treat Depression

Chapter 15

Psychotomimetic Drugs of Abuse

LSD-Type Hallucinogens
Psychomotor Stimulants
Miscellaneous Psychotomimetic
    Drugs

Chapter 16

Antiepileptic Drugs

Types of Epilepsy
Drugs Used to Control Epilepsy
Drugs Used in the Treatment of
    Absence Seizures
Treatment of Status Epilepticus
Use of Antiepileptic Drugs During
    Pregnancy
Antiepileptic Drug Interactions

Chapter 17

Antiparkinson Drugs

Neurotransmitters Affecting the
    Basal Ganglia
Drug Therapy

Chapter 18

General Anesthetics

General Anesthesia
Use of General Anesthetics

Chapter 19

Opioid (Narcotic) Analgesics

Pain Opioid Analgesics
Site and Mechanism of Action
Pharmacological Effects
Absorption and Metabolism
Adverse Effects

Acute Opioid Poisoning
Opioid Antagonists
Special Considerations
Drug Interactions

Chapter 20

**Nonopioid Analgesics,
Antiinflammatory, and Antigout Drugs**

Inflammation
Nonopioid Analgesics
Salicylates
Acetaminophen
Drugs Useful in Treating Gout
Drug Interactions

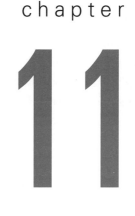
INTRODUCTION TO THE CENTRAL NERVOUS SYSTEM

Key Terms

basal ganglia: extrapyramidal system; part of the brain that regulates motor activity.

cerebellum: part of the brain that coordinates body movements and posture and helps maintain body equilibrium.

cerebral cortex: part of the brain that controls the body's voluntary activities.

cerebral medulla: part of the brain that conducts nerve impulses to and from different areas of the brain.

cerebrum: uppermost part of the brain that controls higher intellectual abilities.

electroencephalogram (EEG):   a recording of the electrical activity of the cortex.

hypothalamus: part of the brain that controls many body functions.

limbic system: neural pathway connecting different brain areas involved in regulation of behavior and emotion.

medulla oblongata: part of the brain that controls cardiac, vasomotor, and respiratory functions.

pons: part of the brain that serves as a relay station for nerve fibers traveling to other brain areas.

reticular formation: network of nerve fibers that travel throughout the brainstem and cerebrum; regulates level of wakefulness.

thalamus: part of the brain that regulates sensory impulses traveling to the cortex.

CHAPTER FOCUS

This chapter describes the major structural and functional features of the brain. It also describes how different parts of the brain regulate specific body functions.

CHAPTER OBJECTIVES

After studying this chapter, you should be able to

- describe the three major parts of the brain.
- list the main parts of the brainstem and discuss the functions associated with each part.
- describe the reticular formation and the limbic system and discuss the importance of each.

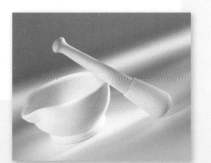

INTRODUCTION

The central nervous system (CNS) is composed of the brain and spinal cord. The primary functions of the CNS are to coordinate and control the activity of other body systems. Distinct nerve pathways in the CNS interconnect different areas of the brain that serve the same function. Neurons in these pathways are linked together by synapses. These neurons release neurotransmitters, which regulate transmission across the synapses. In this way, nerve impulses are conducted to different areas of the brain to influence the levels of activity.

There are a significant number of neurotransmitters—including acetylcholine (ACH), norepinephrine (NE), dopamine, and serotonin—that have been identified in the brain. Some mental illnesses and pathological conditions are associated with abnormal changes in the amount or activity of a specific neurotransmitter. Many of the drugs that act on the CNS do so by affecting neurotransmitter concentrations and activity. While there are a large number of different neurotransmitters in the brain, the function and activities of each are similar to the functions of the neurons and nerve endings (adrenergic, cholinergic) previously discussed with the autonomic nervous system.

Generally, a neuron releases one specific type of neurotransmitter that crosses the synapse and binds to its receptor located on the dendrities of the next adjoining neuron. Neurotransmitters can be either excitatory or inhibitory. Excitatory receptor stimulation generates action potentials that flow along the nerve axon to stimulate release of the neurotransmitter from the nerve endings of that neuron . . . and so on. Inhibitory neurotransmitters produce actions on the next adjoining neuron that inhibit the generation of action potentials. In this manner, neurotransmitters function to either generate nerve impulses that transmit information among the different brain centers or function to inhibit the flow of action potentials, which reduces neural activity. The released neurotransmitters are inactivated by metabolism or reuptake into their respective nerve endings. Figure 11:1 illustrates the synaptic connections of a typical brain neuron.

In the CNS, neurons having the same functions are generally grouped together. The cell bodies of these neurons form control centers for the various body functions. Consequently, the CNS is anatomically divided into different parts. In order to understand how drugs affect the CNS, the main structures and functions of the CNS will be reviewed.

PARTS OF THE BRAIN

The brain may be divided into three main parts: the cerebrum, brainstem, and cerebellum. Each of these parts will be described in the following sections. The main structures of the brain are illustrated in Figure 11:2.

Cerebrum

The **cerebrum** is the largest and uppermost part of the brain. All of the higher intellectual abilities of human beings are controlled by the cerebrum. Anatomically, the cerebrum is divided into right and left cerebral hemispheres. Each hemisphere is composed of an outer cerebral cortex and an inner cerebral medulla.

Cerebral Cortex

The **cerebral cortex** contains the cell bodies of neurons (gray matter) that control voluntary activities of the body. The cortex is subdivided into four main lobes. The cortical lobes are named after the skull bones and include the frontal, parietal, temporal, and occipital lobes. The frontal lobe is responsible for control of muscle movement, the motor components of speech, abstract thinking, and problem solving activity. The parietal lobe is responsible for the sensory sensations of touch, pressure, pain, temperature,

Illustration of the Synaptic Connections Between Brain Neurons

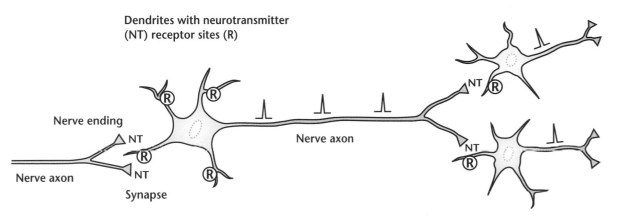

Dendrites with neurotransmitter (NT) receptor sites (R)

Nerve ending

Nerve axon

Synapse

Nerve axon

Nerve ending from one neuron releases neurotransmitter (NT), which crosses synapse to bind to NT receptor (R) on dendrites of next neuron. Receptor stimulation generates an action potential (⋀) that travels down nerve axon to stimulate the release of NT from nerve endings.

FIGURE 11:2

The Main Structures of the Brain

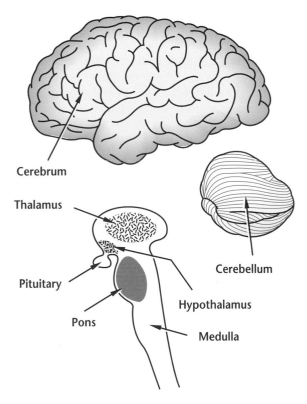

Cerebrum

Thalamus

Pituitary

Pons

Cerebellum

Hypothalamus

Medulla

and vibration. The temporal lobes are involved in memory and language functions. The occipital lobes function in vision. There are neural connections between the lobes and each area of the brain that allow communication,

coordination, and integration of neural function. An **electroencephalogram (EEG)** is a recording of the electrical activity of the cortex. The EEG is useful in diagnosing various brain disorders.

Cerebral Medulla

The inner **cerebral medulla** is composed of the myelinated axons (white matter) of the neurons. The axons conduct nerve impulses to and from different areas of the nervous system. Also, there is a group of cell bodies (gray matter) in the medulla known as the basal ganglia.

Basal Ganglia

The **basal ganglia** are involved in the regulation of motor activity. The basal ganglia are sometimes referred to as the extrapyramidal system. Degeneration of certain neurons within the basal ganglia is responsible for Parkinson's disease and Huntington's chorea.

Brainstem

The brainstem is continuous with the spinal cord and extends up to the cerebrum. The brainstem controls many body functions that are not under conscious control. The main parts of the brainstem include the thalamus, hypothalamus, pons, and medulla oblongata.

Thalamus

Located at the top of the brainstem, the **thalamus** regulates sensory impulses (pain, temperature, and touch) traveling to the cortex.

The thalamus evaluates sensory information and directs it to the appropriate centers in the cortex. Some tranquilizers and analgesic drugs affect sensory information by interfering with the function of the thalamus.

Hypothalamus

Located below the thalamus, the **hypothalamus** controls many body functions including temperature, water balance, appetite, sleep, the autonomic nervous system, and certain emotional or behavioral responses. The pituitary gland is attached to the hypothalamus. Referred to as the master gland of the body, the pituitary gland regulates the function of many other endocrine glands. The pituitary gland and the pharmacology of the endocrine system will be considered in Chapter 35.

Pons

Located below the hypothalamus, the **pons** is involved in the regulation of respiration and serves as a relay station for nerve fibers traveling to other brain areas.

Medulla Oblongata

The **medulla oblongata** lies just above the spinal cord. Within the medulla oblongata are the three vital centers: cardiac (heart), vasomotor (blood pressure), and respiratory (breathing). Normal functioning of the vital centers is essential for life support. Injury to the medulla oblongata frequently results in death. Overdose with drugs, such as alcohol or barbiturates, causes death by depressing the function of the vital centers. Several important reflexes are also regulated by the medulla oblongata, including swallowing, coughing, vomiting, and gagging.

Cerebellum

The **cerebellum** lies behind the brainstem and below the cerebrum. The major functions of the cerebellum, which is divided into right and left cerebellar hemispheres, are to coordinate body movements and posture and to help maintain body equilibrium. Drugs that depress the cerebellum, such as alcohol, usually decrease body coordination and reaction time.

Spinal Cord

The spinal cord is a collection of nerve axons that travel to and from the brain. Nerve axons traveling from the peripheral parts of the body (skin, muscle, visceral organs) to the brain carry sensory information (touch, pain, hot and cold sensations, etc.). Nerve axons traveling from the brain to the peripheral organs and skeletal muscle carry motor impulses that direct organ activity and muscle movement. Drugs that act on the spinal cord, mainly anesthetics, analgesics, and muscle relaxants, are primarily used to alter pain sensation and reduce the tone and activity of skeletal muscle.

FUNCTIONAL COMPONENTS

In addition to the main anatomical parts of the brain just described, several other functional neuronal pathways are located within the brain. These components form diffuse nerve networks that connect many different areas of the brain together; the reticular formation and the limbic system are two such components.

Reticular Formation

The **reticular formation** is a network of nerve fibers that travel throughout the brainstem and cerebrum. It is composed of two types of fibers: excitatory and inhibitory.

When the excitatory fibers are stimulated by various external stimuli (noise, bright light, or danger), the degree of alertness increases, preparing the body for a situation that requires action. The excitatory fibers are usually referred to as the reticular activating system.

When there is a lack of external stimuli, the inhibitory fibers become more active, decreasing the activity of this system and, consequently, the degree of arousal or alertness. This decrease normally occurs during periods of rest or sleep. Consequently, the reticular formation helps regulate the degree of alertness or wakefulness of the nervous system.

The reticular formation is sensitive to the effects of many drugs. Alcohol, barbiturates, and other depressant drugs decrease its activity and may induce sleep or unconsciousness. Stimulants, such as amphetamines and caffeine, increase the activity of the reticular formation and are usually used or abused to maintain wakefulness.

Limbic System

The **limbic system** refers to a collection of neurons and brain areas that form a specific neural pathway. Most of the structures of the limbic system are located around the hypothalamus and lower portions of the cerebrum. The limbic system appears to be involved with the emotional and behavioral responses of the body associated with reward and punishment, sexual behavior, anger or rage, fear, and anxiety; therefore, the limbic system appears to be important to mental health. The functions of the limbic system are not completely understood. However, certain drugs, such as the antianxiety agents, exert a selective effect on the limbic system and are useful for the treatment of certain behavioral and emotional disorders.

The area of pharmacology that deals with drugs affecting the CNS is known as neuropharmacology. In the following chapters, the major classes of drugs that affect the CNS will be considered.

Chapter Review

Understanding Terminology

Match the description in the left column with the appropriate part of the brain in the right column.

___ **1.** Coordinates body movements and posture, helps maintain equilibrium.

___ **2.** Regulates motor activity.

___ **3.** Conducts nerve impulses to and from different areas of the nervous system.

___ **4.** Uppermost part of brain that controls higher intellectual abilities.

___ **5.** Regulates sensory impulses traveling to the cortex.

___ **6.** Controls cardiac, vasomotor, and respiratory functions.

___ **7.** Controls the body's voluntary activities.

a. basal ganglia

b. cerebellum

c. cerebral cortex

d. cerebral medulla

e. cerebrum

f. medulla oblongata

g. thalamus

Acquiring Knowledge

Answer the following questions in the spaces provided.

1. What are the main functions of the central nervous system? _____

_____

2. List some of the neurotransmitters found in the brain. What is the function of a neurotransmitter? _____

_____

_____

3. Where are the basal ganglia located and what function is associated with them? _____

_____

4. List the main structures in the brainstem. _____

_____

_____

5. List the main functions of the hypothalamus and the medulla oblongata. _____

_____

_____

6. Why are the vital centers important? What are the consequences of injury to the medulla oblongata? _____

_____

7. What is the reticular formation? How does it function to regulate the level of wakefulness or arousal?

_____

_____

8. What is the limbic system? What functions are associated with this system? _____

_____

_____

Applying Knowledge—On the Job

Use your critical thinking skills to answer the following questions in the spaces provided.

1. As patient liaison in a large metropolitan hospital, one of your duties is to educate patients and their families about their illnesses and treatments. For the following cases, explain why the patients present with the signs and symptoms that they do.

   a. Patient A, a 16-year-old female, took an overdose of *Amytal* and was brought to the emergency room (ER) by her parents. She presents in the ER with a heart rate of 45, blood pressure of 85 over 55, and slow, irregular breathing.

   _____

   _____

   b. Patient B took an accidental overdose of *Biphetamine* and presents at the ER in a state of excitability, with rapid breathing, heart palpitations, excessive perspiration, anxiety, and irritability.

   _____

   _____

   c. Patient C is an 18-year-old male who has had a few beers once or twice a month since he turned 18. He has never consumed hard liquor until tonight, when he attended a party where he participated in a drinking contest. At that time, he drank several ounces of whiskey in a few minutes. He passed out and could not be awakened. A sober friend brought him to the ER, still unconscious. His heart rate is slow, his blood pressure down, and his breathing is irregular.

   _____

   _____

2. Assume a patient of the doctor you assist has Parkinson's disease. He and his wife think his problem is in his muscles. Explain to them what is really affected and why he has the symptoms he does.

   _____

   _____

Additional Reading

Hanson, H. R. 1995. Clinical evaluation of cranial nerves I through VII. *Hospital Medicine* 31 (10):37.

Pellegrin, T. R. 1997. A faster, focused neurologic exam. *Emergency Medicine* 29 (6):68.

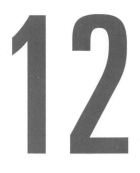

chapter

12

SEDATIVE-HYPNOTIC DRUGS AND ALCOHOL

CHAPTER FOCUS

This chapter describes the pharmacology of drugs used to produce sedation and hypnosis (sleep). It also describes the sleep cycle, how hypnotic drugs affect the stages of the sleep cycle, and the pharmacology of alcohol, a central nervous system (CNS) depressant drug.

CHAPTER OBJECTIVES

After studying this chapter, you should be able to

- name three barbiturate hypnotic drugs and describe their mechanism of action and effect on the sleep cycle.

- describe the adverse effects of barbiturates, the addiction liability, and treatment of barbiturate overdose.

- name three benzodiazepine hypnotic drugs and explain the mechanism by which they produce hypnotic effects.

- list four advantages of using benzodiazepines over barbiturate drugs.

- explain the major pharmacologic effects and adverse reactions of ethyl alcohol.

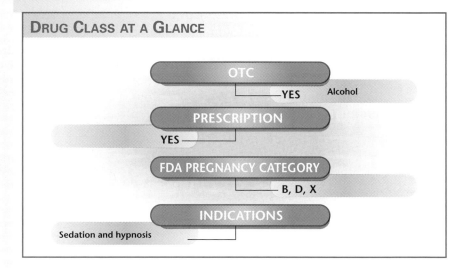

DRUG CLASS AT A GLANCE

OTC — YES Alcohol

PRESCRIPTION — YES

FDA PREGNANCY CATEGORY — B, D, X

INDICATIONS

Sedation and hypnosis

Key Terms

automatism: drug-induced confusion that can cause increased drug consumption.

barbiturate: CNS depressant drug possessing the barbituric acid ring structure.

benzodiazepine: class of drugs used to treat anxiety and sleep disorders.

GABA: gamma-aminobutyric acid, an inhibitory neurotransmitter in the CNS.

hypnotic: drug used to induce and maintain sleep.

nonbarbiturate: refers to hypnotic drugs that do not possess the barbituric acid structure, such as benzodiazepines.

NREM sleep: stages of sleep characterized by nonrapid eye movement (NREM).

REM sleep: stage of sleep characterized by rapid eye movement (REM) and dreaming.

sedative: drug used to produce mental relaxation and to reduce the desire for physical activity.

INTRODUCTION

The central nervous system coordinates and controls the activity of all other body systems. As a result, anything that directly affects the CNS ultimately influences the overall function of the body. With increased CNS stimulation, a person responds by becoming more alert, anxious, and occasionally more irritable. Excessive CNS stimulation can cause convulsions or various forms of abnormal behavior. Abuse of amphetamines or cocaine can cause these effects. In contrast, depression of the CNS reduces both physical and mental activity. Excessive CNS depression can produce unconsciousness, coma, and death. CNS depression is frequently related to abuse of barbiturates and alcohol.

Sedatives and hypnotics (drugs to induce sleep) are used therapeutically to decrease CNS activity. **Sedatives** are used to reduce the desire for physical activity. Usually a sedative will be prescribed after a heart attack or some other condition when overexertion may be harmful. Various emotional or medical situations can cause anxiety and tension to interfere with sleep. When an individual is unable to sleep (insomnia), excessive tiredness can contribute to greater anxiety and make any situation worse. In this instance, **hypnotic** drugs may be prescribed to induce and maintain sleep (Figure 12:1).

Use of hypnotics should be intermittent and only when really needed. Regular use should be limited to 2 to 4 weeks at any one time. Tolerance develops to the hypnotics and effectiveness decreases after several weeks of continuous use.

Several different drug classes are used as sedatives and hypnotics. These drugs are generally classified as the barbiturates and the nonbarbiturates. The **nonbarbiturates** include several miscellaneous drugs and the class of drugs known as the benzodiazepines. Table 12:1 on page 121 lists the most frequently prescribed sedative-hypnotic drugs. Before discussing the pharmacology of the sedatives and hypnotics, a brief review of the sleep cycle will be presented.

SLEEP CYCLE

Although sedative-hypnotic drugs are primarily used to induce and maintain sleep, many of these drugs alter the normal sleep cycle. The normal sleep cycle is divided into two different states: nonrapid eye movement **(NREM)** and rapid eye movement **(REM)** sleep.

NREM has been divided into four stages. Progression from Stage 1 to Stage 4 is characterized by a deeper level of sleep and usually takes 60 to 90 minutes. After Stage 4, individuals normally enter REM sleep for approximately 20 minutes. Dreaming usually occurs during REM sleep. After a period of REM sleep, individuals return to NREM sleep and repeat the cycle. Depending on the length of sleep, most individuals usually go through four to six sleep cycles per night.

Stage 1 NREM

Individuals are somewhat aware of surroundings but relaxed. Stage 1 normally lasts a few minutes and occupies 4 to 5 percent of total sleep time.

Stage 2 NREM

Individuals become unaware of surroundings but can be easily awakened. Stage 2 occupies about 50 percent of total sleep time.

Stages 3 and 4 NREM

Stages 3 and 4 are referred to as "slow-wave sleep" because of the high-amplitude, low-frequency delta waves observed on the electroencephalogram (EEG). These deep stages of sleep are believed to be particularly important for physical rest and restoration. They occupy approximately 20 to 25 percent of total sleep time.

FIGURE 12:1 The Emotional Reaction to the Gradual Depression of the Central Nervous System (CNS)

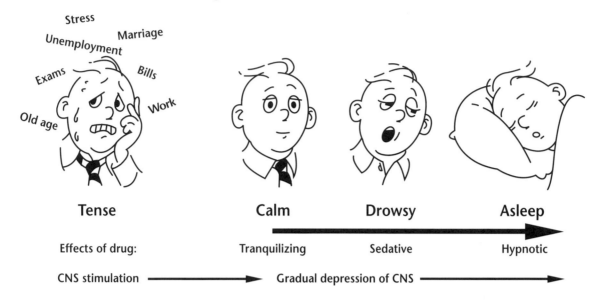

REM

The REM stage is characterized by bursts of rapid eye movement (REM), increased autonomic activity, and dreaming. It is believed to be essential for mental restoration. During REM sleep, daily events are reviewed and information is integrated into memory. Like Stages 3 and 4, REM is a deep state of sleep and occupies about 20 to 25 percent of total sleep time.

BARBITURATE SEDATIVES AND HYPNOTICS

The barbiturates are among the oldest of drugs in the sedative-hypnotic class. These drugs have a number of disadvantages to their use and have in large part been replaced by newer drugs. All of the **barbiturates** are structurally similar to the parent compound, barbituric acid. The barbiturates produce a dose-dependent depression of the CNS. At higher doses, all barbiturates can produce general anesthesia. The barbiturates discussed in this chapter are used primarily for sedation and hypnosis. Barbiturates that are used as anticonvulsants and general anesthetics will be discussed in Chapters 16 and 18, respectively.

Mechanism of Action

Barbiturates are believed to have two mechanisms of action. At lower doses, barbiturates increase the

inhibitory actions of gamma-aminobutyric acid (GABA). **GABA** is an inhibitory neurotransmitter in the CNS that reduces neuronal excitability, especially in the reticular activating system. Increasing the effects of GABA reduces brain activity and promotes sleep.

At higher doses, barbiturates also cause a general depression of the entire CNS that is similar to the actions of the general anesthetics (Chapter 18). This action of the barbiturates is not well understood but may be related to the ability of the barbiturates to dissolve in neuronal membranes, where they interfere with the normal function and movement of ions that regulate neuronal excitability and the release of excitatory neurotransmitters.

The main sites of action of the barbiturates for sedation and hypnosis are the reticular formation and the cerebral cortex. Inhibition of the reticular activating system reduces excitatory stimulation of the cerebral cortex. As a result, individuals become sedated and, with further CNS depression, become sleepy. The dose of barbiturate required to produce hypnosis is usually two to three times greater than the dose required to produce sedation.

Barbiturates usually increase Stage 2 sleep but decrease slow-wave sleep (Stages 3 and 4). In addition, barbiturates suppress REM sleep. When barbiturates are discontinued, patients often spend excess time in REM sleep during the next night or two as to make up for the lost REM sleep (REM rebound effect). During the rebound period, there is increased dreaming that may cause restlessness, anxiety, and nightmares.

| TABLE 12:1 | Doses for Sedation and Hypnosis of the Most Frequently Employed Sedative-Hypnotic Drugs |

| DRUG (TRADE NAME) | DURATION | COMMON DAILY DOSAGE RANGE | |
		SEDATION	HYPNOSIS
Barbiturates:			
amobarbital	Intermediate	50–300 mg	100–200 mg
butabarbital *(Butisol)*	Intermediate	50–120 mg	50–100 mg
pentobarbital *(Nembutal)*	Intermediate	30 mg TID, QID	100 mg
phenobarbital *(Luminal)*	Long	30–120 mg	100–200 mg
secobarbital *(Seconal)*	Short	—	100 mg
Nonbarbiturates:			
chloral hydrate *(Noctec)*	Short	250 mg	500–1000 mg
zaleplon *(Sonata)*	Short	—	5–10 mg
zolpidem *(Ambien)*	Short	—	5–10 mg
Benzodiazepines:			
estazolam *(ProSom)*	Intermediate	—	1–2 mg
flurazepam *(Dalmane)*	Long	—	15–30 mg
quazepam *(Doral)*	Long	—	7.5–15 mg
temazepam *(Restoril)*	Intermediate	—	7.5–30 mg
triazolam *(Halcion)*	Short	—	0.125–0.5 mg

Pharmacokinetics

The barbiturates are well absorbed following oral administration. Once in the circulation, these drugs are readily distributed to all tissues. Symptoms of CNS depression occur within 30 to 60 minutes following oral administration. The drug microsomal metabolizing system (DMMS) in the liver is responsible for inactivation of the barbiturates.

When taken regularly for more than several days, barbiturates begin to induce the microsomal enzymes. Induction refers to an increase in the amount of drug-metabolizing enzymes in the liver. Induction results in faster metabolism of the barbiturate. Consequently, the duration of action is decreased, and patients must take larger doses of the drug to attain the same pharmacological effect as before. When this occurs, patients are said to have developed tolerance.

When induction of the metabolizing enzymes occurs, all of the drug-metabolizing enzymes are increased. Therefore, any other drugs taken at the same time are also metabolized faster. This effect is responsible for a number of drug interactions. Barbiturates are eliminated mostly by the urinary system.

Barbiturate Drugs

Phenobarbital *(Luminal)*

Phenobarbital is classified as a long-acting barbiturate, with a duration of 6 to 12 hours. When used as a hypnotic, phenobarbital may produce a "hangover effect," where individuals feel drugged the next morning because of the prolonged duration of action. For this reason, phenobarbital is used primarily as a sedative where one dose is to produce sedation for most of the day. Phenobarbital is also used in the treatment of epilepsy (Chapter 16).

Pentobarbital (Nembutal)

Pentobarbital is classified as an intermediate-acting sedative-hypnotic, with a duration of 4 to 6 hours.

Amobarbital

Amobarbital is similar to pentobarbital. In addition, both of these barbiturates can be used parenterally to stop convulsions.

Secobarbital (Seconal)

Secobarbital is a short-acting hypnotic, with a duration of 2 to 4 hours. It is particularly useful in individuals who have difficulty falling asleep but not staying asleep.

Adverse Effects

The side effects associated with the sedative-hypnotic drugs are an extension of their therapeutic action (CNS depression). Drowsiness, dry mouth, lethargy, and incoordination occur most frequently. These adverse effects are more annoying than harmful. However, depressed reflexes and impaired judgment may contribute to serious accidents if patients operate motor vehicles or heavy machinery while taking these drugs.

Elderly patients are particularly sensitive to CNS side effects, especially mental confusion and memory difficulties. When memory is impaired due to CNS depression, patients may not remember when the drug was last taken. As a result, more drug may be consumed within a short time. This phenomenon, known as **automatism,** may lead to drug intoxication and death. Mild overdosage of the sedative-hypnotic drugs resembles alcohol intoxication (inebriation). Slurred speech, ataxia, impaired judgment, irritability, and psychological disturbances are characteristic of intoxication.

Addiction Liability

Prolonged and excessive use of barbiturates results in tolerance and physical dependence. In addition, cross-tolerance (resistance) develops to the depressant effects of other CNS depressants, such as alcohol and benzodiazepines.

The mechanism for the production of tolerance and dependency has not yet been clearly determined. Physical dependency usually develops when greater therapeutic dosages are taken on a regular basis for more than 1 to 2 months. Once physical dependence develops, the drug must be used continuously to avoid the onset of withdrawal symptoms. Withdrawal symptoms include anxiety, insomnia, cramping, tremors, paranoid behavior, delirium, and convulsions. The abstinence syndrome (withdrawal) associated with sedative-hypnotics is especially dangerous. If withdrawal is not conducted within an adequately supervised medical center, death may occur.

Barbiturate Poisoning

Overdose with the barbiturates results in extensive cardiovascular and CNS depression. In large doses, these drugs depress all brain activity, including that of the vital centers in the medulla oblongata. Inhibition of vasomotor centers in the medulla oblongata removes sympathetic control of the blood vessels, and dilation of the blood vessels contributes to the production of hypotension and shock.

In the presence of hypotension, kidney function decreases. There is little or no production of urine (oliguria or anuria) to remove the toxic products from the body. Medullary respiratory centers are also depressed, leading to irregular breathing and hypoxia (cyanosis). Severe intoxication with the barbiturates usually leads to coma, respiratory depression, and death.

There is no antidote for barbiturate overdose. Treatment of comatose patients includes supportive therapy to maintain respiration and blood pressure. Endotracheal intubation and artificial respiration may be employed. Also, sympathomimetic (alpha-adrenergic) drugs and intravenous (IV) fluids may be administered to elevate blood pressure. Osmotic diuretics administered intravenously may stimulate urine production so that renal excretion of the drug can occur. In addition, alkalinization of the urine (pH 7.0 or above) will increase the excretion of the more acidic barbiturates, like phenobarbital. Hemodialysis or peritoneal dialysis may be required when kidney function is depressed.

Cautions and Contraindications

The barbiturates are the drugs most frequently used for attempted suicide. Because of their rapid action, the short-acting drugs are particularly dangerous. Many patients die before medical treatment can be administered. To prevent hospitalized patients from hoarding medication, always make sure they have swallowed the sedative-hypnotic at the scheduled time. Never leave pills lying on the nightstand to be taken at discretion.

Most of the barbiturates are contraindicated in patients who have acute intermittent porphyria.

In this condition, an overproduction of hemoglobin (porphyrin) precursors accumulate in the liver. Sedative-hypnotics like the barbiturates stimulate and increase the production of porphyrins that can precipitate an attack (may cause nerve damage, pain, paralysis) in patients prone to this condition.

Pregnancy

The barbiturates are designated as Food and Drug Administration (FDA) Pregnancy Category D, which indicates that they can cause harmful effects to the fetus. Consequently, these drugs should be avoided during pregnancy.

Drug Interactions

Sedative-hypnotic drugs undergo extensive interactions with other drugs. Sedative-hypnotic agents will potentiate the actions of other CNS depressant drugs, leading to greater CNS and respiratory depression. Sedative-hypnotics and alcohol can be a deadly combination and should never be taken together.

Because barbiturates cause enzyme induction, other drugs may be metabolized more rapidly in their presence. This rapid metabolism results in a decreased pharmacological effect of drugs such as the oral anticoagulants and oral contraceptives. Most of the sedative-hypnotic drugs are bound to plasma proteins; therefore, they compete with other drugs for protein-binding sites. Protein-binding displacement usually leads to a potentiation of the pharmacological effect of the drug displaced.

BENZODIAZEPINES

The **benzodiazepines** are a class of drugs widely used in the treatment of anxiety. They are commonly referred to as the antianxiety drugs. The general pharmacology of the benzodiazepines is presented more fully in Chapter 13. However, in addition to producing antianxiety effects, benzodiazepines also depress the reticular activating system to produce sedation and hypnosis. Several benzodiazepines are marketed specifically as sedatives and hypnotics, and these drugs are included in this chapter (Table 12:1).

Mechanism of Action

The benzodiazepines produce sedative and hypnotic effects by increasing the inhibitory activity of gamma-aminobutyric acid (GABA), a neurotransmitter in the CNS. When GABA is released by certain neurons, it binds to GABA receptors and this leads to a reduction in neuronal excitability. The benzodiazepines bind to receptor sites (named benzodiazepine receptors) that are in close relationship to the GABA receptors. When benzodiazepines bind to their receptors, there appears to be an additional increase in the inhibitory activity of GABA, which further decreases neuronal excitability. In the reticular activating system, this depression produces sedation or hypnosis, depending upon the dose of drug administered.

Pharmacokinetics

Benzodiazepines are lipid-soluble drugs that readily enter the CNS. They are well absorbed after oral administration. The benzodiazepines are metabolized by the drug microsomal enzymes. Some of the benzodiazepines are metabolized to active metabolites, which also produce sedation and hypnosis and prolong the duration of action. Unlike the barbiturates, the benzodiazepines do not cause induction of the microsomal metabolizing enzymes at therapeutic doses. Elimination is mainly by way of the urinary tract.

Flurazepam *(Dalmane)*

Flurazepam is classified as a long-acting benzodiazepine. It forms several active metabolites, some of which have long half-lives. For this reason, the sedative and antianxiety effects of flurazepam are usually evident the day following a hypnotic dose. This prolonged action can be useful in anxious patients when sedating drug effects are desired during the following day. On the other hand, daytime sedation and drowsiness may interfere with employment or other activities.

Temazepam *(Restoril)*

Temazepam is an intermediate-acting hypnotic that does not form any important active metabolites. The duration of hypnotic action is 8 to 10 hours, and there are usually little or no drug effects evident the following day. One preparation of temazepam is marketed in a hard gelatin capsule that gives a delayed onset of action. This drug dosage form should be taken 1 to 2 hours before sleep is desired.

Triazolam *(Halcion)*

Triazolam is a short-acting hypnotic with no active metabolites. This hypnotic does not usually cause residual effects the day following a hypnotic dose. However, the short duration of action may cause early morning awakenings.

Effects on Sleep Cycle

All benzodiazepines produce similar effects on the sleep cycle. NREM Stage 2 is increased while NREM Stage 4 is usually decreased. The benzodiazepines do not significantly suppress REM sleep and therefore do not usually cause REM rebound when discontinued.

Advantages of Benzodiazepine Hypnotics

The benzodiazepines generally do not interfere with REM sleep. They produce less tolerance and therefore are effective for a few weeks longer than are the barbiturates. They also do not induce microsomal metabolizing enzymes significantly. When abused, the benzodiazepines generally cause less physical dependence than do barbiturates. These factors, along with the low incidence of adverse effects, give the benzodiazepines a number of advantages over the barbiturates for both sedation and hypnosis.

Adverse Effects

The benzodiazepine hypnotics are well tolerated and produce few adverse effects when used properly. Flurazepam, because of its longer half-life, may cause sedation or a "hangover effect" the following day. Triazolam, which has a very short duration of action, has been associated with rebound insomnia. This involves insomnia occurring over several days following abrupt discontinuance of the drug. In addition, triazolam has been associated with increased daytime anxiety. The adverse effects of the benzodiazepines are further discussed in Chapter 13.

Cautions and Contraindications

Pregnancy

Benzodiazepine hypnotic drugs have been shown to cause harmful effects during pregnancy. They are designated as FDA Pregnancy Category X and, therefore, should not be used during pregnancy.

Drug Interactions

The benzodiazepines potentiate the actions of other CNS depressant drugs, such as alcohol and barbiturates. Such drugs should never be taken together unless specifically ordered by a physician.

The metabolism of the benzodiazepines has been shown to be inhibited by cimetidine (Tagamet), a drug used in the treatment of intestinal ulcers. Consequently, using these drugs together may increase the duration of action of the benzodiazepines.

MISCELLANEOUS NONBARBITURATES

The nonbarbiturate sedative-hypnotics (see Table 12:1) are a diverse group of drugs with differing chemical structures and pharmacologic characteristics. A number of these drugs, such as methaqualone, have been removed from the market by the FDA because they produced tolerance, drug dependency, and were frequently abused. Two newer hypnotic drugs, zolpidem and zaleplon, have become popular because they do not appear to disrupt the normal stages of the sleep cycle. In addition, these drugs appear to be at low risk for the development of drug tolerance, dependency, and withdrawal reactions. Only chloral hydrate, zolpidem, and zaleplon will be discussed.

Chloral hydrate (Noctec, SK-Chloral)

Choral hydrate is related in a general way to alcohol. In the liver, it is metabolized by alcohol dehydrogenase to trichloroethanol, which also produces hypnotic effects (active metabolite). The main use of chloral hydrate is as a hypnotic, particularly in the elderly. Chloral hydrate produces less suppression of REM sleep than do the barbiturates. Side effects usually involve excessive CNS depression and gastric irritation. Although capable of producing tolerance and addiction, chloral hydrate is not particularly popular with drug abusers.

Zolpidem (Ambien)

Zolpidem is not a benzodiazepine, but acts on GABA in a manner that is similar to the actions of the barbiturates and benzodiazepines. The drug is used only as a hypnotic and does not have useful anticonvulsant or skeletal muscle relaxing properties. Zolpidem does not appear to disrupt the normal stages of the sleep cycle nor is it associated with the development of drug dependency and withdrawal reactions. The drug has a short half-life (2–3 hours) and is excreted in the urine. Adverse effects are infrequent and usually limited to dizziness, headache, nausea, and diarrhea. Zolpidem is designated FDA Pregnancy Category B.

Zaleplon (Sonata)

Zaleplon is a relatively new hypnotic drug that closely resembles zolpidem in its action. Like zolpidem, zaleplon increases the inhibitory actions of GABA. The drug is rapidly absorbed from the intestinal tract and provides a short duration of action. Zaleplon is particularly useful for individuals having difficulty falling asleep. Adverse effects include dizziness, headache, and gastrointestinal disturbances. Some individuals, especially the elderly, may experience some mental confusion and problems with memory. As with zolpidem, the development of tolerance and drug dependency with zaleplon appears to be less than observed with the barbiturate and benzodiazepine hypnotic drugs. Zaleplon is designated FDA Pregnancy Category C.

ALCOHOL

Alcohol (ethanol, whiskey, ethyl alcohol, or grain alcohol) is probably the most widely used (self-prescribed) nonprescription sedative-hypnotic and antianxiety agent.

Pharmacological Effects

Alcohol has many pharmacological effects that are seen throughout the body, including the CNS, heart, gastrointestinal tract, and kidneys.

CNS Effects

The CNS is extremely sensitive to the depressant action of alcohol. As with other sedative-hypnotic drugs, alcohol produces a dose-dependent depression of the CNS. After drinking alcoholic beverages, people usually feel "stimulated," uninhibited, and less self-conscious. However, this stimulation is actually due to an initial depression of inhibitory areas within the brain. As the level of alcohol in the brain increases, excitatory and inhibitory fibers are progressively depressed, leading to sedation, hypnosis, and possibly coma. Unlike the other sedative-hypnotic drugs, alcohol produces some analgesia and antipyresis (reduces fever). The mechanisms of alcohol's action in the CNS have not been fully established, but alcohol also appears to increase the inhibitory effects of GABA.

Vascular Effects

In low to moderate amounts, alcohol does not produce any direct deleterious effects on the heart.

Patient Administration and Monitoring

Monitor vital signs and patient response when barbiturates and benzodiazepines are administered parenterally.

Explain the potential drug side effects: excessive drowsiness, mental confusion, and a drug hangover effect the following day.

Explain to patients the dangers of activities such as driving while under the influence of sedative and hypnotic drugs.

Explain to patients the dangers of combining alcohol and other CNS depressant drugs with sedatives and hypnotics.

Remind patients that these drugs should not be used for more than 2 weeks at a time unless otherwise instructed.

Warn patients of the potential for drug dependency when hypnotics are used continuously for prolonged periods.

However, alcohol may induce dilation of the blood vessels in the skin (cutaneous), producing a warm, flushed sensation. The dilation of blood vessels may lead to a rapid loss of body heat, so that body temperature begins to fall. Depression of vasomotor centers in the CNS is most likely responsible for producing the peripheral vasodilation.

Gastrointestinal Effects

Alcohol stimulates the secretion of saliva and gastric juices (acid and pepsin). Overall, this action usually results in an increased appetite. However, ingestion of strong concentrations of alcohol may irritate the gastric mucosa, causing a local inflammation (gastritis). Increased acid secretion coupled with gastritis may lead to gastrointestinal (GI) ulceration in sensitive patients.

Renal Effects

Alcohol promotes an increased excretion of urine (diuresis), which is partly due to the increased fluid intake that accompanies the ingestion of alcoholic beverages. In addition, alcohol blocks the pituitary secretion of anti-diuretic hormone (ADH), which decreases the renal reabsorption of water. Therefore, the water is excreted into the urine. Alcohol inhibits the renal secretion of uric acid by an unknown mechanism that allows uric acid to build up in the blood. In susceptible patients (with gout or gouty arthritis), this elevation in uric acid levels may lead to attacks of joint inflammation.

Nutritional Effects

Besides its direct effects on the various organs, alcohol exerts a profound influence on the nutritional state of individuals. Alcohol is a natural product that possesses calories. For this reason, many people often substitute alcohol for nutritionally rich foods, such as protein. Over a period of time, individuals who consume moderate to large amounts of alcohol in conjunction with a poorly balanced diet may suffer from vitamin and amino acid deficiencies. In particular, deficiency of the B vitamins leads to abnormal growth and function of nervous tissue. Therefore, multiple nutritional deficiencies associated with alcohol consumption produce various conditions such as neuropathies, dermatitis (pellagra), anemia, and psychosis.

Metabolism of Alcohol

Alcohol is readily absorbed throughout the entire GI tract following ingestion. Subsequently, alcohol is distributed to all tissues. However, the CNS receives a significant concentration of alcohol because of its rich blood supply. The concentration of alcohol in the brain is proportional to the concentration of alcohol in the blood.

Unlike other drugs, alcohol is metabolized at a constant rate in the liver. No matter how much alcohol is consumed, only 10 to 15 ml of pure alcohol per hour is metabolized, which is the amount of alcohol in one beer, a glass of wine, or an average-size cocktail. This limits the amount of alcohol that can be consumed without producing intoxication. Alcohol is metabolized primarily to acetaldehyde, which the body can use in the synthesis of cholesterol and fatty acids. Overall, alcohol is efficiently metabolized (about 95 percent) to useful biochemical products and water.

Enzyme induction develops during chronic use of alcohol. Therefore, habitual drinkers often experience shorter durations of action of other drugs metabolized by the microsomal system of the liver (oral anticoagulants and many others).

Adverse Effects

The adverse effects associated with the use of alcohol are separated into acute and chronic effects. Acute intoxication (inebriation) produces extensive CNS depression. Individuals may exhibit ataxia, impaired speech, blurred vision, and loss of memory, similar to the symptoms of intoxication caused by other sedative-hypnotic drugs.

When CNS depression is severe, stupor and coma may result. The skin is cold and clammy, the body temperature falls, and the heart rate may increase. Treatment is usually directed at supporting respiration, so that the brain remains well oxygenated. Even while patients are unconscious, their body tissues can metabolize alcohol until the blood level is safely reduced.

Chronic consumption of alcohol is associated with progressive changes in cell function. Elevated blood alcohol levels for long periods result ultimately in drug tolerance and physical dependence. The abstinence syndrome associated with alcohol addiction is similar to that described for the other sedative-hypnotic drugs. In addition, chronic use of alcohol produces alterations in body metabolism, some of which may be due to the development of malnutrition. Alcohol-induced malnutrition and vitamin deficiency can cause a number of neurological disorders such as Wernicke's encephalopathy and Korsakoff's psychosis. In addition, malnutrition and alcohol contribute to the production of fatty liver and cirrhosis of the liver.

Cautions and Contraindications

The symptoms of alcohol intoxication often resemble those associated with diabetic coma, head injuries, and drug overdose (other sedative-hypnotics). Patients who appear intoxicated should always be kept for observation until an accurate diagnosis is made. If possible, the blood alcohol level should be determined to confirm the suspected diagnosis.

Alcohol should never be combined with other CNS depressant medications. Potentiation occurs with any central-acting depressants, including muscle relaxants, anesthetics, analgesics, and antianxiety drugs. Alcohol is absolutely contraindicated in patients who have hepatic or renal disease, ulcers, hyperacidity, or epilepsy.

Pregnancy

The consumption of alcohol has been associated with harmful fetal effects and should be avoided during pregnancy. Alcohol readily crosses the placenta and distributes to all tissues of the fetus. Infants who were exposed to circulating levels of alcohol *in utero* have shown depressed respiration and reflexes at birth. Babies born to alcoholic mothers are unusually small, are frequently premature, and may be mentally retarded. It is not unusual for a newborn of an alcoholic mother to undergo withdrawal symptoms after birth. Fetal alcohol syndrome is the term used to describe the fetal abnormalities that may include low IQ, microcephaly, and a variety of facial abnormalities.

Clinical Indications

When applied to the skin, alcohol produces a cooling effect, due to rapid evaporation from the skin surface. For this reason, it is used as a sponge bath to reduce elevated body temperature. Also, 70 percent alcohol applied to the skin acts as a bactericidal agent (disinfectant). There is very little medicinal value associated with the consumption of alcohol. However, many over-the-counter (nonprescription) cold remedies and cough syrups contain a significant amount of alcohol; the alcohol present in these preparations is sufficient to produce sedation and hypnosis. Therefore, exposure of patients to alcohol may occur without their knowledge.

Disulfiram (Antabuse)

Disulfiram is a drug used to treat chronic alcoholism. It interferes with the metabolism of alcohol. Alcohol is metabolized through a series of steps to acetaldehyde, which is then converted into acetyl coenzyme A (CoA).

```
alcohol
   ↓
acetaldehyde
   ↓
acetyl coenzyme A
```

Disulfiram slows the conversion of acetaldehyde to acetyl coenzyme A. Therefore, acetaldehyde accumulates in the blood, producing nausea, vomiting, headache, and hypotension. This is known as a disulfiram reaction. Any drug that is metabolized through a similar biochemical pathway, such as paraldehyde, also produces a disulfiram reaction in the presence of disulfiram. Patients taking disulfiram are instructed not to ingest any alcoholic beverages, including cough syrups, special wine sauces, and fermented beverages (cider). As long as a patient is taking disulfiram, even a small amount of alcohol (1 ounce) will produce the unpleasant effects. In this manner, the disulfiram therapy acts as a reinforcing deterrent to alcohol consumption.

Chapter Review

Understanding Terminology

Answer the following questions in the spaces provided.

1. Differentiate between REM sleep and NREM sleep. _____

    _____

2. What is the difference between a sedative and a hypnotic? _____

    _____

3. Explain the meaning of *automatism*. _____

    _____

4. Differentiate between barbiturates and nonbarbiturates. _____

    _____

5. What is GABA an abbreviation for? _____

Acquiring Knowledge

Answer the following questions in the spaces provided.

1. What is the major indication for the use of sedatives and hypnotics? _____

    _____

2. Explain the mechanism of action of barbiturate hypnotics. What are the main sites of action to produce this effect? _____

    _____

3. List the different stages of sleep and the characteristics of each. _____

    _____

    _____

4. How do barbiturates alter the normal sleep cycle? _____

    _____

5. What is the importance of enzyme induction caused by sedative-hypnotic drugs? _____

    _____

    _____

6. What adverse effects are caused by barbiturates? _____

    _____

    _____

7. How does GABA normally function? _____

    _____

    _____

8. Explain the mechanism of action of the benzodiazepine hypnotics. _____

    _____

    _____

9. How do benzodiazepine hypnotics alter the sleep cycle? _____

    _____

10. What is the main difference between flurazepam *(Dalmane)* and triazolam *(Halcion)*? _____

    _____

    _____

11. What are the advantages of the benzodiazepines over the barbiturate hypnotics? _____

_____

12. List some of the effects that alcohol produces on the different body systems. _____

_____

_____

13. Explain how disulfiram (*Antabuse*) is used in the treatment of alcoholism and describe the disulfiram reaction. _____

_____

_____

Applying Knowledge—On the Job

Use your critical thinking skills to answer the following questions in the spaces provided.

1. An 82-year-old woman has been taking a sleeping pill for the past 6 months to help her fall asleep. What can you tell her about the use of hypnotic drugs?

_____

_____

2. Mary's husband John occasionally takes *Dalmane* when he has trouble sleeping. He came home late last night after a banquet and a few too many drinks; he took a *Dalmane* capsule because he wasn't tired and he had to get up early for an important meeting. At 8 A.M., John was sound asleep and Mary couldn't seem to wake him up. What do you think may have happened?

_____

_____

3. You receive a phone call at the doctor's office from Mr. Smith who has a prescription for *Antabuse.* He complains that he feels terrible and has been vomiting. He claims to have just developed a chest cold and has taken a spoonful of *Vicks* cough syrup. Mr. Smith doesn't think the vomiting has anything to do with the cold. What do you think?

_____

_____

4. A young man with a history of occasional drug abuse is in the doctor's office complaining of difficulty sleeping. The physician is writing a prescription for a hypnotic with no refills. Which hypnotic agent might be the best choice for this patient?

_____

_____

5. While undergoing a stressful divorce, John was prescribed 50 mg per day of *Butisol* as a sleep aid. After a week on this regimen, the *Butisol* became less effective, so his doctor increased the dosage to 75 mg a day. After 4 weeks, John finished his prescription, and now his sleep is troubled by nightmares. His doctor refuses to renew the prescription for the *Butisol,* saying it's habit forming. While John was taking the *Butisol,* the *Coumadin* that he takes for thrombosis appeared to have a decreased therapeutic effect. He also had dry mouth and feelings of lethargy.

  a. Why has the *Butisol* affected John as it has, and why is it important that he discontinue taking the drug?

_____

_____

  b. Why might switching to a benzodiazepine drug, like *Dalmane,* help John?

_____

_____

c. If John was taking *Tagamet* for an ulcer, what effect would it have on the dosage of *Dalmane*?

_____

_____

Use the appropriate reference books if needed for the following questions.

6. June is a 36-year-old alcoholic. She has unsuccessfully attempted to quit drinking multiple times. Her physician has decided to initiate disulfiram therapy. What should June be told before taking this medication?

_____

_____

7. John is a healthy 29-year-old who has recently had trouble sleeping. His physician has prescribed *Dalmane* 30 mg. While talking with John, he tells you how happy he is to know that he is going to get a good night's sleep. He works in a high-energy office and was concerned that he might be in danger of losing his job due to his recent lack of energy. Do you think this should be brought to the physician's attention? Why? Would you expect the drug therapy to change? If so, which medication do you think it might be changed to?

_____

_____

8. Julie has never had trouble sleeping until the past month. She is going through a stressful period and is having difficulty falling asleep. Once asleep, she usually sleeps through the night. Her care provider had prescribed *Ambien* 5 mg in a quantity to last 2 weeks. Do you feel this is appropriate? Why?

_____

_____

Internet Connection

Visit the **MedicineNet** website at (http://www.medicinenet.com). Under *Diseases and Treatments,* click on the letter "A" and find the topic *Alcohol, Pregnancy.* Under this heading click on *Fetal Alcohol Syndrome.* How is this condition diagnosed, and what are the main problems, causes, and features of this syndrome? Also, under *Diseases and Treatments,* click on *Sleep* and explore the various headings related to insomnia, snoring, and sleep apnea.

Another search engine is the **National Clearinghouse for Alcohol and Drug Information** (http://www.health.org). Click on *Alcohol and Drug Facts* and familiarize yourself with the topics and information available. This information may be useful for preparing reports on alcohol abuse and prevention.

Additional Reading

Ancoli-Israel, S. 1997. Sleep problems in older adults: Putting myths to bed. *Geriatrics* 52 (1):20.

Lewis, D. C. 1997. Alcoholism in the elderly. *Hospital Practice* 32 (3):211.

Mahowald, M. W. 1995. Initial evaluation of the patient with insomnia. *Hospital Medicine* 31 (2):50.

Mahowald, M. W. 1995. Update on treating insomnia. *Hospital Medicine* 31 (3):31.

Schneider, D. L. 2002. Insomnia: Safe and effective therapy for sleep problems in the older patient. *Geriatrics* 57 (5):24.

Warmer, T. M. 1995. New strategies for treating alcohol withdrawal syndrome. *Hospital Medicine* 31 (3):54.

ANTIPSYCHOTIC AND ANTIANXIETY DRUGS

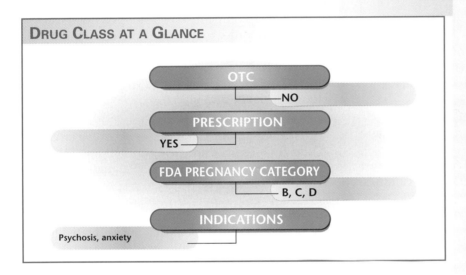

DRUG CLASS AT A GLANCE

OTC
— NO

PRESCRIPTION
YES —

FDA PREGNANCY CATEGORY
— B, C, D

INDICATIONS
Psychosis, anxiety

Key Terms

akathisia: continuous body movement in which an individual is restless or constantly paces about.

antianxiety drug: drug used to treat neurosis and anxiety; these drugs are also referred to as anxiolytics.

antipsychotic: drug used to treat schizophrenia and other psychotic conditions.

dystonic reaction: reaction characterized by muscle spasms, twitching, facial grimacing, or torticollis.

neuroleptic: another term for antipsychotic drug.

neurosis: abnormal behavior characterized by increased anxiety, tension, and emotionalism.

parkinsonism: disease or drug-induced condition characterized by muscular rigidity, tremors, and disturbances of movement.

psychosis: form of mental illness that produces bizarre behavior and deterioration of the personality.

schizophrenia: major form of psychosis; behavior is inappropriate.

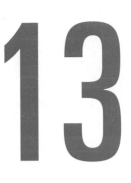

CHAPTER FOCUS

This chapter describes the pharmacology of drugs used to treat some forms of mental illness. It explains how antipsychotic drugs suppress the symptoms of schizophrenia and other psychotic conditions, and it explains the numerous adverse effects that these drugs produce. It also explains how antianxiety drugs reduce the nervousness and hyper emotionalism that accompany various neurotic conditions and tells why these same drugs are useful in the treatment of convulsive seizures, skeletal muscle spasticity, and insomnia.

CHAPTER OBJECTIVES

After studying this chapter, you should be able to

- list three different classes of antipsychotic drugs and describe the main pharmacologic effects they produce.
- describe the common adverse effects and the specific neurological conditions caused by antipsychotic drugs.
- explain the mechanism of action and uses of benzodiazepine antianxiety drugs and name the four areas of the CNS where they exert their actions.
- list five adverse effects associated with antianxiety drugs.

131

tardive dyskinesia: drug-induced involuntary movements of the lips, jaw, tongue, and extremities.

tranquilization: mental state characterized by calmness and peace of mind.

INTRODUCTION

The term *mental illness* refers to a number of emotional and mental disturbances that involve abnormal changes in personality and behavior. These changes may affect the ability of individuals to communicate with other people or to function in normal activities.

TYPES OF MENTAL ILLNESS

There are many different forms of mental illness, but the two basic categories are the psychoses and the neuroses. In both conditions, there is often increased CNS stimulation usually displayed by hyperactivity, agitation, and occasionally violent behavior. Drugs sometimes referred to as tranquilizers are used in the treatment of these conditions. **Tranquilization** is a mental state that is characterized by calmness and peace of mind but without significant sedation or mental confusion.

Psychoses

Psychosis is a mental disorder that involves a breakdown of the personality. Thought patterns and physical actions appear unrelated to real-life situations. Individuals suffer a loss of contact with reality, and normal conversation and communication may be impossible.

The two major forms of psychosis are schizophrenia and severe depression. In **schizophrenia,** individuals are usually withdrawn, and behavior is inappropriate and highly unpredictable. Delusions or hallucinations may also occur. Some patients with schizophrenia may have to be institutionalized. Treatment involves a combination of drug administration and psychotherapy. The drugs used to treat psychosis are referred to as antipsychotic drugs.

In severe depression, there are serious disturbances of mood, with the depressed individuals feeling that everything is hopeless. Depression and its treatment will be discussed in Chapter 14.

Neuroses

Many situations in life give rise to feelings of fear or anxiety. Fear is a particular type of response to a known danger. The sympathetic nervous system is activated, accompanied by other psychological changes. In order to deal with these situations, individuals either overcome the fear or avoid the cause of it. In any case, the physical and behavioral changes associated with fear are no longer brought into play.

The discovery that one has a serious medical problem or disease often causes excessive anxiety. Subconscious psychological conflicts and other emotional situations can generate anxiety where the underlying cause is unknown or consciously denied. Even though the cause of the anxiety may be unknown, the same physiological and behavioral changes occur that are generated by fearful situations. In addition to increased sympathetic effects, there is also hyperarousal of the reticular formation and cortex, which can interfere with sleep and appetite. Increased tenseness and skeletal muscle tone contribute to tiredness and fatigue.

Neurosis, then, is an accumulation of anxiety and tension that leads to emotional changes and abnormal behavior. Treatment involves psychotherapy to determine the cause of the anxiety and drug therapy to relieve the symptoms of anxiety. Drugs used to treat neurosis or anxiety are known as antianxiety drugs.

ANTIPSYCHOTIC DRUGS

Antipsychotic drugs, also referred to as **neuroleptics,** are used to suppress the symptoms of schizophrenia and other psychotic conditions. The antipsychotic drugs have a selective action on subcortical areas of the brain. The thalamus and limbic system, which regulate behavior, appear to be the major sites of action of the antipsychotic drugs.

The cause of psychosis is not clearly understood. However, there does appear to be a disturbance in the function of brain neurotransmitters. Dopamine appears to be particularity important, and drugs that block or reduce the effects of dopamine are effective in treating psychosis, especially schizophrenia. In psychosis, there is apparently excessive dopaminergic activity. The mechanism of action of antipsychotic drugs is thought to involve the ability of these drugs to block dopamine receptors. This reduces dopaminergic activity by preventing dopamine from binding to and activating its receptors.

Serotonin is another brain neurotransmitter that is involved in psychotic behavior. A few of the newer antipsychotic drugs have actions to block serotonin receptors. These drugs, such as clozapine and risperidone, are referred to as "atypical" antipsychotic drugs because their main actions do not affect dopamine like most of the antipsychotic drugs.

Several classes of drugs are used for their antipsychotic effects. Previously, these drugs were referred to as major tranquilizers, but this terminology is no longer popular. The most important antipsychotic drug classes are phenothiazines, butyrophenones, thioxanthenes, and other related drugs.

Phenothiazines

The term *phenothiazine* refers to the basic chemical structure of a large number of drugs similar in structure and pharmacological action. Although some of these drugs are more effective than others, all produce the same pharmacological effects. The first phenothiazine, chlorpromazine, was discovered in the early 1950s. Within a few years, chlorpromazine had revolutionized the treatment of mental illness. Many patients who were previously institutionalized were able to return home and assume more active roles in society. Within a few years, the number of patients in mental institutions was cut almost in half.

The phenothiazines are a very active group of drugs. In addition to an antipsychotic effect, they possess anticholinergic, antihistaminic, alpha-adrenergic blocking, and antiemetic effects. These additional effects allow the phenothiazines to be used for treating nausea, vomiting, pruritus, and certain allergic reactions. The phenothiazines are administered orally (PO) and parenterally (IM and IV). Doses must be individually adjusted, but they usually range from 200 to 1200 mg per day PO for chlorpromazine in the treatment of psychosis. Table 13:1 on page 134 lists the phenothiazines and their main uses.

Antipsychotic Effects

The main effects of the antipsychotic drugs are to reduce the bizarre behavior, hallucinations, and irrational thought disorders of psychosis without significantly depressing other intellectual functions. The antipsychotic effects usually require 1 to 2 weeks to develop fully. With drug therapy, patients usually demonstrate decreased interest in the surroundings and less behavioral activation. However, routine daily activities can be carried out, and patients are able to communicate more rationally. Although the psychosis is not cured, it is possible to control it adequately with the proper medication. In addition, patients are usually more amenable to psychotherapy and other treatment measures.

Adverse Effects

Common adverse effects, such as dry mouth, constipation, visual disturbances, and sedation, are due to anticholinergic and antihistaminic actions. Because antipsychotic drugs block the effects of dopamine, a number of neurological side effects involving the basal ganglia can occur. Dopamine functions as a neurotransmitter in the basal ganglia of the brain. The basal ganglia are important in the regulation of skeletal muscle tone and movement (see Chapter 17).

Three neurological conditions can occur as a result of taking phenothiazine drugs. **Dystonic reactions** are characterized by muscle spasms, twitching, facial grimacing, and torticollis (wryneck). **Akathisia** refers to continuous body movement in which the individual is restless or constantly paces about. **Parkinsonism,** sometimes referred to as extrapyramidal symptoms, involves development of muscular rigidity, tremors, and other disturbances of movement. Reducing the dosage, stopping the drug, or administering centrally acting anticholinergic drugs usually improves these three neurological conditions.

Tardive dyskinesia is a more serious condition that may develop after long-term antipsychotic therapy. This condition involves involuntary movements of the lips, jaw, tongue, and extremities. The symptoms of tardive dyskinesia often appear when antipsychotic drug treatment is stopped. The symptoms can be suppressed by reinstituting the drug or by increasing the dose of the antipsychotic drug. However, this worsens the condition. The symptoms of tardive dyskinesia are frequently irreversible and unresponsive to treatment.

A serious and potentially fatal condition, neuroleptic malignant syndrome (NMS), is also

TABLE 13:1   Antipsychotic Drugs and Their Main Clinical Uses

DRUG (TRADE NAME)	MAIN USE	COMMON DAILY DOSAGE RANGE
Benzisoxazoles:		
risperidone *(Risperdal)*	Antipsychotic	2–6 mg
Butyrophenones:		
haloperidol *(Haldol)*	Antipsychotic, antimanic	5–80 mg
Dibenzapines:		
clozapine *(Clozaril)*	Antipsychotic	12.5–450 mg
loxapine *(Loxitane)*	Antipsychotic	20–250 mg
olanzapine *(Zyprexa)*	Antipsychotic	5–20 mg
quetiapine *(Seroquel)*	Antipsychotic	50–750 mg
Dihydroindolones:		
molindone *(Moban)*	Antipsychotic	15–225 mg
Diphenylbutylpiperidine:		
pimozide *(Orap)*	Tourette's syndrome	1–10 mg
Phenothiazines:		
chlorpromazine *(Thorazine)*	Antipsychotic, antiemetic	50–1200 mg
prochlorperazine *(Compazine)*	Antiemetic	5–50 mg
promethazine *(Phenergan)*	Antihistaminic (colds, motion sickness)	25–50 mg
thioridazine *(Melleril)*	Antipsychotic	50–800 mg
trifluoperazine *(Stelazine)*	Antipsychotic	5–60 mg
triflupromazine *(Vesprin)*	Antipsychotic, antiemetic	50–150 mg
Thioxanthenes:		
thiothixene *(Navane)*	Antipsychotic	5–30 mg

associated with the use of antipsychotic drugs. This syndrome is characterized by hyperthermia, muscular rigidity, catatonia (patient appears frozen in position), and autonomic nervous system instability. Treatment is immediately required and involves stopping antipsychotic drug administration and symtomatic treatment of the symptoms.

Drug allergy is an infrequent but potentially dangerous complication of phenothiazine therapy. Allergic symptoms usually involve skin rashes and photosensitivity, blood disorders, and liver toxicity (cholestatic jaundice). Other miscellaneous adverse effects include skin pigmentation, ocular deposits (lens and cornea), and various endocrine disturbances.

Butyrophenones

The butyrophenones are a group of compounds that differ chemically from the phenothiazines but that produce the same type of antipsychotic effects. The main drug of this group is haloperidol *(Haldol)*.

Actions

On a milligram basis, the butyrophenones are more potent than are the phenothiazines. The usual oral dose of haloperidol is 2 to 15 mg per day. The butyrophenones produce fewer peripheral effects (adrenergic blockade, anticholinergic, and antihistaminic), but greater movement disturbances. Haloperidol is especially useful in the treatment of highly agitated and manic patients.

Adverse Effects

The adverse effects of the butyrophenones are similar to those of the phenothiazines. However, there is a greater incidence of extrapyramidal symptoms with the butyrophenones.

Thioxanthenes

Thioxanthenes have chemical structures very similar to those of phenothiazines. Like phenothiazines and butyrophenones, thioxanthenes exert antipsychotic effects by blocking dopamine in the brain. The most important thioxanthene is thiothixene *(Navane)*.

Actions

Thioxanthenes are said to exert a more selective action than do other antipsychotic drugs because the thioxanthenes do not usually produce as many of the other pharmacological effects (sedation or inhibition of acetylcholine, norepinephrine, and histamine) as do the phenothiazines and butyrophenones.

Adverse Effects

The most frequent adverse effects of the thioxanthenes include drowsiness and postural hypotension. Patients who become allergic to these drugs may develop dermatitis, obstructive jaundice, or blood disorders (anemia and leukopenia). Like other antipsychotic drugs, the thioxanthenes may cause parkinsonian symptoms and other disturbances of movement.

Other Antipsychotic Drugs

There is an increasing number of other chemical drugs that produce pharmacologic and adverse effects that are similar to those of the phenothiazines. The major features of these drugs are given here. Assume that the pharmacologic features are, in general, similar to those of the phenothiazines unless otherwise noted.

Loxapine (Loxitane)

Loxapine is several times more potent than chlorpromazine but otherwise produces similar effects. Sedation and hypotensive effects are low. Adverse effects and toxicities are similar to those of the phenothiazines.

Molindone *(Moban)*

Molindone is very similar to loxapine in potency, pharmacology, and adverse effects.

Clozapine *(Clozaril)*

Clozapine is a low-potency drug that is classified as "atypical." Atypical refers to the antipsychotic mechanism of action of drugs that block receptors in the brain in addition to dopamine receptors. Clozapine has significant serotonin receptor blocking activity. Sedation, hypotension, and anticholinergic effects are prominent. Clozapine has been associated with reductions in the number of granulocytes and weekly blood counts are usually required. Unlike most other drugs, clozapine does not cause extrapyramidal effects such as parkinsonism or tardive dyskinesia.

Risperidone *(Risperdal)*

Risperidone is an "atypical" antipsychotic drug with good receptor blocking activity against both dopamine and serotonin. Sedation, hypotension, and anticholinergic effects are low. Extrapyramidal effects may occur with higher doses.

Pimozide *(Orap)*

Pimozide is a potent antipyschotic drug that is associated with a high incidence of extrapyramidal effects. The main use of pimozide is in the treatment of *Gilles de la Tourette's syndrome* (Tourette's disorder). In this condition there are motor abnormalities such as tics and outbursts of inappropriate (foul) language. Pimozide has also been associated with incidences of cardiac arrhythmias and has the potential to cause sudden death.

Olanzapine *(Zyprexa)*

Olanzapine is a new dibenzapine derivative that causes few or no extrapyramidal symptoms. Like clozapine, the antipsychotic effect is due to the antagonism of both dopamine and serotonin receptors in the brain. The drug is administered on a once-a-day schedule without regard to meals. The most common adverse reactions associated with olanzapine are dry mouth, sleepiness, dizziness, constipation, and weight gain.

Patient Administration and Monitoring

Monitor vital signs and patient response frequently when these drugs are administered parenterally, especially blood pressure and heart activity.

Explain to patient the common side effects: dry mouth, sedation, sleepiness, dizziness, blurred vision.

Instruct patient to report tremors, muscular rigidity, fever, disturbances of movement, visual disturbances, excessive weakness or feelings of faintness, and difficulties with urination and defecation.

Inform patients not to take other medications unless they check with their physician or pharmacist; there are many drug interactions with antipsychotic drugs.

Cautions and Contraindications

Pregnancy

Most antipsychotic drugs are designated either Food and Drug Administration (FDA) Pregnancy Category B or C; a few of the drugs have not been rated. As always, the use of drugs during pregnancy should be avoided if at all possible and used only when the benefits outweigh the risks.

Drug Interactions

As previously discussed, the antipsychotic drugs produce anticholinergic, alpha-blocking, antihistaminic, and central nervous system (CNS) depressing effects. Therefore, these drugs will interact with all other drugs that also produce these pharmacologic effects.

Anticholinergic drugs (atropine-like) decrease the activity of the urinary and intestinal tracts and increase cardiac activity. They also tend to cause CNS depression and mental disturbances, especially in the elderly. Remember also that anticholinergic drugs are *contraindicated* or used with caution in individuals with glaucoma, prostate hypertrophy, and urinary and intestinal obstruction (see Chapter 7). Many antihistamine drugs possess anticholinergic activity and also cause sedation. Consequently, other anticholinergic drugs taken together with antipsychotic drugs will increase the frequency and severity of anticholinergic adverse reactions.

Alpha-blocking activity (blocks alpha effects of norepinephrine and epinephrine) produces a lowering of blood pressure. Individuals taking alpha-blockers for hypertension, or taking other antihypertensive medication, may experience hypotension, orthostatic hypotension, fainting, and the other adverse effects of alpha blockade (see Chapter 6).

The CNS depressant effects of antipsychotic drugs will be increased by all other drugs that also cause sedation, hypnosis, and depression. These include alcohol, barbiturates, benzodiazepines, antihistamines, tricyclic antidepressants, anticholinergics, and narcotics. When taken together these drugs may cause excessive CNS depression leading to coma, respiratory depression or arrest, and death.

ANTIANXIETY DRUGS

Anxiety, tension, and nervousness are effects caused by uncertainty and various situations that are interpreted as being threatening or potentially dangerous. The perceived dangers may be real or due to personal insecurities or unconscious psychological conflicts. Physiologic and behavioral changes—trembling, sweating, nausea, loss of appetite, rapid heartbeat, and emotionalism—are caused by activation of the sympathetic nervous system and areas of the brain, such as the limbic system, that control and regulate emotions and behavior.

When an anxiety condition is prolonged, there are significant behavioral and emotional changes. These changes can result in a type of mental illness known as neurosis. **Antianxiety** drugs, also referred to as anxiolytics, are used to calm individuals and reduce the unpleasant aspects of anxiety and neurotic behavior. In addition, the benzodiazepine antianxiety drugs are also used as sedatives, hypnotics, anticonvulsants, and skeletal muscle relaxants.

Benzodiazepines

The most important antianxiety drugs belong to a chemical class known as the benzodiazepines. Diazepam *(Valium)* and chlordiazepoxide *(Librium)* are benzodiazepines that have been used for more than 40 years. Additional benzodiazepine drugs have been introduced, and these are listed in Table 13:2.

TABLE 13:2 Benzodiazepine Antianxiety Drugs

DRUG (TRADE NAME)	MAIN USE	USUAL DOSE
Long Acting:		
chlordiazepoxide *(Librium)*	Antianxiety, alcohol withdrawal	5–10 mg TID
clonazepam *(Klonopin)*	Anticonvulsant	0.5 mg TID
clorazepate *(Tranxene)*	Antianxiety	7.5 mg TID
diazepam *(Valium)*	Antianxiety, pre-op medication, alcohol withdrawal, anticonvulsant, muscle relaxer	2–10 mg TID
flurazepam *(Dalmane)*	Hypnotic	15–30 mg at bedtime
prazepam *(Centrax)*	Antianxiety	10 mg TID
Short Acting:		
alprazolam *(Xanax)*	Antianxiety	0.25–0.5 mg TID
halazepam *(Paxipam)*	Antianxiety	30 mg TID
lorazepam *(Ativan)*	Antianxiety	0.5–1.0 mg TID
oxazepam *(Serax)*	Antianxiety	15–30 mg TID
temazepam *(Restoril)*	Hypnotic	15–30 mg at bedtime
triazolam *(Halcion)*	Hypnotic	0.25–0.5 mg at bedtime

Mechanism of Action

The benzodiazepines decrease the excitability and the functional activity of specific areas of the brain and spinal cord. Gamma-aminobutyric acid (GABA) is an inhibitory neurotransmitter in the CNS that, when released from nerve endings, binds to receptors (called GABA receptors) located on the membranes of other neurons. GABA appears to allow more chloride ions (Cl^-) to pass into the neurons, which makes the inside of the neuron more negatively charged (hyperpolarization). Hyperpolarization of the neuron reduces neuronal excitability and consequently produces a depressant effect on those neurons.

The benzodiazepine drugs also bind to neuronal membranes at receptor sites (referred to as the benzodiazepine receptors) that are actually a part of the GABA receptors. When both GABA and a benzodiazepine drug are bound to their receptors, more chloride ions pass into the neuron than when only GABA is bound alone. Consequently, a greater degree of hyperpolarization and neuronal depression is produced. Simply stated, benzodiazepines are believed to increase the inhibitory actions of GABA, which results in reduced activity (depression) of specific areas of the CNS.

Sites of Action

There are four main areas of the CNS where the benzodiazepines exert their depressant effects: the limbic system, reticular formation, cerebral cortex, and spinal cord. The major functions of these areas were previously discussed in Chapter 11.

The limbic system is involved with regulation of emotional and behavioral responses. Any emotional or anxiety-producing situation increases the activity of the limbic system. GABA normally functions to inhibit excess stimulation of the limbic system. When anxiety becomes excessive and contributes to neurotic behavior, benzodiazepines are prescribed to decrease the activity of the limbic system. Anxious individuals usually calm down, are less emotional, and are in a better mental state to deal with the situations that cause the anxiety. This is referred to as the antianxiety effect.

The reticular formation regulates the degree of wakefulness and alertness. Amphetamines and other CNS stimulants increase the activity of norepinephrine in the reticular formation, which causes increased wakefulness and hyperactivity. GABA normally functions to decrease the activity of the reticular formation. Benzodiazepines, which increase the inhibitory actions of GABA, are used to produce sedation and hypnosis (sleep). A few of the benzodiazepines, those previously discussed in Chapter 12, are used primarily as sedatives and hypnotics.

Excessive stimulation of the cerebral cortex can cause convulsions and other types of seizures. When administered parenterally, benzodiazepines exert an anticonvulsant effect on the cerebral cortex and are very effective in stopping convulsions. They are believed to exert the anticonvulsant effect by increasing the inhibitory actions of GABA. Diazepam (Valium) and clonazepam (Klonopin) are the benzodiazepines that are considered to be the drugs of choice to stop convulsions.

GABA has an important function in the spinal cord. It helps regulate the degree of skeletal muscle tone and the responsiveness of spinal reflexes that also maintain skeletal muscle activity. By increasing the inhibitory actions of GABA, benzodiazepines decrease skeletal muscle tone. Relaxation of skeletal muscle is helpful in treating back injuries, spinal cord injuries, muscular dystrophy, and cerebral palsy, where muscle spasticity is usually present. Relaxation of skeletal muscle is also believed to contribute to the antianxiety effect, since increased muscle tension is a common finding in anxious individuals.

Pharmacokinetics

Benzodiazepines are well absorbed from the GI tract, and oral administration is the normal route. Diazepam, chlordiazepoxide, and lorazepam can also be given IM or IV when a rapid response is required. The main differences among the various benzodiazepines are in the duration of action. The benzodiazepines are divided into two groups: the long acting and the short acting (Table 13:2).

The long-acting benzodiazepines have half-lives of more than 20 hours. Also, during metabolism by the liver, they form active metabolites, which generally have long half-lives. When taken on a daily basis, these drugs produce effects that can last several days, due to accumulation of active metabolites in the body. Eventually, the active metabolites are conjugated with glucuronic acid. This step inactivates them and allows them to be excreted in the urine.

The short-acting benzodiazepines have half-lives that range from 5 to 20 hours. Either they do not form active metabolites, or, if they do, the active

metabolites do not contribute significantly to the pharmacological effect.

Clinical Indications

The antianxiety drugs are used to relieve nervous tension and anxiety caused by neuroses or other life situations. Patients are made calm and relaxed without being excessively sedated. This state of mind is desirable before surgery, and antianxiety drugs are widely used as preoperative medications. The antianxiety drugs also are used to produce skeletal muscle relaxation in various musculoskeletal disturbances, as anticonvulsant and antiepileptic drugs, and as sedatives and hypnotics. Diazepam and chlordiazepoxide are also used in alcohol withdrawal, where they prevent the withdrawal syndrome and aid in the treatment of alcoholism.

Adverse Effects

The most frequent side effects are drowsiness, confusion, ataxia, minor GI disturbances (nausea and constipation), and rashes. Patients should be warned that performance in operating machinery may be impaired, especially driving an automobile.

Elderly individuals are more susceptible to the CNS depressant effects of these drugs. Other adverse effects, which occur with less frequency, include menstrual irregularities, changes in libido, agranulocytosis, and changes in liver function.

Excessive use of benzodiazepines also has been associated with retrograde amnesia (interference

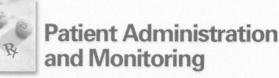

Patient Administration and Monitoring

Monitor vital signs and patient response during parenteral administration.

Explain to patient the common side effects: sedation, dry mouth, mental confusion, and GI disturbances.

Warn patient not to drive or attempt hazardous activities during treatment.

Warn patient not to take alcohol, barbiturates, and other CNS depressants unless authorized by his or her physician.

Instruct patients to report excessive sedation, mental disturbances, or loss of memory.

with memory while under the influence of drug) and psychotic changes. The psychiatric effects have involved, in some cases, aggressive behavior resulting in violent acts.

Drug Dependency

There is increasing recognition of the liability of patients to become dependent on the antianxiety drugs. This dependence takes the form of habituation rather than physical addiction. This problem occurs with patients who have been taking an antianxiety drug for a long time and for whom use is abruptly terminated. An important point to remember is that antianxiety drugs are not curative. They only allay the symptoms and help patients manage until the real cause of the anxiety is discovered and eliminated. Too often, antianxiety drugs are used as a crutch to avoid the discomforts of stress or personal unhappiness.

Abuse of the benzodiazepines on a regular basis, with larger than therapeutic doses, is associated with the development of physical addiction. The withdrawal syndrome is usually not as severe as that with the barbiturates. Also, the withdrawal reaction with the long-acting drugs may not occur until 7 to 10 days after use is ended. With long-acting benzodiazepines, it may also require 1 to 2 weeks to eliminate all of the drug and active metabolites from the body.

Cautions and Contraindications

Pregnancy

The benzodiazepines used for the treatment of anxiety have been designated FDA Pregnancy Category D, and should be avoided during pregnancy.

Drug Interactions

Additive effects occur with other CNS depressants, such as the barbiturates and in particular with alcohol. Several cases of coma and permanent brain damage have occurred after the simultaneous ingestion of diazepam and alcohol.

Cimetidine *(Tagamet)* inhibits the microsomal drug metabolizing enzymes and has been shown to inhibit the metabolism of diazepam and other benzodiazepines. When taken together, the effects of the benzodiazepines are increased and prolonged.

Use of Flumazenil *(Romazicon)*

Flumazenil is a benzodiazepine receptor antagonist that may be administered intravenously to reverse the depressant effects of the benzodiazepine drugs. It can be used in the management of benzodiazepine overdose to antagonize the effects of excessive CNS and respiratory depression. Flumazenil may also be used in cases where one of the benzodiazepines has been administered to induce anesthesia. Midazolam *(Versed)* is an injectable benzodiazepine anthesthetic (see Chapter 18) often used for induction of general anesthesia or for short medical procedures like endoscopy where the state of "conscious sedation" is desired. In this condition, the patient is awake but sedated to the point where unpleasant procedures can proceed without discomfort. Flumazenil is then used to reverse the effects of midazolam after the procedure is completed.

In individuals who are dependent on benzodiazepine drugs (chronic use or abuse), flumazenil may precipitate a withdrawal reaction and, in some cases, seizures.

Azapirones

The azapirones are a new class of antianxiety drugs that also produce antidepressant effects. The first and currently the only drug of this class drug on the market is buspirone *(BuSpar)*, which is primarily used as an antianxiety drug. Although the mechanism of action is still unclear, buspirone appears to produce its antianxiety effect by acting on serotonin receptors. Serotonin is a neurotransmitter in the brain involved in the regulation of anxiety. Anxiety is increased by high levels of serotonin. By binding to certain serotonin receptors, buspirone reduces the activity of serotonin and the level of anxiety.

In comparison to the benzodiazepines, buspirone does not possess sedative, anticonvulsant, or skeletal muscle relaxant properties. At present, the potential for tolerance and drug dependency appears very low. Common adverse effects include dizziness, lightheadedness, rash, and fatigue.

In general, buspirone is well tolerated and there appear to be few contraindications for its use. It serves as a suitable alternative to the benzodiazepines, especially when drug dependence and drug abuse problems with the benzodiazepines are an issue.

Chapter Review

Understanding Terminology

Answer the following questions in the spaces provided.

1. Explain the terms *psychoses* and *neuroses*. _____
   _____

2. What is the difference between fear and anxiety? _____
   _____

3. Define the term *tranquilization*. _____
   _____

Match the definition or description in the left column with the appropriate term in the right column.

___ **4.** A condition characterized by muscular rigidity, tremors, and disturbances of movement.

___ **5.** A major form of psychosis.

___ **6.** A condition causing individuals to have continuous body movement.

___ **7.** Drug-induced involuntary movements of the lips, jaw, tongue, and extremities.

___ **8.** Drugs used to treat schizophrenia.

___ **9.** Drugs used to calm and reduce excessive nervousness.

___ **10.** An inhibitory neurotransmitter in the CNS.

a. akathisia

b. antianxiety drugs

c. antipsychotic drugs

d. GABA

e. parkinsonism

f. tardive dyskinesia

g. schizophrenia

Acquiring Knowledge

Answer the following questions in the spaces provided.

1. List the two main types of psychosis. _____
   _____
   _____

2. What is the mechanism of action of the antipsychotic drugs? _____
   _____
   _____

3. List the three main classes of antipsychotic drugs and give an example of each. _____
   _____
   _____

4. What pharmacological properties do the phenothiazines possess, and how do these properties relate to clinical use and adverse effects?_____
   _____
   _____

5. Describe a few of the more serious adverse effects of the phenothiazine drugs. _____
   _____
   _____

6. List the major sites of action of the benzodiazepines and the clinical effects produced at each site.

_____

_____

7. Describe the clinical uses of diazepam *(Valium).* _____

_____

_____

8. List the adverse effects and drug interactions that may occur with the antianxiety drugs. _____

_____

_____

Applying Knowledge—On the Job

Use your critical thinking skills to answer the following questions in the spaces provided.

1. For each adult patient described, identify a suitable drug for treatment.

   a. Patient A has been diagnosed as manic-depressive and has been brought to the emergency room (ER) exhibiting extremely agitated behavior.

   _____

   b. Patient B is in intensive care following an episode of bizarre delusions and hallucinations.

   _____

   c. Patient C has suffered severe anxiety ever since being diagnosed with a terminal illness.

   _____

   d. Patient D is experiencing uncontrolled Tourette's syndrome.

   _____

   e. Patient E just presented at the ER with grand mal epileptic convulsions in progress.

   _____

   f. Patient F has open-heart surgery scheduled for tomorrow and is experiencing presurgical anxiety.

   _____

   g. Patient G is in alcohol withdrawal in the local Veterans Administration (VA) hospital detoxification unit.

   _____

2. Each of the following patients is suspected of having adverse effects to a drug prescribed for psychosis or neurosis. Identify the type of drug most likely involved in each case.

   a. Patient A has been experiencing dry mouth, constipation, and muscle spasms.

   _____

   b. Patient B presents with postural hypotension and complains of excessive drowsiness.

   _____

   c. Patient C complains of a rash, nausea, drowsiness, confusion, and poor coordination (ataxia).

   _____

   d. Patient D presents with high fever and appears unable to move.

   _____

Use the appropriate reference books to answer the following questions.

3. What is the standard dosage schedule for clozapine? _____

_____

_____

4. What is the standard dosage schedule for thioridazine when used for an adult with psychotic manifestations?

_____

_____

5. a. What is the standard dosage schedule for pimozide?

_____

b. Christopher weighs 66 pounds. What is the maximum daily dose for him?

_____

c. Jack weighs 198 pounds. What is the maximum daily dose for him?

_____

Internet Connection

Visit the **MedicineNet** website at (http://www.medicinenet.com). Under *Diseases and Treatments,* click on the letter "A" and find *Anxiety (Panic Disorder)* and read about this condition. Also click on the letter "P" and find *Psychosis* and learn about this condition and its treatment.

Additional Reading

Benzodiazepines: How safe are they. 1996. *Emergency Medicine* 28 (9):62.

Bottom, T. N. 2002. Neuroleptic malignant syndrome: A brief review. *Hospital Physician* 38 (3): 58.

Dossey, B. 1996. Help your patient break free from anxiety. *Nursing* 26 (10):52.

Dugue, M., and Neugroschl, J. 2002. Anxiety disorders: Helping patients regain stability and calm. *Geriatrics* 57 (8): 27.

Eison, M. S. 1990. Azapirones: Mechanism of action in anxiety and depression. *Drug Therapy Supplement* Aug:3.

Feighmer, J. P., and Boyer, W. F. 1990. Buspirone in the treatment of depression. *Drug Therapy Supplement* Aug:9.

Flaum, M. 1996. Making sense of schizophrenia. *Hospital Practice* 31 (11):51.

Katerndahl, D. A. 1995. Streamlining your approach to panic disorder. *Hospital Medicine* 31 (10):27.

ANTIDEPRESSANTS, PSYCHOMOTOR STIMULANTS, AND LITHIUM

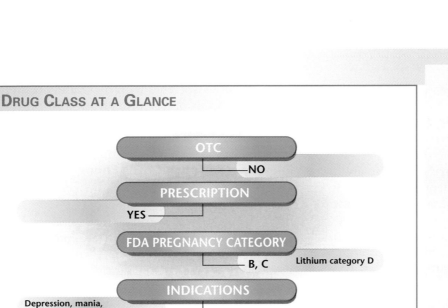

DRUG CLASS AT A GLANCE

OTC
— NO

PRESCRIPTION
YES —

FDA PREGNANCY CATEGORY
— B, C   Lithium category D

INDICATIONS
Depression, mania, and bipolar disorder

Key Terms

depression: mental state characterized by depressed mood, with feelings of frustration and hopelessness.

endogenous depression: a more serious depression that usually requires psychotherapy and drug treatment.

exogenous, or reactive, depression: depression caused by external factors; not as serious as endogenous depression.

lithium: an element similar to sodium that is used in the treatment of mania and bipolar mood disorder.

mania: mental state of excitement, hyperactivity, and excessive elevation of mood.

monoamine oxidase (MAO): enzyme that inactivates norepinephrine and serotonin.

Monoamine Theory of Mental Depression: theory that mental depression is caused by low brain levels of norepinephrine and serotonin (monoamines).

psychomotor stimulant: amphetamine or related drug that increases mental and physical activity.

CHAPTER FOCUS

This chapter describes the pharmacology of drugs used to treat depression and other mood disorders. It explains how these drugs alter the levels of certain neurotransmitters in the brain and how these actions relate to the Monoamine Theory of Mental Depression.

CHAPTER OBJECTIVES

After studying this chapter, you should be able to

- describe how MAO inhibitors, tricyclic antidepressants, and selective serotonin reuptake inhibitors act to provide relief from mental depression.

- name two MAO inhibitors and describe the adverse effects and dietary restrictions relating to these drugs.

- explain the main pharmacological effects produced by antidepressants and describe their adverse effects.

- discuss the use of psychomotor stimulants in the treatment of narcolepsy, hyperkinetic syndrome, and obesity.

- explain the use of lithium in mania and the adverse effects associated with its use.

TYPES OF DEPRESSION

There are several different types of depression. Depression that is caused by external factors (death or unemployment) is referred to as **exogenous, or reactive, depression.** Usually, there is a period of shock and depression, which is followed by a period of readjustment and a resolve that life must go on. In this sense, a reactive depression is self-limiting and usually does not require drug therapy. The love and understanding of family or friends support the individual through the crisis.

The second major type of depression is referred to as **endogenous depression.** Endogenous depression is frequently more serious and usually requires both psychotherapy and drug treatment. This type of depression originates from within the individual and may not be associated with easily recognized causes. Psychological disturbances and maladjustments or biochemical defects in the brain are thought to be involved. Episodes of endogenous depression may occur at intervals throughout one's lifetime.

In some cases of depression, there are alternate periods of hyperexcitability and elation known as mania. Individuals who experience these alternating cycles of depression and mania are classified as manic-depressive. Another term for this condition is bipolar mood disorder.

DRUGS USED TO TREAT DEPRESSION

An important advance in understanding depression occurred with the discovery that the levels of norepinephrine and serotonin (5-HT) in the brain can influence mental behavior. Low levels of norepinephrine and/or serotonin are associated with mental depression, while high levels of norepinephrine and/or serotonin may be involved in mania. This concept involving norepinephrine and serotonin (referred to chemically as monoamines) is known as the **Monoamine Theory of Mental Depression.**

Drugs that can increase the level of norepinephrine or serotonin in the brain are useful in the treatment of mental depression. They are referred to as antidepressants, or mood elevators. The major antidepressant drug classes include the monoamine oxidase inhibitors (MAOIs), the tricyclic antidepressants (TCAs), and the selective serotonin reuptake inhibitors (SSRIs).

The psychomotor stimulants are generally amphetamines or amphetamine-like drugs that produce a generalized CNS stimulation, usually increased wakefulness and alertness. These drugs are not true antidepressants and have limited therapeutic uses.

Lithium is referred to as a mood stabilizer and is used to treat individuals who experience wide shifts of mood, mania, or the alternating cycles of depression and mania (bipolar mood disorder).

Monoamine Oxidase Inhibitors

Monoamine oxidase (MAO) is an enzyme found in most body cells but particularly in the adrenergic nerve endings. The normal function of MAO is to break down norepinephrine and serotonin into metabolites that are then excreted by the kidneys. MAO prevents the buildup of excessive levels of norepinephrine and serotonin in the brain and other body tissue.

In mental depression, there appears to be an abnormal decrease in the levels of brain norepinephrine and serotonin. Drugs that inhibit, or block, MAO are called appropriately MAO inhibitors. By inhibiting MAO, these drugs decrease the amounts of norepinephrine and serotonin that are destroyed. Consequently, the MAO inhibitors permit the levels of norepinephrine and serotonin in the brain to increase. This increase is usually accompanied by clinical improvement of the depression. The MAO inhibitors require 2 to 4 weeks to produce their maximum effect. After a week or so of treatment, there is usually an improvement in appetite and sleep, followed by an elevation of mood and an overall improvement in mental state. These effects continue for approximately 2 weeks after termination of treatment.

The MAO inhibitors are involved in many drug interactions. Caution must be exercised if other drugs, especially other antidepressants, are administered during administration of MAO inhibitors and while MAO inhibitors remain in the system. Serious drug interactions can occur.

Dietary Restrictions

One of the main disadvantages of MAO inhibitor therapy is the dietary restrictions. Many foods contain a substance known as tyramine, which causes the release of norepinephrine from storage granules located inside the adrenergic nerve endings. When MAO is inhibited, tyramine may produce a massive release of norepinephrine, which can result in serious consequences, such as hypertensive crisis or cerebral stroke. Foods that normally contain tyramine include wine, beer, herring, and certain cheeses. In addition, certain sympathetic drugs used in the treatment of cold symptoms (decongestants and bronchodilators) interact with the MAO inhibitors, causing potentiation of the effects of the sympathetic agents. Patients receiving MAO inhibitors must be thoroughly instructed with regard to the foods and other medications to avoid. The most frequently used MAO inhibitors are listed in Table 14:1.

Adverse Effects

The MAO inhibitors, which are capable of producing a wide variety of adverse effects, appear to interfere with nerve transmission in the autonomic ganglia. Consequently, many of the adverse effects are similar to those produced by the ganglionic blockers. Side effects resulting from ganglionic blockade include postural hypotension, dry mouth, constipation, urinary retention, blurred vision, and impotency in males. The MAO inhibitors may produce central nervous system (CNS) stimulation resulting in insomnia, tremors,

TABLE 14:1	Monoamine Oxidase (MAO) Inhibitors	
DRUG (TRADE NAME)	**USUAL DAILY (MAINTENANCE) DOSE**
isocarboxazid (Marplan)	10–20 mg PO
phenylzine (Nardil)	15–75 mg PO
tranylcypromine (Parnate)	10–30 mg PO

or convulsions. In addition, they can produce a type of liver damage that may be fatal. Because of the high incidence of adverse effects, many physicians believe that these drugs should be reserved for patients who do not respond to other antidepressant drugs.

Tricyclic Antidepressants

Tricyclic antidepressant drugs are so named because of the characteristic triple-ring structure that they possess. Recently, some new antidepressants, which produce pharmacological effects similar to those of the tricyclics, have been introduced with two rings (bicyclics), four rings (tetracyclics), and others with quite different chemical structures (nontricyclics). The chemistry of these antidepressants is beyond the scope of this book. However, a simple method of classification involves the chemical substitutions (usually methyl groups) on the nitrogen molecule, which is present in all of the drugs. Most of the drugs can then be classified as being either secondary amines (two substitutions on the nitrogen) or tertiary amines (three substitutions on the nitrogen). Another interesting generalization is that secondary amines mainly increase brain levels of norepinephrine more than serotonin while the tertiary amines mainly increase brain levels of serotonin more than norepinephrine. The key to effective therapy is to identify which neurotransmitter should be increased in each patient; however, this step is not always easy. Frequently, several drugs must be tried with each patient before the most effective drug is found.

Mechanism of Action

The main action of the tricyclics and related antidepressant drugs is to block the reuptake of norepinephrine and serotonin back into the

TABLE 14:2   Tricyclic and Related Antidepressants

DRUG (TRADE NAME)	SEDATION	USUAL DAILY ORAL DOSAGE RANGE
Secondary Amines:		
amoxapine *(Asendin)*	Moderate	150–300 mg
desipramine *(Pertofrane)*	Moderate	75–200 mg
maprotiline *(Ludiomil)*	Moderate	75–225 mg
nortriptyline *(Aventyl)*	Moderate	50–150 mg
protriptyline *(Vivactil)*	None, may cause CNS stimulation	15–40 mg
Tertiary Amines:		
amitriptyline *(Elavil)*	Marked	75–200 mg
doxepin *(Sinequan)*	Marked	75–150 mg
imipramine *(Tofranil)*	Marked	75–200 mg
trimipramine *(Surmontil)*	Marked	100–300 mg

neuronal nerve endings. As a result there is an accumulation of these neurotransmitters in the synaptic clefts. This action restores the level of neuronal activity of norepinephrine and serotonin back toward normal, and alleviates the symptoms and dysfunction of depression.

The pharmacological actions occur within a few hours of administration. However, the full antidepressant effect requires 2 to 4 weeks to develop. Consequently, it is believed that tricyclics and related antidepressant drugs produce a long-term effect that is not yet completely understood. A suggestion is that these drugs may change the sensitivity of the adrenergic (norepinephrine) and serotonergic (serotonin) receptor sites, leading to an increase in the activity of these neurotransmitters, which is the desired neurotransmitter effect that relieves depression.

Pharmacological Actions

In addition to the antidepressant effect, the tricyclics and related drugs produce varying degrees of sedation, anticholinergic effects, and alpha-adrenergic blockade. The degree of sedation among the various drugs is compared in Table 14:2. Generally, the tertiary amines produce more sedation than do the secondary amines. Sedation is often a valuable effect, especially in patients who suffer insomnia along with their depression. The anticholinergic and alpha-blocking effects are associated with many of the side effects of these drugs.

Like the MAO inhibitors, the tricyclics also require 2 to 4 weeks for maximum effect. The antidepressant effects of the tricyclics also continue for approximately 2 weeks after drug administration is terminated. Therefore, extreme caution should be exercised when patients are switched from MAO inhibitors to tricyclics, or vice versa, to prevent drug interaction.

The tricyclics are considered to be among the most effective drugs for the treatment of endogenous depression. Compared to the MAO inhibitors, the tricyclics are safer and produce a lower incidence of adverse effects. Tricyclic and related antidepressants are listed in Table 14:2.

Adverse and Toxic Effects

The tricyclics possess significant anticholinergic activity, which is responsible for many of the common side effects. The side effects include dry mouth, constipation, urinary retention, rapid heartbeat, postural hypotension, blurred vision, and drowsiness. Like the MAO inhibitors, the tricyclics stimulate the CNS and may produce restlessness, tremors, convulsions, or mania.

In addition, the tricyclics may produce toxic effects in the heart and liver. In the heart, the effects can be detected by an electrocardiogram. Alterations in the T wave and ST segment, which may lead to serious cardiac arrhythmias, are the most common changes. In the liver, the tricyclics may cause an obstructive type of jaundice, which is relieved when drug treatment ends.

TABLE 14:3   Drug Interactions of Tricyclic Antidepressants

TRICYCLICS WITH	RESPONSE
Alcohol	Increased sedation
Amphetamines	Increased CNS stimulation
Anticholinergics, antihistamines	Dry mouth, constipation, urinary retention, blurred vision
Anticonvulsants	Increased possibility of seizures
Barbiturates	Increased metabolism of tricyclics (decreased effectiveness), increased sedation
MAO inhibitors	Increased CNS stimulation, hyperpyrexia, seizures
Phenothiazines	Anticholinergic effects, CNS depression

Drug Interactions

The tricyclic antidepressants interact with a number of other drugs, as indicated in Table 14:3.

Selective Serotonin Reuptake Inhibitors

Newer antidepressant drugs have been discovered that have pharmacological actions that are distinct from those of the tricyclics. These drugs are subdivided into two classes: the selective serotonin reuptake inhibitors (SSRIs) and several miscellaneous drugs that are usually classified as "atypical" antidepressants.

The SSRIs are a group of drugs that have a very selective action to block the reuptake and inactivation of serotonin in the brain. This causes an increase in serotonin activity in the brain that is believed to produce the antidepressant effect. Unlike the tricyclic antidepressants, the SSRIs have little action to block cholinergic, adrenergic, or histamine receptors. Consequently, SSRIs produce fewer side and adverse effects, and currently have become the most widely used antidepressant drugs. Fluoxetine (*Prozac*) was the first drug of this class to be introduced and will be discussed in more detail; the other SSRIs are listed in Table 14:4.

Fluoxetine is well absorbed after oral administration. It is metabolized in the liver into an active metabolite that has a half-life that ranges from several days to a week or more. The metabolites are primarily excreted in the urine. Fluoxetine has also been shown to be an inhibitor of the metabolism of other drugs such as anticoagulants and benzodiazepines.

TABLE 14:4   Selective Serotonin Reuptake Inhibitors

DRUG (TRADE NAME)	USUAL DAILY ORAL DOSAGE RANGE
citalopram *(Celexa)*	20–40 mg
escitalopram *(Lexapro)*	10 mg
fluoxetine *(Prozac)*	20–40 mg
fluvoxamine *(Luvox)*	50–200 mg
paroxetine *(Paxil)*	20–40 mg
sertraline *(Zoloft)*	50–200 mg

Clinical Indications

In the treatment of depression, fluoxetine has been shown to be as effective as the tricyclic drugs. Fluoxetine is also indicated for the treatment of obsessive-compulsive disorders (OCD). In this condition, individuals have repetitive and excessive impulses to perform some physical or behavioral action. These impulses can interfere with and disrupt the normal daily routine of work and living.

Adverse Effects

The most common side effects involve the central nervous system (CNS) and gastrointestinal (GI) tract. CNS effects include headache, nervousness, insomnia, and tremors. Gastrointestinal disturbances include nausea, diarrhea, dry mouth, and anorexia. Unlike the tricyclics that may cause weight gain, the SSRIs tend to cause weight loss and are being used by some physicians for this purpose.

The most common symptoms of overdosage include nausea, vomiting, agitation, restlessness, and other signs of CNS excitation; seizures have also been reported. Unlike many of the tricyclics, the SSRIs do not cause sedation.

Atypical Antidepressants

The atypical antidepressant drugs also produce effects that are distinctly different than the tricyclics. Like the SSRIs, they have little effect in blocking cholinergic, adrenergic, or histamine receptors. The atypical drugs affect serotonin and other neurotransmitters such as norepinephrine and dopamine.

The atypical drugs include bupropion (*Wellbutrin*), which is associated with a high incidence of seizures; nefazodone (*Serzone*) and trazodone (*Desyrel*), which may cause sedation and hypotension; and venlafaxine (*Effexor*), whose pharmacologic effects are most similar to those of SSRIs.

Psychomotor Stimulants

The **psychomotor stimulants** include the amphetamines and other closely related drugs, which are really not classified as antidepressants. Their role in the treatment of depression is extremely limited. Because of the delayed therapeutic effects of MAO inhibitors and tricyclics, psychomotor stimulants are occasionally used during the first few weeks of treatment to elevate mood and increase psychomotor activity.

Amphetamines are also used to treat narcolepsy (uncontrolled tendency to fall asleep) and hyperkinesis in children. Amphetamines stimulate the reticular formation, which increases wakefulness and alertness and reduces the number of attacks of narcolepsy. In hyperkinetic children, amphetamines increase alertness and attention span, which are important in improving learning ability. Also, amphetamines seem to calm down the hyperactivity. This result is opposite to what would be expected and is referred to as a paradoxical effect. The reason for this effect is not fully understood.

In addition to mental stimulation, amphetamines stimulate motor, or physical, activity. This stimulation causes individuals who are trying to delay fatigue and stay awake to use amphetamines inappropriately. Amphetamine

TABLE 14:5	Psychomotor Stimulant Drugs
DRUG (TRADE NAME)	**COMMON DAILY DOSAGE RANGE**
amphetamine	10–60 mg
dexmethylphenidate (*Focalin*)	5–20 mg
dextroamphetamine (*Dexedrine*)	5–30 mg
methamphetamine (*Desoxyn*)	5–20 mg
methylphenidate (*Ritalin*)	10–30 mg

stimulation of the CNS is also associated with a decrease in appetite, and weight reduction presents another area of amphetamine abuse. Because the therapeutic benefits of amphetamines are low and the abuse potential high, there are very few situations where use of amphetamines is warranted.

Mechanism of Action

The amphetamines stimulate the CNS by increasing the activity of norepinephrine and dopamine in the brain. Amphetamines increase neurotransmitter activity by several different mechanisms. They act directly to stimulate norepinephrine and dopamine receptors, they stimulate the release of norepinephrine and dopamine from the nerve endings, and they inhibit the reuptake of these neurotransmitters back into the nerve endings. These actions produce CNS stimulation and an elevation of mood. Psychomotor stimulants are listed in Table 14:5, but it should be emphasized that the psychomotor stimulants are not true antidepressant drugs and their use as such is extremely limited.

Amphetamines have the disadvantage of producing drug tolerance and drug dependence. The amphetamines are among the leading "street drugs" that are abused and illegally marketed. Drug abuse of amphetamines is discussed in Chapter 15.

Adverse and Toxic Effects

The psychomotor stimulants increase the activity of the sympathetic nervous system, producing dry mouth, rapid heartbeat, increased blood pressure, restlessness, and insomnia. Toxic doses may produce severe agitation and a paranoid type of psychosis.

Antimanic Drugs

Lithium is the most commonly used drug for the treatment of mania. It is often used in combination with antidepressant drugs in the manic-depressive or bipolar form of psychosis. In mania, there appears to be an excess of norepinephrine and possibly other monoamines (opposite to the situation in depression) in the brain, which produces excitement, hyperactivity, and excessive elevations of mood. **Mania** is characterized by periods of hyperactivity and excitement combined with excessive elevations of mood. Manic individuals are usually very talkative, but their thoughts and ideas are most often unrealistic. Lithium appears to reduce the hyperactivity and the excitement and also allows better organization of thought patterns.

Mechanism of Action

Lithium is an element similar in chemical properties to sodium. The body utilizes lithium as if it were sodium. Both lithium (Li^+) and sodium (Na^+) exist in body fluids as charged particles, or ions. However, whereas Na^+ is normally required for conduction of nerve impulses, Li^+ interferes with nerve conduction. As a result, there is a decrease in the excitability of nerve tissue.

Lithium also appears to increase the reuptake of norepinephrine and dopamine, and also decrease the release of these neurotransmitters. Both of these actions reduce the amount of norepinephrine and dopamine that is free to produce effects in the synaptic clefts. These effects are opposite to those produced by the tricyclic antidepressants, which further strengthens the validity of the Monoamine Theory of Mental Depression.

Pharmacokinetics

Lithium is administered as a salt, lithium carbonate, in the form of capsules (*Eskalith*) or controlled release and slow-release tablets (*Eskalith CR, Lithobid*). Usually 1 to 2 weeks of treatment is required before therapeutic effects are observed.

Lithium can be an extremely toxic drug. Therefore, blood levels are periodically measured to prevent the development of excessive levels of lithium in the body. Lithium and sodium ions compete with each other for renal elimination. Adequate sodium intake is necessary for proper urinary excretion of lithium. Decreased sodium intake and hyponatremia (low sodium levels) promote the retention of lithium and can lead to toxicity.

Patient Administration and Monitoring

Explain to patient that therapeutic drug effects may require 1 or 2 weeks of treatment.

Explain to patient that side effects are common and usually include nausea and tremors.

Explain to patient that lithium is a salt and that increased thirst and frequency of urination are common.

Instruct patient on the importance of adequate fluid and sodium intake.

Instruct patient to report excessive nausea or vomiting, excessive CNS stimulation, dizziness, abnormal muscle movements, low blood pressure, ringing in the ears.

Explain to patient that periodic drug blood levels may be required.

Adverse and Toxic Effects

Side effects are common with lithium, even at therapeutic doses. Initially, most patients experience some nausea or tremors that usually disappear with continued treatment. With overdose, vomiting, diarrhea, drowsiness, loss of equilibrium, ringing in the ears, and frequent urination are common. At toxic levels, the heart and kidneys may be damaged, leading to the development of cardiac arrhythmias or nephritis. Therefore, extreme caution is observed when treating cardiac or renal patients. In addition, lithium occasionally produces disturbances of the thyroid gland, and it is therefore contraindicated in patients with an existing thyroid condition. In acute overdoses, muscle fasciculations, convulsions, and circulatory collapse leading to death are possible. Treatment is aimed at increasing the excretion of lithium by forcing fluids and increasing the intake of sodium.

Cautions and Contraindications

Pregnancy

Lithium has been designated FDA Pregnancy Category D and therefore should not be used during pregnancy.

Chapter Review

Understanding Terminology

Answer the following questions in the spaces provided.

1. Differentiate between mania and depression. _____
    _____

2. Explain the Monoamine Theory of Mental Depression. _____
    _____

3. List the two main types of depression and define each. _____
    _____
    _____

Acquiring Knowledge

Answer the following questions in the spaces provided.

1. What neurotransmitters are deficient in mental depression? _____

2. How do the MAO inhibitors increase the levels of norepinephrine and serotonin in the brain?
    _____
    _____

3. Explain the mechanism of action of the tricyclic antidepressants. _____
    _____
    _____

4. What are the main pharmacological differences between the secondary and tertiary amine antidepressants?
    _____
    _____

5. What adverse effects are associated with the tricyclic antidepressants? __
    _____
    _____

6. How do the selective serotonin reuptake inhibitors produce their antidepressant effect?
    _____
    _____

7. What are the adverse effects of the selective serotonin reuptake inhibitors? __
    _____
    _____

8. What is lithium, and when is its use indicated? _____
    _____

9. Explain the mechanism of action of lithium. _____
    _____
    _____

10. List the adverse effects of lithium. _____

Applying Knowledge—On the Job

Use your critical thinking skills to answer the following questions in the spaces provided.

1. Assume that one of your duties in the mental health clinic where you work is to note for each patient any contraindications or potential drug interactions for current medications. You also assist with drug overdose emergencies.

   a. Patient A has been diagnosed with endogenous depression. He's been taking *Elavil* for several weeks, but it makes him excessively drowsy, so his medication is being changed to an MAO inhibitor. The patient also is taking a prescription decongestant for allergies. What should you note on the patient's chart regarding adverse effects and drug interactions?

   _____

   _____

   b. Patient B appeared at the clinic suffering from a possible overdose of lithium. She appeared drowsy and complained of dizziness and ringing in her ears. What should be done to help rid her body of the excess lithium?

   _____

   _____

2. Joe works as a volunteer on a depression hotline. What type of depression is experienced by each of the following anonymous callers?

   a. Caller A says he has no particular reason to feel down, but he's feeling really depressed anyway. He says he gets down-and-out a lot but it doesn't usually get quite this bad. He wonders if there's any kind of treatment or drug for how he feels.

   _____

   _____

   b. Caller B says she's usually a happy-go-lucky sort of person, but she's been feeling depressed since her mother died last month. She thinks she should be over the worst of her grief by now and wonders if she should get counseling.

   _____

   _____

3. Janet has just been prescribed lithium for her manic states. What should be included in her medication counseling?

   _____

   _____

4. Sue has called your office for advice. She has been taking *Elavil* for depression for about 8 months. She has a severe cold and purchased the decongestant *Sudafed*. When she got home, she read the warnings on the back of the box. It warns not to take this medication if you are taking MAO inhibitors for depression. Can she take this medication?

   _____

   _____

5. Robyn's physician has just prescribed *Nardil* for severe depression. What foods does Robyn need to avoid and why?

   _____

   _____

Internet Connection

Visit the **MedicineNet** website at (http://www.medicinenet.com), under *Diseases and Treatments* click on the letter "D" and read the information about *Depression*. Also under *Diseases and Treatments* click on the letter "B" and read the information on *Bipolar Disorder*. Under the *Pharmacy and Drugs* heading, you can select the first letter of any of the drugs used to treat depression for additional pharmacologic information.

Additional Reading

Buffum, M. D., and Buffum, J. C. 1997. The psychopharmacologic treatment of depression in elders. *Geriatric Nursing* 18 (4):144.

Kurlowicz, L. H. 1997. Nursing standard of practice protocol: Depression in elderly patients. *Geriatric Nursing* 18 (5):192.

Miller, C. A. 1997. Keeping up with new developments in antidepressants. *Geriatric Nursing* 18 (4):180.

Reynolds, C. F. 1996. Depression: Making the diagnosis and using SSRIs in the older patient. *Geriatrics* 51 (10):28.

Sable, J. A, Dunn, L. B., and Zisook, S. 2002. Hate-life depression. *Geriatrics* 57 (2):18.

Travis, L. A., and Lyness, J. M. 2002. The psychiatric consultant: Minor depression. *Geriatrics* 57 (5):65.

15

PSYCHOTOMIMETIC DRUGS OF ABUSE

This chapter describes the pharmacology of the psychotomimetic drugs of abuse. It explains the main effects produced by these drugs and how abuse can lead to drug dependency and other serious complications.

CHAPTER OBJECTIVES

After studying this chapter, you should be able to

- list the psychotomimetic drugs of abuse and their main pharmacological effects.
- describe the development of tolerance and drug dependency associated with psychotomimetic drugs.
- explain the consequences of drug dependency and intoxication and discuss the treatments that are usually administered.

Key Terms

cannabinoid: pharmacologically active substance obtained from the marijuana plant.

cross-tolerance: drug tolerance common to similar drugs; doses of one drug taken shortly after another drug produce decreased effects.

dependency: requirement of larger doses to prevent onset of withdrawal symptoms.

designer drug: chemically altered form of an approved drug that produces similar effects and that is sold illegally.

flashback: phenomenon occurring long after the use of LSD in which the hallucinogenic effects are relived in some type of memory flash.

hallucinogenic drug: a drug or plant substance that produces sensory distortions.

hashish: resin from the marijuana plant that contains higher levels of THC.

psychotomimetic drug: drug or substance that can induce psychic and behavioral patterns characteristic of a psychosis.

synesthesia: distortion of sensory perception; usually associated with the use of LSD.

tetrahydrocannabinol (THC):   active ingredient of the marijuana plant.

tolerance: requirement of larger doses to be consumed in order to obtain the desired effects.

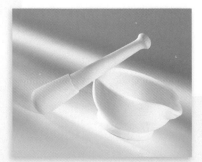

INTRODUCTION

The widespread abuse of psychoactive drugs has become an unfortunate reality in today's society. Whereas most drugs are used to alleviate disease and human suffering, a few drugs are abused for their mind-altering effects. Although they may provide pleasure, they are not solutions to life's problems and can cause other health or social problems.

Initially, the use of a psychoactive drug can provide the novelty of an experience that is often interpreted as pleasurable and exciting. After initial experimentation, many individuals realize the dangers of continued drug consumption and avoid further abuse. For other individuals, drug abuse appears to provide "the answer" for which they have been searching. With continued drug use, some individuals focus all of their attention and available resources on obtaining and consuming illicit drugs. They begin to feel that as long as they have the drug, nothing else really matters or is important. As drug abuse continues, **tolerance** develops and larger doses must be consumed in order to attain previous drug effects. The euphoria and good feelings that were the reason for abusing the drug are no longer experienced. As drug **dependency** develops, consumption of larger doses is necessary to prevent the onset of psychological and physical withdrawal symptoms, forming a vicious cycle from which it is difficult to escape without professional help and a major personal decision to avoid further drug abuse.

This chapter examines the pharmacology of the common drugs of abuse. The narcotic analgesics and barbiturate drugs were presented in other chapters. The remaining drugs of abuse have few therapeutic uses and do not form a distinct drug class. Psychoactive drugs of abuse can be divided into the lysergic acid diethylamide (LSD-type) hallucinogens; the psychomotor stimulants, which include the amphetamines, cocaine, and related designer drugs; and a miscellaneous group of drugs that includes phencyclidine (PCP) and marijuana.

LSD-Type Hallucinogens

Lysergic acid diethylamide (LSD) is a synthetic drug that was first prepared in 1938. It remains one of the most potent hallucinogenic drugs yet discovered. LSD and other **hallucinogenic, or psychotomimetic, drugs** produce similar pharmacological effects. At one time, LSD and other hallucinogenic drugs were investigated for the treatment of alcoholism and mental illness. Currently, these drugs have no therapeutic uses and are classified as Schedule I drugs under the Controlled Substances Act. The prototype of this group is LSD, and it will be discussed in greater detail.

Mechanism of Action

How LSD produces its hallucinogenic effects is not exactly known. Recent evidence suggests that LSD and the other hallucinogens stimulate serotonin receptors in certain areas of the brain, which disrupts normal brain activity and contributes to the sensory distortions and hallucinogenic effects.

Pharmacological Effects

Lysergic acid diethylamide (LSD) is readily absorbed from the gastrointestinal tract. The average hallucinogenic dosage ranges from 50–100 μg. The psychic effects of LSD usually last about 12 hours, with peak effects occurring 1 to 2 hours after oral administration.

Common psychotomimetic effects include sensory distortions and pseudohallucinations. Moving objects appear to be followed by a stream of color or appear as vividly colored geometric patterns. **Synesthesia** may occur, where individuals perceive they are "seeing sounds" or hearing visual images. Perceptual distortions in the size of objects and parts of the body are common. Feelings of separation of part of the body, or loss of a part of the body, or failure to recognize a part as one's own body also occur.

In addition to the psychotomimetic effects, hallucinogenic drugs are potent stimulants of the central nervous system. Piloerection, pupillary dilation, and increased neuromuscular reflex activity can be observed. Cardiovascular effects include tachycardia and increased blood pressure.

NOTE TO THE HEALTH CARE PROFESSIONAL

LSD and similar hallucinogens produce a sequence of dose-related effects that have been divided into three phases:

- The somatic phase occurs initially after absorption, and it consists of CNS stimulation and autonomic changes that are predominantly sympathomimetic in nature.
- The sensory phase is characterized by sensory distortions and pseudohallucinations (the user knows the hallucinations are not real), which are the effects desired by the drug user.
- The psychic phase signals a maximum drug effect. Disruption of thought processes, depersonalization, and true hallucinations (the user believes the hallucinations are real) and psychotic episodes may occur. Experiencing this phase would be considered a "bad trip."

Lysergic acid diethylamide is also associated with the occurrence of flashbacks. A **flashback,** which can occur at any time after exposure to LSD, is characterized by many of the psychotomimetic effects of LSD without readministration of the drug. Flashbacks often occur after use of other psychoactive drugs, which somehow trigger flashback episodes.

Tolerance and Physical Dependency

Tolerance develops rapidly to the psychotomimetic effects of LSD, usually within a few doses of continuous use. Also, **cross-tolerance** exists between LSD and the other drugs of this group, so subsequent doses of one drug taken shortly after another drug produce decreased effects. The tolerance is not accompanied by physical dependency, and abrupt discontinuance after chronic use does not precipitate withdrawal symptoms.

Intoxication and Treatment

The signs and symptoms of LSD intoxication include elevated body temperature and blood pressure, tachycardia, hyperreflexia, dilated pupils, anxiety, hallucinations, and psychotic behavior. LSD has a high therapeutic index, and virtually no known causes of death have been related to overdose toxicity by LSD alone. Consequently, treatment is aimed at protecting patients from accidental injury until the drug effects subside. Individuals should be placed in a quiet, nonthreatening environment and given reassurance that everything will be all right. Benzodiazepine antianxiety agents or barbiturates can be used for their sedative effects. This approach to treatment is considered standard therapy for most hallucinogenic drug intoxication.

Other LSD-Type Hallucinogens

In addition to LSD, two other categories of drugs produce similar effects.

Tryptamine Derivatives

Psilocybin and N,N-dimethyltryptamine (DMT) are obtained from natural sources. Psilocybin is found in the *Psilocybe* mushroom species, which have been eaten ceremonially by native cultures for centuries. Psilocybin is converted to an active metabolite, psilocin, which is believed to be responsible for the majority of psychotomimetic effects. The hallucinogenic dose of psilocybin is approximately 25 mg, which produces effects lasting 3 to 6 hours.

N,N-dimethyltryptamine (DMT) occurs in many plants and has been used as a snuff by various Native American cultures. It is ineffective when taken orally; it must be inhaled or administered parenterally. The usual hallucinogenic dose given by injection is 1 mg per kg of body weight, which produces psychotomimetic effects lasting approximately 1 hour.

Phenethylamine Derivatives

Mescaline and 2,5-dimethoxy-4-methylamphetamine (DOM) are phenethylamine derivatives similar in structure to norepinephrine and amphetamine. Central nervous system stimulation and sympathomimetic effects are prominent features of both drugs. Mescaline, found in the peyote cactus, is among the least potent of the hallucinogenic drugs. It is readily absorbed from the gastrointestinal (GI) tract and produces effects that last about 6 hours. DOM, or STP ("Serenity, Tranquility, Peace"), is a synthetic compound. The usual hallucinogenic dose is 3–5 mg, which produces effects lasting 6 to 8 hours.

PSYCHOMOTOR STIMULANTS

Amphetamine and cocaine are potent CNS stimulants that are widely used. At higher doses, these drugs produce prominent psychotomimetic effects. The central actions and pharmacological effects of these drugs are very similar. A number of drugs related to the amphetamines are known as "designer drugs." A **designer drug** is a slightly altered derivative of an approved drug, such as amphetamines or narcotics. The effects are similar to those of the approved drug, but they are usually more intense and mind-altering. Designer drugs are synthesized by illegal laboratories and sold "on the street" for great profit.

The major actions of amphetamines and cocaine occur within the brain. Both increase the amounts of norepinephrine (NE) and dopamine (DA) within the brain. The increased levels of NE produce prominent peripheral and central sympathomimetic effects. The higher levels of DA influence behavioral activity, particularly that involving the limbic system. The behavioral actions account for the ability of these drugs to act as potent reinforcers of behavior. This reinforcement acts to compel drug abusers to take the drug repeatedly.

Amphetamines

A number of drugs are referred to as "amphetamines." These include amphetamine itself, dextroamphetamine, methamphetamine ("speed"), and a few related drugs. The amphetamines are basically sympathomimetic amines with chemical structures very similar to NE and DA. There are, however, some important pharmacokinetic differences between the drugs and the neurotransmitters. The structures of norepinephrine and amphetamines are compared in Figure 15:1.

Pharmacokinetics

In comparison to NE and DA, the amphetamines are lipid soluble and are not affected by the enzymes and inactivation mechanisms that quickly terminate the effects of the neurotransmitters. Consequently, the amphetamines are well absorbed orally, readily pass into the brain, and produce effects lasting

Comparison of the Structures of Norepinephrine and Amphetamine

Norepinephrine

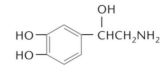

Amphetamine

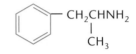

several hours. Intravenous injection of amphetamines, especially methamphetamine ("speed"), has become a significant problem. Large amounts are often injected over several days, and during these sustained high-dosage bouts, the psychotomimetic effects of the drug frequently occur.

Pharmacological Effects

Abuse of amphetamines is based on the action of these drugs to influence physical performance and psychological mood. After oral administration, people feel more confident, alert, talkative, and generally hyperactive. Amphetamines increase endurance and reduce feelings of fatigue. Following intravenous administration, users experience the initial "rush," which has been described as orgasmic. The euphoria and excitement produced by amphetamines are important reinforcing properties on behavior. Compulsive behavior drives users to repeat the drug again and again in order to maintain the good feelings, the "reward."

After discontinuance of the drug, profound sleep usually occurs. Upon awakening, users experience disagreeable, depressed feelings ("crash") and want to resume drug taking immediately.

Initially, the hyperactivity may stimulate users to be more industrious and diligent, but eventually, performance deteriorates. Activity may continue for hours, but it may also become compulsive and highly stereotyped. Users gets "hung up" doing one thing over and over again. As amphetamine usage increases and dosages become larger, the psychotomimetic effects become apparent and can lead to psychotic behavior. Amphetamine psychosis is similar to paranoid schizophrenia. Although users may feel elated, they appear glum, depressed, and withdrawn. Suspicion, hostility, and aggressive behavior may lead to violent acts. Sensory illusions, auditory and visual hallucinations, and distortions of body image may occur. Psychosis can occur after only a few doses, but it usually occurs after chronic use of high doses.

Tolerance and Dependency

Tolerance to amphetamines, especially after prolonged intravenous administration, develops rapidly, and larger amounts are usually administered with continuous use. Tolerance develops to the euphoria and to the appetite suppressant effect. Abrupt discontinuance of amphetamines after chronic use results in mild to moderate physical withdrawal symptoms. Withdrawal effects appear to be predominantly psychological in nature and include extreme fatigue, mental depression, and a strong desire for the drug.

Intoxication and Treatment

A number of adverse effects and potential complications are caused by overstimulation of the sympathetic and central nervous systems. The psychotomimetic effects of the paranoid psychosis have already been described. Sympathetic stimulation produces hyperthermia and profuse sweating, respiratory difficulties, tremors, and various cardiovascular effects. Intense cardiovascular stimulation results in tachycardia, arrhythmias, and hypertension, which may contribute to intracranial hemorrhage and sudden death. After prolonged intravenous use, severe fatigue and exhaustion may be followed by convulsion, coma, and death. Chronic intoxication can produce all of these conditions, and, in addition, there may be extreme weight loss from lack of appetite.

Treatment of amphetamine intoxication is aimed at supporting vital functions and providing symptomatic therapy. Acidifying the urine will increase excretion. Adrenergic blockers and vasodilators can be administered to control excessive sympathetic and cardiovascular stimulation. Diazepam is generally preferred to control seizures and can also be used for sedation when necessary. Highly agitated individuals can be given antipsychotic drugs, which reduce psychotic symptoms by antagonizing the actions of DA and NE.

Cocaine

Cocaine was isolated from the leaves of *Erythroxylon coca* in 1855. Native Indians of South America have chewed coca leaves for centuries to ward off fatigue and hunger. In the late nineteenth century, cocaine was considered a "wonder drug" and advocated for treatment of numerous medical conditions, including morphine and alcohol addiction. After recognizing the potential dangers of cocaine abuse, the government enacted legislation in 1914 that restricted and controlled the use of cocaine. Cocaine was "rediscovered" in the 1970s, when the phenomenon of recreational drug use dramatically increased. In recent years, the widespread abuse of cocaine has generated major social and medical problems.

The pharmacological effects of cocaine are similar to those of the amphetamines. However, cocaine possesses a number of features that make it more popular with drug users. Cocaine is prepared in different forms, that can be administered by a variety of methods. The intensity and duration of drug effects are highly dependent on the preparation used and the route of administration.

Preparations of Cocaine

Cocaine base is extracted from coca leaves and converted to a water-soluble hydrochloride salt. It is in this form that cocaine is exported and adulterated with other substances, such as sugars and local anesthetics. Cocaine hydrochloride can be administered orally, intranasally, and intravenously. It is destroyed, however, by the high temperatures generated during smoking. Several methods exist for conversion of cocaine hydrochloride back into free-base (without hydrochloride) form. Free-base cocaine possesses greater lipid solubility and a lower melting point. Consequently, it can be smoked, which allows almost instantaneous delivery of cocaine to the brain in a concentrated bolus. The intensity of effect is greatly increased. One form of free-base cocaine, "crack," is prepared by an alkalinization-water process that forms a crystalline, rocklike substance that makes a cracking sound when it is smoked.

Pharmacokinetics

Cocaine is absorbed from the intestinal tract and from all mucous membranes. Pharmacological effects are delayed (30 to 60 minutes) and are less intense after oral administration, compared to other routes. Drug effects are detectable 3 to

5 minutes after intranasal administration, peak in 20 to 30 minutes, and last 60 to 90 minutes. Plasma levels measured an hour or more after oral or intranasal administration are comparable; however, it is the concentration of cocaine in the brain that is important. Intranasal administration provides higher drug levels in the brain within a shorter period of time; therefore, the effects are more intense. Intravenous injection and smoking both provide immediate effects of high intensity but of shorter duration. Peak effects by these routes occur in minutes and last about 20 minutes. Smoking cocaine is the most popular route of administration; it is more convenient than making injections, and there is less nasal irritation (and no septal perforation) than when taken intranasally. The half-life of cocaine is about 30 to 40 minutes; the metabolites of cocaine are excreted in the urine.

Pharmacological Effects

Cocaine is a powerful CNS stimulant, producing marked euphoria, self-confidence, and heightened feelings of physical and mental ability. These ego-reinforcing effects can lead to delusions of grandeur, which have been referred to as "cocainomania." The positive psychological effects are followed by dysphoria, anxiety, and feelings of depression as the drug effect wears off, creating a desire in users to repeat the drug again, which often leads to prolonged binges where cocaine use becomes compulsive. This is similar to the situation that develops with amphetamines. However, the duration of action after smoking or injecting cocaine is only 20 to 30 minutes, compared to several hours with amphetamines. Consequently, cocaine must be administered much more frequently in order to maintain the good feelings. This frequency contributes to the reinforcing properties of cocaine on behavior and leads to drug dependency.

As dosages of cocaine are increased, CNS stimulation becomes excessive. Tremors and myoclonic jerks develop and may progress to clonic-tonic convulsions. Peripheral sympathomimetic effects increase, and cardiovascular stimulation resulting in hypertension, tachycardia, and arrhythmias may progress to serious complications and sudden death. A toxic psychosis, similar to that caused by amphetamines, can develop after high dosages or prolonged use. Symptoms include hostility, social withdrawal, paranoia, hallucinations, delusions, and violent behavior.

Tolerance and Dependency

The question of tolerance to cocaine is not entirely clear. Acute tolerance does develop to the sympathomimetic and psychological effects when cocaine is used frequently within short periods of time. Before widespread abuse in the 1970s, cocaine was considered a relatively safe drug that did not cause physical dependency. However, with the technique of free basing, where higher doses are administered frequently on a daily basis, the evidence suggests that cocaine does produce some degree of physical dependency. There is a mistaken perception by many that substances that only cause psychological dependency are generally safe. Cocaine is one of the most psychologically habituating drugs known, and individuals who become dependent on it suffer fates similar to those of individuals addicted to alcohol, narcotics, and other physically addicting drugs. The symptoms of withdrawal from cocaine include craving for the drug, dysphoria, irritability, anxiety, depression, tremors, eating and sleeping disturbances, and thoughts of suicide.

Intoxication and Treatment

Depending on the dosage and time since administration, users may be euphoric and excited or dysphoric, anxious, and depressed. After prolonged binges of cocaine use, extreme fatigue, exhaustion, hyperthermia, seizures, and coma may occur. The most serious effects of acute cocaine poisoning are in the CNS and cardiovascular system, leading to convulsions and cardiac complications. Tachycardia and arrhythmias may precipitate ventricular fibrillation and sudden death. CNS stimulation is followed by severe CNS depression, resulting in respiratory failure and cardiovascular collapse. Individuals with underlying cardiovascular disease are at greater risks of complication and sudden death. The psychotic reactions that usually occur after prolonged use are similar to those observed with amphetamines.

Treatment of cocaine intoxication is similar to that for amphetamine poisoning, supportive and symptomatic. Diazepam is useful to control seizures and for sedation. Since the half-life of cocaine is short, the greatest danger in acute intoxication occurs within the first few hours. Antipsychotic drugs, such as chlorpromazine and haloperidol, are useful because of their multiple effects to antagonize DA and NE.

Treatment of cocaine dependency usually involves education of individuals to the dangers of continued use and behavioral modification to control compulsive desires for the drug. A newer approach to control cocaine dependency is the use of tricyclic antidepressants (TCAs). Treatment with TCAs has been reported to lessen the euphoric effects of cocaine and to reduce cravings for continued use of the drug.

Designer Drugs

Several of the designer drugs are derivatives of the amphetamines. These include methylenedioxyamphetamine (MDA, or the "love drug"), methylenedioxymethamphetamine (MDMA, "Adam," or "Ecstasy"), and methylenedioxyethamphetamine (MDEA, or "Eve"). These drugs are usually taken orally.

Pharmacological Effects

These amphetamine derivatives produce CNS stimulation, euphoria, and visual distortions. Larger doses produce anxiety, panic, excessive sympathetic stimulation, and paranoia. Chronic abuse often produces hallucinations and psychotic disturbances resembling schizophrenia.

Treatment

Treatment of intoxication with these drugs is similar to that for amphetamines and cocaine.

MISCELLANEOUS PSYCHOTOMIMETIC DRUGS

Phencyclidine

Phencyclidine (PCP) was investigated for use as a general anesthetic in humans. However, because of a high incidence of emergence delirium, it was dropped from further consideration for this purpose. Phencyclidine is still used in veterinary practice to immobilize primates. Because of its psychotomimetic effects, the drug has gained wide popularity as a drug of abuse.

Mechanism of Action

The pharmacology of PCP is complex. Phencyclidine produces multiple pharmacological actions, including CNS stimulation, CNS depression, peripheral autonomic effects, analgesia, and anticonvulsant activity. The psychotomimetic effect that occurs at nonanesthetic doses is varied and is the result of mixed CNS stimulant and depressant actions exerted at multiple brain sites. Phencyclidine interacts with several neurotransmitters, and these interactions are known to account for many of the actions of PCP.

Pharmacokinetics

Phencyclidine can be administered by various routes, including inhalation (smoking), oral, insufflation (snorting), and intravenous injection. Like other anesthetics, PCP is lipid soluble and widely distributed to peripheral tissues, where it accumulates in fat, which accounts for the prolonged duration of action.

Pharmacological Effects

The effects of PCP vary significantly with increasing dosage. At low doses, there is CNS stimulation, euphoria, and sympathetic stimulation similar to the effects produced by amphetamines. With increasing dosage, thought processes become disoriented and speech is slurred. This is followed by paresthesia, slowed reflexes, and ataxia. Disorders of body image are common, with both elongation and shrinkage of extremities. This state may last 4 to 6 hours, after which a depressive state occurs, along with a paranoid behavior pattern. It may take several days before the affected individual returns to normal. In acute toxicity, individuals exhibit marked anxiety, agitation, hallucinations, and occasionally violent behavior. This may progress to dysphoria, catatonia, muscle rigidity, convulsions, nystagmus, hypertensive crisis, coma, and death.

Treatment of Intoxication

Initial treatment is similar to that with LSD-type hallucinogens: a nonstimulating environment and reassurance. Propranolol to control excess sympathetic stimulation and diazepam for sedation may be administered when deemed necessary. Acidification of the urine to pH 5.5 will increase excretion of PCP and shorten the half-life.

Tolerance and Dependency

Tolerance develops fairly rapidly to the behavioral and toxic effects of PCP during chronic use. PCP has been demonstrated to be a positive reinforcer of behavior. This indicates the development of some degree of dependency. The drug dependency appears to be predominantly psychological rather than physical. Withdrawal symptoms, when present, include a craving for the drug, increased anxiety, and mental depression.

Marijuana

The source of marijuana is a species of hemp plant, *Cannabis sativa*. The flowering tops of the female plant are particularly rich in a sticky resin in which the psychoactive principals are found in the highest concentrations. The resin can be extracted from the plant and is known as **hashish.** Marijuana generally refers to the dried, chopped plant (seeds, flowers, twigs, leaves), which is smoked like tobacco. The pharmacologically active substances in marijuana are compounds referred to as **cannabinoids.** The major active cannabinoid present in the plant is **tetrahydrocannabinol (THC).** The resin, hashish, usually contains about 10 percent THC.

Pharmacokinetics

The cannabinoids are highly lipid-soluble compounds. The most common route of administration of marijuana is smoking, which provides bioavailability of 10 to 25 percent, depending on the efficiency of smoking technique. Effects after smoking begin within 5 to 15 minutes, peak at 30 to 90 minutes, and generally last 3 to 4 hours. Tetrahydrocannabinol is widely distributed throughout the body, and the highly lipid-soluble THC is taken up by peripheral body compartments and sequestered in adipose tissue. Biotransformation of THC occurs predominantly in the liver by the microsomal enzyme system. Metabolic degradation is complex, with approximately 80 different metabolites already identified. The primary metabolite is active and equipotent with THC. This compound is subsequently biotransformed to a number of inactive metabolites, which are then eliminated, via the bile, into the feces, with the remainder excreted in the urine.

Mechanism of Action

The mechanism of action of the cannabinoids is not well understood. However, a receptor was recently identified in the brain that is believed to bind cannabinoids. The receptor is referred to as the cannabinoid receptor. In addition, an endogenous substance, named anandamide, has been identified in the brain that is believed to bind to the cannabinoid receptor. This suggests that there may be cannabinoid-like substances that play some role in activities of the brain. These findings may lead to a better understanding of the actions of the cannabinoids in the future.

Pharmacological Effects

Conjunctival reddening and increases in heart rate have been the most consistently reported effects of marijuana. Heart rate increases of 20 to 50 beats per minute may occur and are dose-related. Tolerance develops to this effect with chronic use. After one marijuana cigarette, the user usually experiences physical and mental relaxation, feelings of euphoria, and increased sociability. These feelings come and go as if in waves. Conversation and ideas tend to concentrate on the "here and now" and not on past or future circumstances. There is a sense that time is passing slowly. With moderate intoxication, there may be drowsiness, lapses of attention, and impairment of short-term memory. At high levels of intoxication, reflexes are slowed, muscle coordination decreases, ataxia is evident, and speech and the ability to concentrate become more difficult. Performance of a variety of tasks deteriorates. The more complex the task, the greater the degree of disruption produced. Dreamlike states with alterations of auditory and visual perceptions reflect the psychotomimetic actions of marijuana. Psychic effects may also include dysphoria, acute panic-anxiety reactions, and psychotic episodes. Marijuana psychosis may, in part, be caused by unmasking of latent psychiatric disorders. It appears to occur under conditions of unusually heavy drug use. Symptoms are delirium, disorientation, and schizophrenic-like behavior.

Chronic use of marijuana in the young has frequently been related to the development of an "amotivational syndrome." This is a highly controversial issue. Many studies have concluded that the lack of interest and motivation demonstrated by many heavy users of marijuana was present before drug use and that amotivation is not a specific effect of marijuana. However, students who frequently use marijuana during school and study time are certainly limiting their academic and future potential.

At low doses, marijuana produces a slight bronchodilation. However, marijuana smoke contains higher concentrations of tar and some carcinogens than does tobacco smoke. Chronic use can produce hoarseness, cough, and bronchitis. Heavy use results in increased airway resistance and has been associated with precancerous changes in the respiratory epithelium.

Marijuana alters the plasma levels of some reproductive hormones. In males, lower testosterone levels decrease the sperm count and motility. In females, levels of luteinizing hormone (LH) and prolactin are suppressed, resulting in sporadic ovulation and irregular menstrual cycles. Tetrahydrocannabinol readily crosses the placenta, and teratogenic effects have been demonstrated in animal studies. Specific birth defects have not been observed in humans, but lower birth weights have been recorded in mothers who smoked marijuana during pregnancy.

Experimental studies have shown marijuana to cause a mild, transitory immunosuppressant effect. Decreased levels of T-lymphocytes have been observed in some chronic users. The clinical significance of this effect has not been determined.

Tolerance and Dependency

Tolerance to marijuana—that is, diminished response to a given dose when repeated—has been demonstrated. However, the development of tolerance usually occurs only after prolonged use of higher amounts of marijuana. The tolerance is variable and develops to a greater degree for some effects, such as tachycardia, CNS depression, and euphoria. Tolerance is rapidly reversed after cessation of marijuana use. Some of the tolerance may be metabolic in origin and caused by induction of microsomal enzymes. As with chronic tobacco smoking, tars and residues in marijuana smoke stimulate the drug microsomal enzyme system. However, this effect on metabolism does not explain all of the tolerance that develops. Cross-tolerance with other psychoactive drugs has not been demonstrated.

Abrupt cessation of marijuana after prolonged use has indicated some dependency. The dependency appears to be more psychological than physical and of considerably less intensity than that observed with cocaine and amphetamines. Withdrawal symptoms are mild and not unlike those observed in individuals who quit the tobacco habit. Symptoms include dysphoria, anxiety, tremors, eating and sleeping disturbances, and increased sweating.

Intoxication and Treatment

The most common intoxication reaction requiring treatment is acute panic-anxiety reaction, where users appear to lose control and feel as if they are losing their mind. This reaction occurs most frequently with inexperienced users, who are unfamiliar with the effects of marijuana. The effects rarely last more than a few hours. Diazepam may be administered to individuals who are particularly agitated. Psychotic reactions, which were discussed previously, occur after high doses or prolonged use and may require hospitalization and treatment with antipsychotic drugs.

Therapeutic Potential of THC

Tetrahydrocannabinol and various derivatives are currently undergoing clinical investigation in the treatment of glaucoma and as an antiemetic for cancer patients who are receiving chemotherapy. Dronabinol (Marinol) is a drug formulation of THC approved for use as an antiemetic to combat the nausea and vomiting associated with chemotherapy. Dronabinol (Marinol) has recently been approved for the stimulation of appetite and prevention of weight loss in patients with a confirmed diagnosis of acquired immunodeficiency syndrome (AIDS).

Chapter Review

Understanding Terminology

Match the definition or description in the left column with the appropriate term in the right column.

___ **1.** Because of this, doses of one drug taken shortly after another drug produce decreased effects.

___ **2.** Because of this, one consumes larger and larger doses of a drug in order to get the desired effects.

___ **3.** Pharmacologically active substance found in the marijuana plant.

___ **4.** Because of this, larger and larger doses of a drug are necessary to prevent withdrawal.

___ **5.** A distortion of sensory perception that occurs with the use of LSD.

___ **6.** Hallucinogenic effect of LSD relived long after the use of LSD.

a. cannabinoid

b. cross-tolerance

c. dependency

d. flashback

e. synesthesia

f. tolerance

Acquiring Knowledge

Answer the following questions in the spaces provided.

1. Briefly describe the psychotomimetic syndrome. _____

_____

2. List the pharmacological effects produced by LSD. What is synesthesia? _____

_____

3. Describe the development of tolerance to LSD. What does the term *cross-tolerance* refer to?

_____

_____

4. What is the usual treatment for LSD and other hallucinogenic drug intoxication? _____

_____

5. What mechanism of action is common to both amphetamines and cocaine? _____

_____

6. Characterize the development of tolerance and dependency with the psychomotor stimulants.

_____

_____

7. Describe the pharmacological effects produced by phencyclidine (PCP). _____

_____

8. What do the terms *marijuana, cannabinoid, tetrahydrocannabinol (THC),* and *hashish* refer to?

_____

_____

9. List the common pharmacological effects produced by marijuana. _____

_____

10. What adverse effects are associated with the chronic use of marijuana? _____

_____

Match the descriptions in the left column with the appropriate phase of hallucinogen use in the right column.

___ **11.** Produces the effects desired by the user.

___ **12.** Occurs right after absorption of the hallucinogen.

___ **13.** A "bad trip."

___ **14.** Consists of CNS stimulation and autonomic changes that are predominantly sympathomimetic in nature.

___ **15.** Produces sensory distortions and pseudohallucinations.

___ **16.** Characteristic of a maximum drug effect.

___ **17.** Produces disruption of thought, depersonalization, hallucinations, and psychotic episodes.

a. psychic phase

b. sensory phase

c. somatic phase

Applying Knowledge—On the Job

Use your critical thinking skills to answer the following questions in the spaces provided.

1. Mark works in an emergency room (ER) that gets lots of illicit-drug-overdose cases. How do you think he should deal with the following patients?

   a. Patient A presents with LSD toxicity, experiencing anxiety, paranoia, and real hallucinations (as opposed to pseudohallucinations, which the individual knows are not real).

   _____

   _____

   b. Patient B presents with signs and symptoms of morphine intoxication, including hyperthermia, profuse sweating, respiratory difficulty, an abnormal electrocardiogram (EKG), and hypertension.

   _____

   _____

   c. Patient C presents with cocaine intoxication, following a prolonged binge on the drug. She has had a mild seizure and shows psychotic behavior, hyperthermia, and exhaustion.

   _____

   _____

2. Assume you work a drug abuse hot line. What aspect of drug abuse does each of the following callers exhibit?

   a. Caller A says he needs help quitting cocaine. His main reason for wanting to quit is that he can no longer afford to buy the amount of cocaine he needs to get high. He says it seems that he uses more every day, and he still doesn't get as high as he did when he first started using the drug.

   _____

   b. Caller B says he thinks he needs to get medical help with his cocaine problem. He's been using cocaine for months now, and he needs larger and larger doses just to keep from feeling sick and strung out. He can't imagine going without the cocaine, but he knows things can't go on this way, either.

   _____

3. A coworker confides in you that working full time, going to school, and taking care of a child and husband is exhausting, so occasionally she takes amphetamines to help her get through it all. She doesn't feel it is a problem because she only uses them when she needs to. What do you do?

   _____

   _____

4. You are over at a coworker's house and she brings out some marijuana. What do you do?

_____

_____

5. A coworker suffers from chronic sinus problems. After many months, this coworker confides in you that she indulges in recreational use of cocaine. What do you do?

_____

_____

Internet Connection

The following Internet websites provide extensive information on many aspects of drug abuse and drug abuse education that may be of use to you for preparing reports and presentations:

American Council for Drug Education (http://www.ACDE.org) **National Institute on Drug Abuse** (http://www.nida.nih.gov) **National Clearinghouse for Alcohol and Drug Information** (http://www.health.org)

Visit the last website listed and click on _Alcohol and Drug Facts._ Under this heading are subheadings for: _Cocaine, Crack, Hallucinogens, Marijuana, Methamphetamine, Ice,_ and others. Search these headings for additional information on the drugs of abuse that were presented in this chapter.

Additional Reading

Abraham, H. D., and Aldridge, A. M. 1993. Adverse consequences of lysergic acid diethylamide. _Addiction_ 8:1327.

Des Jarlais, D. C., and Friedman, S. R. 1994. AIDS and the use of injected drugs. _Scientific American_ 270 (2):82.

Evanko, D. 1991. Designer drugs. _Postgraduate Medicine_ 89 (6):67.

Hannan, D. J., and Adler, A. G. 1990. Crack abuse. _Postgraduate Medicine_ 88 (1):141.

Hess, D., and DeBoer, S. 2002. Ecstasy. _American Journal of Nursing_ 102 (4):45.

Understanding drug addiction: Implications for treatment. 1996. _Hospital Practice_ 31 (10):47.

Zafar, H., Vaz, A., and Carlson, R. W. 1997. Acute complications of cocaine intoxication. _Hospital Practice_ 32 (2):167.

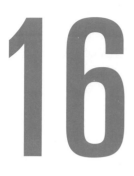

16

ANTIEPILEPTIC DRUGS

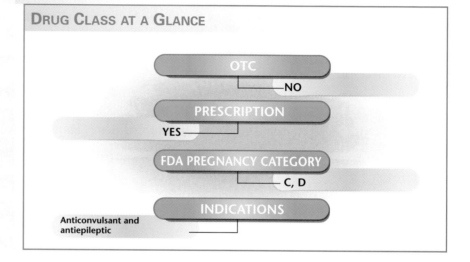

DRUG CLASS AT A GLANCE

OTC — NO

PRESCRIPTION — YES

FDA PREGNANCY CATEGORY — C, D

INDICATIONS — Anticonvulsant and antiepileptic

Key Terms

absence seizure: generalized seizure that does not involve motor convulsions; also referred to as petit mal.

anticonvulsant: drug that prevents or stops a convulsive seizure.

antiepileptic: drug used to prevent epileptic seizures.

clonic: convulsive spasm in which rigidity and relaxation alternate in rapid succession.

epilepsy: condition characterized by periodic or recurrent seizures or convulsions.

generalized seizure: seizure originating and involving both cerebral hemispheres.

grand mal: generalized seizure characterized by full-body tonic and clonic motor convulsions.

partial seizure: seizure originating in one area of the brain that may spread to other areas.

seizure: abnormal discharge of brain neurons that causes alteration of behavior and/or motor activity.

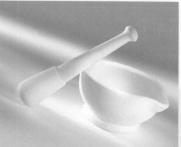

status epilepticus: continuous series of grand mal convulsions.

tonic: convulsive spasm characterized by sustained muscular contractions.

INTRODUCTION

Epilepsy is a condition involving periodic seizures that may lead to motor convulsions. A **seizure** is defined as an abnormal electrical dicharge of brain neurons that leads to alterations in behavior and motor (muscle) activity. This abnormal discharge causes the nerve cells to become hyperexcitable, so that they fire uncontrollably. The result is usually an impairment or temporary loss of consciousness that may be accompanied by some form of muscular twitching or motor convulsion.

When the cause of epilepsy cannot be determined, the epilepsy is referred to as idiopathic epilepsy. When the cause can be associated with specific factors—such as brain tumors, birth defects, or infectious diseases—the epilepsy is referred to as symptomatic epilepsy.

TYPES OF EPILEPSY

There are many different types of epilepsy, and proper diagnosis is essential to selection of proper treatment. An important diagnostic tool aiding in the detection of epilepsy is the electroencephalogram (EEG), which records the electrical activity of the brain. Specific types of epilepsy produce characteristic electrical patterns. These patterns can be readily recorded by the EEG and identified. Classification of the different epilepsies is based on a neurological examination and EEG evaluation. The most common types of epilepsy will be briefly described.

Generalized Seizures

Generalized seizures originate in and involve both cerebral hemispheres. They are classified as: tonic-clonic, myoclonic, and absence seizures.

Tonic-Clonic Seizures

These seizures produce full-body motor convulsions and are also referred to as **grand mal** seizures. **Tonic** convulsions are convulsive spasms characterized by sustained muscular contractions. **Clonic** convulsions are convulsive spasms in which rigidity and relaxation alternate in rapid succession. Uncontrolled urination and defecation may also occur in grand mal. An attack usually lasts 1 to 2 minutes. Following the convulsions, individuals experience confusion, fatigue, and muscle soreness.

A series of grand mal seizures without cessation is referred to as **status epilepticus.** Status epilepticus is a major medical emergency and demands immediate treatment if death is to be avoided.

Myoclonic Seizures

Myoclonic seizures produce motor convulsions that are usually brief and often confined to one part of the body; however, these seizures may spread and become generalized.

Absence Seizures

Absence seizures are generalized seizures that are usually confined to a brief impairment of consciousness. This may involve a form of staring or rapid eye blinking that lasts anywhere from 10 seconds to 2 minutes. Although there is impairment of consciousness, individuals usually do not fall or experience motor convulsions. After a seizure, activity often continues as if nothing had happened. This type of epilepsy is also known as petit mal.

Partial Seizures

Partial seizures are classified as either simple or complex.

Simple Partial Seizures

Simple partial seizures may be sensory or motor in nature. These seizures usually involve a limited area of the brain and are often manifested by a sensory change (numbness) or muscular twitch that is confined to one body part. The seizures are brief in duration and usually there is no loss of consciousness.

Complex Partial Seizures

Complex partial seizures involve a loss of consciousness, usually not longer than 2 minutes, and are accompanied by some type of characteristic movement. These movements have been described as "purposeless" because they are not goal-directed and involve such things as lip smacking. The term *psychomotor* is also used to describe these seizures. Following the attack, the individual usually has no memory of what occurred during the seizure. Complex partial seizures may spread and include other areas of the body, or may also become tonic-clonic and involve the entire body.

DRUGS USED TO CONTROL EPILEPSY

All of the primary drugs used to treat epilepsy possess anticonvulsant properties. An **anticonvulsant** is defined as a drug, usually administered IM or IV, that prevents or arrests convulsive seizures. The term **antiepileptic** infers that the drug, usually administered orally, can be used prophylactically to reduce or prevent epileptic seizures. Not all drugs with

anticonvulsant activity can be used in epilepsy; many anticonvulsant drugs produce a significant degree of sedation that interferes with performance of daily activities.

Antiepileptic drugs decrease the excitability of brain cells and, consequently, reduce the incidence and severity of seizures. This action enables affected individuals to have greater control over their daily lives. Several different drug classes possess antiepileptic properties. Each of these will be discussed in relationship to the type of epilepsy for which it is used. The most frequently used antiepileptic drugs and their main indications are summarized in Table 16:1.

Barbiturates

The barbiturates, previously discussed with respect to their sedative and hypnotic properties, are excellent anticonvulsant drugs. All barbiturates have anticonvulsant properties, but only a few, such as phenobarbital and mephobarbital, have the additional property of being antiepileptic. They have a selective effect at lower doses to prevent seizures. Sedation and hypnosis are common pharmacological effects produced by barbiturates. However, in the treatment of epilepsy, excessive sedation or hypnosis is an unwanted side effect. Fortunately, tolerance to the sedative and hypnotic effects develops with chronic use. The barbiturates are used alone or in combination with other antiepileptic drugs.

TABLE 16:1 Commonly Used Antiepileptic Drugs With Main Indications

DRUG (TRADE NAME)	MAIN INDICATION	COMMON ADULT ORAL MAINTENANCE DOSAGE RANGE
carbamazepine *(Tegretol)*	Partial and generalized tonic-clonic seizures	800–1200 mg
phenobarbital *(Luminal)*	Partial and generalized tonic-clonic seizures	60–200 mg
phenytoin *(Dilantin)*	Partial and generalized tonic-clonic seizures	300 mg
valproic acid *(Depakene)*	All generalized and partial seizures	200–400 mg
clonazepam *(Klonopin)*	Myoclonic, absence, and akinetic seizures	1.5–10 mg
ethosuximide *(Zarontin)*	Absence seizures	750–1500 mg
trimethadione *(Tridione)*	Absence seizures	900–1800 mg
diazepam *(Valium)*	Status epilepticus	Slow IV injection, 5–10 mg
felbamate *(Felbatol)*	Partial Seizures	1200–3600 mg
gabapentin *(Neurontin)*	Partial Seizures	300–1800 mg

Mechanism of Action

As previously discussed in Chapter 12, one of the actions of the barbiturates is to increase the inhibitory effects of the inhibitory neurotransmitter gamma-aminobutyric acid (GABA). In the brain, this suppresses the excitability of epileptogenic neurons and makes them less likely to discharge and initiate a seizure. The effect on GABA occurs at lower doses and therefore limits the sedative and depressant effects of the barbiturates.

Clinical Indications

Barbiturates, like phenobarbital, are mainly used in the treatment of all types of partial seizures and in the control of tonic-clonic seizures.

Sudden discontinuation of barbiturates can produce convulsions. Therefore, when barbiturate withdrawal is desired, a patient's dose should be gradually reduced over the course of 1 to 2 weeks.

Hydantoins

The most important drug from this class is phenytoin *(Dilantin)*. Phenytoin is a very potent antiepileptic drug, and it can be used in several types of epilepsy. It is probably the most important antiepileptic drug available. A significant advantage of phenytoin is that it produces little sedation. Ethotoin *(Peganone)* and fosphenytoin *(Cerebyx)* are other hydantoins.

Mechanism of Action

The mechanism of action of phenytoin and the other hydantoins involves an effect on sodium ions in brain cells. In epilepsy, there appears to be a disturbance in the distribution of ions that are involved in the electrical activity of the brain. Phenytoin decreases the level of sodium (Na^+) ions inside nerve cells. This change decreases the hyperexcitability of the nerve cells involved in initiating the epileptic seizure. Consequently, the incidence of seizures is dramatically reduced in most epileptic patients.

Clinical Indications

Phenytoin is used for all types of partial seizures and for tonic-clonic generalized seizures.

Adverse Effects

The adverse effects of the individual hydantoins are similar. Mephenytoin causes the greatest incidence of adverse effects, whereas ethotoin causes the least. The most common adverse effects involve the cerebellum. The symptoms are dizziness, visual disturbances, and postural imbalance. Other adverse effects include skin rashes, hirsutism, and gingival hyperplasia. Good dental hygiene may prevent the overgrowth of the gums.

Carbamazepine (Tegretol)

Carbamazepine is structurally related to the tricyclic antidepressants. The mechanism of action is similar to that of phenytoin and involves an action to block sodium ion channels.

This action decreases the amount of sodium ions inside of nerve cells and inhibits high-frequency and repetitive firing of neurons. Carbamazepine also possesses analgesic properties. The analgesia is useful in the treatment of trigeminal neuralgia and related conditions.

Clinical Indications

Carbamazepine is used in the treatment of all types of partial seizures and generalized tonic-clonic seizures.

Adverse Effects

Common side effects include nausea, vomiting, diplopia, drowsiness, and dizziness. More serious effects involve liver disturbances, jaundice, and bone marrow depression, which may lead to aplastic anemia. In overdosage, carbamazepine may cause convulsions and respiratory depression.

Valproic Acid *(Depakene)*

Valproic acid is one of the few drugs that can be used in all types of epilepsy. Its mechanism of action is related to its ability to increase levels of GABA, the inhibitory neurotransmitter in the central nervous system (CNS). Valproic acid has little effect on causing sedation.

Adverse Effects

The most common side effects of valproic acid are nausea, vomiting, diarrhea, and tremor. The most serious problem with valproic acid has been the development of a potentially fatal liver toxicity, especially in young patients. The cause of the liver toxicity has been linked to the metabolites of valproic acid, which are hepatotoxic.

Primidone (Mysoline)

Primidone is chemically related to the barbiturates. Most of the drug is metabolized and converted in the body into phenobarbital, which is believed to account for most of its antiepileptic effects. Uses and adverse effects are similar to phenobarbital.

Drugs Used in the Treatment of Absence Seizures

Succinimides

The succinimides are a group of compounds that are only used in the treatment of absence seizures. The most important and most widely used succinimide is ethosuximide (*Zarontin*). Ethosuximide has a long half-life that usually allows twice-a-day dosing. The mechanism of action is related to the ability of ethosuximide to decrease specific calcium currents (T currents) in the thalamus. These calcium currents are believed to play an important role in absence seizures.

The succinimides commonly produce GI disturbances such as nausea, vomiting, and diarrhea. In addition, some drowsiness and dizziness may occur. Occasionally, blood disorders, such as leukopenia, develop.

Oxazolidiïnediones

The oxazolidinediones are another class of drugs used primarily in petit mal. The two main drugs of this class are trimethadione (*Tridione*) and paramethadione (*Paradione*). Trimethadione is more effective than paramethadione, but it also produces a greater incidence of adverse effects. The mechanism of action of these drugs is not well understood.

The oxazolidinediones are considerably more toxic than the succinimides. One of the adverse effects characteristic of the oxazolidinediones is hemeralopia, or "snow blindness," a visual disturbance in which patients seem to be looking at everything as if through a snowfall. Hypersensitivity reactions, such as rashes and blood disorders, usually necessitate alternate therapy. In addition, cases of liver and kidney damage have been reported.

Benzodiazepines

As discussed in Chapter 13, the benzodiazepines possess anticonvulsant activity. These drugs act by increasing the inhibitory effects of GABA. Diazepam (*Valium*), clonazepam (*Klonopin*), and lorazepam (*Ativan*) are the drugs used as anticonvulsants. Diazepam and lorazepam are usually administered intravenously to stop seizures that are in progress, usually the grand mal type seizures. Although these drugs have fairly long half-lives, the anticonvulsant effect only lasts about 30 to 60 minutes. Therefore, these drugs may have to be readministered. Clonazepam is also used as an antiepileptic drug in the treatment of myoclonic and akinetic seizures, and in cases of absence seizure unresponsive to ethosuximide. The main side effect of these drugs in the treatment of seizures is sedation. The adverse effects of the benzodiazepines were presented in Chapter 13.

Newer Antiepileptic Drugs

Felbamate (*Felbatol*)

Felbamate is a relatively new drug indicated for the treatment of partial seizures. Its mechanism of action has been related to its ability to interfere with sodium ions, similar to the actions of phenytoin. Unfortunately, felbamate has been associated with the development of aplastic anemia and liver failure. Consequently, the drug is reserved for patients who do not respond to other drugs and whose epilepsy is so severe that the benefits of therapy outweigh the risks of developing these serious adverse effects.

Gabapentin (Neurontin)

Gabapentin is similar in structure to GABA and was designed to act in a similar manner. However, the drug appears to act by other mechanisms that are not currently well understood. Gabapentin is used in patients over 12 years of age in combination with other antiepileptic drugs in the treatment of partial seizures. The most common adverse effects include sleepiness, ataxia, fatigue, nausea, and dizziness.

Lamotrigine (Lamictal)

Lamotrigine is unrelated to other antiepileptic drugs. Its mechanism of action is not well understood but is believed to involve interference with sodium ions. The drug is used in combination with other antiepileptic drugs in the treatment of partial seizures. The most common adverse effects include dizziness, ataxia, sleepiness, headache, visual disturbances, and rash.

Levetiracetam (Keppra)

Levetiracetam is unrelated to other antiepileptic drugs and its mechanism of action is poorly understood. The main indication is adjunctive therapy in the treatment of partial seizures in adults. The drug may be taken without regard to meals. The most frequently reported adverse effects include sleepiness, dizziness, headache, and nervousness.

Tiagabine (Gabitril)

Tiagabine is believed to block the reuptake of the inhibitory transmitter GABA, allowing more GABA to be available for receptor stimulation. The drug is indicated for the treatment of partial seizures. Tiagabine should be taken with food. Common adverse effects include nausea, GI disturbances, abdominal pain, dizziness, tremors, nervousness, mental confusion, and cough.

TREATMENT OF STATUS EPILEPTICUS

Diazepam is currently the preferred drug for the treatment of status epilepticus. It is administered intravenously to stop seizures that are in progress. Because of its short anticonvulsant duration of action, repeated administration of diazepam may be required. Other antiepileptic drugs, such as phenytoin, that have longer durations of action and that are used in the chronic control of epilepsy are often administered at the same time.

USE OF ANTIEPILEPTIC DRUGS DURING PREGNANCY

Seizure activity often increases during pregnancy in women with epilepsy. Epileptic seizures, especially if frequent and severe, can produce harmful effects to the developing fetus. Both epilepsy and the drugs used to treat epilepsy have been associated with an increased risk for infant mortality and teratogenic effects (fetal malformations). Antiepileptic drugs are designated Food and Drug Administration (FDA) Pregnancy Categories C and D. The risk appears to increase with the number of drugs used. The general practice, if possible, is to avoid the use of drugs during pregnancy unless maternal seizures pose a serious health threat. If antiepileptic drug therapy is required, the practice is to limit drug use to one drug at the lowest dose that will provide an acceptable level of control. Carbamazepine, phenytoin, valproate, and especially trimethadione are the drugs most commonly associated with fetal malformations. The malformations most often include craniofacial defects, neural tube defects such as spina bifida, and other developmental delays. Folic acid deficiency has also been associated with the development of spina bifida and current practice is to recommend folic acid supplementation during pregnancy.

ANTIEPILEPTIC DRUG INTERACTIONS

There are a variety of drug interactions involving the antiepileptic drugs. When used in combination, these drugs often produce drug interactions with each other. Carbamazepine, phenobarbital, and phenytoin cause microsomal enzyme induction and increase the rate of metabolism of any other drug requiring microsomal metabolism. This results in reduced drug effects and duration of action of the drugs requiring metabolism. Valproic acid inhibits the microsomal enzymes and will therefore increase the effects of drugs requiring microsomal metabolism. Cimetidine (*Tagamet*) and other drugs that inhibit microsomal enzymes will increase the concentrations and effects of anticonvulsant drugs requiring microsomal metabolism, especially carbamazepine.

Most antiepileptic drugs are highly plasma protein bound. They can displace and be displaced by other drugs that are also highly protein bound. This increases the free drug concentration (unbound fraction) of the drug displaced and produces greater pharmacologic effects.

Patient Administration and Monitoring

Monitor vital signs when anticonvulsant drugs are administered intravenously, especially when treating seizures in progress.

Explain to patient the common side effects of most drugs: nausea, dizziness, ataxia, and sedation.

Caution patients about the dangers of engaging in hazardous activities, such as driving while under the influence of drugs.

Instruct patients to take medications with meals if nausea or GI disturbances are excessive, especially with carbamazepine, ethosuximide, and phenytoin.

Explain to patient the importance of taking drugs as prescribed and the dangers of missing doses since this may precipitate seizures.

Instruct patients to report seizures and other significant adverse effects.

Instruct patients not to take other drugs unless they check with their physician or pharmacist.

Chapter Review

Understanding Terminology

Match the definition or description in the left column with the appropriate term in the right column.

___ **1.** Drug that prevents or stops a convulsive seizure.

___ **2.** Drug that prevents epileptic seizures.

___ **3.** Condition characterized by periodic seizures or convulsions.

___ **4.** Generalized seizure only involving a brief impairment of consciousness.

___ **5.** Seizures characterized by full-body tonic and clonic convulsions.

___ **6.** Continuous series of grand mal convulsions.

___ **7.** Seizure characterized by some purposeless body movement or sensory change.

a. anticonvulsant

b. antiepileptic

c. epilepsy

d. grand mal

e. absence seizure

f. complex partial seizure

g. status epilepticus

Acquiring Knowledge

Answer the following questions in the spaces provided.

1. Describe what occurs to the brain cells in epilepsy. _____

_____

2. List the common types of epilepsy and describe the characteristics of each. _____

_____

3. In what types of epilepsy are the barbiturates and hydantoins most useful? _____

_____

_____

4. What is the mechanism of action of phenytoin (*Dilantin*)? _____

_____

_____

5. List the adverse effects of phenytoin. _____

_____

_____

6. What drug classes are used primarily to treat absence seizures? _____

_____

_____

7. List the adverse effects of trimethadione (*Tridione*). _____

_____

_____

8. What is the drug of choice for treating status epilepticus? _____

_____

_____

Applying Knowledge—On the Job

Use your critical thinking skills to answer the following questions in the spaces provided.

1. Assume that you assist with medications in a busy neurological practice and you've been asked to deal with each of the following cases.

   a. Patient A is a 14-year-old female who frequently has short periods when she loses consciousness. After each seizure, she continues what she was doing as though nothing happened. How would you characterize the type of epilepsy this patient has?

   _____

   _____

   b. Patient B has absence epilepsy. Name at least two different drugs that could be prescribed to treat this type of epilepsy.

   _____

   _____

   c. How would you advise Patient C about adverse effects for the antiepileptic drug trimethadione?

   _____

   _____

   d. Patient D has tonic-clonic convulsions in progress. What should be done? _____

   _____

2. Assume you are a health educator for a health maintenance organization (HMO). You've just been assigned the task of designing a brochure or poster giving cautions for epilepsy patients regarding adverse effects of the most widely used antiepileptic drugs: the barbiturates and hydantoins. Use a separate sheet of paper to show the design of your brochure or poster.

   _____

   _____

3. An epileptic patient has come into his regular pharmacy at 8:30 P.M. He has just returned from vacation and his luggage was lost, including his *Dilantin* and phenobarbital. He has no refills available. Do you think it would be appropriate for the pharmacist to give him an emergency supply, enough to last the patient until the pharmacy can reach the physician?

   _____

   _____

4. Freddy suffers from absence seizures. *Zarontin* has not adequately controlled them. His physician has decided to add a benzodiazepine to his drug therapy. Which one would be appropriate? What is the average dosage range?

   _____

   _____

5. Which of the antiepileptic drugs also has an additional indication other than epilepsy? What is that indication?

   _____

   _____

Internet Connection

Contact the **MedicineNet** search engine (http://www.medicinenet.com) and click on *Diseases and Treatments;* then highlight the letter "E" and find *Epilepsy.* Read additional information about epilepsy and additional sources of information.

Additional Reading

Bhagwath, G., and DiSalle, M. 2001. Carbamazepine-induced generalized pustular eruption. *Hospital Physician* 37 (6):59.

Harder, A., Tuchek, J. M., and Harder, S. 1996. Seizure control: How to use the new antiepileptic drugs in older patients. *Geriatrics* 51 (9):42.

Pourmand, R. 1997. Seizures and epilepsy in older patients: Evaluation and management. *Geriatrics* 51 (3):39.

Shantz, D., and Spitz, M. 1993. What you need to know about seizures. *Nursing* 23 (11):34.

17

ANTIPARKINSON DRUGS

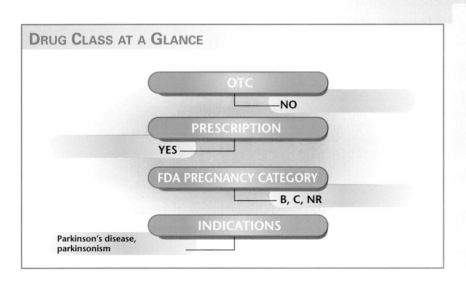

DRUG CLASS AT A GLANCE

OTC
— NO

PRESCRIPTION
YES —

FDA PREGNANCY CATEGORY
— B, C, NR

INDICATIONS
Parkinson's disease, parkinsonism

Key Terms

acetylcholine (ACH): excitatory neurotransmitter in the basal ganglia.

basal ganglia: group of cell bodies located in the cerebral medulla that regulates skeletal muscle tone and body movement.

dopamine: inhibitory neurotransmitter in the basal ganglia.

dyskinesia: involuntary body movements.

dystonia: weak and slow body movements.

parkinsonism: symptoms of Parkinson's disease, which include resting tremor, muscle rigidity, and disturbances of movement and postural balance.

Parkinson's disease: disorder of the basal ganglia, usually characterized by a deficiency of dopamine.

CHAPTER FOCUS

This chapter explains the causes and symptoms of Parkinson's disease, which affects the basal ganglia. It also describes the pharmacology of drugs used to treat this disease.

CHAPTER OBJECTIVES

After studying this chapter, you should be able to

- list the major symptoms of Parkinson's disease.
- explain the relationship between dopamine and acetylcholine in the basal ganglia.
- describe the action of drugs that increase dopamine or decrease acetylcholine levels in the basal ganglia.
- discuss the actions and adverse effects of four different types of antiparkinsonian drugs.

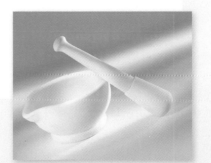

INTRODUCTION

The **basal ganglia** are a group of cell bodies (gray matter) located in the medulla (white matter) of the cerebrum. The major function of the basal ganglia is to help regulate skeletal muscle tone and body movement. The most common disease involving the basal ganglia is **Parkinson's disease.** In this disease, cell damage to the basal ganglia produces symptoms of **parkinsonism.** These symptoms include resting tremors, muscle rigidity, and disturbances of movement and postural balance.

It is believed that Parkinson's disease is caused by an accelerated aging and destruction of the neurons in the basal ganglia that produce dopamine. Some of the conditions that may contribute to Parkinson's disease are viral infections, brain tumors, and arteriosclerosis. Certain antipsychotic drugs, like chlorpromazine and haloperidol, are prone to causing the symptoms of Parkinson's disease. This is referred to as parkinsonism. This occurs because the mechanism of action of antipsychotic drugs is to block dopamine receptors in certain areas of the brain. Unfortunately, the antipsychotic drugs also block dopamine receptors in the basal ganglia.

Parkinson's disease is treated mainly by drug therapy. Although drug treatment is effective in reducing the symptoms of the disease, the disease continues to progress because of the continued destruction of the neurons that produce dopamine. Individuals may become physically disabled and bedridden in the later stages of the disease.

NEUROTRANSMITTERS AFFECTING THE BASAL GANGLIA

Normal function of the basal ganglia depends mainly upon the interaction between two neurotransmitters: **acetylcholine (ACH)** and dopamine. ACH and dopamine help regulate the activity of the motor nerves that control voluntary muscle movements. ACH is an excitatory neurotransmitter in the basal ganglia that increases muscle tone and activity, while **dopamine** is an inhibitory neurotransmitter in the basal ganglia that decreases muscle tone and activity.

Normally, the activity of ACH and dopamine are balanced, allowing smooth and well-controlled body movements. The deficiency of dopamine in Parkinson's disease disturbs the balance between ACH and dopamine in favor of ACH. The increased activity of ACH produces excessive motor nerve stimulation, resulting in tremors, muscle rigidity, and the other symptoms of Parkinson's disease.

DRUG THERAPY

Several different classes of drugs are used to treat Parkinson's disease. The aim of drug therapy is to influence the activity of the specific neurotransmitters that affect the basal ganglia. The rationale is to either increase the level of dopamine by administering levodopa (precursor of dopamine) or increase dopaminergic activity by administering drugs that stimulate dopamine receptors. In addition, anticholinergic drugs are used to reduce the activity of ACH. Drugs that act to increase the activity of dopamine are summarized in Table 17:1.

Levodopa (Dopar, Larodopa)

In Parkinson's disease, there is a deficiency of dopamine in the basal ganglia. Dopamine does not readily cross the blood-brain barrier. However, the precursor of dopamine, l-dihydroxyphenylalanine (levodopa), does cross the blood-brain barrier into the brain. In the basal ganglia, levodopa is converted to dopamine. As the level of dopamine increases, there is lessening of parkinsonian symptoms and a significant improvement in physical mobility. Many patients are able to resume normal physical activities. Although not all patients respond to levodopa, it is the most effective drug available.

Levodopa is administered orally in rather large doses. The initial dose is 0.5 to 1.0 g per day. This dose is gradually increased until the usual dose of 4 to 8 g per day (divided doses) is reached.

TABLE 17:1 Antiparkinson Drugs That Increase the Effects of Dopamine

DRUG (TRADE NAME)	MECHANISM OF ACTION
amantadine *(Symmetrel)*	Stimulates release of dopamine from nerve terminals
bromocriptine *(Parlodel)*	Dopamine receptor agonist
carbidopa *(Lodosyn)*	Inhibits peripheral conversion of l-dopa to dopamine
levodopa *(Dopar, Larodopa)*	Converted to dopamine in basal ganglia
levodopa\carbidopa *(Sinemet)*	Combination that inhibits peripheral conversion of l-dopa to dopamine and allows more l-dopa to pass into the brain
pramipexole *(Mirapex)*	Dopamine receptor agonist
ropinirole *(Requip)*	Dopamine receptor agonist
selegiline *(Eldepryl)*	Monoamine oxidase B inhibitor that increases dopamine levels by inhibiting the metabolism of dopamine in the brain

Mechanism of Action

A large amount of the levodopa given is rapidly converted to dopamine before passing into the brain and basal ganglia. In order to minimize this premature conversion, levodopa is usually given along with another drug, carbidopa. Carbidopa *(Lodosyn)* inhibits the enzyme that converts levodopa to dopamine so that more levodopa passes into the brain before being converted to dopamine. Carbidopa does not cross the blood-brain barrier and, therefore, does not prevent the conversion of levodopa to dopamine in the basal ganglia. A combination of levodopa and carbidopa is available under the trade name of *Sinemet,* and is the most widely used drug preparation.

Adverse Effects

The most common adverse effects of levodopa are nausea, vomiting, and loss of appetite (anorexia). In the brain, high levels of dopamine interfere with cardiovascular reflexes that maintain blood pressure. Consequently, some patients experience orthostatic hypertension or fainting. Since dopamine can stimulate beta-1-adrenergic receptors (Chapter 6), some patients may experience rapid or irregular heartbeat, especially if large amounts of levodopa are converted to dopamine in the peripheral circulation. Increased formation of dopamine in the limbic system and thalamus may also cause various behavioral and psychotic-like disturbances.

Several side effects related to movement disorders are common during antiparkinson therapy. **Dystonias,** described as weak and slow body movements, occur when the levels of dopamine are low and the levels of ACH high in the basal ganglia. Dystonias are associated with insufficient levodopa dosage or when the drug effect is wearing off. The wearing off effect is also referred to as the "end-of-dose effect." In contrast, when dopamine levels are higher than ACH levels, there are excessive and involuntary body movements. These movements are referred to as **dyskinesias** and are characterized by uncontrolled movements of the head, neck, and trunk. Dyskinesias usually occur when levodopa dosages are too high or they may occur for a brief period of time after drug administration when peak levodopa concentrations are attained in the basal ganglia. Although these effects are usually not life-threatening, they are a source of embarrassment and frustration to patients.

Another effect that may occur as drug treatment progresses is the "on-off" phenomenon. This is characterized by alternating periods of improvement and periods of worsening of parkinsonian symptoms during drug therapy. The on-off phenomenon is not well understood but is believed to involve fluctuating levels of dopamine in the basal ganglia. Smaller doses taken at more frequent intervals appears to help. In addition, limiting and controlling the dietary intake of proteins also appears to reduce this phenomenon. The amino acids in protein can compete with and decrease the amounts of levodopa that gain entry into the brain.

Drug Interactions

A number of drugs interfere with the action of levodopa. The antipsychotic drugs (phenothiazines and reserpine) decrease the effectiveness of levodopa because they block dopamine receptors. This may cause symptoms of Parkinson's disease (parkinsonism). Vitamin B_6, or pyridoxine, may increase the rate of metabolism of levodopa. When used as a vitamin supplement, vitamin B_6 may decrease the effectiveness of levodopa.

Selegiline (Eldepryl)

Selegiline is a drug that primarily inhibits the metabolism of dopamine in the brain. Dopamine is metabolized by the enzyme, monoamine oxidase B. By inhibiting monoamine oxidase B, selegiline increases the concentration and prolongs the duration of action of dopamine that is formed in the brain. The drug is used alone, early in Parkinson's disease, to slow progression of the disease. It is more commonly used in combination with levodopa to increase and prolong the effects of levodopa.

Adverse Effects

Adverse effects of selegiline are associated with increased dopamine levels and are similar to those of the dopamine agonist (see Dopamine Agonists section), but occur with less frequency and intensity. At very high doses selegiline can also inhibit monoamine oxidase (MAO) A. This is the enzyme that primarily metabolizes norepinephrine, epinephrine, and serotonin. Serious drug interactions may occur when selegiline is administered together with either the MAO inhibitors or *the* selective serotonin reuptake inhibitors (SSRIs) used to treat mental depression (Chapter 14).

COMT Inhibitors

Catechol-O-methyltransferase (COMT) is an enzyme that normally is involved in the metabolism of dopamine. Drugs such as tolcapone *(Tasmar)* and entacapone *(Comtan)* inhibit COMT in both the brain and the periphery. These drugs are administered with levodopa to prolong the duration of action.

Adverse effects caused by these drugs are due mostly to the increased levodopa and dopamine levels and include nausea, mental disturbances, and dyskinesias. Tolcapone has also been reported to cause liver toxicity.

Dopamine Agonists

Dopamine agonists bind to and stimulate dopamine receptors in the basal ganglia. These drugs are particularly useful as Parkinson's disease progresses and the ability of the basal ganglia to produce dopamine is severely affected.

Bromocriptine (Parlodel)

Bromocriptine is a dopamine receptor agonist. The dopamine agonists are generally less effective than levodopa, but are particularly useful as the disease progresses and the ability of the basal ganglia to produce dopamine decreases. Bromocriptine may be added to therapy in patients already receiving levodopa. The adverse effects are similar to those for dopamine: nausea, vomiting, mental disturbances, postural hypotension, and dyskinesia.

Bromocriptine also inhibits the secretion of prolactin from the pituitary gland by stimulating dopamine receptors there. It can be used in the treatment of galactorrea and to prevent lactation after childbirth.

Pergolide (Permax)

Pergolide is a dopamine receptor agonist structurally related to bromocriptine. The drug is more potent than bromocriptine but otherwise similar in pharmacological and adverse effects. Pergolide is usually reserved for treatment of the later stages of Parkinson's disease.

New Dopamine Agonists

Two new dopamine receptor agonists have recently been approved. Like bromocriptine, these drugs stimulate dopamine receptors in the basal ganglia. Pramipexole *(Mirapex)* and ropinirole *(Requip)* have been approved by the Food and Drug Administration (FDA). Both drugs can be used alone early in Parkinson's disease or in combination with levodopa as the disease progresses and requires greater drug therapy.

Adverse effects of both drugs are similar and include nausea, dizziness, somnolence, and central nervous system (CNS) disturbances such as hallucinations. Most of these effects are related to excess stimulation of dopamine receptors.

Amantadine (Symmetrel)

Amantadine is an antiviral drug that was accidentally discovered to be beneficial in treating Parkinson's disease.

Mechanism of Action

The mechanism of action of amantadine is associated with the release of dopamine from its neuronal storage sites in the brain. As a result, the activity of dopamine in the basal ganglia is increased. Amantadine, in oral doses of 100 to 200 mg per day, appears to work best when it is used in the early stages of the disease and in combination with other antiparkinson drugs.

Adverse Effects

The main adverse effects of amantadine are dry mouth, gastrointestinal (GI) disturbances, and a number of CNS effects, usually visual disturbances, dizziness, and confusion. In addition, some patients experience a peculiar type of skin discoloration that clears up when the drug is stopped. The discoloration is referred to as *livido reticularis*.

Anticholinergic Drugs

Over a century ago, it was observed that anticholinergic drugs, such as atropine and scopolamine, relieved some of the symptoms of Parkinson's disease. Before the discovery of levodopa, anticholinergic drugs were the main treatment for parkinsonism. When there is a deficiency of dopamine in the basal ganglia, there is excess ACH (cholinergic) activity. By blocking ACH actions, the anticholinergic drugs decrease the level of cholinergic activity, reducing tremors, muscle rigidity, and postural disturbances.

Atropine and scopolamine produce a high incidence of peripheral anticholinergic side effects. Newer anticholinergic drugs that act primarily in the brain and that produce a lower incidence of peripheral side and adverse effects are the drugs used. These include benztropine *(Cogentin)*, trihexphenidyl *(Artane)*, and others. The anticholinergic drugs are listed in Table 17:2.

Clinical Indications

Anticholinergic drugs are less effective than levodopa and the dopamine agonists. In some patients, the combination of levodopa and an anticholinergic drug provides improved results. Anticholinergic drugs are also used in patients treated with antipsychotic drugs who develop parkinsonism. By blocking cholinergic receptors in the basal ganglia, these drugs lower the effects of acetylcholine and help restore the acetylcholine/dopamine balance that is important for normal basal ganglia function. The basic pharmacology of the anticholinergic drugs was previously discussed with the parasympathetic nervous system in Chapter 7. It might be helpful to review this information at this time.

Adverse Effects

The main adverse effects associated with anticholinergic drugs are caused by a decrease in parasympathetic activity. They include dry mouth, constipation, urinary retention, rapid heartbeat, and pupillary dilation (mydriasis).

Antihistaminic Drugs

Histamine is a substance that is released from certain cells in the body (mast cells), usually in response to irritation or injury. After being released, histamine produces many of the symptoms associated with allergy and inflammatory reactions. Drugs that block the action of histamine are known as antihistamines. The pharmacology of the antihistaminic drugs will be discussed in Chapter 31.

Mechanism of Action

Many of the antihistamines produce anticholinergic effects, and these effects are believed to provide the antiparkinson action. The antihistamines are used in the early stages of the disease and in combination with other antiparkinson drugs. The antihistaminic drug most frequently used is diphenhydramine *(Benadryl)*.

Adverse Effects

The most common side effect of the antihistamines is CNS depression, which usually produces drowsiness and sedation. In addition, dry mouth and GI disturbances may occur because of the anticholinergic activity.

TABLE 17:2	Anticholinergic Drugs Used in Parkinson's Disease

DRUG (TRADE NAME)	COMMON DAILY ORAL DOSAGE RANGE
benztropine *(Cogentin)*	0.5–4 mg
biperiden *(Akineton)*	6–10 mg
procyclidine *(Kemadrin)*	7.5–15 mg
trihexyphenidyl *(Artane)*	1–10 mg

Patient Administration and Monitoring

Measure vital signs when possible to detect decreases in blood pressure or increases in heart rate caused by drugs that act through dopamine.

Instruct patients on the importance of following dosing schedules and that missed doses will result in movement difficulties and an increase in parkinsonian symptoms.

Explain to patient the expected side effects of drugs that increase dopamine activity: nausea, dizziness, sleepiness, and occasionally CNS disturbances such as vivid dreams or hallucinations.

Explain to patient the side effects of anticholinergic drugs: dry mouth, constipation, visual disturbances, difficulties with urination. Remember that these drugs are used with caution in patients with glaucoma, prostate hypertrophy, and in the elderly.

Warn patients about the end-of-dose effect and the on-off phenomenon that may occur, and to report these occurrences since adjustments in dosage or diet may be helpful.

Warn patients to be extremely careful when engaged in activities where impairment or temporary loss of movement could endanger their safety.

Chapter Review

Understanding Terminology

Answer the following questions in the spaces provided.

1. How are the terms *parkinsonism* and *Parkinson's disease* related? _____

_____

2. Define the terms *dyskinesia* and *dystonia.* _____

Acquiring Knowledge

Answer the following questions in the spaces provided.

1. What two neurotransmitters normally control the activity of the basal ganglia? What happens in Parkinson's disease?

_____

_____

_____

2. Describe the main symptoms of Parkinson's disease. _____

_____

3. What is the mechanism of action of levodopa? Carbidopa? Selegiline? _____

_____

4. List the adverse effects associated with levodopa. _____

_____

5. What drug interactions are possible with levodopa therapy? _____

_____

6. Why are anticholinergic drugs useful in the treatment of Parkinson's disease? _____

_____

7. What side effects are produced by anticholinergic drugs? By antihistaminic drugs? _____

_____

8. What is the mechanism of action of amantadine *(Symmetrel)?* _____

_____

_____

9. Describe the mechanism of action of bromocriptine *(Parlodel).* _____

_____

_____

Applying Knowledge—On the Job

Use your critical thinking skills to answer the following questions in the spaces provided.

1. The local university hospital has a neurological clinic that treats many patients with Parkinson's disease. Why might each of the following patients treated this week at the clinic be prescribed a drug other than *Sinemet?*

   a. Patient A has been taking *Sinemet* for 2 weeks and complains of fainting when getting out of bed, a racing heart, and loss of appetite.

_____

   b. Patient B is a self-confessed "health nut" who takes multiple vitamin supplements every day, including all of the B vitamins.

   c. Patient C is taking *Marplan* for depression.

2. Why might each of the following patients be prescribed a drug other than *Artane?*

   a. Patient A has been taking *Artane* for a week and presents with nausea, constipation, rapid heartbeat, and fever.

   b. Patient B is taking haloperidol for Tourette's syndrome.

3. Explain how the "unbalancing" of dopamine and acetylcholine levels in the basal ganglia can cause dystonias and dyskinesias.

4. Explain why the combination product *Sinemet* is so commonly used in treating Parkinson's disease.

5. How do you think taking the combination tablet *Sinemet* would increase patient compliance over taking *Dopar* and *Lodosyn* separately?

6. What is another indication for *Parlodel* other than Parkinson's disease? How does it work?

Internet Connection

Contact the **MedicineNet** search engine (http://www.medicinenet.com) and click on *Diseases and Treatments,* then highlight the letter "P" and find *Parkinson's Disease.* Provided is additional and very useful background information on Parkinson's disease and the drugs used to treat this condition. Also highlight the letter "D" and find *Dystonia.* Organize a short presentation concerning the description, causes, and treatments for dystonia. What is the relationship of this condition to Parkinson's disease? You can also click on the *Pharmacy and Drugs* heading to acquire additional information on any of the drugs mentioned in these articles.

Additional Reading

Danisi, F. 2002. Parkinson's disease: Therapeuptic strategies to improve patient function and quality of life. *Geriatrics* 57 (3):46.

Jenner, P. 1995. The rationale for the use of dopamine agonists in Parkinson's disease. *Neurology* 45:S6.

Kieburtz, K., Shoulson, I., and McDermott, M. 1997. Safety and efficacy of pramipexole in early Parkinson's disease. *Journal of the American Medical Association* 278:125.

GENERAL ANESTHETICS

DRUG CLASS AT A GLANCE

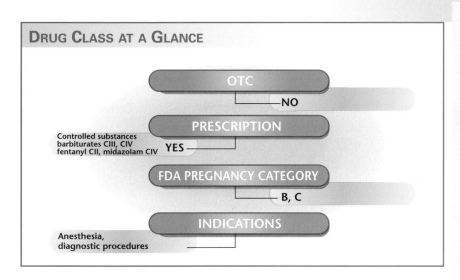

OTC
— NO

PRESCRIPTION

Controlled substances
barbiturates CIII, CIV
fentanyl CII, midazolam CIV — YES

FDA PREGNANCY CATEGORY
— B, C

INDICATIONS

Anesthesia,
diagnostic procedures

Key Terms

adipose tissue: tissue containing fat cells.

analgesia: decreased response to pain; condition in which painful stimuli are not consciously interpreted (perceived) as hurting.

dissociative anesthesia: form of general anesthesia in which patients do not appear to be unconscious.

euphoria: feeling of well-being or elation; feeling good.

general anesthesia: deep state of unconsciousness in which there is no response to stimuli, including painful stimuli.

halogenated hydrocarbon: compound that contains halogen (chlorine, fluorine, bromine, iodine) combined with hydrogen and carbon.

hypothalamus: center of the brain that influences mood, motivation, and the perception of pain.

hypoxia: reduction of oxygen supply to tissues below the amount required for normal physiological function.

CHAPTER FOCUS

This chapter describes drugs that reduce patient response to painful stimuli by altering patient consciousness.

CHAPTER OBJECTIVES

After studying this chapter, you should be able to

- identify the various stages of general anesthesia and describe the physical responses as the central nervous system (CNS) functions are depressed.

- name two classes of general anesthetics by their routes of drug administration.

- explain why more than one anesthetic may be administered to provide muscle relaxation without totally depressing the brain.

- describe how general anesthetics are excreted from the body and how this differs from the way local anesthetics are excreted.

- explain what an adjunct to anesthesia is and cite two examples of drug adjuncts used with general anesthetics.

- list three side effects that may be associated with anesthetic use.

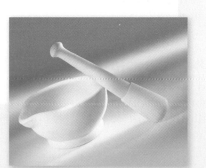

induction of general anesthesia: time required to take a patient from consciousness to Stage III of anesthesia.

maintenance of general anesthesia: ability to keep a patient safely in Stage III of anesthesia.

medullary depression: inhibition of automatic responses controlled by the medulla, such as breathing or cardiac function.

medullary paralysis: condition in which overdose of anesthetic shuts down cardiovascular and respiratory centers in the medulla, causing death.

neuroleptanalgesia: condition in which a patient is quiet, calm, and has no response to pain after the combined administration of an opioid analgesic and fentanyl.

neuroleptanesthesia: state of unconsciousness plus neuroleptanalgesia produced by the combined administration of nitrous oxide, fentanyl, and droperidol.

synergistic: when the action resulting from a combination of drugs is greater than the sum of their individual drug effects.

INTRODUCTION

Mild inhibition of cortical activity reduces anxiety, whereas more intense depression of the limbic and reticular systems produces sleep. Sleep is a state of unconsciousness in which stimulation such as yelling or shaking will arouse an individual. **General anesthesia** is a deeper state of unconsciousness (sleep), in which an individual cannot respond to stimulation.

GENERAL ANESTHESIA

Drugs discussed in the previous chapters selectively depress the central nervous system (CNS). During general anesthesia, all sensations are inhibited. Because sensations are suppressed, general anesthesia is used primarily to prevent the reactions to painful stimuli associated with surgery. General anesthesia agents are CNS depressants that abolish pain by inhibiting the function of the CNS through an unknown mechanism.

The extent of CNS depression under general anesthesia is much greater than that produced by other CNS depressant drugs (tranquilizers, sedatives, and hypnotics) at therapeutic doses. All of the major areas of the CNS are suppressed except for the medullary centers that regulate the vital organs (heart and lungs). An anesthesiologist controls the delicate balance between the beneficial effects of anesthesia and **medullary depression,** which can result in medullary paralysis and death.

Signs and Stages of Anesthesia

General anesthesia is produced by gradually depressing the CNS. The sequence of depression is divided into four stages, as illustrated in

Figure 18:1. During Stage I, the cerebral cortex is gradually inhibited. This stage is characterized by a decreased response to pain **(analgesia),** a feeling of **euphoria** (well-being or elation), and a loss of consciousness (sleep).

Once the cerebral cortex is fully depressed, the **hypothalamus** assumes control of body functions (Stage II). Stage II is known as the "excitement phase," because there is an overall increase in sympathetic tone. Blood pressure, heart rate, respiration, and muscle tone increase during this stage. During Stage II, cardiac arrhythmias may occur. Eventually, however, the hypothalamus is depressed, and patients enter Stage III.

Stage III is usually referred to as surgical anesthesia, because surgery is most efficiently performed at this level of general anesthesia. Stage III is divided into four planes (1–4) that reflect the progressive depth of CNS depression. During this stage, cardiovascular and respiratory functions return to normal, spinal reflexes are inhibited, and skeletal muscles are relaxed. Surgical incisions can be made throughout Stage III without producing pain or skeletal muscle contraction.

Stage IV is the phase of **medullary paralysis.** This stage represents an overdose of general anesthetic, in which cardiovascular and respiratory centers in the medulla are inhibited and death occurs.

FIGURE 18:1 Signs and Stages of Anesthesia Associated with CNS Depression

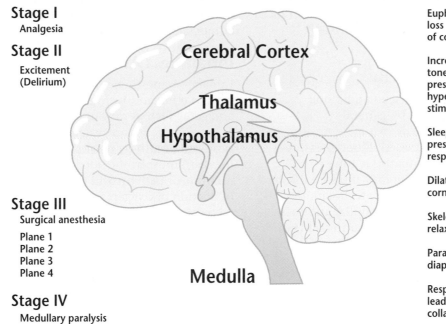

Stage I
Analgesia

Stage II
Excitement
(Delirium)

Cerebral Cortex

Thalamus

Hypothalamus

Stage III
Surgical anesthesia
Plane 1
Plane 2
Plane 3
Plane 4

Medulla

Stage IV
Medullary paralysis

Euphoria, giddiness, loss of pain, loss of consciousness

Increased sympathetic tone: elevated blood pressure and heart rate, hyperreaction to stimulation

Sleep, normal blood pressure and respiration

Dilated pupils, loss of corneal reflex

Skeletal muscle relaxation

Paralysis of the diaphragm, hypotension

Respiratory paralysis leads to circulatory collapse and death

The clinical signs associated with each stage of general anesthesia vary with the general anesthetic being used. Some anesthetics produce excellent analgesia at Stage I, while others do not produce any analgesia until Stage III. However, most anesthetics used today are capable of producing Stages III and IV anesthesia as just described. An anesthetic that produces all stages of general anesthesia (I, II, III, and IV) is a *complete* anesthetic.

Induction and Maintenance

Induction of general anesthesia is the time required to take a patient from consciousness to Stage III. **Maintenance of general anesthesia** is the ability to keep a patient safely in Stage III. The ideal general anesthetic would produce rapid induction and slow maintenance without entering Stage IV anesthesia. In addition, recovery from the ideal general anesthesia would occur rapidly without side effects.

Unfortunately, there is no ideal general anesthetic. Some anesthetics are excellent for induction (nitrous oxide, thiopental, and fentanyl citrate-droperidol), whereas others are better for maintenance of general anesthesia. Also, all anesthetics are associated with side effects. Today, anesthesiologists usually employ a combination of anesthetics to meet the needs of surgeons and to minimize patient reaction. Rapid, smooth induction with well-controlled maintenance is the key to good general anesthesia.

Route of Administration

General anesthetics are administered by inhalation or intravenous injection. These routes provide rapid delivery of the drug into the blood, which facilitates smooth induction of general anesthesia. Unlike other drugs, most of the general anesthetics do not bind to plasma proteins. General anesthetics dissolve in the blood before they are distributed to other tissues. Eventually, general anesthetics are carried to the CNS, where the primary pharmacological effect is produced. The degree of CNS depression is related to the concentration of the anesthetic in the brain. However, the level of drug necessary to produce general anesthesia varies with each anesthetic. Induction and duration of general anesthesia also vary with each anesthetic and are related to the physical properties of the drug.

Physiological Effects

Although the primary action of anesthetics is on the CNS, anesthetics also influence a variety of other tissues. Selection of the proper anesthetic may depend on the drug's alteration of cardiac, bronchial, or hepatic function.

Central Nervous System

In general, all nervous tissue is depressed by general anesthetics. Voluntary (motor) and involuntary (autonomic) systems are inhibited.

Respiratory function is depressed through a central action. However, oxygen deprivation does not occur because ventilation is controlled by the anesthesiologist. Some anesthetics cause pituitary secretion of antidiuretic hormone (ADH), resulting in postoperative urinary retention, especially in elderly patients.

Cardiovascular System

The myocardium (heart muscle) and blood pressure may be depressed by general anesthetics. However, the degree of depression varies with the anesthetic used. Blood pressure may decrease because sympathetic tone is inhibited, whereas heart rate may increase due to vagal inhibition. Occasionally, catecholamines are secreted from the adrenal medulla, and these circulating catecholamines may counteract the myocardial depression. On the other hand, some anesthetics sensitize the heart to the catecholamine stimulation, and ventricular arrhythmias may occur.

Salivary and Bronchial Secretions

Inhalation anesthetics irritate the mucosal lining of the respiratory tract and salivary glands. This irritation leads to the secretion of mucus, coughing, and spasms of the larynx in unconscious patients.

Skeletal Muscle

Depression of pyramidal systems and spinal reflexes causes skeletal muscle relaxation in Stage III (Plane 3) anesthesia (page 185). However, certain anesthetics produce additional skeletal muscle relaxation by inhibiting neuromuscular function. Usually, acetylcholine is blocked from interacting with the skeletal muscle membrane in these situations.

Gastrointestinal Tract

Nausea and vomiting are the most common side effects associated with the use of general anesthetics. These effects frequently occur during recovery, making patients uncomfortable. Decreased intestinal motility may lead to postoperative constipation.

Liver

Halothane, enflurane, and chloroform, in particular, are suspected of producing liver damage (hepatotoxicity). Repeated exposure to these agents may cause altered enzyme production, jaundice, or hepatic necrosis. Patients with liver damage, jaundice, or known sensitivity to these anesthetics should not be exposed to them.

USE OF GENERAL ANESTHETICS

General anesthetics include inhalation anesthetics and injectable anesthetics. In addition, there are adjuncts to general anesthesia.

Inhalation Anesthetics

Inhalation anesthetics include volatile liquids such as ether and **halogenated hydrocarbons** and gases such as nitrous oxide (see Table 18:1). These anesthetics are usually inhaled through the nose and mouth by means of a face mask. Air (oxygen) must be included in the anesthetic mixture, or patients will rapidly develop **hypoxia** (reduction of oxygen supply to tissues below the amount required for normal physiological function). Anesthesiologists control the mixture and rate of delivery of anesthetic throughout the surgical procedure. When the face mask is removed, patients quickly exhale inhalation anesthetics. As a result of exhalation, the blood drug level falls, and the patients begin to recover from the general anesthesia.

Most general anesthetics are excreted through the lungs. However, a small percentage of the halogenated hydrocarbons (halothane, enflurane, isoflurane, and methoxyflurane) are metabolized in the liver. All of the inhalation anesthetics except nitrous oxide (it is not potent enough to maintain Stage III, Plane 3 anesthesia) produce all stages of general anesthesia; therefore, they can be used for induction and maintenance of general anesthesia. Nitrous oxide ("laughing gas") can be used only for induction of general anesthesia. However, nitrous oxide produces such good analgesia that it is frequently used alone for dental procedures or in combination with other anesthetics.

Injectable Anesthetics

Injectable anesthetics include the barbiturates (methohexital, thiamylal, and thiopental), etomidate *(Amidate)*, ketamine *(Ketalar)*, midazolam *(Versed)*, propofol *(Diprivan)*, and a combination of fentanyl citrate and droperidol *(Innovar)* (see Table 18:1 for a display of injectable anesthetic effects). The barbiturate anesthetics can be used for induction or maintenance of general anesthesia. These drugs are usually administered intravenously because extravascular injections cause pain, swelling, and ulceration.

Thiopental, an ultrashort-acting barbiturate, induces general anesthesia within 30 seconds, but the tissue levels fall slowly. Barbiturate anesthetics are highly fat soluble and thus are redistributed to fatty tissues. The drug accumulates in **adipose (fat) tissue** and leaves the tissue so slowly that it takes a long time for these anesthetics to become metabolized and excreted into the urine. As the anesthetic leaves the adipose tissue, it is redistributed to other organs. Redistribution of the drug leads to residual CNS depression (hangover), mental disorientation, and nausea during the recovery period.

Barbiturate anesthetics are associated with the same side effects and contraindications as other barbiturates (their adverse effects were discussed in Chapter 12). Barbiturate anesthetics may cause laryngospasm or bronchospasm during the postoperative recovery period. It is important to observe patients carefully because they may choke or aspirate fluid into the lungs. An absolute contraindication to the use of thiopental or methohexital as anesthetics is a history or predisposing evidence of *status asthmaticus*.

Etomidate (*Amidate*) and propofol (*Diprivan*) are hypnotic drugs used for intravenous induction of

TABLE 18:1	Side Effects and Uses of General Anesthetics			
ANESTHETIC (TRADE NAME)	**USE**	**EFFECT ON RESPIRATORY SYSTEM**	**NAUSEA & VOMITING**	**POTENTIALLY HEPATOTOXIC**
Inhalation Anesthetics—Volatile Liquids:				
chloroform	Obsolete	Seldom	Moderate	Yes
ether	Maintenance	Frequently, increases secretions	High	—
enflurane (*Ethrane*)	Maintenance	Seldom	—	Yes
isoflurane (*Forane*)	Maintenance	Seldom	Low	Yes
halothane (*Fluothane*)	Maintenance	Seldom	Low	Yes
methoxyflurane (*Penthrane*)	Maintenance	Seldom	Low	Yes
Inhalation Anesthetics—Gases:				
nitrous oxide	Induction	—	Low	Yes
Injectable Anesthetics:				
etomidate (*Amidate*)	Induction	Bronchospasm	Low–moderate	—
fentanyl citrate and droperidol (*Innovar*)*	Induction	Seldom secretions, laryngospasms	Low	—
ketamine (*Ketalar*)	Induction and maintenance	Salivation and laryngospasm	High	—
methohexital (*Methohexital*)***	Induction and maintenance	Bronchial secretions	Moderate	—
midazolam (*Versed*)***	Preoperative sedation and induction	Salivation and bronchospasm	—	—
propofol (*Diprivan*)	Induction and maintenance	Salivation	Low–moderate	—
thiamylal (*Surital*)**	Induction	Bronchial secretions	Moderate	—
thiopental (*Pentothal*)**	Induction	Seldom	Low–moderate	—

*Schedule II drug.
**Schedule III drug.
***Schedule IV drug.

general anesthesia. Etomidate has no analgesic activity and exerts less depressant effects on the heart and respiratory centers than do the barbiturates. Because of its cardiorespiratory profile, this drug may be advantageous for use in high-risk surgical patients who cannot tolerate tissue depression. Propofol is used in combination with other anesthetics for induction or maintenance of general anesthesia.

Midazolam (*Versed*) is a short-acting CNS depressant related to the benzodiazepines (diazepam—*Valium*—and chlordiazepoxide—*Librium*) but more potent. Midazolam is frequently administered intravenously prior to short diagnostic or endoscopic procedures to produce conscious sedation. Patients are awake but do not fight against the intubation procedures. Midazolam is also used for induction of general anesthesia before administration of other anesthetics or to supplement nitrous oxide. Because of the CNS depressant action of midazolam, preanesthetic opioid medications will potentiate the hypnotic effect of midazolam.

Ketamine (*Ketalar*) is a short-acting nonbarbiturate **dissociative anesthetic** that produces good analgesia and loss of memory but does not relax skeletal muscles. Therefore, patients appear to be awake but do not respond to stimulation. Ketamine is thought to act primarily upon the limbic system so that very little respiratory and cardiovascular depression is produced. In fact, blood pressure and heart rate may be elevated during the anesthesia. This short-acting anesthetic is rapidly metabolized in the liver. It can be given intramuscularly or intravenously to induce anesthesia. Vivid dreams and hallucinations usually occur during the recovery period. In a small percentage of patients, delirium occurs. Severe reactions are treated with short-acting barbiturates. Ketamine is not a restricted drug; however, it is chemically related to phencyclidine, a hallucinogen of high abuse potential.

When *Innovar*, a mixture of an opioid analgesic (fentanyl) and a tranquilizer (droperidol), is administered, **neuroleptanalgesia** is produced. This type of anesthesia provides excellent analgesia while patients remain conscious. This combination cannot produce unconsciousness **(neuroleptanesthesia)** unless a third anesthetic (nitrous oxide) is added. Fentanyl and droperidol are eventually metabolized by the liver. Unusual side effects that occur with the use of droperidol are extrapyramidal symptoms. Occasionally, a parkinsonian syndrome—uncontrolled movements of the tongue and head—occurs. The fentanyl-droperidol product may be administered intramuscularly or by slow intravenous injection. If an opioid analgesic is prescribed following this kind of anesthesia, the dose of the opioid may be significantly reduced to one-fourth of the recommended dose, because these drugs have a **synergistic** action on the CNS.

Adjuncts to General Anesthesia

In addition to the anesthetic agents, a variety of different drugs are routinely used before and after surgical procedures, as outlined in Table 18:2. Preanesthetic and postanesthetic medications are administered to aid induction of general anesthesia, counteract the side effects of anesthetics, or make recovery more comfortable for patients. Many people approach surgery with fear and apprehension; usually there is intense anxiety about the existing medical problem and concern about the outcome of the operation. Some individuals also experience severe pain as a result of their medical condition. Anxiety and CNS stimulation tend to counteract a smooth induction into anesthesia. Therefore, CNS depressants, such as opioid analgesics, tranquilizers, or sedative-hypnotics may be administered before surgery. Often, these adjunct medications are given the evening before so that patients are groggy and unaware of the preparations being carried out prior to surgery.

Most general anesthetics that take patients into Stage III, Plane 3 anesthesia produce skeletal muscle relaxation. However, it may be advantageous in certain operations (abdominal and thoracic) to have skeletal muscle relaxation for a long time with minimal CNS depression. For this purpose, neuromuscular blocking drugs, such as tubocurarine or succinylcholine, may be administered during surgery. These drugs produce adequate skeletal muscle relaxation while patients are maintained in early Stage III anesthesia.

Anticholinergic drugs may be used as preanesthetic medications to prevent the salivary and bronchial secretions induced by some anesthetics. Bronchial secretions of mucus usually line the respiratory tract and may impair the transfer of oxygen and anesthetic across the lungs. If the secretions are not controlled, hypoxia may develop.

Cautions and Drug Interactions

Many patients are not aware of possible drug reactions, allergies, or hypersensitivities that they have. This lack of awareness is especially likely if

TABLE 18:2   Adjunct Medications Used With Anesthetics

PHARMACOLOGICAL CLASS	ADMINISTRATION	REASON FOR USE
Analgesics (opioid)	Preanesthesia, postanesthesia	Relieve pain and produce sedation
Antianxiety agents	Preanesthesia	Decrease apprehension
Antiarrhythmic drugs	During surgery	Control arrhythmias
Antibiotics	Preanesthesia	Decrease infection
Anticholinergics	Preanesthesia, during surgery	Decrease salivary and bronchial secretions, prevent bradycardia
Cholinergic drugs	Postanesthesia	Relieve urinary retention
Sedative-hypnotic drugs (short-acting agents)	Preanesthesia	Decrease apprehension
Skeletal muscle relaxants	During surgery	Sustain skeletal muscle relaxation
Tranquilizers	Preanesthesia, postanesthesia	Sedate, control nausea and vomiting

Note: Not all drugs can be mixed in the same syringe without compromising the activity of the active components. Some drug combinations result in discoloration of the solution, haze formation, or even precipitation. These are signs of drug incompatibility that should alert medical personnel to discard the solution and avoid such combinations in the future.

patients have not previously encountered surgery or preanesthetic medications. Therefore, patients should be carefully observed for any unusual reactions to medications before and after general anesthesia.

Most of the problems that arise following general anesthesia result from residual depression of the CNS. Patients frequently feel "hung over," dizzy, or nauseous, and should be assisted, since mental disorientation may lead to impaired judgment and incoordination. Postanesthetic medications such as analgesics, muscle relaxants, and tranquilizers will potentiate the residual CNS depression of general anesthetics. Antibiotics, such as streptomycin, kanamycin, and erythromycin, will potentiate the skeletal muscle relaxation to produce muscle weakness and fatigue.

Several of the inhalation anesthetics and surgical adjuncts (skeletal muscle relaxants) produce malignant hyperthermia in certain individuals. This acute toxicity is due to a genetic defect.

Solution Incompatibilities

The injectable anesthetics, as their name implies, must be prepared as solutions to facilitate parenteral administration. Frequently, parenteral medications are given in combination for convenience and efficient drug handling and to minimize patient discomfort by reducing the number of injections. Considering the variety of drugs that may be used during an operation, it is understandable why combining medications might be useful. Drug admixture may be performed by adding solutions to an existing intravenous line or by mixing two or more drugs in the same syringe prior to injection.

Neither the fentanyl-droperidol product nor ketamine should be combined in the same syringe with a barbiturate, because drug precipitation results. Methohexital and thiopental have been reported to be incompatible with several antibiotics, antihistaminics, and opioid analgesics. Examples of drugs that should not be combined with the barbiturate anesthetics are chlorpromazine, kanamycin, lidocaine, promazine, streptomycin, tetracycline, methicillin, methyldopa, and prochlorperazine. Thiopental should not be combined with amikacin, codeine, meperidine, morphine, penicillin G, promethazine, succinylcholine, and tetracycline because precipitation will occur.

Solutions containing barbiturates are usually alkaline (pH greater than 10). As a rule, these alkaline solutions should not be mixed with acid solutions because the barbiturate will precipitate. Such incompatible acid solutions include atropine, scopolamine, and succinylcholine. Methohexital undergoes a specific interaction with silicone and rubber, which dictates that it should never be in contact with rubber stoppers or parts of syringes that have been treated with silicone.

Special Considerations

With the use of any complete anesthetic, patient vital signs should be monitored frequently before, during, and after anesthesia. During the postoperative recovery period, patients' airways must be kept unobstructed. It is important to check patients for signs of hypoxia (skin discoloration), laryngospasm, or gagging, which can precipitate aspiration of fluid into a patient's lungs. Patients should be positioned so that the potential for aspiration of secretions is minimized.

Intravenous fluids and vasopressor drugs should be kept available for the treatment of hypotensive episodes. Patients should be monitored and positioned to avoid redistribution of anesthetic to the CNS, which may precipitate severe hypotension and respiratory arrest during the recovery period.

Overdose occurs most often as a result of too much anesthetic administered or because the rate of administration is too fast. With supportive therapy, fluid replacement, mechanical support of respiration, the effects usually reverse once the anesthetic is stopped. The patient is continually monitored until the vital signs return to an acceptable stable level.

Postoperative nausea often associated with the barbiturate anesthetics may be lessened or avoided by having patients fast prior to receiving the drug. Patients have experienced mental confusion following ketamine anesthesia. Since drugs such as ketamine may be used as adjuncts in diagnostic procedures, patients should be cautioned not to drive or operate hazardous machinery for 24 to 36 hours after recovering from general anesthesia.

Patient Administration and Monitoring

Patients are usually exposed to these drugs in an operating room environment. For such procedures it is expected that the patient will be closely monitored during and after surgery to assure adverse reactions are minimized. Even for diagnostic procedures, the patient is kept for observation until it is clear there is no immediate risk. The opportunity for adverse effects is more likely to occur when information on patient medical history is inadequate prior to the selection of the anesthetics and premedication regimen. Patient history is extremely important to ascertain which drugs are most appropriate. Patient interview will provide information that is critical to minimizing adverse reactions to anesthesics.

Alcohol consumption, blood pressure medication, antibiotic, and OTC product use should be thoroughly reviewed. Midazolam will be potentiated by CNS depressants, including alcohol in cough/cold preparations.

Midazolam is contraindicated in patients with acute narrow-angle glaucoma, although it may be used in open-angle glaucoma.

Ketamine is not the drug of choice in patients where a significant increase in blood pressure would be hazardous.

Hypersensitivity to anesthetics and/or premedications from previous exposure, or knowledge of a family member experiencing difficulty during surgery, may provide evidence of a contraindication to specific anesthetics. This is especially valuable as an indication of predisposition to malignant hyperthermia.

Chapter Review

Understanding Terminology

Answer the following questions in the spaces provided.

1. Name the brain center that influences mood, motivation, and the perception of pain.

   _____

   _____

2. Differentiate among *analgesia, general anesthesia, dissociative anesthesia, medullary depression,* and *medullary paralysis.*

   _____

   _____

3. Explain the difference between induction of anesthesia and maintenance of anesthesia.

   _____

   _____

Acquiring Knowledge

Answer the following questions in the spaces provided.

1. How does general anesthesia differ from sleep?

   _____

   _____

2. How is general anesthesia produced?

   _____

   _____

3. How do the effects of general anesthetics on the CNS differ from those of lesser anesthetics?

   _____

   _____

4. What do the various stages of anesthesia represent?

   _____

   _____

5. What effects do general anesthetics have on the cardiovascular and respiratory systems?

   _____

   _____

6. How may the general anesthetics produce skeletal muscle relaxation?

   _____

   _____

7. How do the inhalation anesthetics differ from the injectable anesthetics?

   _____

   _____

8. What is neuroleptanesthesia?

   _____

   _____

9. For what purpose are the various adjunct medications administered?

_____

_____

10. What types of drug interactions may occur in postsurgical patients?

_____

_____

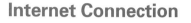

Internet Connection

Web pages that present information on anesthetics include sites directed at parents and health care providers. These sites explain procedures in order to help patients understand the unfamiliar environment of the operating room. The material is expected be read by the general public and is therefore user friendly.

Enter health.howstuffworks.com (no www is needed). A list of hyperlinked topics are presented and include, how anesthesia works, and specific drugs such as inhaled anesthetics and injectable anesthetics. The information at the website is provided by an anesthesiologist in the department of Anesthesiology at Johns Hopkins Medical School.

Additional Reading

Birka, A. 1999. New perspectives on the use of propofol. _Crit Care Nurse_ 19 (4):18.

Haslego, S. S. 2002. Malignant hyperthermia: How to spot it early. _RN 65_ (7):31.

Hazen, S. E. 1997. Elder care—general anesthesia and elderly surgical patients. _Association of Operating Room Nurses Journal_ 65 (4):815.

Humphries, Y. 1997. Superiority of oral ketamine as an analgesic and sedative for wound care procedures in the pediatric patient with burns. _Journal of Burn Care and Rehabilitation_ 18 (1):34.

McAuliffe, M. S. 1997. Anesthetic drug interactions. _CRNA—the Clinical Forum for Nurse Anesthetists_ 8 (2):84.

Moore, J. L. 1992. Malignant hyperthermia. _American Family Physician_ 45 (5):2245.

Powell, R. M. 2000. Ondansetron given before induction of anesthesia reduces shivering after general anesthesia. _Anesth Analg._ 90 (6):1423.

Reimann, F. M. 2000. Synergistic sedation with low-dose midazolam and propofol for colonoscopies. _Endoscopy 2000_ 32 (3):239.

Stewert-Amidei, C. 2002. Pharmacology advances in the neuroscience intensive care unit. _Crit Care Nurs Clin North Am_ 14 (1):31.

19

OPIOID (NARCOTIC) ANALGESICS

DRUG CLASS AT A GLANCE

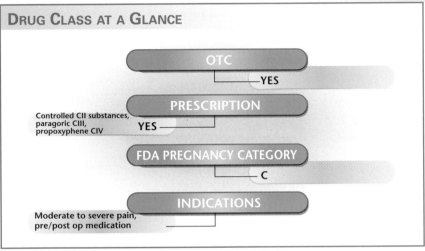

OTC
— YES

PRESCRIPTION
Controlled CII substances, paragoric CIII, propoxyphene CIV   YES

FDA PREGNANCY CATEGORY
— C

INDICATIONS
Moderate to severe pain, pre/post op medication

Key Terms

addiction: a chronic neurobiologic disease in which genetic, psychosocial, and environmental factors induce changes in the individual's behavior to compulsively use drugs despite the harm that may result.

agonist: drug that attaches to a receptor and initiates an action.

analgesia: relief from pain.

analgesic: substance (synthetic or naturally occurring) that inhibits the body's reaction to painful stimuli or perception of pain.

antagonist: drug that attaches to a receptor, does not initiate an action, but blocks an agonist from producing an effect.

antidiuretic hormone (ADH): substance produced in the pituitary gland that decreases urine production by allowing the kidneys to reabsorb water.

antitussive: able to suppress coughing.

anuria: no formation of urine.

dysphoria: feeling of discomfort or unpleasantness.

CHAPTER FOCUS

This chapter describes drugs that minimize the response to (reaction to or perception of) intense pain without altering consciousness. Opioid analgesics are not general or local anesthetics. This chapter also discusses addiction.

CHAPTER OBJECTIVES

After studying this chapter, you should be able to

- describe the sources of opioid analgesics.
- discuss the pharmacological effects of these drugs.
- discuss absorption and metabolism of these drugs.
- list the adverse effects of these drugs.
- explain acute opioid poisoning.
- discuss the actions of opioid antagonists.
- discuss special considerations in the use of opioid analgesics and list drug interactions.

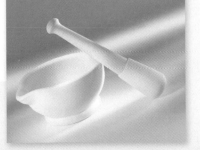

emesis: vomiting.

endogenous: naturally occurring within the body.

endorphins: neuropeptides produced within the CNS that interact with opioid receptors to produce analgesia.

expectorant: substance that causes the removal (expulsion) of mucous secretions from the respiratory system.

hyperalgesia: an abnormally painful response to a stimulus.

narcotic (opioid): a substance extracted or derived from opium, or a synthetic substance that acts on the brain receptors like opiates to relieve pain and induce partial consciousness (stupor).

narcotic (opioid) antagonist: a drug that attaches to opioid receptors and displaces the opioid analgesic or opioid neuropeptide.

neuropathic pain: pain resulting from a damaged nervous system or damaged nerve cells.

nociceptor: specialized peripheral nerve cells sensitive to tissue injury that transmit pain signals to the brain for interpretation of pain.

nonopioid analgesic: formerly known as nonnarcotic analgesics, such as NSAIDs and COX-2 inhibitors.

oliguria: smaller than normal amount of urine produced.

opiate: drug derived from opium and producing the same pharmacological effects as opium.

opioid: drug that produces the same pharmacological effects as opium and its family of drugs or the neuropeptides (enkephlin, endorphin) produced by the body.

opioid analgesics: chemically related to morphine or opium but are used to relieve pain.

peripheral nerve: part of the nervous system that is outside the central nervous system (the brain or spinal cord), usually near the surface of the tissue fibers or skin.

phlegm: secretion from the respiratory tract; usually called mucus.

physical dependence: condition in which the body requires a substance (drug) not normally found in the body in order to avoid symptoms associated with withdrawal, or the abstinence syndrome.

referred pain: origin of the pain is in a different location than where the individual feels the pain.

spasmogenic: causing a muscle to contract intermittently, resulting in a state of spasms.

synthetic drug: drug produced by a chemical process outside of the body.

tolerance: ability of the body to alter its response (to adapt) to drug effects so that the effects are minimized over time.

INTRODUCTION

Pain functions primarily as a protective signal. Pain may warn of imminent danger (fire) or the presence of internal disease (appendicitis or tumors). On the other hand, pain may be part of the normal healing process (inflammation). Relief from pain is desirable when the duration and intensity of pain alters the ability of an individual to function efficiently. In such situations, analgesic drugs are useful, because these agents relieve pain without producing a loss of consciousness.

There are two major classes of analgesics: the opioid analgesics and the nonopioid analgesics. Opioid analgesics are usually referred to as strong analgesics, whereas nonopioid drugs are considered mild analgesics. This classification suggests the type of pain that can be alleviated by each group. Opioid analgesics are capable of inhibiting pain of any origin. However, these drugs are used primarily to relieve moderate to severe pain of trauma, pain associated with myocardial infarction, pain associated with terminal illness, and postoperative pain.

PAIN

The sensation of pain is comprised of at least two elements: the local irritation (stimulation of **peripheral nerves)** and the recognition of pain (within the CNS). Free nerve endings called **nociceptors** are located in the skin, muscle, joints, bones, and viscera. Nociceptors respond to tissue injury. When there is no injury, there is no pain stimulus, so the nociceptors are quiet. When a pain generating event happens, biochemical changes occur within the localized area of the injury. Usually, prostaglandins, histamine, bradykinins, serotonin, and Substance P are among the peripheral neurotransmitters released that trigger nociceptors to wake up. Nociceptors alert the brain to the intensity of the pain by increasing the frequency of signals sent to specialized areas within the CNS.

The signals travel through the spinal cord into the area called the dorsal horn (DH) where they are routed to the appropriate area of the brain that can interpret the intensity and quality of pain present. Pain signals are sent up A-delta nociceptor and C-nociceptor fibers in the ascending pathways to the brain (Figure 19:1). If the signal is passed through the A-delta fibers (myelinated), the pain is consciously experienced as sharp. If the signal is passed through C fibers (unmyelinated), dull, aching pain is felt.

Pain management and selection of the most appropriate analgesic depends on the type and duration of pain. **Nociceptive pain** can only occur when all neural equipment (nerve cells, nerve endings, spinal cord, and brain) is working properly. When pain results from abnormal signals or nerves damaged by entrapment, infection (Herpes zoster or HIV), amputation, or diabetes, it is called **neuropathic pain.**

Pain duration is either acute or chronic. Acute pain usually appears in association with an observable injury (e.g., sunburn, broken foot, muscle sprain, or headache) and disappears when the injury heals. Chronic pain persists for weeks, months, or years even with analgesic therapy. Nociceptive pain can be either acute or chronic, while neuropathic pain is chronic, even though it may be intermittent. If an injury doesn't heal or the pain is not adequately inhibited, nociceptors get "really irritated," a condition known as peripheral sensitization, and send so many signals through the CNS that the patient overresponds to even normal stimuli, such as a feather or brush touched to the area. In neuropathic conditions sensitization can also occur within the spinal

FIGURE 19:1 Site of Action for Drugs that Relieve Pain

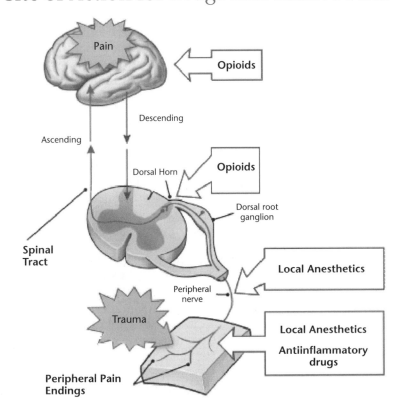

neurons observed as over responsiveness **(hyperalgesia),** prolonged pain, or the spread of pain to an uninjured area **(referred pain).**

No matter what type of pain is present, relief from pain **(analgesia)** is the therapeutic goal. The specialized medical discipline of pain management has changed the spectrum of therapy and the types of drugs used, especially to achieve satisfactory analgesia as soon as possible. Inadequate control of pain can delay healing. With chronic pain, psychological and emotional changes occur that cause the patient to become tired and irritable; patients develop insomnia, significant stress responses such as increased heart rate and blood pressure, depression, impaired resistance to infection, and even increased sensitization to pain. The psychological component associated with the inability to permanently relieve the pain intensifies the response to pain by stimulating the CNS.

In other chapters, pain relief (analgesia) has been shown to be the primary therapeutic action of local anesthetics and nonsteroidal antiinflammtory drugs (NSAIDs). By inhibiting sodium and potassium ion movement through the nerves, local anesthetics block nerve conduction and the sensation of pain is avoided. Analgesia is also produced by interrupting the metabolic pathway of inflammation, such as inhibition of prostaglandins by NSAIDs. Local anesthetics and NSAIDs act at the site of injury or at the level of the peripheral nerves (Figure 19:1). Because some antiepileptic drugs and tricyclic antidepressants depress neuronal excitability and suppress abnormal discharges, these drugs play an important adjunct role in pain management. While local anesthetics and antiepiletic drugs are used to reduce or ameliorate pain, the NSAIDs, acetaminophen, and COX-2 inhibitor drugs are most often referred to as the **nonopioid analgesics.**

Although the terminology used to describe the mechanism of analgesia is relatively new, the drugs discussed in this chapter, **opioid analgesics,** in their natural plant form, have been medicinally used for 5000 years.

OPIOID ANALGESICS

Until recently, drugs that were extracted from opium **(opiates)** or synthetic chemicals that produced the same pharmacological effects as opium were called **narcotic** analgesics. While this name still applies to the laws that govern the use of this class of drugs, current medical and research terminology refer to these drugs as **opioid** analgesics. The naturally occurring opiates (derivatives of opium) include morphine and codeine. Morphine is the largest component of the chemicals (alkaloids) extracted from the poppy plant. The term **opioids** is used today for any molecule, whether natural or **synthetic,** that acts on opioid receptors. Morphine is the prototype or standard opioid analgesic. Because it has been used for centuries as a medicinal drug, its clinical effects are well established and its dose-response has been well documented. This allows morphine to be the standard by which the potency of all the other opioid analgesics is measured.

It is held that opioid analgesics can relieve virtually any type of pain. Certainly, all opioid analgesics relieve moderate to severe acute and chronic pain. Opioid analgesics are the drug of choice in treating acute postoperative pain, including dental pain (oral analgesia), without incurring an increased risk of bleeding (as with NSAIDs). Opioid analgesics are first line therapy for pain associated with procedures (bone marrow biopsy), pain due to trauma (burns, vehicular accident), and cancer or visceral pain (pancreatitis, appendicitis). The opioids vary in their potency, onset of action, and incidence of opioid side effects (Table 19:1).

A select group of opioids are used for another therapeutic effect besides analgesia. Codeine, hydrocodone, and dextromethorphan are **antitussive** which means they effectively suppress the cough reflex. Dextromethorphan and codeine are the most commonly used antitussives and are considered to be much less potent than morphine and to possess a lower addiction liability.

Tolerance and physical dependence are factors that influence drug use. **Tolerance** develops to all opioids, although the onset and the altered drug effect may vary. When tolerance develops to the annoying side effects of the drug (sedation), it is considered a therapeutic benefit. However, when tolerance results in the need for a larger dose of drug to produce a CNS action (euphoria, analgesia), that is not considered to be a beneficial outcome. **Physical dependence** develops with long-term daily use of all strong opioids. Physical dependence means that with sustained use the body reacts (withdrawal syndrome) to sudden removal or rapid dose reduction of the drug. This reaction can be minimized or avoided by gradual dose reduction over several days to a week when the medication is to be discontinued.

Pharmacological Effects of Opioid Analgesics

DRUG	ADDICTION POTENTIAL	ANALGESIC POTENCY	ANTITUSSIVE ACTIVITY**	INCIDENCE OF NAUSEA AND VOMITING**	RESPIRATORY DEPRESSION**
alfentanil	*	Same as morphine	not rated	not rated	not rated
codeine	Low	Less than morphine	3	1	1
heroin	Highest	Greater than morphine	?	1	2
hydrocodone	Low	Less than morphine	3	?	1
hydromorphone	High	Greater than morphine	3	1	2
levorphanol	High	Same as morphine	2	1	2
meperidine	High	Same as morphine	1	2	2
methadone	Low	Same as morphine	2	1	2
morphine	High	Good	3	2	2
oxycodone	High	Same as morphine	3	2	2
oxymorphone	Highest	Greater than morphine	1	3	3
pentazocine	Moderate	Less than morphine	not rated	2	2
propoxyphene	Low	Less than morphine	not rated	1	1
sufentanil	*	Greater than morphine	not rated	not rated	not rated

**3 = high; 2 = moderate; 1 = low. *not rated

Physical dependence is not the same as addiction. **Addiction** is a complex interaction of genetic, psychological, and socio-environmental factors that describe behaviors in the individual that include compulsive drug use, craving, and lack of control over drug use. Treatment of pain with opioids, especially under adequate medical supervision, does not mean all treated individuals will become addicts.

Because of the potential for abuse, opioid analgesics are federally restricted controlled substances. These drugs can be obtained only by prescription from a physician registered and licensed with the Drug Enforcement Agency (DEA). Because of their high abuse potential, most opioids used as analgesics or adjuncts to anesthesia are restricted to controlled Schedule II. Schedule II (CII controlled substances) requires that listed drugs must have a new prescription written for each refill. Opioids with less abuse potential, such as codeine, appear in Schedules III and V according to the strength (amount of codeine) of the preparation. Opioids with the least

abuse potential such as dextromethorophan and opiates used as antidiarrheals are Schedule V drugs. Dextromethorphan does not require a prescription for cough preparation sold over-the-counter. The classification schedules (C1 to CV) associated with various opioid controlled substances are indicated in Table 19.2 along with the usual adult doses for analgesia.

Opiates come from cultivated plants or are chemically synthesized from morphine. In the late nineteenth century, morphine was chemically converted into heroin under the good intention of producing an analgesic that was less addicting than morphine. Unfortunately, heroin is 3 times more potent than morphine and more rapidly addicting. Heroin is fully restricted to Schedule I (CI) because it has a high abuse potential and no medically sanctioned use in the United States. This means it cannot be legally prescribed in the United States. The enforcement of laws that affect the distribution of controlled substances, even those with significant medical value, comes under the Drug Enforcement Agency. This agency

TABLE 19:2   Analgesic Doses of Centrally-Acting Analgesics

DRUG (TRADE NAME)	SCHEDULE	ADULT DOSE ANALGESIA	INTRAMUSCULAR ONSET (MIN)	ADMINISTRATION DURATION (HR)
Opiates:				
codeine	II	15–60 mg PO, SC, IM, IV*	15–30	4–6
heroin	I	No recognized medicinal value in the United States		
hydromorphone (*Dilaudid*)	II	2 mg PO, 1–2 mg SC, IM, IV*	15–30	4–5
morphine	II	5–20 mg IM, SC**	15–20	3–7
opium tincture	II	0.6 ml QID	—	—
oxycodone (*Roxicodone*)	II	5 mg PO*	15–30	4–6
oxymorphone (*Numorphan*)	II	1–1.5 mg IM, SC*; 0.5 mg IV	5–10	3–6
pantopon	II	5–20 mg IM, SC**	15–20	6–8
paregoric	III	5–10 ml PO (0.25–0.5 mg/kg for child) QD–QID	—	—
Opioids:				
alfentanil (*Alfenta*)	II	8–75 µg/kg IV	—	60
buprenorphine (*Buprenex*)	V	0.3 mg IM, IV*	—	—
butorphanol(*Stadol*)***		0.5–2 mg IM**, IV	10	3–4
butorphanol nasal spray (*Stadol NS*)		1 mg (1 spray in one nostril); repeat if needed in 90 min	—	—
dezocine (*Dalgan*)	II	5–20 mg IM, IV**	30	2–4
fentanyl (*Sublimaze*)	II	0.05–0.1 mg/kg IM	5–15	1–2
fentanyl transdermal (*Duragesic*)	II	Individualized dose		
fentanyl transmucosal (*Actiq*)	II	200–1800 mcg lozenge on a stick	—	—
levorphanol (*Levo-Dromoran*)	II	2–3 mg PO, SC	30–90	6–8
meperidine (*Demerol*)	II	50–150 mg PO, SC, IM**	10–15	2–4
methadone (*Dolophine, Methadone*)	II	2.5–10 mg PO, IM, SC**	10–15	4–6
nalbuphine (*Nubain*)***	IV	10 mg/70 kg SC, IM, IV*	15	3–6
pentazocine (*Talwin*)***	IV	50–100 mg PO; 30 mg IM, SC**	20	3
propoxyphene (*Darvon, Dolene*)	IV	65 mg PO**	15–30	4–6
remifentanil (*Ultiva*)	II	Continuous infusion		
sufentanil (*Sufenta*)	II	8–30 µg/kg IV	—	—
Central analgesic (nonopioid receptor active)				
tramadol (*Ultram*)		50–100 mg PO*	15–30	2–4

*Dose repeated every 6 hours.
**Dose repeated every 3–4 hours.
***These drugs are partial antagonist analgesics.

monitors the potential for abuse and "street value" associated with these drugs when sold for non-medicinal purposes.

SITE AND MECHANISM OF ACTION

Recognition of pain involves a component that intensifies the response to pain because the CNS anticipates how painful the injury will be. This recognition leads to anxiety and apprehension (CNS stimulation), which heightens the reaction to pain. Opioid analgesics are called central analgesics because they selectively act within the CNS to reduce the reaction to pain. Opioid analgesics do not impair the function of peripheral nerves. The pain is still present (especially in chronic conditions), but patients either can tolerate the pain or "don't care."

Several different types of opioid receptors have now been identified within the spinal cord and brain. Morphine was thought to interact with membrane-bound receptors as long as 40 years ago. However, it wasn't until the 1970s that evidence for an opioid receptor in the body was confirmed by the discovery of the endogenous peptides. These peptides include endorphin, enkephlin, dynorphin, and the newest ones, nociceptin and nocistatin. The word **endorphin** is derived from the words *endo*genous and m*orphine*. These peptides are believed to be important for survival because, when released, they provide pain relief that allows the injured person to move away from the harmful stimulus. Endorphins have been shown to be more than four times more potent than intravenous morphine. Eventually, the peptides are metabolized, levels decrease, and the pain signal returns causing the person to seek help to reduce the continuing pain.

Three opioid receptors are the most clinically important—**mμ, kappa,** and **delta.** Each of the peptides has a preference for one of the opioid receptors. Endorphins are produced within the pituitary and hypothalamus and are selective for mμ receptors. Enkephlins, produced throughout the CNS and peripheral nerve endings, prefer delta receptors, while dynorphins, primarily found in pain nerve endings, interact with kappa receptors. Reduction in the awareness and reaction to pain is controlled through a combination of mμ, kappa, and delta receptors within the brain.

Morphine and the other opioid analgesics act by binding to opioid receptors and mimicking **(agonist)** the effects of the analgesic peptides. The therapeutically important opioid analgesics interact with mμ and kappa receptors, inhibit neurotransmitter release such as Subtance P, inhibit nociceptor signals from reaching the spinal cord, reduce nerve excitability, and alter pain perception. All of these **agonist** actions contribute to pain relief. Most of the traditional opioids (morphine, oxymorphone, oxycodone, methadone, fentanyl) are pure agonists referred to as mμ agonists. This means they bind to the receptor and produce a response. Agonists for different opioid receptors are believed to relieve different types of pain. This would explain why morphine may not work as well for pancreatic pain, but another opioid analgesic does.

Other opioids (nalbuphine, butorphanol) are partial agonists because they initiate kappa receptors but block mμ receptors. Finally, drugs like naloxone, are pure **antagonists.** These drugs do not produce effects but bind to the receptor so that other agonists cannot and, in this way, reverse the mμ effects of opioids.

PHARMACOLOGICAL EFFECTS

Like the endogenous opioids, opioid analgesics produce effects on a variety of tissues. Opioid receptors are also widely distributed outside of the CNS, such as in the gastrointestinal and urinary tract. In addition to modifying pain perception, the endogenous peptides modify mood, and regulate cardiovascular, respiratory, and endocrine function. This explains how the opioid analgesics produce their classic side effects of sedation (mμ, kappa) euphoria (mμ), dysphoria (kappa), constipation (mμ), urinary retention (mμ), miosis (mμ, kappa), and respiratory depression (mμ).

Effects on CNS

Opioid analgesics may influence CNS function by increasing or decreasing certain CNS activity. For example, opioid analgesics do not cause a loss of consciousness at therapeutic doses. However, these drugs do alter mental behavior. In particular, opioid analgesics produce changes in mood and decrease mental alertness. Some individuals experience a feeling of well-being—a warm glow—known as euphoria. This pleasant experience may entice the individuals to use the drug continually, thus contributing to the development of drug dependency. This is a highly variable response because other individuals may experience **dysphoria,** an unpleasant reaction, which enhances anxiety and fear. Dysphoric individuals are less likely to abuse these drugs.

Vomiting Reflex: Pathway between the Chemoreceptor Trigger Zone (CTZ), the Vomiting Center (VC), and the Stomach

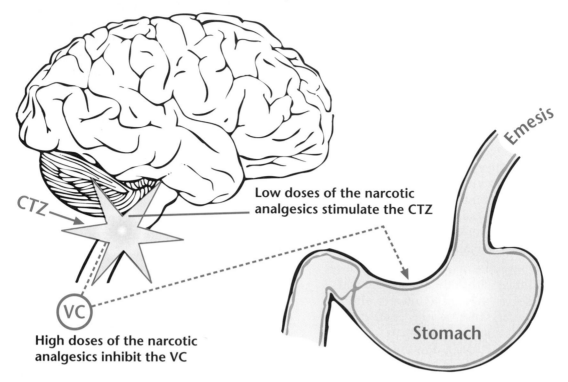

Low doses of the narcotic analgesics stimulate the CTZ

CTZ

Emesis

Stomach

High doses of the narcotic analgesics inhibit the VC

In low doses, most opioid analgesics produce nausea and vomiting. **Emesis** (vomiting) is a direct result of CNS stimulation of the chemoreceptor trigger zone, which in turn leads to direct stimulation of the vomiting center in the medulla. In some individuals, the frequency of vomiting increases when the patient is standing. As the dose of opioid is increased, the drug exerts a depressant action on the vomiting center. Therefore, at large doses, opioid analgesics counteract their emetic response by inhibiting the vomiting center (Figure 19:2).

One of the most important CNS effects produced by these analgesics is respiratory depression. All dose levels of opioid analgesics depress respiratory activity by **mµ receptors** directly inhibiting the respiratory centers in the medulla and the pons. Respiratory rate and volume are reduced so that carbon dioxide (CO_2) is retained in the blood. Mild retention of CO_2 may produce headaches, because CO_2 increases cerebral fluid pressure and intracranial pressure. As respiratory depression increases, so does CO_2 retention. However, the suppressed medulla cannot respond to CO_2 stimulation, and hypoventilation persists. The depth of respiratory depression increases as the dose of the drug increases. Death due to opioid poisoning is usually attributed to respiratory arrest.

Antitussives

Although only a few opioid analgesics are used as antitussives, most of these analgesics suppress the coughing reflex at therapeutic doses. The antitussive effect is produced by direct inhibition of the coughing center in the medulla. These drugs do not cure the underlying cause of the irritation; they merely decrease the intensity and frequency of the cough. Once the cough reflex has been suppressed, patients become less irritable, less anxious, and are usually able to sleep comfortably.

Among the antitussive drugs, codeine, hydrocodone, hydromorphone, and noscapine are natural derivatives of opium whereas dextromethorphan is a synthetic product. Dextromethorphan or very small amounts of codeine have a recognized therapeutic value associated with a low addiction potential when used in recommended doses for short periods. Codeine, in analgesic doses in particular, has come under close scrutiny because of its potential for misuse. Codeine-containing products can no longer be sold without a prescription. In analgesic doses, codeine alone is considered Schedule II (recognized medical benefit although associated with high abuse potential with severe dependence liability). Hydrocodone (*Dicodid*) and

TABLE 19:3 — Comparison of Doses and Schedule Classification of Opioid Antitussive Drugs

TRADE NAME	SCHEDULE	ANTITUSSIVE DOSE	OTHER ACTIVE INGREDIENTS
Bromotuss with codeine	V	10 mg codeine	12.5 mg bromodiphenhydramine
codeine Sulfate Tablets	II	15 mg codeine sulfate	—
Detussin Liquid	III	5 mg hydrocodone	60 mg pseudoephedrine, 5% alcohol
Hycodan tablets and syrup	III	5 mg hydrocodone	1.5 mg homatropine methylbromide
Nucofed Capsules	III	20 mg codeine phosphate	60 mg pseudoephedrine
promethazine with codeine	V	10 mg codeine phosphate	6.25 mg promethazine
Tuss-Ornade Liquid	—	6.7 mg caramiphen edisylate	12.5 mg phenylpropanolamine, 5% alcohol, menthol

hydromorphone (*Dilaudid*) are also Schedule II drugs available only by prescription because of their greater potential for addiction.

The adult antitussive dose of codeine is 10 to 20 mg every 4 to 6 hours. For dextromethorphan, a dose of 15 to 30 mg is recommended over the same time interval. For children 6 to 12 years of age, one-half the adult dose is usually recommended. Table 19:3 compares antitussive doses for the opioid antitussive drugs. These drugs are considered effective for the treatment of a nonproductive cough that is unable to mobilize **phlegm** (mucus). Dextromethorphan is frequently found as the principal drug in over-the-counter cough and cold preparations.

The more potent antitussive drugs (hydromorphone, hydrocodone) are seldom the sole ingredient in over-the-counter cough suppressant remedies. Cough suppression may be only one objective in relieving the symptoms of a cold. Additional objectives of therapy include relieving nasal congestion, reducing pain and fever, and promoting bed rest through sedation. It is not surprising, therefore, that agents such as expectorants, antihistaminics, sympathomimetics, and alcohol are present in various combinations in over-the-counter cold and cough preparations. When codeine or hydrocodone is present, the over-the-counter preparation may be classified as Schedule V because other active ingredients (for example, antihistaminics, sympathomimetic amines) may counteract the potential for abuse.

Expectorants (ammonium chloride, guaifenesin, and terpin hydrate) are often combined with antitussive drugs to alter the volume and viscosity of mucus retained in the respiratory tract. Expectorants promote the discharge of mucus from the respiratory tract, thus reducing chest irritation and congestion. Sympathomimetic amines (ephedrine, phenylephrine, phenylpropanolamine, and pseudoephedrine) are combined with antitussive drugs to produce nasal decongestion by constricting nasal blood vessels. The antihistamines that are H_1-antagonists, such as chlorpheniramine and pyrilamine, exert an anticholinergic action, which may decrease secretion of mucus, whereas alcohol may act as a CNS depressant.

It is not unusual to find that liquid preparations contain alcohol, some in excess of 15 percent. (Consider the possible CNS interactions that may occur when these products are used in addition to other prescription medications.) Table 19:4 on page 202 lists examples of combination over-the-counter preparations that contain an opioid antitussive as the principal active drug. Note the concentration of the antitussive product as well as the types of additional pharmacological agents in each preparation. Although this is not an exhaustive list of available products, notice the various amounts of alcohol present in even pediatric liquid preparations. No wonder some of these products are recommended for bedtime use; they certainly can promote sleep.

Combination Over-the-Counter Preparations Containing Opioid Antitussive Drugs*

TRADE NAME	ANTITUSSIVE	LIQUID CONCEN-TRATION	OTHER INGREDIENTS	AMOUNT OF ALCOHOL
Benylin Cough	10 mg dextromethorphan	2.0 mg/ml	Ammonium chloride, sodium citrate	5%
Children's Nyquil	5 mg dextromethorphan**	1.0 mg/ml	Pseudoephedrine, chlorpheniramine	—
Cheracol D	10 mg dextromethorphan	2.0 mg/ml	Guaifenesin	4.8%
Dimacol Caplets	10 mg dextromethorphan	—	Guaifenesin, pseudoephedrine	—
Multisymptom Tylenol Cold	15 mg dextromethorphan	1.0 mg/ml	Chlorpheniramine, pseudoephedrine	—
Naldecon-DX Child's Syrup	10 mg dextromethorphan	1.0 mg/ml	Guaifenesin, phenylpropanolamine	5%
Novahistine DH Liquid	10 mg codeine***	0.4 mg/ml	Pseudoephedrine, chlorpheniramine Guaifenesin	5%
Novahistine DMX Syrup	10 mg dextromethorphan	2.0 mg/ml	Pseudoephedrine	10%
Nyquil Nighttime Colds Medicine	5 mg dextromethorphan**	1.5 mg/ml	Pseudoephedrine, doxylamine, acetaminophen	25%
Robitussin A-C	10 mg codeine**	2.0 mg/ml	Guaifenesin	3.5%
Robitussin-CF Liquid	10 mg dextromethorphan**	2.0 mg/ml	Guaifenesin, phenylpropanolamine	4.8%
Tylenol Cold Medication, Non-Drowsy	15 mg dextromethorphan	—	Pseudoephedrine, acetaminophen	—
Vicks Formula 44D	10 mg dextromethorphan**	2.0 mg/ml	Pseudoephedrine	10%
Vicks Formula 44M	10 mg dextromethorphan**	1.5 mg/ml	Pseudoephedrine, chlorpheniramine acetaminophen	—

*Not an all-inclusive list of available products.
** Dose of dextromethorphan reduced from earlier formulation.
***Dose of codeine increase from earlier formulation.

Effects on Smooth Muscle

Most of the other pharmacological effects produced by the opioid analgesics are a result of their **spasmogenic** activity. Opioid analgesics increase smooth muscle tone, resulting in periodic muscle contractions or spasms. When spasms occur within the intestinal smooth muscle, peristalsis is inhibited. In addition, these analgesics inhibit parasympathetic stimulation of the intestines by blocking the release of acetylcholine. Both of these effects can result in constipation, which frequently occurs with the use of opioid analgesics. Only one opioid derivative, diphenoxylate, is used in the treatment of persistent diarrhea. Diphenoxylate will be discussed further in Chapter 34.

Many opioid analgesics, especially morphine, produce spasm of the common bile duct, which causes pressure to increase in the gallbladder. Usually, this effect is accompanied by intense pain. However, in the presence of an opioid, the painful warning may be eliminated, although the pressure continues to increase. For this reason, opioids such as morphine should be used with caution in patients with possible biliary obstruction.

Urine formation and urination are both decreased by opioid analgesics, since these drugs stimulate the secretion of **antidiuretic hormone (ADH),** which allows the kidneys to reabsorb water. This decreases the volume of urine produced. In addition, spasmogenic activity (mμ receptors) of the ureters and sphincter muscles inhibits urine from passing out of the bladder. The combination of these effects usually produces **oliguria** (a smaller than normal amount of urine) rather than **anuria** (no formation of urine).

Opioid analgesics affect bronchial smooth muscle by two actions. In addition to their spasmogenic action, these analgesics cause the release of histamine, which directly constricts the bronchioles (see Chapter 31). Constriction of the bronchioles narrows the respiratory passages, making breathing more difficult. This response is dangerous in individuals who already have respiratory difficulties, such as chronic bronchitis, obstructive lung disease, and asthma. Asthmatic patients may be unusually sensitive to histamine release, to the point that opioid analgesics may induce an asthmatic attack.

Effects on Cardiovascular System

Opioid analgesics do not depress cardiac function in therapeutic doses. This lack of effect is important, because it allows these drugs to relieve the pain accompanying myocardial infarction without worsening the condition. Although the cardiac muscle is not affected, bradycardia may occur via mμ receptors. Hypotension may occur due to histamine release and medullary vasomotor depression. Hypotension is frequently encountered when changing from a sitting position to a standing position (orthostatic hypotension).

Effects on Eyes

Most opioid analgesics produce miosis. This effect is caused by stimulation of the mμ receptors in the brain. Most opioid analgesics produce pinpoint pupils in toxic doses. However, meperidine produces mydriasis (dilation). Therefore, the pupil size cannot be used to determine what drug was used by unconscious (overdose) patients.

ABSORPTION AND METABOLISM

Since these analgesics are weak bases, these drugs are not well absorbed in the acid environment of the stomach. They are absorbed in the intestines, where the pH is more alkaline. Regardless of the route of administration, metabolic inactivation of the opioid eventually occurs in the hepatic drug microsomal metabolizing system. Heroin is a particularly unusual drug because it is not metabolized to an inactive product. Heroin is rapidly changed into morphine. Several of the opioids are metabolized to products that produce analgesia. Therefore the circulating active metabolites increase the duration of analgesic activity.

Eventually, the kidneys excrete the metabolic products. Anything that causes the urine to become alkaline, such as alkalosis and diuretics (see Chapter 24), increases tubular reabsorption of the opioids. This action elevates the concentration of drug in the blood and increases the risk of developing drug toxicity.

ADVERSE EFFECTS

The most common effects produced by these analgesics include mental confusion, nausea, vomiting, dry mouth, constipation, and urinary retention. In sensitive individuals, histamine release produces hypotension and allergic reactions ranging from itching, skin rashes, and wheals to anaphylaxis. Therefore, it is important to determine whether patients are allergic to any opioid before administering one.

The effects associated with the chronic use of opioid analgesics are the development of tolerance and physical dependence. Tolerance develops to the euphoria, analgesia, sedation, and respiratory depression produced by the opioid analgesics. Tolerance does not develop equally to all opioid effects. When tolerance develops to sedation, drowsiness, or respiratory depression, this is a beneficial response. If, however, the degree of pain has not changed, but the dose of drug must be increased to achieve relief of pain, this represents analgesic tolerance. (If pain increases, as occurs with cancer patients and the dose of opioid is increased to cover the escalating pain, this is not tolerance.) At sufficiently large doses, even tolerant individuals will die from severe respiratory depression (arrest). The onset of tolerance varies with the analgesic. On the other hand, tolerance seldom develops to the annoying spasmogenic effects such as constipation and urinary retention.

Cancer patients usually take larger doses of opioids and may experience intolerable opioid side effects. Opioid rotation is a term used to indicate a change of opioid analgesic that may produce fewer side effects. Therefore, cross-tolerance to opioid effects is relative to the patient's condition and the specific opioid.

Physical dependence upon any opioid usually develops with chronic use of the analgesic. Many people, including medical professionals and patients who have access to opioid drugs (especially meperidine), develop physical dependence. Even infants who are exposed to opioids through the placental blood can be born physically dependent upon these drugs. Controlled gradual tapering of the medication over time enables the person to move off the medication with little withdrawal effect.

The mechanism by which addiction occurs is not fully understood; however, it is now considered a primary disease rather than a side effect of drug usage. Once addiction is established, the opioid is required to avoid the onset of withdrawal (abstinence syndrome).

The abstinence syndrome associated with these analgesics gradually develops over the 72 hours following the last exposure. During the initial period of withdrawal, sweating, yawning, restlessness, insomnia, and tremors occur. As the syndrome reaches its peak, blood pressure and irritability increase, accompanied by vomiting and diarrhea. Excessive sweating, gooseflesh, chills, and skeletal muscle cramps develop toward the end of the withdrawal period. Individuals who are addicted to these analgesics usually survive the withdrawal period. Administration of an opioid at any time during the withdrawal period will suppress the abstinence syndrome. Other CNS drugs such as barbiturates, alcohol, or amphetamines cannot suppress opioid withdrawal.

Methadone is particularly useful in the treatment of addiction because it satisfies an addict's opioid hunger so that the individual actually becomes acclimated to methadone. Methadone does not produce severe withdrawal symptoms and the symptoms occur gradually during the 6- to 7-week maintenance compared to 72 hours for other opioids. Since oral methadone is half as potent as parenteral methadone, it is easier to withdraw patients from methadone gradually without incurring a severe abstinence syndrome. Levomethadyl acetate is another drug which is only used for the management of opiate addiction.

ACUTE OPIOID POISONING

Opioid overdose, or acute poisoning, frequently occurs from accidental ingestion (children), attempted suicide, or exposure of a fetus during pregnancy. The symptoms of poisoning include coma, decreased respiration, cyanosis, hypotension, and a fall in body temperature. Once patients are adequately ventilated with a respirator, the poisoning can be treated with specific opioid antagonists such as naloxone.

OPIOID ANTAGONISTS

Opioid antagonists are drugs that attach to the opioid receptors and displace the analgesic. Displacement rapidly reverses life-threatening respiratory depression. There are two types of antagonists—pure antagonists and partial antagonists (Table 19:5). Pure antagonists, such as naloxone and nalmefene, are competitive blocking drugs. Naloxone occupies the opioid receptors but has no agonist activity (stimulation). Naloxone inhibits the analgesic from attaching to the receptors but does not produce any pharmacological action of its own. Partial antagonists, such as butorphanol, nalbuphine, and pentazocine, have two actions on the respiratory system. These drugs produce weak morphine-like effects in normal individuals, resulting in respiratory depression. In cases of acute opioid poisoning, however, partial antagonists reverse the respiratory depression. Partial antagonists bind with the receptors and produce little or no stimulation of the receptors which mediate respiratory depression.

Today, the drug of choice in the treatment of acute opioid poisonings is naloxone because it does not produce any respiratory depression.

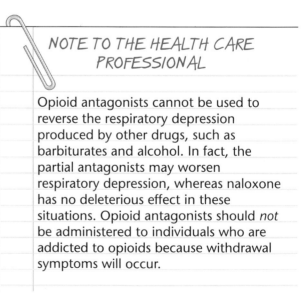

NOTE TO THE HEALTH CARE PROFESSIONAL

Opioid antagonists cannot be used to reverse the respiratory depression produced by other drugs, such as barbiturates and alcohol. In fact, the partial antagonists may worsen respiratory depression, whereas naloxone has no deleterious effect in these situations. Opioid antagonists should *not* be administered to individuals who are addicted to opioids because withdrawal symptoms will occur.

Cautions and Contraindications

Opioid analgesics should not be used in patients with bronchial asthma, heavy pulmonary secretions, convulsive disorders, biliary obstruction, or head injuries. In these cases, opioids may worsen

TABLE 19:5   Opioid Antagonists Used to Treat Opioid Analgesic Respiratory Depression or Addiction

DRUG (TRADE NAME)	TYPE OF ANTAGONIST	ADULT DOSE
Treatment of Respiratory Depression:		
naloxone (*Narcan*)	Pure	0.4–2 mg repeated at 3-min intervals IM, SC, IV
nalmefene (*Revex*)	Pure	Individualized dose by weight
Treatment of Addiction:		
naltrexone (*ReVia*)	Pure	Only after the patient has been opioid-free for 7–10 days; maintenance dose 50 mg every 24 hr
methadone (40 mg)—(*Intensol*)	—	15–20 mg PO initially; 40 mg for those dependent on high opioid doses
methadone diskettes (40 mg)	—	2.5–10 mg PO, IM, SC every 3–4 hr
levomethadyl (*Orlaam*)	—	Maintenance dose 60–90 mg three times a week

the existing condition. Ambulatory and elderly patients should be warned about the drowsiness that may accompany the use of opioid analgesics.

Since opioid analgesics will cross the placental barrier and affect fetuses, use of these drugs during pregnancy should be minimized. Short-term exposure of the fetus at term (from use of these drugs at parturition) presents relatively little potential danger to the newborn.

Opioid analgesics should never be used when a nonopioid analgesic is indicated to relieve the pain. Whenever opioid analgesics are to be administered intravenously, naloxone should be readily available.

Clinical Indications

Opioid analgesics are approved for relief of moderate to severe acute and chronic pain which responds to opioids. Such pain is often associated with myocardial infarction; posttrauma back, head, or neck injury; or cancer. Occasionally the root cause of chronic pain remains unidentified.

The majority of the opioid analgesics are used for the relief of acute and chronic pain. A few, such as fentanyl, alfentanil, and sufentanil, are primarily indicated for preoperative sedation to reduce patient apprehension. In making the patient less apprehensive, physiological mechanisms are no longer poised to fight the anesthesia. As a result, premedication with opioids often reduces the amount of anesthetic required and facilitates induction of anesthesia.

Select analgesics, codeine, dextromethorphan, and hydrocodone, are approved or used alone or in combination to suppress chemical or mechanical stimulated coughing.

SPECIAL CONSIDERATIONS

Opioid analgesics are frequently administered on a repeated schedule (every 4 to 8 hours) to relieve moderate to severe pain. To be effective, these analgesics must be given before intense pain is present. It is important, therefore, that these analgesics be administered on time, as scheduled. Adherence to the prescribed schedule ensures that patients have an adequate blood level of drug to sustain an analgesic effect. If the next dose of drug is significantly delayed, the pain will recur and may be enhanced by psychological factors associated with anticipation of discomfort.

The opioids are available for oral and parenteral administration. Parenteral formulations are used more in surgery and postsurgical recovery. Oral preparations are used to treat acute and chronic pain. Immediate release tablets provide the fastest blood levels from oral absorption. Once the effective analgesic blood level is achieved, the patient may be switched to a controlled release formulation that releases drug over 8 to 12 hours. In this way the duration of analgesia is increased. Even with sustained release formulations, patients often experience breakthrough pain that requires immediate attention. Immediate release

Patient Administration and Monitoring

Although opioid analgesics are frequently used in a controlled environment such as a hospital or rehabilitation center, there is considerable opportunity for outpatient use of prescription as well as over-the-counter analgesics. This potentiates the possibility for adverse reactions and/or drug interactions to occur. Patient vital signs should be monitored, especially respiration rate, to determine whether dose adjustment is required. Elderly patients require careful instruction for identifying adverse effects and contacting the physician. Specific signs such as confusion, drowsiness, forgetfulness, and impaired coordination or vision may be ignored as part of the aging process when, in fact, the degree of debilitation may be caused by the dose, frequency, or combination of medications. Written instructions for contacting the physician should be provided in large easy-to-read type, in a format that can be carried with the patient for easy reference.

Patient Instruction

As a class, these drugs cause drowsiness, sedation, dizziness, and blurred vision in therapeutic doses. Patients should be interviewed to determine whether they perform tasks which require special equipment or machinery (such as operating a sewing machine, drill press, or assembly tools), coordination, or physical dexterity. As coordination and judgment may be impaired during therapy, extra caution must be in place, including identifying a relative, coworker, or on-site medical personnel who is aware of the medication schedule. If necessary, alternate transportation may be advisable, particularly in older patients.

Patients should be instructed to move slowly and cautiously when getting out of bed or walking. Postural hypotension as well as drowsiness may contribute to unsteady conditions, particularly in elderly patients.

Dose Adjustment

Advise patients to check with the physician before taking over-the-counter preparations, particularly cough/cold preparations. Alcohol and CNS depressants enhance the opioid depressant effects.

Advise patients to take the drugs as prescribed. Patients should be advised not to change dose or dose interval unless instructed by the physician. For full analgesic effect, the drug must be taken before intense pain occurs.

---

formulations are required to treat breakthrough pain. All of the oral formulations should be swallowed, never be chewed. The amount of drug that can be released as a burst from chewing the tablet could achieve a higher blood level than expected with an increase in side effects.

Recently there has been a significant change in the attitude and methods regarding the treatment of chronic severe pain. Specialists in pain and symptom management use aggressive drug treatment schedules where dosing is often under the control of the patient. This patient-controlled-analgesia, known as PCA, allows the patient to use the lowest effective dose of opioid before the pain intensity becomes unbearable. In effect, the patient minimizes the opportunity for dependence through lower dose exposure and customized administration schedule.

Drug delivery systems have also improved. A transdermal patch and transmucosal lozenge are now available forms of fentanyl that are used for the treatment of chronic pain. Transmucosal lozenges are sucked rather than swallowed or chewed.

Opioid analgesics are CNS depressants at any dose. It is therefore important to monitor vital signs when patients, especially the elderly, are receiving these drugs. Indications of decreased blood pressure or respiration may be a clue that patients have been overmedicated and are experiencing cardiovascular or respiratory depression.

DRUG INTERACTIONS

A few specific drug interactions occur with these analgesics. Opioid analgesics potentiate the depression of any CNS depressant drug (sedative-hypnotics, alcohol, and general anesthetics). Meperidine undergoes an unusual, potentially

Oral preparations should be swallowed, not chewed, except for fentanyl lozenges which are to be dissolved in the mouth.

Gastrointestinal Effects

If gastrointestinal upset occurs after oral administration, the patient can be advised to take the medication with meals or milk. If nausea, vomiting, or constipation persists, the physician should be notified for further evaluation.

Constipation, a common problem with older patients, may be potentiated with the opioid analgesics, including over-the-counter preparations. The patient should be evaluated to assess bowel function so that appropriate stool softeners or laxatives may be recommended.

Special Formulations

Patients must be instructed on the use of nasal sprays or transdermal patches. Practice preparation and application using these systems is essential to obtaining good compliance, especially in older patients. For transdermal patch application, the area should be clear of hair. Shaving is not the method of choice because it could irritate the skin and promote absorption of greater amounts of drug. Creams, lotions, and soaps which could irritate the skin or prevent patch adhesion should not be used. Fever or high temperatures of climate can cause the patch to release more drug resulting in toxicity. Patients should be instructed to clearly identify those times when they may be in hotter climates than usual so that dose adjustment can be considered.

Notify the Physician

Shortness of breath or difficulty breathing should be reported to the physician immediately. Hypersensitivity to these drugs is a contraindication for their use. Patients with depressed respiratory function such as chronic obstructive pulmonary disorder (COPD), emphysema, or severe asthma will exhibit respiratory distress from opioid-induced respiratory depression.

Any elevation in body temperature, such as fever, which is not associated with flu or cold should be considered as a potential side effect and should be reported to the physician.

Use in Pregnancy

Drugs in this class have been designated Food and Drug Administration (FDA) Pregnancy Category C or NR, not rated. Adequate studies in humans have not been conducted so that safety in pregnancy has not been established. However, these drugs may be used when the potential benefit to the pregnant patient outweighs the risks.

---

fatal, reaction when used in the presence of monoamine oxidase (MAO) inhibitors. Sweating, hypotension, or hypertension may occur in patients taking meperidine with pargyline, phenelzine, or tranylcypromine concomitantly. Dextromethorphan has been reported to undergo a similar interaction with phenelzine. As a result, dextromethorphan should not be given to patients who are receiving MAO inhibitors. Rifampin and phenytoin have been associated with reduction in the plasma concentrations of methadone sufficient to induce withdrawal symptoms.

Certain opioid analgesics may be administered as parenteral solutions; therefore, it is important to be aware of incompatibilities that may result in drug inactivation. Codeine, levorphanol, meperidine, and morphine have been reported to be physically incompatible when mixed in solution with aminophylline, barbiturates, chlorothiazide, heparin, methicillin, phenytoin, sodium bicarbonate, or sulfisoxazole. Pentazocine is incompatible with solutions of aminophylline, barbiturates, glycopyrrolate, and sodium bicarbonate. Meperidine should not be mixed with solutions containing morphine.

Chapter Review

Understanding Terminology

Answer the following questions in the spaces provided.

1. What is an opioid? _____
   _____

2. Describe an antitussive effect. _____

3. Define *opioid antagonist.* _____
   _____

Match the definition or description in the left column with the appropriate term in the right column.

___ 4. The opposite of euphoria.

___ 5. Mucus.

___ 6. Production of only a small amount of urine.

___ 7. Vomiting.

___ 8. Production of no urine.

___ 9. A substance that inhibits one's reaction to pain.

___ 10. Antidiuretic hormone.

a. ADH

b. analgesic

c. anuria

d. dysphoria

e. emesis

f. oliguria

g. phlegm

Acquiring Knowledge

Answer the following questions in the spaces provided.

11. What types of pain are relieved by opioid analgesics? _____
    _____

12. What are the therapeutic uses of opioid analgesics? _____
    _____

13. What is the proposed mechanism of action of opioid analgesics? _____
    _____

14. What effects do the opioid analgesics have on the CNS? _____
    _____

15. How might these effects be involved in other drug interactions? What drugs might potentiate CNS respiratory depression?
    _____
    _____

16. What is the spasmogenic action of the opioid analgesics? _____
    _____

17. Why does urine retention occur with the use of opioid analgesics? _____
    _____
    _____

18. Are all opioid analgesics administered orally? Why or why not? _____

_____

_____

19. What adverse effects are associated with opioid analgesics? _____

_____

_____

Applying Knowledge—On the Job

Use your critical thinking skills to answer the following questions in the spaces provided.

20. One of your jobs as a pharmacy assistant is to alert the pharmacist about patients with potential contraindications or drug interactions. What's wrong with each of the following prescriptions for the patients in question?

   a. Patient A has been prescribed codeine for severe headaches. Pharmacy records indicate that the patient also takes *Metaprel,* a bronchodilator prescribed for bronchial asthma.

_____

_____

   b. Patient B has been prescribed morphine for severe postoperative pain. You note in reviewing his chart that he also takes the drug *Moduretic,* a diuretic, for hypertension.

_____

_____

   c. Patient C has been prescribed *Demerol* for a muscle injury. She's already taking *Nardil* for depression.

_____

_____

21. For each of the following adult patients, how much opioid is needed to produce the desired effect?

   a. Patient A has been prescribed codeine for dental pain. _____

_____

   b. Patient B has been prescribed a cough preparation containing codeine. _____

_____

   c. Patient C has been prescribed *Dilaudid* for pain associated with cancer. _____

_____

   d. Patient D has bronchitis and has been prescribed *Dilaudid* for his painful cough. _____

_____

Use the appropriate reference book(s) if needed to answer the following questions.

22. Plain pentazocine was once available in a tablet form. Naloxone was later added to the tablet. Does this interfere with the pharmacological action of pentazocine when taken orally? Why was this added?

_____

_____

23. For several months Jack has been getting *Vicodin* (hydrocodone 5 mg/acetaminophen 500 mg) from his regular pharmacy. In the last 30 days he has received #280 Vicodin from several different doctors. Would you suspect possible addiction? Would you expect the pharmacy to contact the doctor(s)? Why?

_____

_____

24. It is not uncommon for drug abusers to alter prescriptions for opioids. Common alterations to watch for include changing the quantities (ie; 10 to 40, 30 to 80 or adding a 1 in front of the number—20 to 120) and adding refills where none were indicated. Prescribers can help deter this practice by spelling out the quantities and refills or by writing *no refill* or *non rep* if no refills are desired. Look at the following prescriptions and see if you notice anything that seems out of place. Then explain what, if anything, is out of place and what you think the pharmacy might do.

_____

_____

a. dental—*Vicodin* #42—1 po q6h prn dental pain—refills 4 times. _____

_____

b. bone break—*Tylenol*/codeine 30mg #30—1–2 po q3–4h prn leg pain—refill 4 times.

_____

c. cancer patient—morphine *Intensol* 20mg/ml #120ml—0.25 to 1 ml po q1–2h prn breakthru pain—no refill

_____

d. emergency room—*Demerol* 50mg tablets #110—1 po q4–6h prn migraine pain—0 refills

_____

_____

Internet Connection

Among the best sites providing information on opioid drugs with pictures of natural opiates and synthetic medications used in the management of pain is the National Institutes of Health. This exhibit tells how twentieth century researchers at the National Institutes of Health created new opiate drugs and developed a synthetic source for morphine at www.nih.gov/od/museum/exhibits/opiates/intro-m.html. When you enter the website, select Exhibitions and Galleries. Then select either A Short History of the National Institute of Health Pain Research, or Drugs Used as Medicine, Drugs as Research Tools: Synthetic Opiates and Opioids.

From the National Institute of Drug Abuse (NIDA) several links are presented to medical research centers that explain consequences of opiate use and prevention strategies at www.nlm.nih.gov/medlineplus/prescriptiondrugabuse.html. The alphabetical index allows you to enter a specific area of interest associated with opioids such as treating back pain or nausea and vomiting.

Finally, www.findarticles.com is a site that allows you to enter a topic, word, or phrase such as "opioids" or "treatment of chronic pain" in order to obtain relevant articles from worldwide medical information sources for online review. The articles are usually in English and 1 to 6 pages in length. In addition to renowned journals such as *British Medical Journal* or *Journal of the American Medical Association*, this site provides a fair balance of information from sports medicine and news articles.

Additional Reading

Bedder, M. D. 1996. Epidural opioid therapy for chronic nonmalignant pain: A critique of current experience. *Journal of Pain and Symptom Management* 11 (6):353.

Dejo, R. A. 1996. Drug therapy for back pain. Which drugs help which patients. *Spine* 21 (24):2840.

Goldstein, F. J. 1995, Preemptive analgesia: A research review. *MEDSURG Nursing* 4 (4):305.

Kress, J. P. 1997. Sedating critically ill ventilated patients: A pharmacologic primer. *Journal of Critical Illness* 12 (5):287.

Louie, K. 1992. Management of intractable cough. *Journal of Palliative Care* 8 (4):46.

Parrott, T. 1999. Using opioid analgesics to manage chronic noncancer pain in primary care. *J. Am Board Fam Pract* 12:293–306.

St. Marie, B. 1996. Chemical abuse and pain management. *Journal of Intravenous Nursing* 19 (5):247.

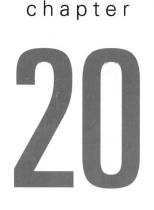

NONOPIOID ANALGESICS, ANTIINFLAMMATORY, AND ANTIGOUT DRUGS

20

DRUG CLASS AT A GLANCE

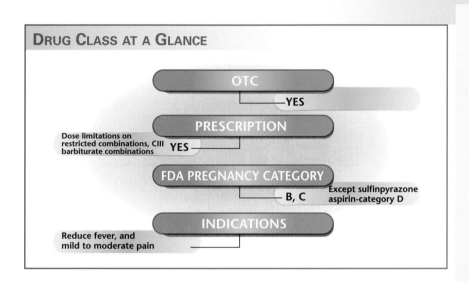

OTC
— YES

PRESCRIPTION

Dose limitations on restricted combinations, CIII barbiturate combinations — YES

FDA PREGNANCY CATEGORY
— B, C   Except sulfinpyrazone aspirin-category D

INDICATIONS

Reduce fever, and mild to moderate pain

Key Terms

analgesia: inhibition of the perception of pain.

anaphylaxis: condition in which the body develops a severe allergic response; this is a medical emergency.

anemia: condition in which the number of red blood cells or the amount of hemoglobin inside the red blood cells is less than normal.

antiinflammatory: minimizing or stopping the response to tissue injury by reducing the pain, localized swelling, and chemical substances released at the site of injury.

antipyresis: reducing an elevated body temperature.

arthralgia: joint pain.

arthritis: inflammation of the joints.

COX: cyclooxygenase, a family of enzymes that produce prostaglandins.

dysmenorrhea: difficult or painful menstruation.

erythema: abnormal redness of the skin, caused by capillary congestion.

CHAPTER FOCUS

This chapter describes drugs that primarily relieve the dull, aching pain associated with joint inflammation, local edema, or minor muscle trauma.

CHAPTER OBJECTIVES

After studying this chapter, you should be able to

- identify situations in which it is appropriate to select a nonopioid drug for pain relief.

- describe the advantage of selecting acetaminophen over aspirin.

- explain why nonopioid analgesics are particularly effective against inflammation.

- describe the primary side effects associated with long-term aspirin and antiinflammatory drug use.

- explain why probenecid and sulfinpyrazone are specifically useful in the treatment of gout.

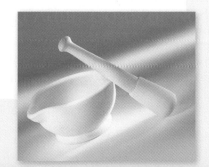

inflammation: condition in which tissues have been damaged, characterized by swelling, pain, heat, and sometimes redness.

intoxication: state in which a substance has accumulated to potentially harmful levels in the body.

ischemia: reduction in blood supply and oxygen to localized area of the body or tissue.

lavage: washing with fluids or flushing of a cavity such as the stomach.

leukopenia: condition in which the total number of white blood cells circulating in the blood is less than normal.

megaloblastic anemia: condition in which there is a large, immature form of the red blood cell, which does not function as efficiently as the mature form.

myalgia: pain associated with muscle injury.

petechia: small area of the skin or mucous membranes that is discolored because of localized hemorrhages.

phagocyte: circulating cell (such as a leukocyte) that ingests waste products or bacteria in order to remove them from the body.

prophylaxis: treatment or drug given to prevent a condition or disease.

prostaglandin: substance naturally found in certain tissues of the body; can stimulate uterine and intestinal muscle contractions and may cause pain by stimulating nerve endings.

rheumatic fever: condition in which pain and inflammation of the joints or muscles are accompanied by elevated body temperature.

salicylism: condition in which toxic doses of salicylates are ingested, resulting in nausea, tinnitus, and delirium.

selective COX-2 inhibitors: drugs that only interact with one of the enzymes in the cyclooxygenase family.

INTRODUCTION

Nonopioid analgesics, also known as mild analgesics, relieve mild to moderate pain without altering consciousness or mental function. In particular, these drugs relieve the low-intensity pain associated with **inflammation,** including that from **arthritis** and gout, and associated with dull aches, including headaches, **arthralgia** (joint pain), and **myalgia** (muscle pain). In addition to reducing mild pain (providing **analgesia),** the nonopioid analgesics reduce fever **(antipyresis)** and reduce inflammation (are **antiinflammatory).** These three pharmacological effects (analgesia, antipyresis, and antiinflammatory) are known as the "three As."

INFLAMMATION

The inflammatory process is a normal response to injury. When tissues are damaged, substances (histamine, bradykinin, prostaglandins, and serotonin) are released that produce vasodilation and increased permeability of the capillary walls. Pain receptors are stimulated, and proteins and fluid leak out of the injured cells. As blood flow to the damaged area increases, **phagocytes** (leukocytes) migrate to the area to destroy harmful substances introduced by the injury. These effects result in the development of the cardinal signs of inflammation: redness, swelling (edema), warmth, pain, and loss of function.

Inflammation is usually considered the first step in the process of healing. However, in some instances, the inflammatory process becomes exaggerated or prolonged, which results in further tissue damage. In these situations, inflammation itself becomes a disease process and requires treatment with antiinflammatory drugs, which interrupt the inflammatory response. These drugs stabilize cell membranes so that the cells become less permeable, thus decreasing the formation of edema. Irritating substances are inhibited from affecting nerve endings, and prostaglandin synthesis is blocked.

Prostaglandins are mediators of the inflammatory response (Figure 20:1). Prostaglandins G_2 and H_2 are capable of stimulating peripheral pain receptors as well as constricting blood vessels. These prostaglandins are further metabolized to PGE_2 and $PGF_{2\alpha}$. Prostaglandin PGE_2 is involved in the production of **erythema** (abnormal redness), edema, and pain that accompany the inflammatory process; $PGF_{2\alpha}$ is associated with uterine contraction and vasodilation.

Figure 20:1 indicates a number of locations where prostaglandin synthesis can be interrupted to minimize the local inflammatory response. The location of prostaglandin inhibition differentiates one antiinflammatory drug from another. In particular, the selectivity of NSAIDs for inhibiting the cyclooxygenase enzymes has been a fairly recent focus of drug development.

Cyclooxgenase **(COX)** is a family of enzymes required to make prostaglandins from arachadonic acid. These enzymes are also called "prostaglandin synthetase," but COX is the newer terminology. The type of prostaglandin produced is dependent upon the specific cell (e.g., platelets versus uterine muscle) and the type of cyclooxygenase present. Two subtypes of cyclooxygenase have been identified: COX-1 and COX-2. COX-1 is believed to always be available in all cells, especially in the platelets, kidneys, and gastrointestinal tract, so that homeostasis in these cells is maintained. COX-2, on the other hand, appears to be manufactured in activated macrophages in response to injury or damage to local tissues.

Nonsteroidal antiinflammatory drugs ease the symptoms associated with inflammation because they inhibit prostaglandin synthesis at many different points in the enzyme pathway.

NONOPIOID ANALGESICS

Nonopioid analgesics differ from opioid analgesics in four ways. First, these analgesics are not chemically or structurally related to morphine (nor are they related to each other by a common structure). Second, they are not effective against severe, sharp (visceral) pain. Third, they produce analgesia through both a central (central nervous system [CNS]) and a peripheral (site of injury) mechanism of action. Fourth, they do not produce tolerance or physical dependency with chronic use.

FIGURE 20:1 Prostaglandin Pathway in Tissue Injury and Inflammation Process

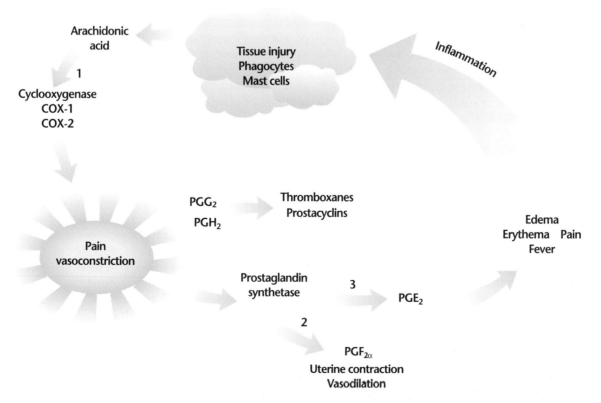

Site 1: Site of inhibition by salicylates (aspirin) and NSAIDs. Site 2: Site of inhibition by ibuprofen. Site 3: Site of inhibition by NSAIDs.

Several nonopioid analgesics are listed in Table 20:1. The salicylates are the oldest and most frequently used nonopioid analgesic drugs.

Nonsteroidal Antiinflammatory Drugs (NSAIDs)

Although many of the drugs listed in Table 20:1 produce the same actions as the salicylates, some drugs are employed for their antiinflammatory effects only. These drugs are also known as nonsteroidal antiinflammatory drugs (NSAIDs) because they are not structurally related to cortisone (adrenal steroid) and produce their antiinflammatory action through a different mechanism. Cortisone is a potent antiinflammatory hormone used in specific inflammatory diseases, often when other nonsteroidal agents have not been effective. The effects of cortisone will be more thoroughly discussed in Chapter 36.

All NSAIDs have the ability to interact with cyclooxygenases. Older NSAIDs like aspirin, ketoprofen, and indomethacin, are considered nonselective—that is, any COX will do. These drugs produce analgesia (COX-1 and COX-2) or decreased platelet aggregation (prophylaxis against clots and stroke, COX-1) that is very beneficial. At the same time, however, these older NSAIDS have a nonbeneficial action on the stomach when COX-1 is inhibited. The COX-1 prostaglandin pathway produces mucus to protect the lining of the stomach from erosion by gastric acid; therefore, when COX-1 is blocked, the protective environment within the stomach is altered, leading to gastric distress and ulcers. Aspirin is unique because it covalently (tight bonding) modifies COX, so that new COX enzyme must be synthesized to replace the bound inactive complex. (This is why relatively small amounts of aspirin affect platelets for more than a day. As aspirin is being absorbed, platelets moving through the intestines have their COX permanently blocked. New COX forms only with the synthesis of new platelets.)

To develop better NSAIDs that relieve pain and inflammation but do not cause gastric problems, drugs were designed that selectively interacted with COX-2. The newest generation of NSAIDs, celecoxib (*Celebrex*), rofecoxib (*Vioxx*), and valdecoxib (*Bextra*), are **selective COX-2 inhibitors.** These drugs alleviate pain and reduce inflammation by inhibiting only COX-2; however, the pain relief is not superior to that of the older NSAIDs. Analgesia is equal to that of the other NSAIDs. While the incidence of ulcers and gastric bleeding is less, patients have reported gastrointestinal effects similar to those of aspirin.

Finally, there is evidence that suggests acetaminophen may inhibit (you guessed it) a COX-3 enzyme. Acetaminophen has been a puzzle because it suppresses pain and fever but has relatively little effect on inflammation or the secretion of stomach acid. Some recent work suggests that it may act on another COX, tentatively called COX-3, that is mainly found in the brain.

Clinical Indications

Nonsteroidal antiinflammatory drugs are approved for the relief of mild to moderate pain where opioids are not indicated or warranted. This includes pain arising from local inflammatory responses including headache, dental extraction, soft tissue injury, sunburn, musculoskeletal, and joint overexertion and strain. Because of the direct action on regional prostaglandin production, NSAIDs are also indicated for the chronic treatment of dysmenorrhea, and for controlling the signs and symptoms of osteo- and rheumatoid arthritis.

Antiinflammatory drugs vary in their ability to reduce all types of inflammation, which may be indicative of a selective interference at enzymatic sites within the prostaglandin synthesis pathway. Sulindac (*Clinoril*), tolmetin (*Tolectin*), meclofenamic acid (*Ponstel*), meclofenamic (*Meclomen*), and piroxicam (*Feldene*) are antiinflammatory drugs used in the treatment of a variety of inflammatory conditions, such as tendinitis, bursitis, rheumatoid arthritis, osteoarthritis, and **dysmenorrhea** (difficult or painful menstruation). For the treatment of osteoarthritis, spondylitis (inflammation of the vertebrae), and gout, aspirin may be the drug of choice. Of the potent antiinflammatory drugs, aspirin overall produces the least serious side effects with chronic use.

The treatment of dysmenorrhea has markedly improved with the advent of the NSAIDs. Also known as menstrual cramps, dysmenorrhea is characterized by uterine contractions, local vasoconstriction **(ischemia),** and pain. In addition, headache, nausea, vomiting, and diarrhea may occur. Evidence suggests that women who suffer the discomfort of dysmenorrhea may have higher levels of uterine prostaglandins, especially $PGF_{2\alpha}$ and PGE_2, than nondysmenorrheic women. Nonsteroidal antiinflammatory drugs are effective in relieving the symptoms of dysmenorrhea and are much better than low doses of aspirin. They appear to inhibit prostaglandin synthetase (see Figure 20:1)

Recommended Adult Doses of Nonopioid Analgesics

DRUG (TRADE NAME)	ANALGESIC AND ANTIPYRETIC (INCLUDING DYSMENORRHEA)	ANTIINFLAMMATORY (OSTEOARTHRITIS, RHEUMATOID ARTHRITIS, ANKYLOSING SPONDYLITIS)
N-acetyl-p-aminophenol:		
acetaminophen (*Datril, Tylenol*)*	325–650 mg every 4 hr 1000 mg TID, QID	Not specifically antiinflammatory; used as short-term adjunct to other therapy
Salicylates:		
aspirin (*Anacin, Bayer, Bufferin, Empirin*)*	325–650 mg every 4 hr	3.2–6 g/day
aspirin (extra strength)	500 mg every 3 hr	1000 mg every 6 hr
diflunisal (*Dolobid*)**	500–1000 mg every 8–12 hr	500–1000 mg/day
salicylic acid (*Amigesic, Disalcid, Arthra-G*)**	1500 mg bid	3 g/day tid
sodium thiosalicylate injectable		50–100 mg/day IM
Synthetic Nonsteroidal Antiinflammatory Drugs:*		
diclofenac (*Cataflam, Voltaren*)**	50 mg TID	100–150 mg/day
etodolac (*Lodine*)**	200–400 mg every 6–8 hr	600–1200 mg/day
fenoprofen (*Nalfon*)**	200 mg every 4–6 hr	300–600 mg TID, QID
flurbiprofen (*Ansaid*)**	Not indicated for this	200–300 mg up to QID
ibuprofen (*Advil, Motrin, Nuprin*)* (available by prescription in 300 mg or more)	200–400 mg every 4–6 hr	300–800 mg QID
indomethacin (*Indocin*)**	Not indicated for this	25–50 mg TID
ketorolac tromethamine (*Toradol*)**	Short-term management of moderate to severe pain 15 mg every 6 hr	
ketoprofen (*Orudis Actron*)*	25–50 mg every 6–8 hr	150–300 mg TID, QID
ketoprofen (*Orudis-KT*)**		12.5–25 mg every 4–6 hrs
meclofenamate (*Meclomen*)**	50–100 mg every 4–6 hr	200–400 mg/day
meclofenamic acid (*Ponstel*)**	250 mg every 6 hr	—
meloxicam (*Mobic*)	Not indicated for this	7.5–30 mg/day
nambumetone (*Relafen*)**	Not indicated for this	1000 mg QD, BID
naproxen (*Aleve*)*	200 mg every 6–8 hr	Repeat dose
naproxen (*Anaprox, Naprosyn*)**	200 mg every 6–8 hr	250–500 mg BID
oxaprozin (*DayPro*)**	Not indicated for this	1200–1800 mg QD
piroxicam (*Feldene*)**	Not indicated for this	20 mg/day
sulindac (*Clinoril*)**	Not indicated for this	300–400 mg/day
tolmetin (*Tolectin*)**	Not indicated for this	400 mg TID up to 1800 mg/day

(continued)

Recommended Adult Doses of Nonopioid Analgesics, *continued*

DRUG (TRADE NAME)	ANALGESIC AND ANTIPYRETIC (INCLUDING DYSMENORRHEA)	ANTIINFLAMMATORY (OSTEOARTHRITIS, RHEUMATOID ARTHRITIS, ANKYLOSING SPONDYLITIS)
Selective COX-2 Inhibitors		
celecoxib (*Celebrex*)	Not indicated for this	200 mg/day
rofecoxib (*Vioxx*)	12.5–50 mg/day	50 mg/day
valdecoxib (*Bextra*)	20 mg BID	10 mg/day

*Available over the counter.
**Available by prescription.
***These drugs are antipyretic and analgesic but are primarily used for their antiinflammatory actions except where doses are noted.

in addition to working at other enzymatic sites. Aspirin primarily affects the cyclooxygenase pathway. Ibuprofen, in particular, has been reported to suppress the release of uterine $PGF_{2\alpha}$ even more than PGE_2. Nonsteroidal antiinflammatory drugs ease the pain, headache, and nausea of dysmenorrhea with minimal risk to patients. Although all of the NSAIDs are effective analgesics, only ibuprofen, ketoprofen, and naproxen are currently available OTC for the treatment of dysmenorrhea.

These nonprescription preparations are also extremely popular with the general public for the treatment of osteoarthritis (mild to moderate pain, including rheumatoid complications). For the same spectrum of indications, these NSAIDs require a prescription for tablet and capsule strengths greater than 300 mg (ibuprofen), 12.5 mg (ketoprofen), and 250 mg (naproxen).

Absorption and Metabolism

The NSAIDs are well absorbed from the stomach following oral administration. Although food may delay drug absorption, it is not uncommon for these drugs to be administered with meals, especially in patients who are susceptible to drug-induced gastric irritation. Following oral administration, most of these drugs exert their analgesic action within 30 minutes, with a 4- to 6-hour duration of action. The NSAIDs are highly (more than 90 percent) bound to plasma proteins. For this reason, these drugs undergo many drug interactions due to displacement of other drugs

from protein-binding sites. Eventually, these drugs are metabolized by the drug microsomal metabolizing system in the liver prior to renal excretion. Acidification of the urine may result in renal reabsorption of these acidic drugs.

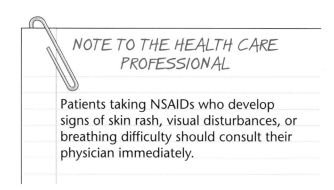

NOTE TO THE HEALTH CARE PROFESSIONAL

Patients taking NSAIDs who develop signs of skin rash, visual disturbances, or breathing difficulty should consult their physician immediately.

Adverse Effects

All antiinflammatory drugs may produce nausea, GI distress, and ulceration. The mechanism of ulceration is not exactly known. However, these drugs are thought to inhibit the synthesis of substances (mucopolysaccharides) that protect the stomach from hydrochloric acid erosion. Although ibuprofen has been reported to produce less gastric distress than do other antiinflammatory drugs, any of these drugs may produce ulceration with chronic use. The most serious complication of ulceration is massive hemorrhage, leading to shock and death.

Through CNS stimulation, antiinflammatory drugs may produce vertigo, vomiting, mental confusion, and headaches. Hypersensitivity reactions may include mild rashes, fever, hepatic damage, and respiratory distress in asthmatic individuals. Anaphylaxis has occurred in aspirin-sensitive patients. Aspirin intolerance may occur in patients with a history of nasal polyps, asthma, or rhinitis. In such patients, angioedema and severe rhinitis result from exposure to aspirin-containing products. **Megaloblastic anemia,** signaled by large, immature red blood cells, has occurred with these drugs because the intestinal absorption of folic acid has been impaired, whereas iron deficiency **anemia** may occur as a result of blood loss through hemorrhage. Bone marrow suppression leading to blood disorders has also been reported to occur in patients who received NSAIDs. Adverse effects are more likely to occur in patients receiving large doses in the chronic treatment of arthritis, especially rheumatoid arthritis. Overdose of the antiinflammatory drugs produces toxicity similar to that described for salicylates. Treatment is primarily supportive because there is no specific antidote for these agents.

Age and underlying condition of the patient do influence the onset of adverse effects. The larger dose in combination with patient age over 65 years appears to predispose to the onset of unwanted effects. The best strategy in elderly patients, therefore, requires using the lowest effective dose. Specific newer potent NSAIDs such as ketorolac tromethamine have a special warning that recommends dosage adjustment for patients over 65 years old and/or less than 110 pounds of body weight. Because ketorolac tromethamine is cleared from the body slowly, this may be exaggerated in older patients and patients with renal impairment, as evidenced by elevated serum creatinine levels.

The selective COX-2 inhibitors exhibit potentially more serious cardiac or renal adverse effects than do other NSAIDs because they focus only on one group of enzymes. Two large clinical studies in 8000 patients each suggest that more patients taking rofecoxib and celecoxib experience an increase in blood pressure (aggravated hypertension), bradycardia, irregular heartbeat, or chest pains than patients taking other NSAIDs. This is exacerbated by the fact that selective COX-2 inhibitors do not have the antithrombotic (clot prevention) protective action of aspirin and other COX-1 inhibitors.

These drugs are at the same risk of contributing to renal insufficiency and alterations in salt and water excretion as other NSAIDs in patients with existing renal problems.

Celecoxib should not be taken by patients who have a history of sensitivity to sulfonamides. All selective COX-2 inhibitors have been associated with exacerbating allergic reactions.

Special Considerations

Nonsteroidal antiinflammatory drugs may be used for short periods (up to 7 days) for the relief of acute inflammation. It is not uncommon, however, for these drugs to be taken for longer periods. In osteoarthritis, a degenerative joint disease, joint movement may be compromised so that movement is painful and difficult (stiff). Pain may occur in the absence of overt signs of inflammation. Although analgesics such as aspirin are indicated, it is still advisable to have patients avoid stressing the involved joints (take weight off the joints and rest).

Rheumatoid arthritis, also a degenerative joint disease, is associated with inflammation of the joint cartilage. Often, inflamed joints are noticeably warm to touch, are difficult to move (especially in the morning), and become immobile or deformed through the course of the disease. The NSAIDs, which include aspirin in large doses (2 to 5 g), will reduce the inflammatory response. At these doses, especially in elderly patients, signs of overdose may be present. Primary signs to watch for include ringing in the ears, gastric upset, and GI bleeding (black, tarry stools). To minimize GI side effects, medication may be given with meals, milk, or antacids. Alcohol should be avoided, since it may enhance the adverse gastric action of these drugs.

SALICYLATES

Salicylates were discovered centuries ago as a natural product of the willow tree bark. Native Americans drank teas and beverages made from willow bark to relieve headaches and toothaches. The salicylates used today include sodium salicylate, aspirin (acetylsalicylic acid), salicylamide, and methyl salicylate. Methyl salicylate (oil of wintergreen, *Ben-Gay, Deep-Heat*) is the only salicylate that is a poison when taken orally. Methyl salicylate is used topically (creams) to produce cutaneous irritation, which increases blood flow and warmth at the site of application. The other salicylates are weak acids that are rapidly absorbed from the stomach and small intestine following oral administration.

Analgesia and Antipyresis

The centers of the brain that regulate pain and temperature are located in the hypothalamus. Nonopioid analgesics, including salicylates, are thought to produce analgesia and antipyresis by selectively affecting the hypothalamic centers, reducing an elevated body temperature but not affecting normal body temperature. The mechanism of the central action involves blockade of prostaglandin stimulation of the central nervous system (CNS). In addition to the central action, these drugs increase peripheral blood flow (vasodilation) and sweating, permitting a greater loss of excess heat from the body.

Analgesia is produced by affecting both the hypothalamus and the site of injury. In response to tissue injury, joint damage, or edema, active substances such as bradykinin, prostaglandins, and histamine are released. **Prostaglandins** and bradykinin, in particular, stimulate peripheral nerve endings, which carry pain impulses to the CNS. Nonopioid analgesics inhibit the synthesis of prostaglandins and prevent bradykinin from stimulating pain receptors. Since prostaglandins also affect hypothalamic centers, nonopioid analgesics inhibit the recognition of pain impulses centrally and peripherally. Aspirin is the most potent inhibitor of prostaglandin synthetase in the salicylate group.

Antiinflammatory Action

Salicylates are excellent antiinflammatory drugs. They are effective in reducing inflammation because they inhibit a primary pathway in prostaglandin synthesis. The development of inflammation and the action of the salicylates upon this response was discussed in the section on Antiinflammatory Drugs.

Gastrointestinal Effects

Salicylates directly irritate the stomach mucosal lining. Many people are sensitive to this action and experience nausea after taking aspirin. In addition, salicylates inhibit prostaglandin synthesis. In the stomach, prostaglandins are an integral part of the normal cytoprotective mechanisms. Prostaglandins mediate secretion of mucus and bicarbonate, which influence the environment of the stomach. In some individuals, vomiting occurs as a result of gastrointestinal (GI) irritation and CNS stimulation. Salicylates stimulate the medullary center known as the chemoreceptor trigger zone. This zone directly excites the vomiting center so that emesis may occur.

Anticoagulant and Cardiovascular Benefit

Aspirin and salicylamide irreversibly inhibit the aggregation of platelets necessary for blood clot formation. As a result, even low doses of aspirin increase bleeding time. In large doses, salicylates may depress the formation of other coagulation factors (prothrombin), thus increasing bleeding time. **Petechial** (localized) hemorrhages that occur in aspirin-sensitive patients are partially due to the anticoagulant actions. With doses of aspirin greater than 6 g per day, prolongation of prothrombin time is clinically significant.

Of therapeutic significance is the fact that aspirin reduces the risk of death and reinfarction following myocardial infarction (MI). While this benefit warrants its prophylactic (daily) use in men, it has not been demonstrated to be of similar value in women. This prophylactic action inhibits platelet aggregation and has no effect once a clot has formed.

These anticoagulant effects increase the potential for hemorrhage in certain patients—that is, those sensitive to salicylates or receiving other anticoagulants or those predisposed to intestinal ulcers. In specific cardiovascular compromised patients where ulcers are present, chronic administration of aspirin may be beneficial to prevent the formation of thromboemboli. While it does appear contradictory, the use of aspirin in such a circumstance would reduce the greater risk of emboli forming or reaching the brain, lung, or heart.

Metabolism and Excretion

Following absorption, salicylates readily bind to plasma proteins (80 to 90 percent). In this way, salicylates are distributed to various tissues, especially the CNS, joint fluids, and kidneys. Eventually, these drugs are metabolized in the liver and excreted into urine. Plasma levels of salicylates are affected by the pH of the urine. Acidic urine permits these weak acids to be reabsorbed by the renal tubules and reenter the blood. In contrast, alkaline urine increases the excretion of salicylates. Urine pH can change in response to acid-base imbalance, drug therapy, or renal impairment.

Adverse and Toxic Effects

In low doses, salicylates relieve pain, aches, and fever. However, to relieve the pain of arthritis, gout, and **rheumatic fever,** salicylates must be used in large doses for long periods of time. Large-dose therapy is more frequently associated with toxic reactions (chronic **intoxication**). However, acute salicylate intoxication may also occur from accidental ingestion of large amounts of drug. Accidental overdose is more likely to occur with children than with adults.

Chronic salicylate intoxication produces nausea, vomiting, or salicylism. **Salicylism** is a series of symptoms that include nausea, ringing in the ears (tinnitus), headache, delirium, and hyperventilation. These effects are due to CNS stimulation and subside when the dose is reduced or the drug is terminated. In addition, hyperglycemia may occur due to increased sympathetic tone.

A cultural contribution to the development of salicylate intoxication may come from the patient's diet. Many foods are known to contain salicylates naturally, such as curry powder, paprika, licorice, prunes, raisins, tea, and gherkins. It has been estimated that the American diet may contain 6 to 200 mg of salicylates per day.

Hypersensitivity to aspirin may produce skin rashes, laryngeal edema, and asthma. Such reactions may be life-threatening, so that hypersensitive patients must avoid all products containing aspirin. Salicylates are readily available as over-the-counter (OTC) drugs, either alone or in combination with other products. Examples of drug mixtures that contain nonopioid analgesics are presented in Table 20:2 on page 220. Such products are present in almost every home, and many times they are found by adventurous children. Attracted by the colored tablets or candy flavor, children often ingest a toxic amount of analgesic.

Acute Toxicity

The dangerous and often fatal reactions of acute salicylate poisoning involve respiratory depression and acidosis. Toxic doses of salicylates depress the medullary respiratory centers so that individuals cannot remove carbon dioxide (CO_2) rapidly, leading to respiratory acidosis. Other acids accumulate in the blood because renal function is impaired. Salicylates and tissue waste products (lactic acid) cannot be cleared from the body. Individuals enter respiratory and metabolic acidosis, and the blood and urine pH values fall. Profuse sweating causes dehydration, and sodium, potassium, and protein excretion in the urine may increase. Cardiovascular function is depressed, resulting in vasodilation and hypotension. The acute lethal dose is estimated to be 10 to 30 g for adults and 4 g for children.

Treatment of salicylate poisoning includes administration of sodium bicarbonate to correct the acidosis and to increase salicylate excretion (increase urine pH). In addition, fluid and electrolytes are infused to correct the hypotension and acid-base balance. Treatment of salicylate poisoning is not always successful. Coma and death may result from dehydration, extensive CNS depression, and renal failure.

Clinical Indications

Salicylates, especially aspirin, are approved for use in mild to moderate pain. This is pain that is not associated with the need for opioids. Inflammation contributing to headache and to muscle and joint pain, including osteoarthritis and rheumatoid arthritis, is reduced and often eliminated by these drugs. Because of the special action on platelet aggregation, aspirin is indicated for use in patients with unstable angina pectoris, transient ischemic attacks (TIAs), stroke, and to reduce the risk of death in men with MI.

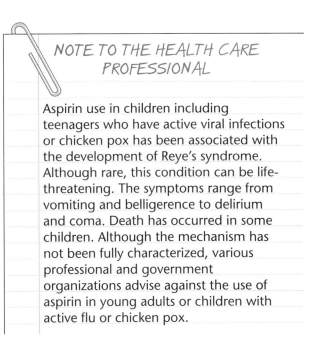

NOTE TO THE HEALTH CARE PROFESSIONAL

Aspirin use in children including teenagers who have active viral infections or chicken pox has been associated with the development of Reye's syndrome. Although rare, this condition can be life-threatening. The symptoms range from vomiting and belligerence to delirium and coma. Death has occurred in some children. Although the mechanism has not been fully characterized, various professional and government organizations advise against the use of aspirin in young adults or children with active flu or chicken pox.

Dose and Formulation Availability

Because of its long-standing use, aspirin has become widely acceptable as safe for use in adults and children. To accommodate the wide spectrum of use, aspirin and salicylates are available in a variety of oral formulations ranging from tablets, capsules, and gum to solutions and liquids more easily swallowed by children. While aspirin is available over-the-counter (OTC) alone or in combination with a wide variety of other active ingredients, a prescription is required for products containing

Drug Mixtures That Contain Nonopioid Analgesics***

TRADE NAME	AMOUNT OF NONOPIOID ANALGESIC	OTHER ACTIVE DRUGS	SCHEDULE
Alka-Seltzer, Ascriptin, Bufferin	325–500 mg aspirin	1700–2085 mg sodium bicarbonate 1000 mg citric acid	—
Bromo-Seltzer	325 mg acetaminophen	2781 mg sodium bicarbonate 2224 mg citric acid	—
*Darvocet-N 50**	325 mg acetaminophen	50 mg propoxyphene	IV
*Darvocet-N 100**	650 mg acetaminophen	100 mg propoxyphene	IV
*Darvon Compound-65**	389 mg aspirin	32.4 mg caffeine, 65 mg propoxyphene	IV
*Equagesic**	325 mg aspirin	meprobamate 200 mg	IV
*Fiorinal**	325 mg aspirin	40 mg caffeine, 50 mg butalbital (barbiturate)	III
Midol IB, Advil, Menadol Pamprin-IB	200 mg ibuprofen	—	—
Maximum Strength Midol PMS Capsules and Gelcaps	500 mg acetaminophen	25 mg *Pamabrom***, 15 mg pyrilamine	—
Pamprin Maximum Cramp Relief	500 mg acetaminophen	*Pamabrom***, pyrilamine	—
Panacet 5/500	500 mg acetaminophen	5 mg hydrocodone	III
Panadol Children's	80 mg acetaminophen	—	
*Percodan**	325 mg aspirin	4.5 mg oxycodone HCl, 0.20 mg oxycodone terephthalate	II
*Percocet**	325 mg aspirin	2.5, 5, 7.5 or 10 mg oxycodone	II
	650 mg aspirin	10 mg oxycodone	II
*Tylenol with Codeine**	300 mg acetaminophen	15 mg codeine	III
*Tylox Capsules**	500 mg acetaminophen	5 mg oxycodone	II
*Vanquish***	204 mg acetaminophen	227 mg aspirin, 33 mg caffeine, magnesium hydroxide and aluminum hydroxide	

*Available by prescription only.
**Over-the-counter diuretic.
***Not an all-inclusive list of available products.

greater than 650 mg of aspirin per tablet (see Table 20:1 for examples). Pediatric dosing is based on age and weight with two 81-mg pediatric tablets (age 2 to 3 years), equal to one-half of a 325-mg adult tablet, every 4 hours. At age 6 to 8 years, the dose is four 81-mg tablets or one adult tablet (325 mg). By age 12 to 14 years, dosing is at the recommended adult level of two (325 mg) tablets (see Table 20:3).

ACETAMINOPHEN

Acetaminophen is often considered an aspirin substitute. However, this assumption is not entirely correct. Acetaminophen (*Datril, Panadol, Tylenol*) produces adequate analgesia and antipyresis but has no proven antiinflammatory

TABLE 20:3	Pediatric Dosing Guidelines for Aspirin and Acetaminophen— Dose Every 4–6 Hours	
AGE	**ACETAMINOPHEN**	**ASPIRIN**
0–3 months	40 mg	—
4–11 months	80 mg	—
1–2 years	120 mg	—
2–3 years	160 mg	162 mg
4–5 years	240 mg	243 mg
6–8 years	320 mg	324 mg
9–10 years	400 mg	405 mg
11 years	480 mg	486 mg
12–14 years	640 mg	648 mg
14 years	650 mg	650 mg

activity. It reduces elevated body temperature by a direct action on the heat regulation centers in the hypothalamus. Acetaminophen is effective against the pain of headache because it inhibits prostaglandin synthetase within the CNS but is not a drug of choice in the treatment of pain associated with muscle aches and inflammation, especially arthritis. Acetaminophen does not significantly inhibit the synthesis of prostaglandins in peripheral systems, which accounts for the lack of antiinflammatory activity. For the relief of headache or the symptomatic relief of cold and flu, aspirin-sensitive patients may substitute acetaminophen because acetaminophen does not produce GI irritation or ulceration in therapeutic doses. Acetaminophen does not affect platelet aggregation or prothrombin response.

Adverse Effects

Although remarkably safe when taken in recommended doses, acetaminophen is not a harmless drug. There are no specific early warning signs of acetaminophen toxicity. The course of poisoning may follow several stages. During the first 24 hours after ingestion, nausea and vomiting may occur. During the next 24 hours, hepatic serum enzymes may rise (SGOT, SGPT, bilirubin, thrombin). Elevations in SGOT may exceed 20,000. Within 36 hours of ingestion of a toxic dose, hepatic damage may result. Deaths have occurred following acetaminophen overdose. Overdose of acetaminophen also produces acidosis and respiratory complications similar to those described for salicylate poisoning.

Treatment for acetaminophen poisoning includes gastric aspiration and **lavage** (washing with fluids) as well as maintenance of fluid balance through conventional measures. Activated charcoal will decrease the absorption of acetaminophen if administered within hours of the ingested overdose. Otherwise, acetylcysteine successfully prevents liver damage when administered intravenously or orally within 10 hours of acetaminophen poisoning. The oral route of administration may be less effective, but intravenous administration has been associated with **anaphylaxis** (severe allergic reaction). Acetylcysteine has been available for years as a mucolytic in cystic fibrosis patients.

Acetaminophen is used in more combination products than any other drug in doses from 160 to 500 mg per dose. When patients take acetaminophen (*Tylenol*) for pain and then use multiple OTC products for relief of cold and flu symptoms, especially in addition to alcohol, there is an increased risk of developing liver toxicity. The FDA has continued to express a concern that adults and children are at risk for developing an acetaminophen toxicity through overdose because flavored medications attract children to these medications and adults frequently take "more than the recommended dose striving to eliminate moderate to severe pain."

Phenacetin, also an analgesic, is not available as a single-entity product. Phenacetin has been associated with serious side effects, including acidosis, methemoglobinemia, and nephritis. Its use has been questioned, and it has been dropped as an ingredient in many combination products. In genetically susceptible individuals (especially those of Mediterranean ancestry), hemolytic anemia may also occur with the use of phenacetin.

Clinical Indications

Acetaminophen is approved to reduce fever, headache, minor musculoskeletal pain, and discomfort associated with the common cold and flu. It is particularly indicated for use in patients allergic to aspirin, those receiving anticoagulant therapy for coagulation disorders, or patients who have upper GI disease and for whom aspirin therapy is not an option. It is recommended for use in patients who experience GI upset from aspirin or nonsteroidal antiinflammatory drugs (NSAIDs); however, it is not interchangeable with these products for chronic therapy of inflammatory conditions such as osteoarthritis. No benefit has been associated with the use of this drug in stroke or infarction.

Dose and Formulation Availability

Acetaminophen is available in OTC products in doses ranging from 80 mg (pediatric) to 650 mg per tablet, capsule, or caplet. Dosing guidelines are available for infants 0 to 3 months (40 mg), 4 to 11 months (80 mg), and 1 to 2 years of age (120 mg). The pediatric and adult doses of 325 mg every 4 hours coincide at the recommendation for 6 to 8 years of age. It is recommended that the adult daily dose not exceed 4000 mg, while the pediatric exposure should not exceed 5 doses in 24 hours (Table 20:3). Because of its acceptability for use in children, acetaminophen is available in a variety of formulations ranging from suppository to solution, elixir, suspension, and syrup. At all doses and formulations, acetaminophen is available without prescription, OTC. For best shelf-life, suppositories should be refrigerated between use.

DRUGS USEFUL IN TREATING GOUT

Gout is a special inflammatory disease. It is associated with the deposition of uric acid in joint fluid (big toe, knees, and elbows) and soft tissue. Uric acid is formed every day from the metabolism of nucleic acids (see Figure 20:2). Humans cannot use uric acid, so it is normally secreted into the urine by the renal tubules. People who suffer from gout usually overproduce uric acid or do not excrete it efficiently. In addition, certain foods, such as beer, wine, cheeses, beans, anchovies, sardines, liver, kidneys, and cream contain a high purine content, which increases the uric acid level of blood (hyperuricemia).

For some unknown reason, uric acid crystals spontaneously accumulate in the joint fluid of gouty individuals. Phagocytes enter the area and attack the uric acid crystals, and this activity leads to a decrease in pH (acid) of the joint fluid, causing more uric acid to accumulate in the joint. This vicious cycle of inflammation produces the edema, redness, and severe pain characteristic of acute gout. In chronic gout, uric acid slowly deposits in soft tissue, causing bulging, deformed joints known as tophi. (Tophaceous deposits may take years to develop.) Uric acid may also accumulate in

FIGURE 20:2 The Metabolic Pathway Leading to the Formation and Excretion of Uric Acid

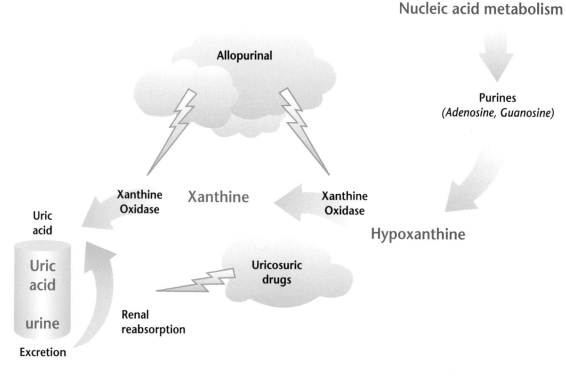

the kidneys, producing urate stones, which may appear in the urine as sand or gravel. Drugs that are useful in the treatment of gout either relieve the acute inflammatory response or reduce the uric acid levels in chronic gout. These agents are listed in Table 20:4.

Treatment of Acute Gout

Antiinflammatory analgesics can be used to reduce the pain and inflammation of acute gouty attacks. In addition, colchicine is extremely useful during the first 48 hours of an acute attack. Colchicine, a drug that comes from the crocus plant, specifically alters the ability of the phagocytes to attack uric acid crystals (Figure 20:3). The pH of the joint fluid does not fall. Therefore, the cycle of uric acid deposition is interrupted, and the gouty attack eventually

subsides. Unfortunately, colchicine frequently produces nausea, vomiting, and diarrhea. Abdominal cramps and blood in the urine (hematuria) may also occur.

Prophylactic Treatment of Gout

Prophylactic therapy involves the long-term use of drugs to prevent the occurrence of gouty attacks and tophi. Two major classes of drugs are used in long-term **prophylaxis**—hypouricemic agents and uricosuric agents.

Allopurinol is a hypouricemic drug. It is also known as an antimetabolite because it resembles the structure of hypoxanthine. Allopurinol inhibits the enzyme xanthine oxidase, which is necessary to turn hypoxanthine into uric acid (see Figure 20:2). Therefore, no uric acid is formed, and hypoxanthine is excreted into the urine. Eventually,

---

TABLE 20:4	Drugs Effective in the Treatment of Gout
DRUG (TRADE NAME)	**ADULT ORAL DOSE**
Antigout (Acute):	
colchicine	0.5–1.2 mg every 1–2 hr* or 0.5–1.8 mg/day**
Antiinflammatory Analgesics:	
aspirin***	3–5 g/day
choline salicylate (*Arthropan*)***	870 mg every 3–4 hr
indomethacin (*Indocin*)	50 mg TID
naproxen (*Naprosyn*)	750 mg followed by 250 mg every 8 hr
sodium thiosalicylate (*Rexolate*)	100 mg every 3–4 hr
sulindac (*Clinoril*)	200 mg BID
Hypouricemic:	
allopurinol (*Zyloprim*)	200–400 mg/day (mild) 400–600 mg/day (severe)
	600–800 mg/day (uric acid nephropathy; neoplasias)
Uricosuric:	
aspirin	Doses greater than 4 g
probenecid	250–500 mg BID
sulfinpyrazone (*Anturane*)	100–200 mg BID
Mixtures:	
colchicine (0.5 mg) and probenecid (500 mg)	One tablet daily for 1 week followed by one tablet BID

*Until pain is relieved.
**Prophylactic dose.
***OTC; prescription required for all others.

FIGURE 20:3 Cycle of Inflammation During an Acute Gout Attack

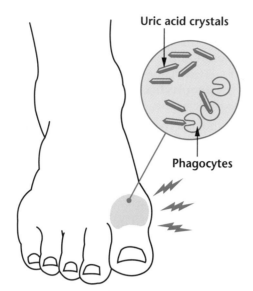

Uric acid crystals are attacked by the phagocytes, resulting in a decrease in the pH (acid) of the joint fluid, which causes more uric acid crystals to accumulate in the joint.

the uric acid in the blood decreases, preventing the future development of tophi and urate stones in the kidneys. Allopurinol can also be used to reduce the hyperuricemia associated with certain malignancies and other drug therapy (thiazide diuretics). The most common side effects associated with the use of allopurinol are fever, rash, and **leukopenia** (low white blood cell count).

Probenecid and sulfinpyrazone are uricosuric drugs. Uricosuric drugs enhance the renal excretion of uric acid without altering the formation of uric acid, leading to a rapid clearance of uric acid from the blood. These agents inhibit the renal reabsorption of uric acid so that it passes into the urine. Probenecid is rapidly absorbed following oral administration. Often, probenecid is administered in combination with colchicine as a preparation called *ColProbenecid,* which reduces the blood urate level, while colchicine protects against the onset of an acute gouty attack.

Probenecid and sulfinpyrazone frequently cause GI disturbances, including nausea and vomiting. It is recommended that these medications be taken with meals, milk, or antacids to avoid GI upset. Other adverse effects reported with probenecid or sulfinpyrazone include skin rash and fever. To reduce the likelihood of developing renal urate

stones, any person taking an antigout drug should drink 10 to 12 8-ounce glasses of water daily. This drug also completely inhibits prostaglandin synthetase, which prevents platelet aggregation.

Clinical Indications

For the treatment of acute gout attacks, relief of pain and interruption of the inflammatory process, colchicine and specific NSAIDs (indomethacin, naproxen) and sodium thiosalicylate are indicated.

For the treatment of hyperuricemia associated with gout and gouty arthritis, probenecid is approved for use. Because of its ability to inhibit the renal tubular secretion of most penicillins and cephalosporins, probenecid elevates and prolongs the plasma levels of these antibiotics. Probenecid is therefore also approved for use as an adjunct to antibiotic therapy.

Sulfinpyrazone is approved for the treatment of chronic and intermittent gouty arthritis and not acute gout. Allopurinol is approved for the management of primary and secondary gout, acute gout attacks, tophi, joint destruction, uric acid stones, or nephropathy. Because of its mechanism of action, it is also recommended for reduction of serum and urinary uric acid resulting from the treatment of malignancies, leukemia, and lymphoma.

DRUG INTERACTIONS

Nonopioid analgesics and antiinflammatory drugs undergo a variety of drug interactions. The major area of interaction includes drug displacement from protein-binding sites. This displacement usually results in an increased toxicity of the displaced drug. Inhibition of uric acid excretion is the next most frequent drug interaction. Since most of these drugs are weak acids, they compete with uric acid for sites of excretion along the renal tubules. This competition may cancel the uricosuric effect desired in the treatment of chronic gout. Of noteworthy importance is the potential for serious interaction with acetaminophen because of its ubiquitous use. The hepatotoxicity associated with acetaminophen may increase with the long term use of drugs that induce microsomal enzymes. The concomitant use of acetaminophen with several drugs ranging from alcohol to sulfinpyrazone is associated with decreased analgesic therapeutic effect to hepatotoxicity. Clinically significant drug interactions among the classes of drugs represented in this chapter are presented in Table 20:5 on page 226.

Patient Administration and Monitoring

The drugs in this class are so widely available as OTC preparations and are used by such a broad group of patients that there is more opportunity for inappropriate use to occur. Children and the elderly may be more susceptible to inappropriate exposure, in part, because the drugs are not seen as harmful—that is, as strong, serious medications. After all, prescriptions are not required for the vast majority of the preparations. Therefore, patients benefit from an opportunity to hear clear instruction about the use of these drugs.

Patient Instructions

Whether the active analgesic or antiinflammatory is OTC or prescription, the potential for adverse effects to occur increases with dose and chronic use. Explain to patients that too frequent readministration of OTC preparations can equal the mg amount available by prescription.

Patients should be clearly instructed to take solid oral formulations with a full glass of water to avoid the possibility of the pill or capsule lodging in the esophagus. Probenecid and allopurinol must be accompanied by 10 to 12 full glasses of water daily in order to maintain a neutral to slightly alkaline urine and prevent the formation of kidney stones. Large doses of vitamin C may acidify the urine and increase the potential for kidney stone formation.

Patients may be told that GI irritation can be reduced by taking the medication with milk or with meals. Sustained-release formulations should not be crushed or chewed because more drug is delivered earlier than the formulation intended.

Notify the Physician

With any of the analgesic, antiinflammatory drugs, the patient should call the doctor if fever continues more than 3 days, if pain persists more than 5 days, or if redness or swelling develops. Severe or recurrent pain, or high or continued fever, may indicate serious illness requiring medical attention.

With any of these drugs, the patient should notify the doctor if ringing in the ears (tinnitus), dizziness, hearing impairment, or dimmed vision occurs and discontinue the medication as directed.

Bronchospasm and/or rhinitis may indicate the development of aspirin intolerance. The physician should be notified for further evaluation. Patients with acute asthma, urticaria, and nasal polyps should avoid aspirin and NSAIDs.

These drugs may cause drowsiness that will reduce the coordination and attention required for driving, operating machinery, or performing tasks requiring manual dexterity. Elderly patients should not exceed the recommended daily doses of NSAIDs; this includes exposure to OTC preparations while taking prescribed NSAIDs.

Special Caution with Aspirin

Aspirin, alcohol, and alcohol-containing products should be avoided during NSAID therapy.

When possible, aspirin should be avoided 1 week prior to surgery because of the possibility of postoperative bleeding. Patients allergic to tartrazine dye should avoid aspirin.

Use in Pregnancy

All of these drugs are designated Food and Drug Administration (FDA) Pregnancy Category B or C except for aspirin (D). Aspirin causes effects in the mother, including anemia, bleeding, and delayed labor. Since salicylates cross the placenta, prostaglandin synthesis in the fetus may be suppressed. The recommendation is to avoid salicylates during pregnancy, especially during the third trimester. Acetaminophen is the alternative analgesic at all stages of pregnancy. It appears safe for short-term use.

Drug Interactions With the Nonopioid Analgesics and Antigout Drugs

PHARMACOLOGICAL AGENTS	INTERACT WITH	RESPONSE
acetaminophen	Alcohol, barbiturates, carbemazepine, hydantoins, isoniazid, rifampin, sulinpyrozone	Increased risk of hepatotoxicity
allopurinol	cyclophosphamide	Increased bone marrow depression
allopurinol	ampicillin	Skin rash has occurred with concurrent use of these drugs
allopurinol	Thiazides, ACE inhibitors	Higher risk of hypersensitivity to allopurinol
aspirin	Antacids, corticosteroids, urinary alkalinizing drugs	Decrease the effects of salicylate by increasing renal excretion, decreasing tubular reabsorption
aspirin (doses > 2 g/day)	Sulfonylureas, insulin	Potentiate glucose lowering effect; hypoglycemia
aspirin	heparin	Increased risk of bleeding
diflusinal	indomethacin	Decreased renal clearance of indomethacin; fatal GI hemorrhage has occurred
NSAIDs	Alcohol	Increased risk for GI ulceration
NSAIDs	lithium	May elevate the plasma level of lithium
indomethacin oxyphenbutazone phenylbutazone salicylates	Anticonvulsants, methotrexate, oral anticoagulants, oral hypoglycemics	Increased bleeding toxicity due to protein binding displacement or additive effect of depressing prothrombin
salicylates	Uricosuric agents	Decreased renal excretion of uric acid
indomethacin	furosemide, thiazide diuretics	Decreased sodium excretion and antihypertensive action
indomethacin	lithium	May elevate plasma lithium concentrations
probenecid	acyclovir, clofibrate, oral hypoglycemics, methotrexate, NSAIDs, penicillins, sulfonamides	Decreases renal excretion, increases plasma concentrations of these drugs
sulfinpyrazone	acetaminophen	Hepatoxicity risk increases with chronic use of sulfinpyrazone
sulfinpyrazone	Oral anticoagulants	Increased anticoagulant action by protein binding displacement; increased bleeding
sulfinpyrazone	verapamil	Increased clearance of verapamil; decreased effect

Abbreviations: ACE, angiotensin-converting enzyme.

Chapter Review

Understanding Terminology

Answer the following questions in the spaces provided.

1. How do the nonopioid analgesics differ from the opioid analgesics? _____
_____
_____

2. Define *analgesia*. _____
_____
_____

3. Explain the term *inflammation*. _____
_____
_____

Match the description in the left column with the appropriate term in the right column.

_____ **4.** Joint pain.

_____ **5.** Pain associated with muscle injury.

_____ **6.** Inflammation of the joints.

_____ **7.** Small area of skin or mucous membrane that is discolored because of localized hemorrhages.

_____ **8.** Condition in which pain and inflammation of joints are accompanied by elevated body temperature.

_____ **9.** Painful menstruation.

_____ **10.** Condition in which toxic doses of salicylates result in nausea, tinnitus, and delirium.

a. arthralgia

b. arthritis

c. dysmenorrhea

d. myalgia

e. petechia

f. rheumatic fever

g. salicylism

Acquiring Knowledge

Answer the following questions in the spaces provided.

1. What are the three major pharmacological effects produced by the salicylates? _____
_____
_____

2. How do the nonopioid analgesics relieve pain? _____
_____
_____

3. Why do some people experience nausea and vomiting after taking aspirin? _____
_____
_____

4. Why do the salicylates potentiate the action of the oral anticoagulant drugs? _____
_____
_____

5. What physiological changes might occur during acute salicylate toxicity? _____

_____

_____

6. Why is acetaminophen recommended for patients who are aspirin sensitive? _____

_____

_____

7. How do antiinflammatory drugs interrupt the process of inflammation? _____

_____

_____

8. Which antiinflammatory drugs should not be administered over long periods of time (such as 2 months)?

_____

_____

9. What metabolic imbalance is associated with the production of gout? _____

_____

_____

10. How does colchicine alleviate the acute inflammatory reaction of gout? _____

_____

_____

11. How do allopurinol and probenecid differ in their antigout mechanism of action? _____

_____

_____

Applying Knowledge—On the Job

Use your critical thinking skills to answer the following questions in the spaces provided.

1. Assume that you work in an emergency room of a hospital. For each of the following patients who come to the ER tonight with a nonopioid drug overdose, determine the probable drug and what should be done to treat the overdose.

   a. Patient A presents with respiratory acidosis, low blood and urine pH values, profuse sweating, vasodilation, and hypotension.

   _____

   _____

   b. Patient B presents with nausea and vomiting. Liver enzymes (AST, ALT, bilirubin, and thrombin) are all high and rising. Liver damage seems imminent.

   _____

   _____

2. For each of the following adult patients, how much nonopioid analgesic drug is required to produce the desired effect?

   a. Patient A wants to take aspirin to relieve the fever, aches, and pains of the flu.

   _____

   _____

   b. Patient B wants to take aspirin as an antiinflammatory agent for osteoarthritis.

   _____

   _____

   c. Patient C wants to take ibuprofen for dysmenorrhea.

   _____

   _____

d. Patient D wants to take ibuprofen for osteoarthritis inflammation.

_____

_____

e. Patient E wants to take naproxen for menstrual pain.

_____

_____

f. Patient F wants to take naproxen for inflammation associated with rheumatoid arthritis.

_____

_____

3. A mother of a 26-month-old child calls. Her child is coughing, has nasal congestion, and is running a fever. She would like to know how much aspirin she should give her child. The child weighs 22 pounds.

_____

_____

4. John is 62 years old and is currently taking _Coumadin, Tenormin,_ and _Micronase._ He wants to know if he can take _Anacin_ for his headache.

_____

_____

5. Your office receives a frantic call from a young mother. Her 1-1/2 year old accidentally got ahold of children's chewable _Tylenol._ She is not sure how many she ate, but thinks there were at least 20 tablets in the bottle, and now it is empty. She feels that her daughter must have gotten into this within the last 1-1/2 hours. What should she do?

_____

_____

Internet Connection

Web pages that present information on arthritis (osteoarthritis, rheumatoid), management of moderate pain, and gout discuss the use of NSAIDs. This material is designed for use by medical associates and consumers and therefore is user friendly to access and comprehend. Go on the Internet and enter www.google.com. At the search box, enter _Pain Management NSAIDs._ Among the links provided will be www.ehendrick.org, which maintains Access Med. _AccessMed_ is a source of online health information of more than 55,000 illnesses, conditions, and procedures. _AccessMed_ contains detailed images and information that is easy to read and understand, with links to drug and disease-related information such as chronic pain management. NSAID toxicity over the long term can be viewed at www.ehendrick.org/healthy/00059590.

The Pain Management Research Center of America is dedicated to helping to find solutions for the millions (86 million in America alone) who suffer from chronic pain. This center maintains a website at www.pain-research.org/cox2.html that provides fair, balanced information on osteoarthritis and the variety of options for management of chronic pain.

The FDA and National Institutes of Health provide up-to-date information through medical and consumer links such as www.healthfinder.gov. This site discusses osteoarthritis—the most common type of arthritis, especially among older individuals. Osteoarthritis symptoms (pain, swelling, and loss of motion) and treatments are covered. It also offers a gout fact sheet that reviews how gout develops and what medications are used to treat it. The government site also provides consumer information on specific drugs such as the COX-2 inhibitors.

Additional Reading

Cohen, M. R. 1997. Medication errors: Pediatric acetaminophen a matter of concentration. *Nursing* 27 (9):22.

Conaway, D. C. 1995. Using NSAIDs safely in the elderly. *Hospital Medicine* 31 (5):23.

Hinton, R. 2002. Osteoarthritis: Diagnosis and therapeutic considerations, *American Family Physician* 65 (5):841. (access online at www.aafp.org)

Jones, A. K. 1997. Primary care management of acute low back pain. *Nurse Practitioner: American Journal of Primary Health Care* 22 (7):50.

Levin, A. A. 1996. New NSAIDs warnings. *Health Facts* 21 (201):2.

Paris, P. M. 1996. Treating the patient in pain. *Emergency Medicine* 28 (9):66.

Rainsford, K. D. 1999. Profile and mechanisms of gastrointestinal and other side effects of nonsteroidal antiinflammatory drugs (NSAIDs). *American Journal of Medicine* 107 (6A):27S.

Wolfe, M. M. 1996. NSAIDs and the gastrointestinal mucosa. *Hospital Practice* 31 (12):37.

part

PHARMACOLOGY OF THE HEART

4

Chapter 21

Cardiac Physiology and Pathology

Cardiac Function
Main Diseases of the Heart

Chapter 22

Cardiac Glycosides and the Treatment of Congestive Heart Failure

Cardiac Glycosides
Diuretic Therapy of CHF

Chapter 23

Antiarrhythmic Drugs

Types of Arrhythmias
Class 1 Antiarrhythmic Drugs
Class 2 Antiarrhythmic Drugs
Class 3 Antiarrhythmic Drugs
Class 4 Antiarrhythmic Drugs
Other Antiarrhythmic Drugs
Special Considerations

Chapter 24

Antianginal Drugs

Nitrites and Nitrates
Beta-Andrenergic Blocking Drugs
Calcium Antagonists
Clinical Indications for Antianginal
Drugs

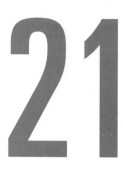

chapter

21

CARDIAC PHYSIOLOGY AND PATHOLOGY

CHAPTER FOCUS

This chapter describes the basic physiological concepts of normal heart function and the diseases that commonly affect the heart. It also explains how these disease states affect cardiac function.

CHAPTER OBJECTIVES

After studying this chapter, you should be able to

- describe normal cardiac function related to contractility, blood flow, and neuronal control.

- explain the consequences of congestive heart failure on the cardiovascular system.

- describe the development and progression of coronary artery disease.

Key Terms

angina pectoris: chest pain caused by insufficient blood flow to the heart.

arteriosclerosis: hardening or fibrosis of the arteries.

atherosclerosis: accumulation of fatty deposits in the walls of arteries.

AV: atrioventricular.

CAD: coronary artery disease.

CHF: congestive heart failure.

conduction system: specialized cardiac tissue that regulates the activity of the heart.

electrocardiogram (ECG): recording of the electrical activity of the heart.

myocardial infarction (MI): heart attack.

myocardium: heart muscle.

SA: sinoatrial.

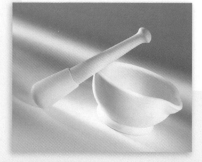

INTRODUCTION

The heart is a muscle whose main function is to generate the force that moves the blood through the circulatory system. Occasionally, efficient cardiac function becomes impaired and results in a life-threatening situation. Fortunately, however, several classes of drugs are therapeutically useful in alleviating many cardiac conditions.

CARDIAC FUNCTION

To understand the action of the different classes of drugs that affect the heart, it is convenient to divide it into three functional parts: cardiac muscle, conduction system, and nerve supply.

Cardiac Muscle

The pumping ability of the heart is due to the arrangement of the heart muscle **(myocardium)** into a system of four chambers. Contraction of the chambers increases pressure within the ventricles and forces the blood through a system of valves and out into general circulation. This is illustrated in Figure 21:1.

The blood supply to the myocardium is routed via the coronary arteries that branch off of the aorta immediately after the aorta leaves the heart. Under normal conditions, blood flow in the coronary arteries is dependent upon the force of myocardial contractions. Any interference with the normal function of the myocardium or with the normal flow of blood to the myocardium results in a decreased capacity of the heart to contract.

Conduction System

The **conduction system** of the heart is composed of a specialized type of muscle tissue that is located in specific areas of the heart. The conduction system is illustrated in Figure 21:2. Conduction tissue has a unique characteristic

FIGURE 21:1 Blood Flow Through the Cardiac Chambers and Valves

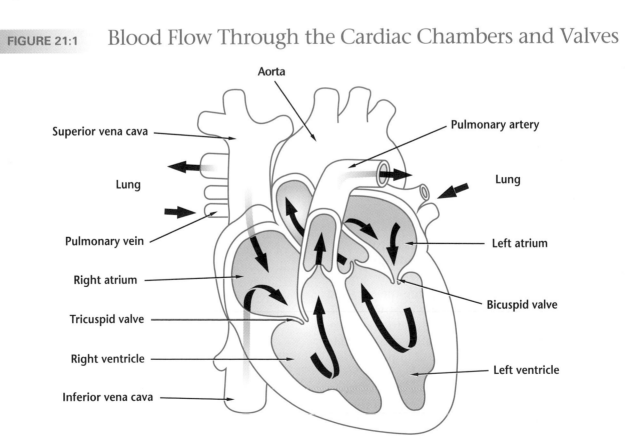

Relationship Between the Cardiac Conduction System and Electrocardiogram

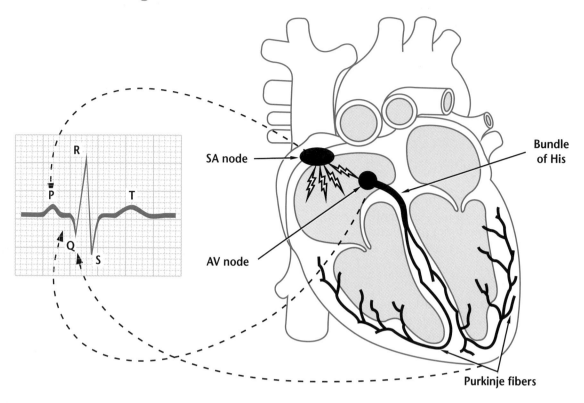

known as *autorhythmicity*. This characteristic enables the heart to initiate its own electrical stimulation. Normally, an electrical impulse is generated within the sinoatrial **(SA)** node. This impulse continues through the atrioventricular **(AV)** node into the common bundle of His, through the left and right bundle branches and Purkinje fibers. This movement results in contraction of the atria followed by contraction of the ventricles. Thus, the conduction system is responsible for coordinating the contractions of the heart chambers.

A recording of the electrical activity of the conduction system results in a characteristic waveform known as the **electrocardiogram (ECG).** The pattern of the ECG reflects depolarization (sodium ions entering the cell) and repolarization (potassium ions leaving the cell) of cardiac tissue. Depolarization of the atria produces the P wave of the ECG. The PR interval is the time required for passage of an electrical impulse from the SA node through the AV node. Depolarization of the ventricles produces the QRS wave (AV node through Purkinje fibers). Repolarization of the ventricles produces the ST segment and the T wave. A normal ECG is shown in Figure 21:2.

Nerve Supply

The heart receives its nerve supply from both divisions of the autonomic nervous system. Since the heart possesses the ability to initiate its own heartbeat, the function of the autonomic nervous system is to regulate the rate and force of contraction of the heart. Sympathetic nerves release norepinephrine at the nerve endings, increasing heart rate (positive chronotropic action) and force of contraction (positive inotropic action). Parasympathetic nerves release acetylcholine at the nerve endings, decreasing heart rate (negative chronotropic action) and force of contraction (negative inotropic action). Each division opposes the other and, depending upon the level of body activity, one division adjusts its activity so that homeostatic conditions are maintained.

MAIN DISEASES OF THE HEART

The two most common diseases affecting the heart are congestive heart failure **(CHF)** and coronary artery disease **(CAD).**

Congestive Heart Failure

In CHF, the contractile ability of the heart to pump blood is decreased so that the heart pumps out less blood than it receives. Blood accumulates inside the chambers, causing enlargement (dilatation) of the heart. Consequently, there is less blood circulating in the blood vessels to supply the body organs. The kidneys—particularly sensitive to a decrease in blood flow—respond by retaining more water and electrolytes, leading to fluid retention and general edema.

When the left side of the heart fails, fluid accumulates in the lungs (pulmonary edema) and interferes with gas exchange, resulting in shortness of breath. When the right side fails, fluid accumulates in the abdominal organs (ascites) and lower extremities. Failure in one side of the heart is usually followed by failure of the other side, resulting in total heart failure. Congestive heart failure is treated with cardiac glycosides, diuretics, and a variety of vasodilator drugs.

Coronary Artery Disease

Coronary artery disease is a general term for several types of cardiac disease. An insufficient flow of blood through the coronary arteries to the heart is a common factor in all these diseases.

Arteriosclerosis

Arteriosclerosis is a disease of the aging process in which there is a hardening (fibrosis) and narrowing of the arteries. These changes result in a decreased blood flow. One type of arteriosclerosis, in which fatty deposits (plaques) accumulate within the walls of the arteries, is known as **atherosclerosis.** The coronary arteries are particularly prone to both conditions and, as stated earlier, any abnormal decrease in coronary blood flow decreases the function of the heart.

Angina Pectoris

Angina pectoris refers to the clinical condition characterized by chest pain caused by insufficient coronary blood flow. Arteriosclerosis, atherosclerosis, and coronary artery spasms appear to be the causes of angina pectoris. Attacks of angina, usually caused by physical exertion or psychological stress, are relieved by rest and a class of drugs known as the vasodilators, or antianginal drugs.

Myocardial Infarction

Heart attack **(myocardial infarction, or MI)** is the leading cause of death in industrialized nations. When an area of the myocardium is deprived of its blood supply (ischemia), the muscle cells die (necrosis), resulting in an area of dead cells known as an infarct. Complete blockage, or thrombosis, of one of the coronary arteries is usually responsible for an MI.

Large infarcts usually result in sudden death, whereas lesser infarcts undergo a healing process in which the dead muscle cells are replaced by connective (scar) tissue. Consequently, after an attack, the amount of contractile tissue of the heart is permanently reduced. Secondary complications commonly involve the development of CHF or disturbances of the conduction system (cardiac arrhythmias). Treatment for a myocardial infarction is aimed at allowing the heart to rest and undergo its normal healing process while treating any complications.

Chapter Review

Understanding Terminology

Answer the following questions in the spaces provided.

1. What is the difference between angina pectoris and myocardial infarction? _____
   _____

2. What do the following abbreviations stand for: AV, CAD, CHF, ECG, SA? _____
   _____
   _____

3. Differentiate between arteriosclerosis and atherosclerosis. _____
   _____

Acquiring Knowledge

Answer the following questions in the spaces provided.

1. Describe the path of blood flow through the cardiac chambers. Which ventricle forces the blood
   into the general circulation (aorta)? _____
   _____

2. How is the blood supplied to the myocardium? _____
   _____
   _____

3. What makes the cardiac conduction system unique? Where is the conduction system located?
   _____
   _____

4. Describe the path of an electrical impulse that is generated at the SA node. _____
   _____

5. Name the characteristic parts of a normal ECG. What can an ECG tell you about cardiac functions?
   _____
   _____

6. What would a lengthened PR interval indicate? What does a widened QRS complex suggest?
   _____
   _____

7. How do the divisions of the autonomic nervous system (ANS) affect cardiac function? _____
   _____
   _____

8. How might congestive heart failure affect the function of the heart? _____
   _____

9. How can coronary heart disease contribute to the development of a myocardial infarction?
   _____
   _____

Applying Knowledge—On the Job

Use your critical thinking skills to answer the questions in the spaces provided.

1. A patient is brought into the emergency room in a collapsed state. She has shortness of breath, low blood pressure, and is making a gurgling sound with each breath.

_____

_____

2. During a scheduled office visit Mrs. Jones explains that after she climbs stairs she has to sit down and rest for a while. One day last week when there was no place to sit she felt some pain and discomfort in her chest.

_____

_____

3. Your grandfather is complaining of extreme weakness and fatigue. You notice that his ankles are swollen and that he can't put his shoes on.

_____

_____

4. Mr. Smith's pulse is irregular and a subsequent ECG reveals that his QRS waves have an abnormal appearance and the T wave is inverted. What part of the heart do you think is affected?

_____

_____

5. The rescue squad brings in a patient who is complaining of a sharp pain radiating down his left arm. He is extremely fatigued, short of breath, and has a very rapid heart rate. The ECG records a serious cardiac arrythmia.

_____

_____

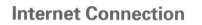

Internet Connection

Contact **MedicineNet** (http://www.medicinenet.com) and find *Heart Attack* (letter *H*) and *Pericarditis* (letter *P*) under the *Disease and Treatment* main heading. Both articles provide extremely useful background information on the causes, symptoms, and treatment options for these common cardiac conditions.

Additional Reading

Caplan, M., and Ranieri, C. 1989. What's his ECG telling you? *RN* Feb:42.

Carelock, J., and Clark, A. 2001. Heart failure: Pathophysiologic mechanisms. *American Journal of Nursing* 101 (12): 26.

Echocardiography: A practical primer. 1996. *Emergency Medicine* 289 (11):83.

Miracle, V., and Sims, J. M. 1996. Normal sinus rhythm. *Nursing* 26 (5):50.

Owen, A. 1995. Tracking the rise and fall of cardiac enzymes. *Nursing* 25 (4):34.

22

CARDIAC GLYCOSIDES AND THE TREATMENT OF CONGESTIVE HEART FAILURE

CHAPTER FOCUS

This chapter describes the pharmacology of the cardiac glycosides that are used to treat congestive heart failure (CHF). It explains how glycosides increase the force of cardiac contractions to relieve the symptoms of heart failure and discusses the roles of diuretic and vasodilator drugs in the management of CHF.

CHAPTER OBJECTIVES

After studying this chapter, you should be able to

- describe the symptoms of CHF.
- list two cardiac glycosides and explain their mechanisms of action.
- differentiate between digitalization and maintenance in relationship to drug administration.
- explain the effects of potassium and calcium on the actions of the glycosides.
- describe five adverse effects caused by glycosides.
- explain the roles of diuretics and vasodilators in the treatment of CHF.

DRUG CLASS AT A GLANCE

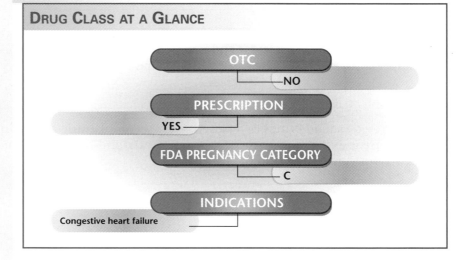

OTC — NO

PRESCRIPTION — YES

FDA PREGNANCY CATEGORY — C

INDICATIONS
Congestive heart failure

Key Terms

adenosine triphosphatase (ATP):   enzyme that energizes the sodium/potassium pump and is inhibited by glycosides.

cardiac glycoside: drug obtained from plants of the genus *Digitalis*.

congestive heart failure (CHF):   condition in which the heart is unable to pump sufficient blood to the tissues of the body.

digitalization: method of dosage with cardiac glycosides that rapidly produces effective drug levels.

ectopic beat: extra heartbeat.

hypercalcemia: high serum calcium.

hyperkalemia: high serum potassium.

hypokalemia: low serum potassium.

maintenance dose: daily dosage of glycoside that maintains effective drug levels in the blood.

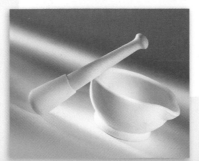

INTRODUCTION

Congestive heart failure (CHF) occurs when the heart is unable to pump sufficient blood to the tissues of the body. Blood accumulates in the heart, lungs, and veins of the lower extremities, which is referred to as congestion. Congestion may cause formation of blood clots in the veins (venous thrombosis), pulmonary edema that interferes with breathing, and cardiac arrhythmias, which can lead to sudden death.

When CHF occurs, the body tries to reverse the effects of heart failure by stimulating compensatory reflexes involving the sympathetic nervous system. Sympathetic reflexes release norepinephrine and epinephrine, which cause vasoconstriction and increase heart rate and force of contractions. These effects are an attempt to increase blood flow and relieve the congestion. Also, the kidneys respond by retaining sodium and water, which increase blood volume and blood pressure. Unfortunately, these compensatory responses do not usually reverse heart failure, and with time, they further weaken the heart. Individuals with CHF usually have the following symptoms: tiredness, fatigue, shortness of breath, rapid heartbeat, and peripheral edema.

Drug therapy involves the use of **cardiac glycosides,** which increase the force of myocardial contractions; diuretics, which eliminate excess sodium and water; and vasodilator drugs, which indirectly increase the amount of blood pumped by the heart (cardiac output).

CARDIAC GLYCOSIDES

The cardiac glycosides are a group of compounds obtained from the plant leaves of *Digitalis purpurea* and *Digitalis lanata*. These compounds, known as glycosides, are similar in chemical and pharmacological properties. Individual glycosides differ mainly in their rates of absorption and durations of action.

Pharmacological Effects

The unique and main pharmacological effect of the glycosides is to increase the force of myocardial contractions in congestive heart failure (CHF) without causing an increase in oxygen consumption. The efficiency of the heart is improved, restoring normal blood circulation. Kidney function increases due to the added blood flow and glomerular filtration rate. This increase results in elimination of the excess fluid and electrolytes associated with edema. The glycosides produce a dramatic relief of the symptoms and hemodynamic disturbances caused by CHF.

The glycosides also decrease heart rate and atrioventricular (AV) conduction. These effects are caused by stimulation of the vagus nerve. In addition, the glycosides have a direct depressant action on the AV node. They produce several characteristic changes in the electrocardiogram (ECG) that can be observed. At therapeutic doses, there is depression of the ST segment and there are changes in the T wave. In addition, there is lengthening of the PR interval, which reflects slower conduction through the AV node. At higher doses, the decreased conduction through the AV node can lead to various degrees of heart block.

Special Considerations

Before administering glycosides, a patient's pulse should be taken to ensure that the heart rate is between 60 and 100 beats per minute. If the rate is below 60 or above 100, the attending physician should be consulted before the drug is given. In addition, the heart rhythm should be normal.

Mechanism of Action

Cardiac glycosides increase the force of myocardial contractions by accelerating the entry of calcium ions inside cardiac muscle cells. First, the glycosides inhibit the enzyme **adenosine triphosphatase (ATP),** which energizes the sodium/potassium pump. Normally, the sodium/potassium pump removes sodium from inside the cell (after depolarization) and brings potassium back into the cell (after repolarization). Inhibition of ATP leads to accumulation of sodium ions inside heart muscle cells. Second, the increase of sodium ions inside heart muscle is believed to stimulate an exchange mechanism whereby cells can get rid of excess sodium ions by exchanging them for calcium ions. Thus, calcium levels increase inside the heart muscle and this increases the formation of actinomyosin, resulting in greater myocardial contraction.

After treatment with the glycosides, a congested heart contracts more forcefully within a shorter period of time. This change increases the amount of blood pumped out of the heart and improves blood circulation, which relieves the congestion of heart failure.

Pharmacokinetics

In acute CHF, the administration of glycosides normally follows a sequence known as digitalization and maintenance. During **digitalization,** glycosides are administered (PO or IV) at doses and intervals that rapidly produce an effective blood level. Subsequent daily **maintenance doses** are lower and adjusted to maintain a therapeutic level of glycoside in the blood.

Digoxin and digitoxin are two of the most widely used preparations. Both can be administered orally or intravenously, depending on the urgency of the situation. Food may delay absorption of the glycosides but usually does not interfere with the extent of absorption. Digoxin is not bound significantly to plasma proteins and is excreted mostly unmetabolized by the urinary tract. The half-life of digoxin is normally 1.5 to 2.0 days, but it may be prolonged in older patients.

Digitoxin is more lipid soluble than is digoxin and requires metabolism by the liver. Digitoxin metabolites are excreted by way of the urinary and gastrointestinal (GI) tracts. The half-life of digitoxin is normally 5 to 7 days.

The cardiac glycosides have a low therapeutic index. When serum levels increase above the therapeutic range, adverse and toxic effects frequently occur. Glycosides also are slowly metabolized and excreted. For these reasons, serum drug levels are routinely performed to measure the amount of drug in patients and adjust the dosage, if necessary. Table 22:1 lists the main glycoside preparations.

Serum Electrolyte Levels and Glycoside Action

Glycosides are affected by changes in the serum electrolytes, particularly potassium and calcium. **Hypokalemia** (low serum potassium) sensitizes the heart to the toxic effects of the glycosides. Decrease in serum potassium may cause an increased incidence of arrhythmias, which can lead to ventricular fibrillation and sudden death. Administration of potassium salts is required to restore normal electrolyte levels during these crises. In contrast, **hyperkalemia** (high serum potassium) antagonizes the therapeutic effects of the glycosides. **Hypercalcemia** (high serum calcium) enhances the action of the glycosides and also can lead to arrhythmias.

Many patients with CHF are also treated with diuretics to reduce the edema associated with this condition. It is important that these patients receive adequate amounts of potassium in their diets to counterbalance the excretion of potassium caused by diuretics. Fruit juices, bananas, and vegetables are good sources of dietary potassium. In addition, there are commercial preparations of potassium supplements such as *K-Lyte* or *Slow-K.*

Adverse and Toxic Effects

The major adverse effects of the glycosides are caused by overdose. Mild symptoms include nausea, vomiting, headache, visual disturbances, and rashes. Dose reduction is usually sufficient to relieve these symptoms. The serious toxic effects involve the development of cardiac arrhythmias. Usually, there is an appearance of extra heartbeats **(ectopic beats).** Most common are premature ventricular contractions (PVCs). An increase in these contractions can lead to ventricular tachycardia, ventricular fibrillation, and cardiac arrest. Treatment involves stopping the glycoside and administering potassium and antiarrhythmic drugs to restore the normal cardiac rhythm.

TABLE 22:1	Commonly Used Cardiac Glycosides		
DRUG (TRADE NAME)	**ROUTE**	**ORAL DOSE FOR MAINTENANCE**	**PEAK EFFECT (HR)**
digitoxin *(Purodigin)*	PO, IV	0.05–0.2 mg	8–12
digoxin *(Lanoxin)*	PO, IV	0.125–0.5 mg	6

In serious cardiac glycoside intoxication, an antidote is available to reduce the severity of toxicity. Digoxin immune fab *(Digibind)* is a preparation of antidigoxin antibodies that is administered parenterally. The antibodies bind up the glycoside drug and make it unavailable for producing its pharmacological effects. The symptoms and severity of toxicity are usually reduced within 30 to 60 minutes. The antibody-glycoside drug complex is eliminated in the urine. The main indication for Digoxin Immune Fab is treatment of life-threatening glycoside intoxication.

Clinical Indications

The main use of cardiac glycosides is the treatment of CHF, to increase the force of contractions. These drugs are also used in some cases of atrial fibrillation and atrial tachycardia. The effect of the glycosides in slowing conduction through the AV node results in fewer electrical impulses reaching the ventricles. Consequently, the ventricular rate decreases toward a normal rhythm.

Drug Interactions

Antacids, laxatives, kaolinpectin *(Kaopectate)*, and cholestyramine *(Questran)* can decrease the absorption of glycosides from the GI tract. The antiarrythmic drug, quinidine, increases glycoside plasma levels. Reduction in glycoside dosage is usually required when these two drugs are used together. The calcium channel blockers, verapamil and diltiazem, and any of the beta-blockers decrease heart rate and force of contraction. These drugs may depress cardiac function and precipitate CHF; this can counteract the therapeutic effectiveness of the glycosides. Diuretics (thiazides and organic acids) and cardiac glycosides cause loss of potassium. When these drugs are used together they may cause hypokalemia and increased glycoside toxicity.

DIURETIC THERAPY OF CHF

The pharmacology of the diuretics is presented in Chapter 25. The main effect produced by diuretics is the elimination of excess sodium and water by the urinary tract. Sodium and water retention is the main cause of excess blood volume and edema, which contribute to the congestion and circulatory disturbances of CHF. Diuretics are used alone or in combination with cardiac glycosides in the treatment of this condition to rapidly decrease excess blood volume and congestion, allowing the heart to function more efficiently. Thiazide diuretics, which give a mild to moderate diuretic effect, are frequently used. The organic acids, such as furosemide *(Lasix)*, are indicated when a more potent diuretic effect is required. In acute CHF, the organic acids are administered parenterally for rapid relief of edema and pulmonary congestion.

Vasodilator Therapy of CHF

The main effect of vasodilator drugs is to relax or dilate blood vessels—both arteries and veins. Vasodilation lowers peripheral resistance and blood pressure. These changes decrease cardiac work and oxygen consumption. The heart is able to pump more blood (increased cardiac output)

Patient Administration and Monitoring

Monitor vital signs during administration of cardiac glycosides, especially during digitalization and parenteral administration. Pay particular attention to heart rate.

Monitor the ECG for cardiac arrythmias and signs of digitalis toxicity such as excessive ST segment and T wave depression or heart block.

Always measure the pulse rate before administering the cardiac glycosides. The physician should be notified when heart rate is below 60 beats per minute.

Instruct patient on the importance of adequate potassium intake and that fruit juices, bananas, and vegetables are good sources.

Explain to patient that common over-the-counter drugs such as antacids and laxatives may reduce drug absorption.

Explain to patient the common side effects: nausea, headache, dizziness, and visual disturbances.

Instruct patient to report excessive vomiting, visual disturbances (halo effect around lights), irregular pulse rates, or heart palpitations.

with less effort. Drugs that primarily dilate arteries or arterioles have a greater effect to lower blood pressure. This effect is referred to as "decreasing the afterload" of the heart, which, simply stated, means that the heart doesn't have to work as hard to pump blood after the blood pressure has been lowered. Drugs that primarily dilate veins (venodilators) mainly decrease venous return of blood back to the heart. This is referred to as "decreasing the preload," and also reduces cardiac work. A few drugs dilate both arteries and veins and produce a "balanced" vasodilation that decreases both pre- and afterload.

Vasodilator therapy of CHF has been shown to be very beneficial, especially with the drug class known as the angiotensin-converting enzyme inhibitors (see Chapter 26). These drugs have become the preferred agents for the treatment of CHF. There is less risk of toxicity with vasodilators than with cardiac glycosides. Vasodilator drugs are used alone and in combination with diuretics and cardiac glycosides. The therapeutic actions of some of the vasodilator drugs are summarized in Table 22:2. More detailed pharmacology of the vasodilators can be found in Chapters 24 and 26.

TABLE 22:2	Vasodilator Drugs Used in Congestive Heart Failure		
VASODILATOR	**MAIN EFFECT**		**EFFECT ON HEART**
Angiotensin-converting enzyme inhibitors captopril (*Capoten*) enalopril (*Vasotec*) linsinopril (*Prinvil, Zestril*)	Decreases formation of angiotensin (potent vasoconstrictor formed in the blood) and produces dilation of arteriolar and venous vessels		Increased cardiac output
hydralazine (*Apresoline*)	Dilates arteriolar more than venous vessels		Increased cardiac output
nitroglycerin	Dilates venous more than arteriolar vessels		Decreased venous return and work of the heart
prazosin (*Minipress*)	Dilates arteriolar and venous vessels		Increased cardiac output
sodium nitroprusside (*Nipride*)	Dilates arteriolar and venous vessels		Increased cardiac output

Chapter Review

Understanding Terminology

Answer the following questions in the spaces provided.

1. Define *CHF.* _____
   _____
   _____

2. What are ectopic beats? _____
   _____

3. Differentiate between hyperkalemia and hypokalemia. _____
   _____
   _____

Acquiring Knowledge

Answer the following questions in the spaces provided.

1. What is the main action of cardiac glycosides on the myocardium? _____
   _____
   _____

2. Explain the effect of digitalis on heart rate. _____
   _____
   _____

3. Explain the clinical importance of digitalization and tell how digitalization differs from
   maintenance. _____
   _____

4. What are the more serious adverse effects of digitalis? Discuss the factors that increase their
   development.
   _____
   _____

5. What precautions should be observed prior to administration of the cardiac glycosides?
   _____
   _____

6. How do the cardiac glycosides differ from each other? _____
   _____
   _____

7. What changes can be observed in an ECG at therapeutic doses? At toxic doses? _____
   _____
   _____

8. What role do diuretics play in the treatment of congestive heart failure? _____
   _____
   _____

9. Explain why vasodilator drugs are beneficial in the treatment of congestive heart failure.
   _____
   _____

Applying Knowledge—On the Job

Use your critical thinking skills to answer the following questions in the spaces provided.

1. Mrs. McNally is a 65-year-old female who presents at the clinic where you're working with complaints of increased shortness of breath and swelling of her feet. Her past medical history includes a diagnosis of hypertension and moderate degree of renal failure. Pertinent laboratory tests show a slightly decreased potassium level of 3.2 M/l (normal 3.5–5 M/l) and an increased serum creatinine of 2.1 mg/dl (normal 0.8–1.5 mg/dl). The physician's diagnosis is acute congestive heart failure. The physician's course of therapy includes doubling Mrs. McNally's dose of hydrochlorothiazide from 25 mg to 50 mg daily and prescribing digoxin 0.25 mg twice daily for 2 days and then 0.25 mg daily.

   a. What is the most likely electrolyte disturbance that may occur in this patient?

   _____

   _____

   b. What are the terms used to describe the administration of the diuretic twice daily for 2 days then once daily thereafter?

   _____

   _____

   c. What does the increased level of serum creatinine suggest about this patient's renal function?

   _____

   _____

2. Outline the steps to be taken in severe cardiac glycoside intoxication. _____

   _____

   _____

3. Explain the rationale behind the use of digoxin in the treatment of atrial fibrillation.

   _____

   _____

Internet Connection

Contact **MedicineNet** (http://www.medicinenet.com) and click on the *Diseases and Treatment* heading. Click the letter *C* and find *Congestive Heart Failure*. This website provides background information on the causes, symptoms and treatment for CHF and also lists additional articles related to CHF.

Additional Reading

Blumenfeld, J. D., and Laragh, J. H. 1997. Diagnosis and management of heart failure. *Hospital Medicine* 33 (3):36.

Fowler, J. P. 1995. When CHF turns deadly. *Nursing* 25 (2):54.

Weeks, S. M. 1996. Caring for patients with heart failure. *Nursing* 26 (3):52.

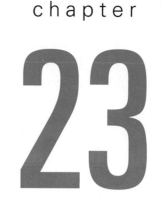

chapter

23

ANTIARRHYTHMIC DRUGS

DRUG CLASS AT A GLANCE

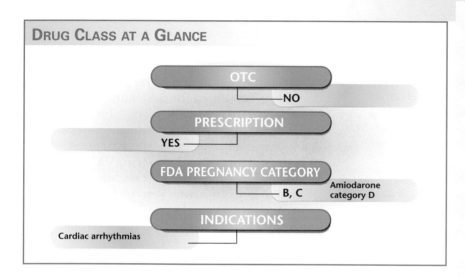

OTC
— NO

PRESCRIPTION
YES —

FDA PREGNANCY CATEGORY
— B, C   Amiodarone category D

INDICATIONS
Cardiac arrhythmias

CHAPTER FOCUS

This chapter describes cardiac arrhythmias and the drugs used to treat these disorders of cardiac conduction. It describes the four major classes of antiarrhythmic drugs and discusses adverse effects produced by these drugs.

CHAPTER OBJECTIVES

After studying this chapter, you should be able to

- describe four commonly occurring arrhythmias.

- discuss the phases of the normal cardiac cycle and the importance of certain ions to cardiac function.

- list four different classes of antiarrhythmic drugs and their mechanisms of action.

- describe three common adverse effects associated with each antiarrhythmic drug class.

Key Terms

antiarrhythmic drug: drug used to restore normal cardiac rhythm.

arrhythmia: disorder of cardiac conduction.

cinchonism: quinidine toxicity, which is characterized by ringing in the ears (tinnitus), dizziness, and headache.

ectopic focus: area of the heart from which abnormal impulses originate.

hyperglycemia: elevated blood glucose level.

nystagmus: involuntary movement of the eyes.

premature atrial contraction: premature contraction of the atria, usually caused by an ectopic focus.

premature ventricular contraction (PVC): premature contraction of the ventricles, usually caused by an ectopic focus.

supraventricular arrhythmia: arrhythmia that originates in the atrial or atrioventricular (AV) nodal area.

ventricular fibrillation: the most serious arrhythmia; can result in cardiac arrest and death.

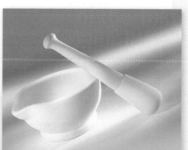

INTRODUCTION

Disorders in cardiac rhythm, referred to as **arrhythmias,** are one of the most commonly occurring pathophysiological conditions. Arrhythmias may develop in a diseased heart (as a result of congestive heart failure, coronary artery disease, or myocardial infarction) or as a consequence of chronic drug therapy. The symptoms of a rhythm disorder may range from mild palpitations to cardiac arrest. The severity of the symptoms determines the overall effect on cardiac function and blood pressure. The clinical management of an abnormal cardiac rhythm involves a group of pharmacological agents that attempt to convert the existing arrhythmia to a normal rhythm.

TYPES OF ARRHYTHMIAS

The atria and the ventricles of the heart develop a variety of arrhythmias when the normal electrical impulse is impaired. Arrhythmias associated with the atria and the ventricles include premature contractions, tachycardia, flutter, and fibrillation. These are illustrated in Table 23:1.

Arrhythmias that originate in the atria and atrioventricular (AV) nodal areas are referred to as **supraventricular arrhythmias** (above the ventricles). Arrhythmias that originate below the

AV node are referred to as ventricular arrhythmias. **Ectopic foci,** areas of abnormal impulse generation, may appear when electrical impulses traveling through the conduction system are delayed or blocked. In this situation, another area of the heart (atria or ventricle) may become excitable and produce an abnormal heartbeat. Ectopic foci that originate in the atria are referred to as **premature atrial contractions** (PACs). Ectopic foci that originate in the ventricles are referred to as **premature ventricular contractions** (PVCs). Figure 23:1 shows the appearance of a PVC produced by an ectopic focus.

TABLE 23:1	Commonly Occurring Arrhythmias and Their ECG Patterns

ARRHYTHMIA	CHARACTERISTIC RATE (BEATS/MINUTE)	ECG
Tachycardia (atrial or ventricular)	150–250	
Atrial flutter	200–350	
Atrial fibrillation	Greater than 350	
Ventricular fibrillation	Uncoordinated contractions	
Premature contraction of the atria	Variable	
Premature contractions of the ventricles	Variable	
Bradycardia	Less than 60	

FIGURE 23:1 Correlation of a Ventricular Ectopic Focus (Premature Ventricular Contraction, PVC) With the ECG

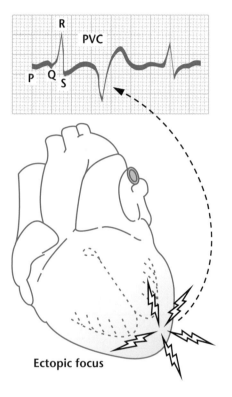

Ectopic focus

The most serious arrhythmia is **ventricular fibrillation,** which constitutes a medical emergency. During fibrillation, the electrical activity of the ventricles is severely disturbed and the ventricles cannot contract efficiently enough to maintain adequate circulation. If not treated immediately, cardiac arrest and death will result.

ECG Monitoring of Arrhythmias

The characteristic pattern of an electrocardiogram (ECG) was reviewed in Chapter 21. Electrocardiograms are extremely valuable for determining abnormalities in cardiac rhythm and conduction. Heart rate can be determined by counting the number of QRS waves that occur in a 1-minute period. In addition, the width of the individual waves indicates malfunctions in the atrial or ventricular conduction systems. Changes in the normal sequence of PQRST . . . PQRST . . . of the ECG pattern indicate abnormalities in normal cardiac conduction. Table 23:1 shows how various arrhythmias appear on ECGs.

FIGURE 23:2 Phases of the Cardiac Action Potential of Ventricular Muscle

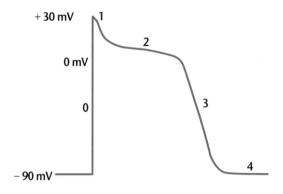

Electrophysiology of the Heart

One of the most important aspects of the heart is the function of several ions that regulate the electrophysiological properties of the heart. The ions are sodium (Na^+), potassium (K^+), and calcium (Ca^{2+}). Each ion has a specific role in the development of the various phases (0 through 4) of the cardiac action potential, shown in Figure 23:2, that leads to contraction of heart muscle. The properties of the heart are listed in Table 23:2 on page 248 and are correlated with the phases of the cardiac action potential and the movement of ions.

When some part of the heart develops an arrhythmia, the properties of the heart and the movement of the ions are disturbed. The therapeutic effects of antiarrhythmic drugs rest in their ability to affect the electrophysiological properties of the cardiac membrane and the movement of ions so that the properties of the heart are restored to normal or are at least improved. When this occurs, the rhythm of the heart (reflected by the ECG) improves, and most important, the ability of the heart to pump blood is restored.

Antiarrhythmic drugs do not cure the underlying causes of an arrhythmia. These agents attempt to restore the normal cardiac rhythm. Some antiarrhythmic agents are useful in several different cardiac disorders, whereas others have a limited clinical use. Successful conversion of an arrhythmia depends on the type of arrhythmia present and the particular drug employed. Currently, the antiarrhythmic drugs are grouped into four classes based on their effects. Table 23:3 summarizes the most commonly used antiarrhythmic drugs and their main uses.

TABLE 23:2 — Correlation of Electrophysiological Properties of the Heart With the Phases of the Cardiac Action Potential and the Movement of Ions

PROPERTY	PHASE	IONIC MOVEMENT
Excitability	0	Na^+ rapidly moves to the inside of the cell, causing reversal of the membrane potential (-90 mV to $+30$ mV)
Refractory period (RP)	1–3	K^+ moves to the outside of the cell, bringing the membrane potential back to its resting level (-90 mV)
Plateau phase	2	Ca^{2+} moves to the inside of the cell and is involved in regulating the force of muscle contraction
Automaticity	4	A latent property of ventricular muscle; in pacemaker cells (SA and AV nodes), there is a slow inward movement of Na^+ and Ca^{2+} and an outward movement of K^+, which "automatically" excites the membrane and begins another membrane depolarization (phase 0)

TABLE 23:3 — Antiarrhythmic Drugs and Their Uses

DRUG (TRADE NAME)	ARRHYTHMIAS TREATED	AVERAGE DOSE
quinidine (*Cardioquin, Quinaglute, Quinidex*)	Supraventricular tachyarrhythmias, ventricular arrhythmias	200–400 mg BID, TID PO
procainamide (*Procanbid*)	Supraventricular tachyarrhythmias, ventricular arrhythmias	250–500 mg QID PO
disopyramide (*Norpace*)	Supraventricular tachyarrhythmias, ventricular arrhythmias	100–200 mg TID, QID PO
lidocaine (*Xylocaine*)	Ventricular arrhythmias	1–2 mg/kg bolus IV, 1–4 mg/min infusion
propranolol (*Inderal*)	Supraventricular and ventricular tachyarrhythmias	40–80 mg TID, QID PO 1.0–3.0 mg twice at 2-min intervals if necessary in any 4-hr period
verapamil (*Calan, Isoptin*)	Supraventricular tachyarrhythmias	80–120 mg TID, QID PO 5–10 mg IV

CLASS 1 ANTIARRHYTHMIC DRUGS

One of the common features of the Class 1 antiarrhythmic drugs is that they possess local anesthetic activity (see Chapter 10). Like local anesthetics, the Class 1 drugs interfere with the movement of sodium ions during excitation and depolarization of nerves, cardiac membranes, and other excitable tissues. Consequently, the excitability of the heart is reduced, particularly any area of the heart that is hyperexcitable and arrhythmogenic (giving rise to arrhythmias). In addition, Class 1 drugs slow conduction velocity, prolong the refractory period, and decrease automaticity of the heart, actions that also contribute to the antiarrhythmic effect.

Quinidine

Chemically related to quinine, quinidine is a natural product obtained from the bark of the cinchona tree. The use of quinidine for cardiac disorders dates back to the eighteenth century, when patients suffering from malaria were treated with extracts of the cinchona bark. The presence of quinidine in these concoctions resulted in improvement in patients in which malaria and atrial flutter occurred simultaneously. Quinidine is used in the treatment of supraventricular arrhythmias, such as atrial flutter and fibrillation, and in various ventricular arrhythmias.

Pharmacologic Effects

Quinidine is a general cardiac depressant because it depresses both the myocardium and the conduction system. Depression of the myocardium decreases the contractile force of the heart. This effect usually occurs at higher dosages. Depression of the conduction system is the desired effect. This action reduces cardiac excitability and slows conduction of electrical impulses through the heart. By these actions, quinidine suppresses the activity of ectopic foci and other abnormal disturbances of conduction associated with cardiac arrhythmias.

The overall effect of quinidine is to slow the heart rate. However, quinidine initially exerts an anticholinergic effect (vagolytic) on the sinoatrial (SA) node. This vagolytic action may result in an initial tachycardia, which may temporarily worsen an existing arrhythmia. However, the overall effect of quinidine at therapeutic concentrations is to decrease heart rate.

Pharmacokinetics

Quinidine is well absorbed from the gastrointestinal (GI) tract after oral administration. Quinidine is metabolized to several active metabolites; excretion is primarily by way of the urinary tract. Occasionally, high levels of quinidine buildup in the blood, causing side effects and toxicities. Patients with renal or liver disease, in particular, may experience increased adverse effects to quinidine because these organs are not functioning properly to metabolize and eliminate quinidine and its active metabolites from the blood.

The factors that make quinidine a valuable drug also make it a cardiac poison when large amounts of quinidine are present in the blood. At high doses, quinidine will depress all cardiac function, leading to the development of arrhythmias, congestive heart failure (CHF), and possible cardiac arrest.

Adverse Effects

The most common noncardiac side effects include nausea, vomiting, and diarrhea due to irritation of

ECG Indications of the Toxic Effects of Quinidine

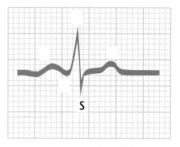

Normal ECG

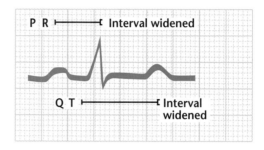

the GI tract. **Cinchonism** is an adverse syndrome produced by quinidine in overdosage or in patients who are sensitive to the drug. This condition is characterized by ringing in the ears (tinnitus), dizziness, salivation, headache, and hallucinations.

Quinidine also depresses smooth and skeletal muscle function. Depression of arteriolar smooth muscle may cause hypotension. Depression of skeletal muscle results in weakness and fatigue, which may interfere with respiration (dyspnea).

Evidence of quinidine's cardiotoxicity can be seen with ECGs. In particular, the PR, QRS, and T intervals widen as a result of decreased conduction through the atrioventricular (AV) node and ventricles as shown in Figure 23:3. These changes may result in premature contractions of the atria or the ventricles. Toxic levels may suppress pacemaker activity and produce cardiac arrest.

Less frequently there may be hypersensitivity reactions involving the development of hepatitis and thrombocytopenia. The latter condition can lead to bleeding problems.

Drug Interactions

Hyperkalemia (high plasma potassium levels) or excessive potassium supplementation can increase quinidine toxicity. In large amounts, potassium itself is a cardiac depressant. Therefore, the combination of excessive potassium and quinidine may cause cardiac depression and various arrhythmias.

Quinidine is contraindicated in patients who have AV block, especially when the nodal blockade is due to digitalis toxicity. In these situations, quinidine will only worsen the AV block, resulting in the development of heart block and ventricular arrhythmias. In addition, quinidine increases digitalis plasma concentrations when these drugs are used together. Consequently, the dosage of digitalis must be lowered in these situations.

Quinidine also inhibits the metabolism of some other drugs, particularly the beta-blockers like propranolol. Dosage adjustments are usually required when these drugs are used together.

Procainamide *(Procanbid)*

A synthetic drug related to procaine (a local anesthetic), procainamide produces the same pharmacological actions as quinidine when used as an antiarrhythmic drug. Although the oral route is most widely used, procainamide may also be administered intravenously. Procainamide has a short half-life and is administered in extended-release tablets (*Procanbid*) that allow a 12-hour dosing interval. The drug forms an active metabolite, N-acetylprocainamide (NAPA), that also contributes to the therapeutic effect.

> ### NOTE TO THE HEALTH CARE PROFESSIONAL
>
> When combined with procainamide or quinidine for the treatment of arrhythmias, lidocaine may produce SA nodal arrest.

Adverse Effects

Procainamide produces relatively few side effects at therapeutic doses; however, nausea, vomiting, anorexia, and skin rashes may occur. Following chronic use of procainamide, some patients develop a red butterfly rash and arthralgia similar to the symptoms seen in lupus erythematosus. Procainamide is also capable of producing changes in ECGs similar to those produced by quinidine. Usually, widening of the PR, QRS, and QT waves occurs, along with the appearance of premature beats. At higher doses procainamide is also a cardiac depressant. A less frequent adverse reaction is agranulocytosis (decrease in granulocyte blood cells), which can increase the incidence of infection.

Disopyramide *(Norpace)*

The actions of disopyramide (*Norpace*) on the heart are similar to those of quinidine and procainamide. Disopyramide produces a decrease in excitability and prolongation of the refractory period. This drug is useful in treating both atrial and ventricular arrhythmias. In addition, disopyramide produces anticholinergic effects that account for the common side effects such as dry mouth, visual disturbances, constipation, and urinary retention. Disopyramide is a general cardiac depressant. At higher doses or with the development of toxicity, it may produce a quinidine-like depression of the heart and CHF in patients with a predisposition to congestive heart failure.

Lidocaine (*Xylocaine*)

A synthetic drug used primarily as a local anesthetic agent, lidocaine (*Xylocaine*) is widely used for ventricular arrhythmias, especially those resulting from a myocardial infarction or arrhythmias occurring during surgery. As a rule, lidocaine is ineffective in atrial arrhythmias and is therefore not recommended for use in these conditions. Although lidocaine suppresses ectopic foci associated with ventricular arrhythmias, it does not depress normal impulse conduction. The main effect of lidocaine, prevention of ventricular arrhythmias, is attributed to its ability to depress automaticity (Phase 4).

Pharmacokinetics

The major disadvantage of lidocaine is that it must be administered parenterally (IV or IM). Since a single administration results in a very short antiarrhythmic response, lidocaine is usually given as an intravenous infusion to maintain the antiarrhythmic action. Usually, a bolus injection of lidocaine (50 to 100 mg) is initially administered over a 2-minute period, followed by continuous infusion at a rate of 1 to 4 mg per minute.

Adverse Effects

Since lidocaine is rapidly metabolized in the liver, impaired liver function will result in elevated blood levels of lidocaine. At higher concentrations, lidocaine produces stimulation of the central nervous system (CNS), which may result in convulsions. Toxic blood levels of lidocaine usually produce CNS depression (anesthetic effect), and possible cardiac and respiratory arrest.

Mexiletine (*Mexitil*) and Tocainide (*Tonocard*)

These are two derivatives of lidocaine that have been structurally modified so that they can be administered orally. They produce cardiac effects similar to lidocaine and are used for treatment of outpatient ventricular arrhythmias.

Phenytoin (*Dilantin*)

Phenytoin finds its greatest use as an antiepileptic drug. However, its ability to alter neural function also permits phenytoin to act as an antiarrhythmic. Phenytoin is recommended for ventricular arrhythmias, especially those induced by digitalis, such as AV block, where phenytoin appears to increase AV conduction and may eliminate the AV block. Both oral and parenteral (IV) uses of phenytoin are possible. Phenytoin is slowly absorbed from the GI tract, metabolized by the liver, and excreted into the urine.

The most common adverse effects include blurred vision, vertigo, and **nystagmus** (involuntary movement of the eyes). Administration of large doses of phenytoin may result in elevated blood glucose levels **(hyperglycemia),** especially in diabetics and patients with renal insufficiency. The hallmark of chronic phenytoin use is gingival hyperplasia, which may be reduced by good oral hygiene and dental care.

Other Class 1 Antiarrhythmic Drugs

Flecainide (*Tambocor*), moricizine (*Ethmozine*), and propafenone (*Rythmol*) are newer drugs that are usually reserved for treatment of arrhythmias that are unresponsive to other antiarrhythmic drugs. The most effective use of these drugs is still undergoing clinical evaluation.

CLASS 2 ANTIARRHYTHMIC DRUGS

The beta-adrenergic blockers are classified as Class 2 antiarrhythmic drugs. Frequently, in heart disease, there is increased sympathetic activity with increased release of norepinephrine and epinephrine. These agents increase heart rate, excitability, conduction velocity, and automaticity, particularly of ventricular muscle. In addition, they shorten the refractory period, all of which can contribute to the development of various arrhythmias.

By antagonizing the effects of norepinephrine and epinephrine at the beta-1 receptors, beta-blockers decrease excitability, conduction velocity, and automatism and prolong the refractory period. Often, these effects eliminate arrhythmias in patients with increased sympathetic activity. The beta-blockers were previously discussed in Chapter 6.

Propranolol (*Inderal*)

Propranolol is the beta-blocker most widely used as an antiarrhythmic drug. In addition to its beta-blocking effect, propranolol produces a quinidine-like depression of cardiac membranes at higher doses. Both supraventricular and ventricular arrhythmias can be treated with propranolol. In addition, propranolol can be used in combination with Class 1 antiarrhythmics when control is not achieved with one drug alone.

The main cardiac effects of propranolol are a slowing of heart rate, a decrease in AV conduction, and a prolongation of the refractory period. Propranolol can be administered orally and intravenously in emergency situations.

The most common cardiovascular adverse effects are hypotension and bradycardia. In overdosage, propranolol, and other beta-blockers, may cause congestive heart failure and possible cardiac arrest. Skin rashes, mental confusion, and visual disturbances may also occur.

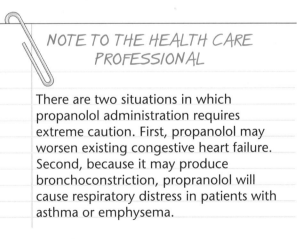

NOTE TO THE HEALTH CARE PROFESSIONAL

There are two situations in which propanolol administration requires extreme caution. First, propanolol may worsen existing congestive heart failure. Second, because it may produce bronchoconstriction, propranolol will cause respiratory distress in patients with asthma or emphysema.

Esmolol (*Brevibloc*)

Esmolol is a selective beta-blocker that mainly affects beta-1 receptors in the heart. It is administered by intravenous infusion in emergency situations when rapid beta-blockade is desired to lower heart rate. The duration of action is very short, only a few minutes, because of rapid metabolism by esterase enzymes in the blood and liver. Excessive bradycardia, delayed AV conduction, and hypotension are adverse effects associated with overdosage.

CLASS 3 ANTIARRHYTHMIC DRUGS

The main antiarrhythmic action of the Class 3 drugs is to interfere with the efflux of potassium ions (K^+) during repolarization phases 1 through 3. This action prolongs the refractory period of the heart and decreases the frequency of arrhythmias.

Bretylium (*Bretylol*)

Bretylium is an adrenergic neuronal blocker (see Chapter 6) that decreases the release of norepinephrine from adrenergic nerve endings. In addition, bretylium prolongs the refractory period of the ventricles. This action is useful in the treatment of resistant ventricular tachycardia and ventricular fibrillation, which are the main indications for the use of bretylium. Administration can be oral; however, because of poor GI absorption, the parenteral route (IM or IV) is preferred. Adverse effects include minor GI disturbances such as nausea and diarrhea, and hypotension.

Amiodarone (*Cordarone*)

Amiodarone is a very potent antiarrhythmic drug that is used mainly when other drugs are not effective. Amiodarone has some local anesthetic activity and, in addition, blocks a number of pharmacological receptors (alpha, beta, calcium). The major antiarrhythmic effect is prolongation of the refractory period. Amiodarone contains iodine and can interfere with thyroid function. The drug has a very long half-life, up to 60 days, and dosage must be carefully regulated. Amiodarone can be administered orally or by intravenous injection.

Adverse Effects

Adverse effects can be serious and include corneal deposits and visual disturbances, dermatitis and skin discoloration, pulmonary fibrosis, and liver dysfunction. Amiodarone is designated Food and Drug Administration (FDA) Pregnancy Category D and should not be used in pregnancy or in nursing mothers.

Sotalol (*Betapace*)

Sotalol is a nonselective beta-blocker that also has Class 3 antiarrhythmic activity. The main effects are prolongation of the refractory period, slowed AV conduction, and decreased automaticity of the heart. Adverse effects are similar to those of other beta-blockers.

CLASS 4 ANTIARRHYTHMIC DRUGS

The Class 4 antiarrhythmic drugs are referred to as the calcium antagonists or calcium channel blockers. These drugs decrease the entry of calcium into cells that have electrophysiological properties, or cells with excitable membranes that develop action potentials. Such cells include those of the heart and blood vessels.

By interfering with calcium, the calcium antagonists produce two major effects on the heart. The first important effect is on the pacemaker cells of the heart (SA and AV nodes). In pacemaker cells, calcium is required for normal activity and heart rate. By interfering with calcium, the calcium antagonists decrease the rate of the SA node (decreased heart rate) and the conduction velocity of the AV node (decreased AV conduction). These effects are particularly useful in treating various types of fast supraventricular tachycardias, often referred to as tachyarrhythmias.

The second major effect of the calcium antagonists is on muscle, both cardiac and smooth muscle. As indicated in Table 23:2, entry of calcium during Phase 2 of the action potential is important for regulating the force of myocardial contractions. Interference with calcium entry into cardiac muscle decreases the ability of the heart to develop forceful contractions and may potentially lead to congestive heart failure. This result is not a desired therapeutic effect. However, the same action occurs in vascular smooth muscle, and here the calcium-blocking effect causes relaxation of smooth muscle and vasodilation. This effect is useful in the treatment of angina pectoris and in the treatment of hypertension. Two of the calcium antagonists, verapamil (*Calan, Isoptin*) and diltiazem (*Cardizem*), are used for their antiarrhythmic actions.

Verapamil (*Calan*)

The major effect of verapamil is on the pacemaker cells of the heart. Verapamil decreases SA node activity, resulting in a slight decrease in heart rate. More important, verapamil decreases AV node conduction. This effect makes it very useful in treating various types of AV nodal arrhythmias and other supraventricular tachycardias. Verapamil is

Patient Administration and Monitoring

Monitor vital signs and ECG recordings frequently during parenteral administration and in newly admitted hospital patients who are still stabilizing and adjusting to therapy.

Explain to patient the common side effects of prescribed drugs:

Quinidine and procainamide—GI disturbances, headache, dizziness

Disopyramide—dry mouth, other anticholinergic effects

Phenytoin—blurred vision, vertigo

Propranolol—tiredness, fatigue, GI disturbances, sedation

Verapamil—headache, dizziness, constipation

Instruct patient to report significant changes or adverse effects, especially related to pulse rate, blood pressure, or breathing; with quinidine the signs of cinchonism; with procainamide the development of rash, arthralgia, or infection; with propranolol extreme weakness, slow pulse, or breathing difficulties.

administered PO (40 to 120 mg TID) and IV (5 to 10 mg) in emergency situations. Verapamil also produces vasodilation and is used in the treatment of angina pectoris (see Chapter 24).

Common adverse effects of verapamil include headache, dizziness, and minor GI disturbances, especially constipation. The vasodilating effect can produce hypotension, especially when patients change position. More serious complications include cardiac depression leading to CHF and various degrees of heart block, especially if verapamil is taken with other cardiac depressant drugs. Verapamil is usually contraindicated in patients with existing SA and AV node disturbances or with CHF.

Diltiazem (*Cardizem*)

Diltiazem is less potent than verapamil as an antiarrhythmic drug but more potent than

verapamil as a vasodilator. The main use of diltiazem is as an antihypertensive drug (see Chapter 26).

OTHER ANTIARRHYTHMIC DRUGS

Adenosine (*Adenocard*)

Adenosine is an antiarrhythmic drug that is only used in emergency and acute situations. Adenosine is the naturally occurring metabolite of adenosine triphosphate (ATP). The drug is administered intravenously to terminate episodes of supraventricular tachycardia. The main effect of adenosine is to decrease AV conduction and, to a lesser extent, SA pacemaker activity. This action slows the rate of the ventricles in cases of acute tachycardia. The duration of action of adenosine is extremely short, 15 to 30 seconds. Adverse effects are brief, but include asystole, dyspnea, and occasionally bronchospasm.

SPECIAL CONSIDERATIONS

The control of arrhythmias can be a difficult task and patients are often in a precarious situation. Sudden changes in ECGs and the development of life-threatening arrhythmias, like ventricular fibrillation, are always a possibility. In the hospital, ECGs constantly monitor heart patients. It is important to be aware of ECG monitors, to check them frequently, and to be alert for sudden changes in the appearance of ECGs or the condition of patients.

Antiarrhythmic drugs are frequently administered in the hospital by IV infusion. Dosages (drips per minute) are carefully adjusted to deliver the proper amount of drug. Other medications frequently are administered through the same IV line; and procedures, like measuring the central venous pressure (CVP), require turning off or adjusting the infusion. It is extremely important that when these other procedures are completed the infusion rate of the antiarrhythmic drug is adjusted back to its proper rate of delivery. Failure to do this can result in serious consequences for patients.

It is important to be aware of the adverse effects of the various antiarrhythmic drugs and to be alert for their appearance. Many of the antiarrhythmic drugs are cardiac depressants and can produce CHF or any variety of cardiac arrhythmias themselves.

Chapter Review

Understanding Terminology

Match the definition or description in the left column with the appropriate term in the right column.

_____ **1.** High level of glucose in the blood.

_____ **2.** A drug used to restore normal cardiac rhythm.

_____ **3.** Involuntary movement of the eyes.

_____ **4.** Premature ventricular contraction.

_____ **5.** The most serious type of arrhythmia.

_____ **6.** Arrhythmia that originates in the atrial or AV nodal area.

_____ **7.** A disorder of cardiac conduction.

a. antiarrhythmic

b. arrhythmia

c. hyperglycemia

d. nystagmus

e. PVC

f. supraventricular arrhythmia

g. ventricular fibrillation

Acquiring Knowledge

Answer the following questions in the spaces provided.

1. When would the use of an antiarrhythmic drug be indicated? _____

_____

2. For what arrhythmias are quinidine and lidocaine used? _____

_____

3. How does quinidine produce a cardiotoxic effect? How does this affect ECGs? _____

_____

4. What pharmacological effect do the Class 1 antiarrhythmic drugs have in common? _____

_____

5. What is cinchonism? _____

_____

6. Describe the procedure for the administration of lidocaine. _____

_____

7. Explain the difference between the mechanism of action of propranolol and that for bretylium.

_____

8. What is the main indication for the use of bretylium? For adenosine? _____

_____

9. Explain two important effects of verapamil on the cardiovascular system. _____

_____

10. What are the adverse effects of each of the classes of antiarrhythmic drugs? _____
_____
_____

Applying Knowledge—On the Job

Use your critical thinking skills to answer the following questions in the spaces provided.

1. Mr. Wise is a 75-year-old, otherwise healthy male who was admitted to the hospital for a total right knee replacement. On postoperative day 2, a ventricular arrhythmia was diagnosed. The cardiologist was consulted and prescribed *Norpace* 150 mg QID. On the fourth day postoperatively, Mr. Wise complains he cannot urinate and is ordered by the house physician to be catheterized. The house physician asks what medications the patient is on. What do you think the physician is thinking about the cause of the urinary difficulties?

_____
_____

2. Mrs. Jones has been taking digoxin for many years. Recently she developed an arrythmia and her cardiologist is considering quinidine. Explain the potential drug interaction that may occur. What needs to be done to avoid this interaction?

_____
_____

3. You are working in a pulmonologist's office when a patient comes in for a refill prescription on her *Proventil* inhaler, which she uses as needed for her asthma. She mentions that her asthma seems to have worsened over the past couple of months. Upon reading her chart, you notice that she was referred to a cardiologist 3 months ago. While waiting for the physician to approve the refill, you ask what the cardiologist said. The patient states that the cardiologist started her on propranolol for an irregular heartbeat. Is this important information to tell the pulmonologist? Explain.

_____
_____

4. Mr. Able has been taking verapamil for treatment of his hypertension. At a recent checkup his family physician noticed that Mr. Able had sustained tachycardia. The physician asks you to get some of those free samples of propranolol that were dropped off by the drug sales representative. Could there be a potential problem if the patient takes these two drugs together?

_____
_____

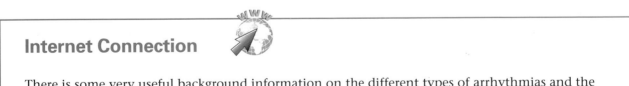

Internet Connection

There is some very useful background information on the different types of arrhythmias and the antiarrhythmic drugs. Contact **MedicineNet** (http://www.medicinenet.com), click on the *Diseases and Treatment* heading and highlight the letter *H*. Click on *Heart Rhythm Abnormalities, Palpitations*.

Additional Reading

Karnes, N. 1995. Adenosine: A quick fix for PSVT. *Nursing* 25 (7):55.

Leibowitz, D. 1993. Sotalol: A novel beta-blocker with class III antiarrhythmic activity. *Journal of Clinical Pharmacology* 33:508.

Palatnik, A. M. 2001. How cardiac drugs do what they do. *Nursing 2001* 31 (5): 54.

Roden, D. M. 1994. Risks and benefits of antiarrhythmic drug therapy. *New England Journal of Medicine* 331:785.

Wilber P. J. 1997. Therapeutic options in atrial flutter and fibrillation. *Hospital Practice* 32 (5):143.

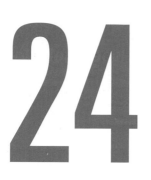

ANTIANGINAL DRUGS

CHAPTER FOCUS

This chapter explains the causes of angina pectoris and discusses the different drug classes used in the treatment of this condition. It also describes the pharmacology of drugs used to treat angina pectoris.

CHAPTER OBJECTIVES

After studying this chapter, you should be able to

- describe the two main types of angina pectoris and the usual cause of each type.

- discuss the mechanisms of action of the three major drug classes used to treat angina pectoris.

- list the different routes of administration for nitrite and nitrate drugs.

- explain the common adverse effects associated with each antianginal drug class.

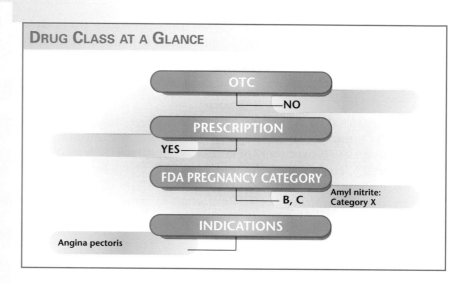

DRUG CLASS AT A GLANCE

OTC — NO

PRESCRIPTION — YES

FDA PREGNANCY CATEGORY — B, C — Amyl nitrite: Category X

INDICATIONS — Angina pectoris

Key Terms

angina pectoris: chest pain due to decreased blood flow to the heart.

coronary artery: artery that supplies blood flow to the heart.

exertional angina: angina pectoris caused by increased physical exertion.

vasospastic angina: angina pectoris caused by vasospasm of the coronary arteries.

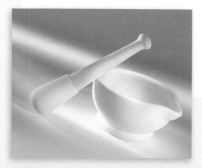

INTRODUCTION

The **coronary arteries,** which supply the heart with blood, are one of the main areas affected by arteriosclerosis (hardening of the arteries) and atherosclerosis (fatty hardening of the arteries). In coronary artery disease the walls of the coronary arteries become thickened and calcified, which results in a decreased blood flow to the heart (ischemia). During physical exertion, when the heart requires more oxygen, ischemia may cause chest pain known as **angina pectoris.** This type of angina is referred to as **exertional angina** because it usually occurs during physical activity. Another type of angina, referred to as **vasospastic angina,** often occurs at rest and is caused by vasospasm of the coronary arteries. Vasospasm decreases blood flow and also causes myocardial ischemia.

Important nondrug components to the treatment of coronary artery disease are diets that limit fat and cholesterol, exercise, elimination of smoking, and weight control. Three major classes of drugs are used to treat angina: nitrites and nitrates, beta-adrenergic blockers, and calcium antagonists.

Nitrites and Nitrates

Nitrites and nitrates were previously known as the coronary dilators, but research has shown that during angina these drugs do not produce significant effects on coronary arteries that are atherosclerotic and hardened by calcification. Since in angina pectoris the coronary arteries are already maximally dilated due to ischemia, the main effect of these drugs is to produce a general vasodilation of systemic veins and arteries, which decreases preload and afterload of the heart (review vasodilator therapy of coronary heart failure [CHF], Chapter 22) and reduces cardiac work and oxygen consumption.

These drugs are used in two ways. First, they are administered during attacks of angina to relieve the intense pain. The most common route of administration is sublingual. The drugs in this group have an almost immediate onset of action, although their duration is short. Second, they are administered prophylactically to prevent attacks of angina. Table 24:1 lists the main drugs in this class.

Mechanism of Action

The mechanism of action of these drugs is to relax vascular smooth muscle. This effect is caused by nitrate and nitrite ions, which are chemically released from these drugs. These nitrate or nitrite ions are converted by enzymes in blood vessels to nitric oxide (NO). Nitric oxide is a potent, but short-acting, vasodilator that relaxes vascular smooth muscle. Venodilation (dilation of veins) is greater than arteriolar dilation at the lower dosage ranges of these drugs.

The main effects produced by vasodilation are a decrease in venous return to the heart (decrease in preload) and a decrease in blood pressure (decrease in afterload). Consequently, cardiac work is reduced. With a reduction in cardiac work, less oxygen is required by the heart, and relief of pain is accomplished. In the vasospastic form of angina, the vasodilating effect of the nitrates is effective in relieving vasospasm of the coronary arteries.

Clinical Use of Nitroglycerin

Nitroglycerin is the most widely used drug of this class and can be administered in several different forms.

Sublingual Nitroglycerin

As a sublingual tablet, nitroglycerin is the drug of choice in the treatment of acute anginal attacks. Patients place the nitroglycerin tablet under the tongue and allow the tablet to dissolve without swallowing. Effects usually occur within 1 to 3 minutes with the peak effect occurring at about 5 minutes.

Nitroglycerin Ointment 2%

The ointment is applied topically to an area of the chest or abdomen and is covered with a plastic dressing. Absorption occurs through the skin, with

Nitrites and Nitrates Used in Angina Pectoris

DRUG (TRADE NAME)	COMMON DOSAGE	ONSET	DURATION
Amyl nitrite			
(*Vaporole*)	0.3 ml inhalation	30–60 sec	10 min
Isosorbide dinitrate			
(*Isordil*)	2.5–10 mg sublingual	2–5 min	2–4 hr
	5–30 mg PO QID	30 min	2–4 hr
Nitroglycerin			
(*Nitro-bid*)	2% ointment	15 min	4–8 hr
(*Nitrostat*)	0.3–0.6 mg sublingual	1–3 min	10–45 min
(*Nitrogard*)	1,2, and 3 mg extended-release tablets	30 min	8–12 hr
(*Transderm-Nitro*)	2.5–15 mg/day transdermal patch	30–60 min	24 hr

an onset of action of 15 minutes and a duration of 4 to 8 hours, depending on the amount applied. Each inch of ointment squeezed from the tube contains approximately 15 mg of nitroglycerin.

Nitroglycerin Extended-Release Tablets and Capsules

Nitroglycerin is available in tablets of 2.6, 6.5, and 9.0 mg and capsules of 2.5, 6.5, and 9.0 mg that release the drug gradually over a prolonged period. Duration of action is 8 to 12 hours. Both nitroglycerin ointment and extended-release capsules and tablets are used two or three times daily to prevent the occurrence of anginal attacks (prophylaxis).

Transdermal Nitroglycerin (*Transderm-Nitro*)

This nitroglycerin is contained within an adhesive patch that is applied on the torso. The nitroglycerin is slowly and uniformly released into the bloodstream over a 24-hour period. Transdermal use is indicated mainly for the prevention of angina.

Nitroglycerin for Intravenous Infusion

Nitroglycerin can be administered intravenously in emergency and surgical situations in the hospital.

Adverse Effects

The main adverse effects of the nitrites and nitrates are related to the vasodilating action.

Cutaneous flushing, dizziness, headache, weakness, and fainting are commonly experienced. Blood pressure usually decreases, and this drop can cause a reflex tachycardia. With frequent use or overuse, tolerance to these drugs can develop, but there is some controversy regarding the clinical significance of this effect.

Nitrites and nitrates may be contraindicated in patients with glaucoma because vasodilation may increase intraocular pressure. At higher doses, these drugs oxidize hemoglobin to methemoglobin, which cannot transport oxygen. Consequently, less oxygen is transported by the blood and symptoms of hypoxia or anemia may develop.

Patient Education

Since anginal attacks are unpredictable, it is important for patients to carry the prescribed medication at all times. Nitroglycerin is volatile, and tablets lose potency if exposed to air or light. Therefore, it is important that tablets be carried in light-resistant, airtight containers. Also, standard practice is not to use nitroglycerin tablets that are more than 6 months old since there may be significant loss of potency.

When patients experience angina, they should be instructed to sit down, place a nitroglycerin tablet under the tongue, and allow it to dissolve without swallowing. Relief should occur within 5 minutes. If it does not, they should repeat the process with another tablet. If there is no relief after three tablets, patients should notify the physician or seek medical assistance.

Patients should be aware of the common side effects, such as cutaneous flushing, headache, and dizziness. They should be advised to lie down if they feel faint. These effects are expected and only last for a few minutes. In addition, patients should become aware of the activities that cause angina (overexertion, emotional upset, or overeating) and try to avoid these situations if possible.

BETA-ADRENERGIC BLOCKING DRUGS

The beta-blockers antagonize or reverse the effects of sympathetic activation caused by exercise and other physical or mental exertions. In the heart, sympathetic stimulation (beta-1 receptors) increases heart rate, force of myocardial contractions, and oxygen consumption. The therapeutic action of beta-blockers in the treatment of angina lies in the ability of these drugs to decrease heart rate and force of contractions. These changes decrease cardiac work and therefore oxygen consumption. Decreasing oxygen consumption often prevents development of myocardial ischemia and pain.

Beta-blockers are indicated for the long-term (chronic) management of angina pectoris. Patients taking beta-blockers usually have less frequent anginal attacks or a delayed onset of pain during physical exertion. This is another way of saying that they have increased work capacity or exercise tolerance. Propranolol (*Inderal*) is the beta-blocker with the longest history of use, but there are a large number of beta-blockers available and most have been shown to be equally effective in the treatment of angina (see Chapter 6, Table 6:5 for a summary of beta-blockers). The usual dose of propranolol is 10 to 90 mg PO, BID, TID, or QID, depending on the patient and the severity of the disease.

Propranolol can also be used in combination with nitrates in patients who require more than one drug to control angina. Information about the adverse effects of propranolol and other beta-blockers can be reviewed in Chapter 6.

CALCIUM ANTAGONISTS

Mechanism of Action

Calcium antagonists, which interfere with the movement of calcium ions through cell membranes, are the newest class of drugs used to treat angina pectoris. Contraction of vascular smooth muscle is very dependent on calcium influx (movement from extracellular to intracellular sites), which normally occurs during membrane depolarization (action potential) of smooth muscle. Drugs that inhibit calcium influx decrease vascular tone and produce a vasodilating effect. As discussed in regard to the nitrites and nitrates, vasodilation decreases venous return and blood pressure, and this decreases cardiac work and oxygen consumption. In addition, calcium antagonists have been shown to dilate the larger coronary arteries, which increases coronary blood flow.

Verapamil (*Calan, Isoptin*)

Verapamil is widely used to treat supraventricular arrhythmias (see Chapter 23). In addition, its vasodilating properties allow it to be considered for the treatment of angina. Because of its prominent effects on the heart, verapamil can also decrease heart rate and the force of myocardial contraction. These actions also decrease cardiac work, but may also decrease cardiac function if the dosage is too large.

Diltiazem (*Cardizem*)

Diltiazem causes fewer effects on the heart than verapamil, usually producing only a slight decrease in heart rate. Diltiazem is a vasodilator of the coronary arteries and usually produces a modest fall in blood pressure.

Nifedipine (*Procardia*)

Nifedipine has minor effects on heart rate and myocardial contraction, but it is a very potent vasodilator and usually lowers blood pressure.

Nicardipine (*Cardene*)

Nicardipine is similar to nifedipine in that the main pharmacological effects are vasodilation and relaxation of coronary artery spasm.

Other Calcium Antagonists

Amlodipine (*Norvasc*), bepridil (*Vascor*), felodipine (*Plendil*), and isradipine (*DynaCirc*) are newer calcium antagonists. With the exception of bepridil, all are similar in action and adverse effect profile to nifedipine. Bepridil can slow heart rate and also possesses antiarrhythmic properties. The major reservations to the use of bepridil lie in the potential of the drug to produce serious cardiac arrhythmias. The uses of bepridil are limited to patients unresponsive to other drug treatments.

Adverse Effects

Common adverse effects of the calcium antagonists include headache, facial flushing, dizziness, hypotension, and minor gastrointestinal (GI) disturbances. Constipation is one of the more common side effects of verapamil. Because nifedipine, nicardipine, and related drugs are potent vasodilators, they may also cause reflex tachycardia if blood pressure drops below normal. Verapamil and diltiazem may slow the heart rate and produce signs of cardiac depression that may lead to CHF.

CLINICAL INDICATIONS FOR ANTIANGINAL DRUGS

The nitrates, beta-blockers, and calcium antagonists are widely used to control exertional angina, whereas calcium antagonists are the preferred drugs for treating vasospastic angina. Various combination therapies with the three classes of antianginal drugs are possible. The major contraindication to combination therapy is with beta-blockers and calcium antagonists (verapamil and diltiazem), which together can cause excessive cardiac depression.

Patient Administration and Monitoring

Monitor vital signs when these drugs are administered during the treatment of acute angina.

Instruct the patient on the proper self-administration of sublingual nitroglycerin or similar preparations.

Explain to patient the common side effects of the drugs that dilate blood vessels: dizziness, headache, flushing, faintness, nausea.

Instruct patient to report excessive changes in blood pressure and pulse rate, or other significant changes.

Explain to patient the importance of weight control, diets low in fats and cholesterol, eliminating smoking, and exercise if approved by the physician.

Help patient to identify the situations or stresses that trigger angina and establish mechanisms for avoidance.

Chapter Review

Understanding Terminology

Answer the following questions in the spaces provided.

1. What are two main types of angina pectoris? How do they differ? _____
_____

2. Write a short paragraph using the following terms: *coronary arteries, atherosclerosis, angina pectoris, exertional angina,* and *vasospastic angina.*
_____

Acquiring Knowledge

Answer the following questions in the spaces provided.

1. What is the mechanism of action of the nitrites and nitrates? _____
_____

2. What are the different routes of administration for nitroglycerin? When is each indicated? _____
_____

3. Explain the mechanism of action of propranolol in the treatment of angina. _____
_____

4. What is the effect of the calcium antagonists on vascular smooth muscle? _____
_____

5. Compare the adverse effects of the nitrates and the calcium antagonist drugs. _____
_____

Applying Knowledge—On the Job

Use your critical thinking skills to answer the following questions in the spaces provided.

1. While doing your afternoon assessment of your patients in cardiac care, you ask Mr. Horn if he has had a bowel movement today. He states he has not moved his bowels in 3 days. You review the chart and see that 4 days ago, on admission, he was started on *Lasix, Transderm-Nitro* patch, verapamil, and a potassium supplement.
   a. Which drug is most likely causing the constipation? _____
   _____
   b. What advice might you likely give your patient? _____
   _____

2. Mrs. George was just started on *Procardia* and *Nitro-Bid* upon her admission to the cardiac care unit. She has also just been allowed to get out of bed. What advice should you give her?
   _____
   _____

3. Instruct Mrs. Smith (or one of your classmates) on the proper procedure for administering sublingual nitroglycerin. What should she do if the first tablet does not provide relief? Second tablet? Third tablet?
   _____
   _____

4. Prepare a short oral presentation for a new angina patient that describes the various nondrug modalities that are important in the control of angina.

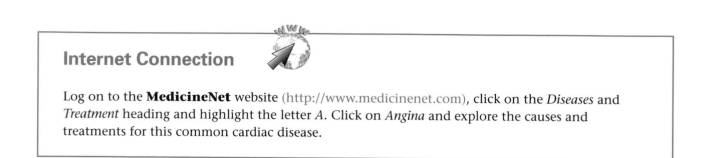

Internet Connection

Log on to the **MedicineNet** website (http://www.medicinenet.com), click on the *Diseases* and *Treatment* heading and highlight the letter *A*. Click on *Angina* and explore the causes and treatments for this common cardiac disease.

Additional Reading

Custer, B. G. 2002. Management of acute myocardial infarction. *Physician Assistant* 26 (5):44.

How reliable is ischemia as a prognostic indicator. 1997. *Emergency Medicine* 29 (6):34.

Lazzara, D., and Sellergren, C. 1996. Chest pain emergencies. Making the right call when the pressure is on. *Nursing* 26 (11):42.

Miracle, V. 1995. Assessing chest pain. *Nursing* 25 (2):51.

PHARMACOLOGY OF THE VASCULAR AND RENAL SYSTEMS

Chapter 25

Diuretics

Renal Physiology
Conditions Associated With Renal
    Dysfunction
Osmotic Diuretics
Carbonic Anhydrase Inhibitors
Thiazide and Thiazide-Like Diuretics
Organic Acid Diuretics
Potassium-Sparing Diuretics
Miscellaneous Diuretics
Special Considerations
Drug Interactions and
    Incompatibilities
Overdose

Chapter 26

Antihypertensive Drugs

Physiological Factors Controlling
    Blood Pressure
Antihypertensive Therapy

Chapter 27

Anticoagulants and Coagulants

Coagulation
Anticoagulant Mechanism of Action

Monitoring Coagulation
Thrombolytic Enzymes
Coagulants/Hemostatics

Chapter 28

Nutrition and Therapy

Nutrients
Vitamins
Fat-Soluble Vitamins
Water-Soluble Vitamins
Body Water
Minerals

Chapter 29

Hypolipidemic Drugs

Liver Metabolism and Lipoproteins
Monitoring Blood Lipid Levels
Bile Acid Sequestrants
HMG-CoA Reductase Inhibitors
Miscellaneous Hypolipidemics
Clinical Indications
Contraindications
Drug Interactions

Chapter 30

Antianemics

Causes of Anemia
Iron Deficiency Anemia
Cyanocobalamin Deficiency
Folic Acid Deficiency
Erythropoetin

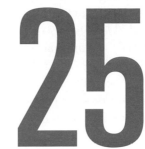

DIURETICS

DRUG CLASS AT A GLANCE

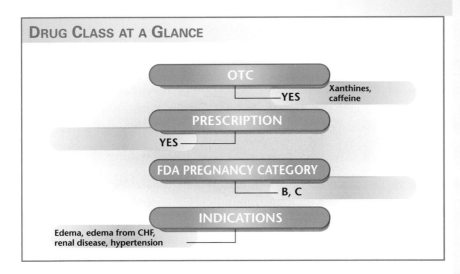

OTC
YES — Xanthines, caffeine

PRESCRIPTION
YES

FDA PREGNANCY CATEGORY
B, C

INDICATIONS
Edema, edema from CHF, renal disease, hypertension

Key Terms

acidification: process that alters the pH to less than 7.

acidosis: pH less than 7.5 or a condition in which the tissues have relatively more acid or acid waste than normal.

alkalosis: pH greater than 7.42 or a condition in which the tissues have less acid than normal.

anuria: condition in which no urine is produced.

aqueous humor: ocular fluid; watery substance that is located behind the cornea of the eye and in front of the lens.

convoluted: coiled or folded back on itself.

distal convoluted tubule (DCT): part of the nephron that is closest to the collecting duct.

diuresis: condition that causes urine to be excreted, usually associated with large volumes of urine.

extracellular: area outside the cell.

hypochloremia: abnormally low level of chloride ions circulating in the blood.

hypokalemia: abnormally low level of potassium ions circulating in the blood.

CHAPTER FOCUS

This chapter describes drugs that remove water from the body. Usually, the water is excreted in the urine along with sodium ions.

CHAPTER OBJECTIVES

After studying this chapter, you should be able to

- explain the role of the kidneys in water excretion.
- describe the difference between renal filtration and renal reabsorption.
- identify two areas of the renal tubules where sodium and water transport are connected.
- explain how the action of osmotic diuretics differs from that of thiazide diuretics.
- explain what happens when a diuretic becomes refractory.
- describe three major side effects of nonrefractory diuretics.

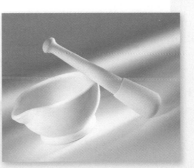

metabolic waste products: substances formed through the chemical processes that enable cells to function; usually, these substances are excreted by the body.

nephritis: inflammation or infection in the kidneys.

oliguria: condition in which very small amounts of urine are produced.

proximal convoluted tubule (PCT): part of the nephron that is closest to the glomerulus.

refractory: unable to produce an increased response even though the stimulation or amount of drug has been increased.

tubular reabsorption: process in which the nephrons return to the blood substances (ions, nutrients) that were filtered out of the blood at the glomerulus.

tubular secretion: process in which the nephrons produce and release substances (ions, acids, and bases) that facilitate sodium ion reabsorption and maintain acid-base balance.

uremia: accumulation of nitrogen waste materials (for example, urea) in the blood.

INTRODUCTION

The primary functions of the kidneys are to maintain water, electrolyte, and acid-base balance. In order to accomplish this, the kidneys receive a large portion of the cardiac output (25 percent). As blood flows through the kidneys, substances are constantly filtered from the blood. Large molecules, such as plasma proteins, cannot pass through renal membranes, so only small molecules (ions, water, and glucose) and cell waste products are cleared from the blood.

However, the body requires ions and water to function efficiently. For example, electrolytes—sodium (Na^+), potassium (K^+), and chloride (Cl^-)—preserve the stability of cell membranes, whereas bicarbonate ions (HCO_3^-) buffer the blood to maintain the pH at 7.34 to 7.42. Therefore, the kidneys must reabsorb the essential elements and eliminate the waste products. This balance between renal reabsorption and excretion results in the formation of urine.

RENAL PHYSIOLOGY

Urine formation is essential for normal body function because it enables the blood to reabsorb necessary nutrients, water, and electrolytes. In addition, **metabolic waste products** are eliminated from the body through the urine. These processes take place in the working units of the kidneys known as the nephrons. The kidneys contain millions of nephrons, and each nephron is composed of several segments: the glomerulus, the **proximal convoluted tubule (PCT),** the loop of Henle, the **distal convoluted tubule (DCT),** and the collecting duct (Figure 25:1). Urine is produced in the nephrons through the processes of filtration, reabsorption, and secretion.

Filtration

Filtration of substances from the blood into the nephrons occurs in the glomerulus. The remaining segments (renal tubules) are involved with reabsorption and secretion. The proximal tubule, loop of Henle, and distal tubule contain specialized transport systems that pull ions out of the nephrons and transport them back into the blood **(tubular reabsorption).** One of the most important tubular reabsorption mechanisms transports sodium ions into the circulation. These segments also secrete substances (ions, acids, and bases) that facilitate sodium ion reabsorption and maintain acid-base balance **(tubular secretion).**

Tubular Reabsorption

Most of the ions and nutrients that are filtered at the glomerulus are reabsorbed by the renal tubules. The renal tubules reabsorb as much sodium as possible (99 percent). Sodium ions are extremely important because they are the principal cations (positively charged ions) in the **extracellular** fluid, and their large extracellular

Sites and Mechanisms of Sodium Reabsorption Along the Nephron

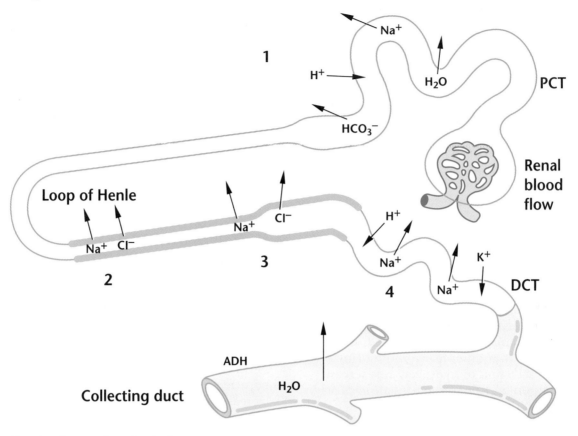

PCT = Proximal convoluted tubule
DCT = Distal convoluted tubule

concentration creates an osmotic gradient that attracts water molecules. Thus, the renal mechanism for water conservation (balance) is directly dependent upon the tubular reabsorption of sodium ions.

Along the nephron, sodium ions are reabsorbed by two mechanisms: cation exchange and chloride ion transport (Figure 25:1). In the proximal and distal convoluted tubules, sodium ions (Na^+) are reabsorbed in exchange for hydrogen ions (H^+). Hydrogen ions are produced in the tubular cells through the action of the enzyme carbonic anhydrase (CA). In the presence of this enzyme, carbon dioxide (CO_2) and water (H_2O) combine to form carbonic acid (H_2CO_3). Carbonic acid rapidly breaks down into hydrogen ions (H^+) and bicarbonate ions (HCO_3^-).

$$CO_2 + H_2O \leftrightharpoons H_2CO_3 \rightarrow HCO_3^- + H^+$$

The hydrogen ions are secreted by the proximal and distal tubules in exchange for sodium ions (see Figure 25:1, sites 1 and 4). Subsequently, the sodium and bicarbonate ions are transported into the blood.

In addition to the hydrogen ion exchange, the distal convoluted tubules secrete potassium ions (K^+) in exchange for sodium. The secretion of potassium ions is primarily controlled by the adrenal mineralocorticoid aldosterone. Within these tubules are aldosterone receptors. By interacting with its receptors, aldosterone causes intracellular potassium ions to enter the tubular fluid (urine). As the potassium ions are secreted, sodium ions are reabsorbed (Figure 25:1, site 4).

In the loop of Henle, sodium ions are reabsorbed, but not through an ion-exchange mechanism. Sodium ions are reabsorbed in the loop of Henle in conjunction with chloride ions (Cl^-). In other words, chloride ions are actively reabsorbed and sodium ions follow (Figure 25:1, sites 2 and 3).

When the renal tubules reabsorb sodium ions through the described mechanisms, an osmotic gradient is established along the nephron. More sodium ions are present in the blood, and fewer sodium ions are present inside the renal tubules. Therefore, water molecules migrate toward the sodium ions and into the blood (water reabsorption). Water is primarily reabsorbed within the proximal convoluted tubules and the collecting ducts. Under the influence of the pituitary hormone antidiuretic hormone (ADH), the pores of the collecting ducts open, and water rushes toward the sodium ions. As a result, water is removed from the urine, and urine volume decreases. The renal reabsorption of sodium and water maintains the plasma volume and water balance.

It is important to understand the mechanisms of tubular reabsorption of sodium ions because these mechanisms are the basis of diuretic action. Diuretics increase urine flow **(diuresis)** by inhibiting the renal tubular reabsorption of sodium ions and water.

Tubular Secretion

The major secretory functions of the nephrons involve the tubular secretion of hydrogen ions, potassium ions, weak acids, and weak bases. Part of the tubular secretory process (cation exchange) has already been mentioned, since it directly results in sodium reabsorption. However, the tubular secretion of hydrogen ions serves another important role in the regulation of acid-base balance. This effect is accomplished through **acidification** of the urine (reducing the pH level to less than 7). Certain renal tubular mechanisms (carbonic anhydrase system) maintain the pH of the blood between 7.34 and 7.42 by altering the pH of the urine. As described, the carbonic anhydrase system produces hydrogen ions (H^+) and bicarbonate ions (HCO_3^-) from CO_2 and water. The bicarbonate is transported into the blood, where it neutralizes (buffers) cell waste products, such as lactic acid. As a result, the pH of the blood remains relatively neutral as long as bicarbonate is available. At the same time, hydrogen ions secreted into the renal tubular fluid acidify the urine (to a pH between 4 and 6). Any condition that impairs the renal production of hydrogen and bicarbonate ions alters the acid-base balance of the body. For example, insufficient bicarbonate production because of carbonic anhydrase inhibition leads to metabolic **acidosis.**

As part of their excretory function, the renal tubules have specialized transport systems that remove weak acids and bases from the blood. Normal cell metabolism produces weak acids (uric acid) and weak bases. Usually, these substances are presented to the kidneys for excretion. The proximal convoluted tubules

secrete weak acids and weak bases into the urine. Many drugs are also weak acids (aspirin, barbiturates, and penicillin) or weak bases (opioid analgesics and antihistamines), which are also secreted into the tubular fluid through the proximal convoluted tubules. Metabolic waste products (weak acids, weak bases) compete for the same transport sites that excrete these drugs. This competition can result in altered drug excretion—for example, accumulation in the blood. As long as the kidneys continue to produce urine, the blood is cleared of waste products and toxic (drug) substances.

CONDITIONS ASSOCIATED WITH RENAL DYSFUNCTION

Renal function may be altered by renal disease or cardiovascular dysfunction. Usually, infection or inflammation in the renal tissues **(nephritis)** reduces renal function. Reduced renal function occurs in glomerulonephritis and pylonephritis. On the other hand, circulatory problems associated with congestive heart failure (CHF), hypertension, and shock decrease renal function by reducing blood flow to the kidneys. Such circulatory disorders are often severe enough to produce renal failure.

Whether the renal tissue is damaged or the blood flow is reduced, the ultimate result is decreased urine flow, decreased urine volume **(oliguria),** or no urine production at all **(anuria).** As a result, the blood is not adequately filtered, and toxic products and ions accumulate. Such an accumulation can lead to uremia, edema, and hypertension.

Uremia (toxemia) is an accumulation of nitrogenous waste products in the blood due to impaired renal filtration. Edema and hypertension are associated with fluid (water) retention in the circulatory system, often as a result of insufficient sodium clearance. Fluid accumulates in the extracellular spaces of the body when too much sodium is retained in the circulation and tissue fluid. Circulating sodium ions create an osmotic gradient, which pulls water molecules into the circulation. This action causes the blood volume to expand, producing an increase in blood pressure (hypertension). The same phenomenon occurs with edema, in that water migration into the tissues causes swelling, especially in the legs and feet. The increased fluid retention and pressure put a greater strain on the failing heart and kidneys.

Clinical Indications

Diuretics are primarily used in the management of anuria, hypertension, and edema. Edema may result from acute or chronic organ disease (for example, CHF, liver cirrhosis) or localized inflammation of specific tissues such as the brain, eyes (glaucoma), and kidneys (nephritis). As long as the kidneys are capable of functioning, urine production and renal excretion of water can be stimulated by increasing the blood flow to the kidneys or by decreasing the renal reabsorption of water. Some diuretics stimulate urine production by increasing glomerular filtration. Other diuretics reduce the excess fluid associated with hypertension and edema by decreasing renal sodium reabsorption. Hence, water reabsorption decreases, and urine flow increases (diuresis).

There are five major classes of diuretics: osmotic agents, carbonic anhydrase inhibitors, thiazide and thiazide-like compounds, organic acids, and potassium-sparing diuretics (Table 25:1). Each of these classes of diuretics produces diuresis by inhibiting water and sodium ion reabsorption in the kidneys. However, these drugs inhibit reabsorption at different sites along the nephrons. Thus, the intensity of the diuresis varies with each class of drugs. In general, the intensity of diuresis is dependent upon the extent to which sodium ions are excreted into the urine.

Osmotic Diuretics

Osmotic diuretics are compounds that can be filtered by the glomerulus but not reabsorbed by the renal tubules.

Mechanism of Action

Since these drugs cannot cross tubular membranes, osmotic diuretics become trapped in the tubular lumen and create an osmotic gradient. Water molecules tend to migrate toward the diuretic molecules. Consequently, this water is not reabsorbed and is excreted into the urine along with the diuretic. Although water reabsorption is inhibited, there is no major alteration of sodium reabsorption. Therefore, this class of diuretics produces a mild diuresis with no alteration in electrolyte or acid-base balance.

Clinical Indications

Mannitol (*Osmitrol*) is the most frequently used osmotic diuretic. Since it cannot penetrate cell membranes, mannitol must be given intravenously (Table 25:2). Once inside the circulation, it acts osmotically, attracting fluid from edematous tissues. The route of administration and low intensity of diuresis produced limit the clinical use of mannitol. Mannitol is used to stimulate urine flow in the treatment of anuria and oliguria before irreversible renal damage occurs. Mannitol may be indicated for acute renal failure or in cardiovascular surgeries in which renal function is severely compromised. Increased urine flow is also valuable in the treatment of drug toxicity or overdose. Mannitol-induced diuresis maintains renal function and keeps the flow of dilute urine so that renal excretion of the toxic substance is achieved. Mannitol is also used in the treatment of cerebral edema and glaucoma. Localized swelling, edema, and pressure (intraocular, cerebral) can be reduced with mannitol. Among the osmotic

TABLE 25:1 Classes of Diuretics

CLASS	DRUGS
Carbonic anhydrase inhibitors	Acetazolamide, dichlorphenamide, methazolamide
Organic acids (loop diuretics)	Bumetanide, ethacrynic acid, furosemide, torsemide
Osmotic (lumenal) diuretics	Glycerin, isosorbide, mannitol, urea
Potassium-sparing diuretics	Amiloride, spironolactone, triamterene
Thiazide and thiazide-like diuretics	Bendroflumethiazide, benzthiazide, chlorothiazide, chlorthalidone, hydrochlorothiazide, hydroflumethiazide, indapamide, methychlothiazide, metolazone, polythiazide, quinethazone, trichlormethiazide
Xanthine derivatives (active ingredients of over-the-counter diuretic products)	Caffeine, pamabrom, theobromine, theophylline

Uses and Dose Range of Osmotic Diuretics and Carbonic Anhydrase Inhibitors

DRUG NAME (TRADE NAME)	USE	ADULT DOSE
Osmotic Diuretics:		
glycerin (*Osmoglyn*)	Reduce intraocular pressure; interrupt acute glaucoma attacks (glaucoma)	1–2.0 g/kg PO 1.5 hr prior to surgery
isosorbide (*Ismotic*)	Reduce intraocular pressure; interrupt acute glaucoma attacks (glaucoma)	1.5 g/kg (1–3 g/kg) BID, QID
mannitol (*Osmitrol*)	Oliguria	20–200 g in 24 hr 20% solution, IV
	Reduce intracranial or intraocular pressure	1.5–2 mg/kg of a 15%, 20%, or 25% solution, IV
	Excretion of toxic substances	5–25% solution infused IV (maximum 200 g)
	Urologic irrigation	2.5% solution IV
urea (*Ureaphil*)	Reduce intracranial or intraocular pressure	30% solution slow IV infusion (maximum 120 g/day)
Carbonic Anhydrase Inhibitors:		
acetazolamide (*Diamox, Dazamide*)	Edema, glaucoma, epilepsy	250–1000 mg/day PO, IV in divided doses every 4 hr
dichlorphenamide (*Daranide*)	Glaucoma	100–200 mg PO followed by 100 mg every 12 hr as needed, 25–50 mg QD, BID, TID maintenance
methazolamide (*Neptazane*)	Glaucoma	50–100 mg PO BID, TID

diuretics in use, mannitol and urea are administered intravenously, while glycerin and isosorbide, administered orally, produce diuresis up to 6 hours.

Adverse Effects

Mannitol is expected to be administered under close observation so that relatively few adverse effects occur. Most often nausea, dizziness, headache, and chills occur. The most serious reaction is an extension of its osmotic effect in the circulation. Mannitol may produce a strain on cardiac function because it increases the plasma volume (expansion). This effect is important in individuals who have impaired cardiac function (CHF). Therefore, mannitol is not recommended for the treatment of chronic edema due to cardiovascular insufficiency.

CARBONIC ANHYDRASE INHIBITORS

Acetazolamide (*Diamox*) is a diuretic that increases sodium and water excretion by inhibiting the enzyme carbonic anhydrase. As explained in the beginning of this chapter, this enzyme produces hydrogen ions and bicarbonate ions from CO_2 and water. This reaction occurs in the proximal and distal convoluted tubules (Figure 25:1, sites 1 and 4). Acetazolamide inhibits the action of carbonic anhydrase so that very little hydrogen and bicarbonate are produced. Therefore, no hydrogen ions are available for exchange with sodium ions (decreased sodium reabsorption). As a result, sodium ions are excreted into the urine along with increased amounts of water.

Additional Renal Effects

Since the hydrogen ion exchange is blocked, the distal convoluted tubules attempt to reabsorb sodium ions by increasing the potassium ion exchange. The increased secretion of potassium ions causes an increased loss of potassium in the urine. Eventually, this loss of potassium leads to **hypokalemia** (decreased potassium ions in the blood). Inhibition of carbonic anhydrase not only inhibits sodium and water reabsorption but also affects the acid-base balance of the body. Since carbonic anhydrase is inhibited, no bicarbonate is produced to buffer the blood. This situation results in metabolic acidosis.

Route of Administration

Acetazolamide is well absorbed following oral administration. It is not metabolized in the body but excreted totally by the kidneys. Since acetazolamide is a weak acid, it is secreted by the proximal convoluted tubules into the urine.

In the presence of metabolic acidosis, acetazolamide excretion is enhanced, and diuresis decreases. Acetazolamide no longer produces diuresis in the presence of acidosis. Because the drug action is inhibited when the acid-base balance is altered, acetazolamide is a **refractory** diuretic. The dose range of acetazolamide for the treatment of edema, glaucoma, and epilepsy is presented in Table 25:2. In some cases, patients are started on the lowest dose and titrated upward until successful results are achieved.

Intramuscular administration should be avoided because the alkaline solution causes pain on injection. However, when rapid relief is required to reduce ocular pressure, the drug can be administered intravenously.

Clinical Indications

Although it produces adequate diuresis, acetazolamide has been largely replaced by other diuretics as an individual treatment of edema. When used today, it is an adjunct treatment in CHF or drug-induced edema. However, acetazolamide is still used for its effects on the ocular tissues. Acetazolamide reduces the pressure and edema associated with chronic simple (open-angle) or narrow-angle (angle-closure) glaucoma principally because ocular fluid **(aqueous humor)** is formed through the action of carbonic anhydrase; hence, acetazolamide inhibits the production of aqueous humor and reduces painful pressure. In the treatment of glaucoma, the intravenous route of administration may be selected to ensure a rapid reduction in intraocular pressure. Carbonic anhydrase inhibitors may be used with miotic and osmotic drugs in patients with chronic simple (open-angle) glaucoma.

Carbonic anhydrase inhibitors are also useful in the treatment of epilepsy. The induction of acidosis apparently decreases the seizure activity in some epileptic states (petit mal and unlocalized seizures).

Acetazolamide has the interesting distinction of being approved for the treatment of acute mountain sickness. This is a response to significant change in altitude with inadequate time for the body to adjust to the change in atmosphere as occurs with mountain climbers and rescue and paramilitary operations. Doses of 500–1000 mg/day taken 48 hours before and after ascent relieve symptoms of oxygen deficit, muscle weakness, cramping, and headache.

Adverse Effects

The most common adverse effects produced by this group include drowsiness, anorexia, gastrointestinal (GI) distress, headache, depression, allergic rash, and acidosis. Hypokalemia and hyperuricemia may also occur. Hyperuricemia, which is too much uric acid in the blood due to impaired urate excretion, is usually a problem only in individuals who are predisposed to gout.

Contraindications

Patients who have metabolic acidosis due to renal failure or severe respiratory acidosis should not receive carbonic anhydrase inhibitors. These drugs aggravate acidosis. Acetazolamide therapy should be avoided in glaucoma patients who have renal disturbances, mental depression, or electrolyte imbalances.

THIAZIDE AND THIAZIDE-LIKE DIURETICS

Thiazide and thiazide-like drugs are the largest group of diuretics. Although they are not chemically related, the thiazide and thiazide-like diuretics produce the same pharmacological action on the renal tubules. Both groups can be administered orally to produce a diuretic response. The thiazide and thiazide-like diuretics differ only in potency and duration of action (see Table 25:3. Commonly used drugs in this class include hydroflumethiazide (*Diucardin*), chlorothiazide (*Diuril*), chlorthalidone (*Hygroton*), and metolazone (*Zaroxolyn*).

TABLE 25:3 — Recommended Doses of Thiazide and Thiazide-like Diuretics

DRUG (TRADE NAME)	DURATION OF ACTION	ADULT ORAL DOSE
Thiazides:		
bendroflumethiazide (*Naturetin*)	6–12 hr	2.5–5 mg/day
benzthiazide (*ExNa*)	6–18 hr	50–200 mg/day
chlorothiazide (*Diuril, Diurgen*)	6–12 hr	500–2000 mg/day
hydrochlorothiazide (*Esidrix, Ezide, HydroDIURIL, Oretic*)	6–12 hr	25–200 mg/day
hydroflumethiazide (*Diucardin, Saluron*)	6–12 hr	25–200 mg/day
methyclothiazide (*Enduron, Aquatensin*)	24 hr	2.5–10 mg/day
polythiazide (*Renese*)	24–48 hr	1–4 mg/day
trichlormethiazide (*Diurese, Metahydrin, Naqua*)	24 hr	1–4 mg/day
Thiazide-like Diuretics:		
chlorthalidone (*Hygroton*)	24–72 hr	50–100 mg/day
indapamide (*Lozol*)	up to 36 hr	2.5–5 mg/day
metolazone (*Zaroxolyn*)	12–24 hr	5–20 mg/day
quinethazone (*Hydromox*)	18–24 hr	50–100 mg/day

Mechanism of Action

This class of diuretics was originally synthesized to produce a potent carbonic anhydrase inhibitor that did not cause acidosis. However, these diuretics are only weak carbonic anhydrase inhibitors. They produce diuresis primarily by inhibiting sodium transport in the distal portion of the nephron. This inhibition causes a substantial loss of sodium and water and produces intense diuresis (Figure 25:1, site 3). The potent mobilization of sodium causes chloride and potassium excretion to increase. As a result, these drugs usually produce **hypochloremic alkalosis** and **hypokalemia.** The thiazide and thiazide-like diuretics are not refractory. As long as these drugs are continually administered, diuresis will occur even in the presence of alkalosis. As an extension of their renal action, thiazide-induced hyponatremia (low sodium level) has been reported to occur in elderly patients.

Adverse Effects

Because thiazide and thiazide-like diuretics rapidly remove water and sodium from the body, the plasma volume may decrease, causing a drop in blood pressure. Patients receiving these diuretics often experience orthostatic hypotension, which is a sudden drop in blood pressure when they quickly change from a sitting position to a standing position. The rapid fall in blood pressure causes individuals to become dizzy, lightheaded, and faint. In addition to hypotension, these diuretics may produce hypokalemia, hyperuricemia, and hyperglycemia. The hyperglycemia may be due to a decreased glucose utilization. Because of the effective mobilization of electrolyte excretion, it is not surprising that the patient may experience muscle spasms or cramps. This effect can upset the blood sugar level in individuals with diabetes mellitus. Hypersensitivity reactions, such as skin rashes, have also been reported with the use of these drugs. These diuretics may produce nausea, diarrhea, constipation, anorexia, headache, impotence, and elevation of blood urea nitrogen or serum creatinine levels. The spectrum and intensity of adverse effects encountered will be related to the general health and condition of the patient. Usually reducing the dose or withdrawing therapy will terminate the adverse effect.

Clinical Indications

Although the thiazide and thiazide-like diuretics are widely used in the treatment of edema with hypertension, they can alleviate edema of any cause, including the chronic edema associated with CHF or renal disease. These diuretics are particularly useful in the management of mild to moderate hypertension because they reduce the plasma volume and relax vascular smooth muscle. While the antihypertension action requires 4 to 6 weeks to establish, the diuretic action begins immediately.

ORGANIC ACID DIURETICS

Bumetanide (*Bumex*), ethacrynic acid (*Edecrin*), furosemide (*Lasix*), and torsemide (*Demedex*) are organic acid, or loop, diuretics (see Table 25:4 on page 274). These drugs are known as loop diuretics because they promote diuresis by inhibiting sodium and chloride ion transport in the loop of Henle. This action results in a tremendous loss of sodium, chloride, and water. The intense diuresis is usually accompanied by hypochloremic alkalosis. The organic acid diuretics continue to produce an increased urine flow in spite of the acid-base changes; therefore, they are not refractory. Hypokalemia may occur with the use of organic diuretics. It is not uncommon for furosemide or ethacrynic acid to be added to other diuretic regimens, especially metolazone. This produces a synergistic diuretic response and increases the opportunity for adverse reactions to occur.

Adverse Effects

The effects produced by organic acid diuretics are similar to those of the thiazide diuretics and include nausea, hypotension, hypokalemia, hyperuricemia, and hyperglycemia. In addition, the organic acid diuretics have produced tone deafness (ototoxicity) in some patients. These diuretics should not be administered in conjunction with aminoglycoside antibiotics (amikacin, kanamycin, neomycin, or streptomycin) because aminoglycoside antibiotics may potentiate the ototoxicity of the loop diuretics.

Clinical Indications

The organic acid diuretics, which have a greater diuretic action than do the thiazides, are often used to relieve edema in patients who have become resistant to the thiazide diuretics. The organic acid diuretics are also useful in severe peripheral edema and pulmonary edema where greater diuretic activity is needed. Otherwise, the primary use is reduction of edema associated with CHF, liver cirrhosis, and renal disease. Parenteral administration is indicated when a rapid response is required or when GI absorption is impaired, making oral administration unfeasible.

POTASSIUM-SPARING DIURETICS

The potassium-sparing diuretics include amiloride (*Midamor*), spironolactone (*Aldactone*), and triamterene (*Dyrenium*) (Table 25:4).

Mechanism Of Action

Following oral administration, these drugs produce diuresis by inhibiting potassium secretion in the distal convoluted tubules (Figure 25:1, site 4). Spironolactone blocks aldosterone receptors located in these tubules. Because aldosterone receptors partially control potassium secretion, the exchange for sodium is inhibited by spironolactone. Although not aldosterone antagonists, amiloride and triamterene inhibit sodium reabsorption by altering the membranes of the distal convoluted tubules so that potassium cannot be secreted. These three drugs produce a mild diuresis without inducing electrolyte changes or acid-base disturbances.

Adverse Effects

The side effects associated with amiloride, spironolactone, and triamterene include nausea, diarrhea, and hyperkalemia. Spironolactone and triamterene also can cause gynecomastia. Unlike the other diuretics, potassium-sparing diuretics promote potassium retention in the blood (hyperkalemia). This effect often occurs in patients who have impaired renal function or who are diabetic. However, the incidence of hyperkalemia is minimized in most individuals receiving spironolactone and triamterene because these drugs are seldom administered alone. Potassium-sparing diuretics are primarily employed as adjuncts to thiazide or loop diuretic therapy. Amiloride, spironolactone, and triamterene inhibit the hypokalemia produced by the other potent diuretics; therefore, these three diuretics conserve potassium.

Clinical Indications

The potassium-sparing diuretics are useful in the management of edema when combined with thiazides and loop diuretics. These diuretics are

Uses and Doses of Organic Acid and Potassium-Sparing Diuretics

DRUGS (TRADE NAME)	DURATION OF ACTION ORAL DOSES	USE	ADULT ORAL DOSE
Organic Acids (Loop Diuretics):			
bumetanide (*Bumex*)	4–6 hr	Edema associated with congestive heart failure, renal disease, or cirrhosis of the liver and nephrotic syndrome; short-term management of ascites	0.5–10 mg/day
ethacrynic acid (*Edecrin*)	6–8 hr		50–200 mg/day > 200 mg/day for refractory patients
furosemide (*Lasix*)	6–8 hr	Also used in the management of hypertension and acute pulmonary edema	20–80 mg/day
torsemide (*Demadex*)	6–8 hr	Same as ethacrynic acid cirrhosis	10–20 mg/day 5–10 mg/day
Potassium-Sparing Diuretics:			
amiloride (*Midamor*)	24 hr	Hypertension	5–20 mg/day
		Adjunctive therapy with thiazide or loop diuretics in congestive heart failure; to restore potassium in hypokalemic patients; prevent hypokalemia	
spironolactone (*Aldactone*)	48–72 hr	Hypertension	50–100 mg/day
		Edema	50–100 mg/day
		Hyperaldosteronism, hypokalemia	100–400 mg/day
spironolactone (50 mg) and hydrochlorothiazide (50 mg) (*Aldactazide*)	48–72 hr	Hyperaldosteronism, edema, hypertension	50–200 mg/day (1–4 tablets/day)
triamterene (*Dyrenium*)	12–16 hr	Edema, hypertension	100–200 mg/day

often used to control potassium depletion in patients who cannot tolerate oral potassium supplements (see "Special Considerations"). Spironolactone also is used in primary hyperaldosteronism to reduce potassium loss.

MISCELLANEOUS DIURETICS

The xanthine derivatives (caffeine, pamabrom, theobromine, and theophylline) are naturally occurring drugs that produce a mild diuretic response. These drugs stimulate urine flow by increasing the blood flow through kidneys, resulting in an increased glomerular filtration rate and urine formation. Most often, xanthine diuretics are used

in combination with other diuretics. Side effects associated with the xanthine diuretics include CNS stimulation, hypotension, and headache. Caffeine is the active ingredient in over-the-counter diuretics.

SPECIAL CONSIDERATIONS

Most of the diuretics, especially the most potent, produce changes in electrolyte and acid-base balance with chronic use. Therefore, the serum electrolytes should be monitored periodically to follow the effects of the diuretics. The serum potassium level is particularly important because changes in potassium can alter cardiovascular and skeletal muscle function. Potassium depletion (hypokalemia) can produce muscle weakness, fatigue, and cardiac arrhythmias.

Hypokalemia

Clinical estimates of diuretic-induced hypokalemia vary between 10 and 40 percent of patients chronically receiving diuretic therapy. To avoid the potassium reduction, or hypokalemia, produced by the potent diuretics, patients usually are encouraged to follow a supplementation schedule. Orange juice and bananas supply a large amount of dietary potassium. These fruits should be eaten daily to compensate for the diuretic-induced potassium loss. Additional foods considered to be potassium rich are dates, figs, prunes, apricots, raisins, sweet and white potatoes, as well as grapefruit and prune juices.

In severe edema, which requires stronger diuretic therapy, oral potassium salt supplements (*K-Lyte* or *Slow-K*) may be required. These potassium supplements often produce GI irritation, which reduces patient compliance. Therefore, the potassium-sparing diuretics are useful as an adjunct drug to reduce potassium depletion during diuretic therapy.

Orthostatic Hypotension and Dehydration

Since diuretics remove salt and water from the circulation, blood pressure may be altered, resulting in orthostatic hypotension. Patients taking a diuretic should be cautioned about potential changes in blood pressure, since the hypotension can lead to dizziness and fainting. The vital signs should be monitored periodically in order to follow effects on circulation and blood pressure.

Often, the use of diuretics is directed toward reducing the sodium level in the blood. Therefore, many patients receiving diuretics must also restrict their dietary sodium intake. As the frequency of urination increases, the urine volume should be recorded to determine the effectiveness of the diuretic. The potent diuretics can produce weight loss and dehydration due to intense removal of water from the body.

Blood Glucose Monitoring

Diabetic patients who require long-term diuretic therapy should have their blood glucose levels monitored periodically. Patients sensitive to sulfonamide drugs may develop allergic reactions to furosemide or thiazide diuretics.

DRUG INTERACTIONS AND INCOMPATIBILITIES

Diuretics are involved in a number of drug interactions because they bind to plasma proteins, alter acid-base balance, and stimulate renal excretion. The most important interaction is the potentiation of digitalis toxicity. Diuretics are frequently used in combination with the cardiac glycosides (digitalis) in the treatment of CHF. Diuretic-induced hypokalemia increases the toxic effect of digitalis on the myocardium, resulting in the production of arrhythmias. Therefore, it is important to maintain the potassium balance during diuretic therapy. Another important interaction occurs when diuretics are used concomitantly with lithium. Diuretics may decrease the renal clearance of lithium, thus increasing the risk of lithium toxicity.

Carbonic anhydrase inhibitors potentiate potassium depletion in the presence of corticosteroids and increase the excretion of acidic drugs.

Alcohol, antihypertensive drugs, barbiturates, and opioid analgesics increase the possibility of orthostatic hypotension when taken with the potent diuretics such as thiazides and organic acids. Diazoxazide potentiates hypotension, hyperglycemia, and hyperuricemia when taken with thiazide diuretics.

Aminoglycoside antibiotics potentiate otoxicity with organic acid diuretics.

Some diuretics can be prepared as solutions for parenteral administration. Usually, the intramuscular route is associated with pain or local irritation, so direct intravenous injection or intravenous infusion is the parenteral route of choice. Since diuretics may be given slowly through the tubing of a running infusion, it is important to avoid mixing solutions that will result in drug incompatibility. Drug incompatibility may be associated with drug precipitation, complex formation, or discoloration of the solution, any of which may alter total drug activity or potency. Mannitol (*Osmitrol*), chlorothiazide (*Diuril*), ethacrynic acid (*Edecrin*), and furosemide (*Lasix*) have been reported to be incompatible with specific solutions or infusions.

Mannitol (*Osmitrol*) should not be mixed with whole blood because agglutination may occur. Advanced premixing of mannitol and cisplatin (antineoplastic drug) may result in complex formation. Chlorothiazide (*Diuril*) has been reported to be incompatible when mixed in solution with amikacin, chlorpromazine, codeine, insulin, methadone, morphine, procaine, promethazine, streptomycin, tetracycline, and vancomycin. Ethacrynic acid has been reported to be incompatible with solutions of drugs with a final pH of less than 5 and should never be mixed with whole blood for infusion. Furosemide may precipitate if combined with ascorbic acid, epinephrine, norepinephrine, or tetracycline solutions.

OVERDOSE

Diuretics will produce an exaggeration of their clinical effects when the dose exposure is greater than therapeutically required. Plasma volume depletion contributes to hypotension, dizziness, and drowsiness. Electrolyte deficiency produces confusion, muscle weakness, and gastrointestinal disturbances. There is no antidote for any diuretic. Gastric lavage and vomiting may be necessary while maintaining hydration and electrolyte balance parenterally, and supporting respiration as necessary.

Patient Administration and Monitoring

The term *diuretic* or "water pill" is so familiar to patients that it may be prudent to remind them how effective these drugs are. Certain unpleasant effects may be annoying, but do not warrant interrupting therapy, while other actions require the doctor's attention. Diuretic activity will begin immediately, so that the pills should be taken early in the day to minimize urinary urgency (nocturia) during sleep. Medication should be taken as directed "even if the patient is feeling well." Body weight should be periodically (even daily) measured, particularly in elderly patients, who are especially susceptible to excessive diuresis.

Drug Administration

Patients who experience GI upset after taking oral diuretics may be advised to take the medicine with meals or milk.

Patient Instruction

Alcohol, including over-the-counter (OTC) preparations for cold/flu and coughs and hay fever which contain alcohol, should be avoided while on diuretics. The alcohol potentiates dehydration, drowsiness, and dizziness, which may occur with the diuretics.

Diabetic patients may experience a change in their blood sugar values during home monitoring or glucose testing. If the patient is seeing another physician or specialist (diabetologist, endocrinologist) for diabetes, remind the patient to have the diuretic added to that medication history.

Special dose adjustment for elderly patients is not necessary; however, patients should be advised to move slowly when rising from bed or chairs because of the orthostatic hypotension.

Photosensitivity may occur with triamterene. Patients should be advised to avoid unnecessary exposure to the sun while on therapy.

Notify the Physician

Patients should notify physician if muscle pain, weakness or cramps, nausea, vomiting, diarrhea, or palpitations occur.

Sudden joint pain should be reported to the physician immediately for further evaluation. This could be indicative of developing gout.

Use in Pregnancy

Drugs in this class have been designated Federal Drug Administration (FDA) Pregnancy Category B or C. Safety for use during pregnancy has not been established. Routine use of diuretics during normal pregnancy is inappropriate. They are not useful in treating toxemia. These drugs are indicated for use during pregnancy only when the underlying conditions of the patient, such as CHF or renal disease, warrant treatment. These drugs will cross the placental barrier and affect the fetus. These drugs should be used only when clearly needed and the potential benefits are greater than the risks.

Chapter Review

Understanding Terminology

Answer the following questions in the spaces provided.

1. Compare the terms *tubular reabsorption* and *tubular secretion*. _____

    _____

    _____

2. What is meant by the term *refractory*? _____

    _____

    _____

3. Explain the difference between the terms *acidosis* and *alkalosis*. _____

    _____

    _____

Match the definition or description in the left column with the appropriate term in the right column.

___ 4. A condition in which no urine is produced.   a. anuria

___ 5. Watery substance behind cornea of the eye and in front of the lens.   b. aqueous humor

___ 6. An inflammation or infection in the kidneys.   c. diuresis

___ 7. A condition that causes very small amounts of urine to be produced.   d. nephritis

___ 8. An accumulation of urea in the blood.   e. oliguria

___ 9. A condition that causes a large volume of urine to be excreted.   f. uremia

Acquiring Knowledge

Answer the following questions in the spaces provided.

1. What are the main functions of the kidneys? _____

    _____

    _____

2. Describe the mechanism of sodium reabsorption from the renal tubules. _____

    _____

    _____

3. What is the mechanism of action of most diuretic drugs? _____

    _____

    _____

4. How does the mechanism of action of the osmotic diuretics differ from that of other diuretic drugs?

    _____

    _____

5. How can acetazolamide produce metabolic acidosis? _____

    _____

    _____

6. What adverse effects are common to both the thiazide and the organic acid diuretics? _____

_____

_____

7. How do amiloride, spironolactone, and triamterene affect potassium secretion by the distal convoluted tubules?

_____

_____

8. When are diuretics used? Why are they useful in the treatment of hypertension? _____

_____

_____

Internet Connection

Go into the www.healthnet.com home page. In the search box, type blood pressure, edema or diuretics to obtain a number of titles.

Click on *Women Matter* to review Conditions and Diseases from the woman's perspective on stroke and heart disease and to familiarize yourself with the relationship between high blood pressure and stroke.

Another website maintained by the American Association of Family Practitioners (www.aafp.org) provides patient information handouts and online search capability for diuretic use, *Treatment of Edema* and *Congestive Heart Failure.* At the AAFP home page, click on the top of the page to enter *Patient Information Handouts.* Then select one of the categories, for example, *Circulatory System,* to reach *Information from Your Family Practitioner.*

At the AAFP home page, type in *Diuretic Use* at the search box. Review the list of abstracts presented. Select *Low Dose Combination Therapy in Hypertension* or *Diuretic Therapy for Older Patients with Type II Diabetes.*

Additional Reading

Holomb, S. S. 1997. Understanding the ins and outs of diuretic therapy. *Nursing* 27 (2):34.

Hoyt, R. E. 2001. Reducing readmissions for congestive heart failure. *American Family Physician* 63 (3): 1593.

Margo, K. 2001. Spironolactone in left-sided heart failure: How does it fit in? *American Family Physician* 64 (8): 1393.

Novak, G. D. 1995. New agents in the treatment of glaucoma. *Ophthalmology World News* 1 (2):1.

Rosholm, J. U. 2002. Hyponatraemia in very old nonhospitalized people: Association with drug use. *Drugs Aging* 19 (9): 685.

Weiss, R. 2002. Changing patterns of initial drug therapy for the treatment of hypertension in a Medicaid population, 1997–2000. *Clinical Therapeutics* 24 (9): 1451.

ANTIHYPERTENSIVE DRUGS

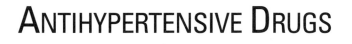

chapter

26

DRUG CLASS AT A GLANCE

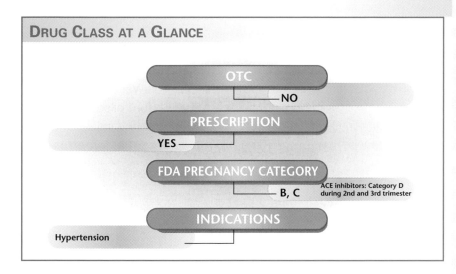

OTC — NO

PRESCRIPTION — YES

FDA PREGNANCY CATEGORY — B, C
ACE inhibitors: Category D during 2nd and 3rd trimester

INDICATIONS
Hypertension

CHAPTER FOCUS

Many different drug classes with important pharmacological and adverse effects are used to treat hypertension. This chapter explains physiological factors involved in hypertension and the effect of drugs on these factors. It also discusses the pharmacology of the drugs used to control hypertension.

CHAPTER OBJECTIVES

After studying this chapter, you should be able to

- describe the major physiological factors that regulate blood pressure.
- understand the role of the kidneys and renin-angiotensin-aldosterone system in blood pressure regulation.
- list five antihypertensive drug classes.
- list two important pharmacological actions of each drug class.
- describe two important adverse effects caused by each drug class.

Key Terms

aldosterone: hormone released from adrenal cortex that causes the retention of sodium.

angiotensin: potent vasoconstrictor.

angiotensin-converting enzyme (ACE) inhibitor: drug that inhibits angiotensin formation.

blood pressure (BP):   the pressure of the blood within the arteries; depends primarily on the cardiac output and the peripheral resistance.

cardiac output (CO):   amount of blood pumped by the heart per minute.

essential hypertension: major form of hypertension, for which the cause is unknown.

heart rate (HR):   number of heartbeats per minute.

hypertension: abnormally high blood pressure.

malignant hypertension: condition of hypertensive crisis when BP is over 210/120.

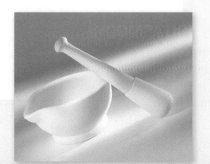

peripheral resistance (PR):   resistance generated by the flow of blood through the arteries.

renin: substance released by the kidneys into the bloodstream; stimulates the formation of angiotensin.

secondary hypertension: form of hypertension in which the cause is known.

stroke volume (SV):   amount of blood pumped per heartbeat.

INTRODUCTION

Hypertension, a condition in which blood pressure (BP) in the arterial system is abnormally high, is one of the leading causes of cerebral strokes, heart attacks, and kidney disease. An estimated 10 percent of the American population has hypertensive disease. The symptoms of hypertension usually appear years later after the disease is well established and permanent organ damage has occurred.

It is estimated that only half of the people with hypertension are aware of their disease, and many of those are not receiving proper treatment. This situation is difficult to understand, since the detection of high blood pressure is relatively easy. Newer treatment methods are also available, and most cases of hypertension can now be controlled.

In the majority of hypertensive cases (approximately 90 percent), the cause of hypertension is unknown. This type of hypertension is referred to as **essential hypertension.** When the cause of hypertension is known, the hypertension is referred to as **secondary hypertension.** Since the cause of essential hypertension is unknown, the goal of drug therapy is to lower the blood pressure back to the normal range to prevent or at least reduce the serious consequences of chronic hypertension.

PHYSIOLOGICAL FACTORS CONTROLLING BLOOD PRESSURE

Blood pressure is mainly determined by two factors: cardiac output (CO) and peripheral resistance (PR).

Cardiac Output

Cardiac output (CO) is the amount of blood that is pumped out of the heart per minute. Two factors determine cardiac output: the **heart rate (HR)** in beats per minute, and the **stroke volume (SV),** the amount of blood pumped per beat. The formula for cardiac output (CO) is:

$$CO = HR \times SV$$

Peripheral Resistance

The **peripheral resistance (PR)** is the resistance or friction that the arterioles have against the flow of blood. The main factor that increases the peripheral resistance is vasoconstriction. Vasoconstriction and a rise in BP are produced by sympathetic stimulation (norepinephrine, epinephrine), angiotensin, and other vasoactive factors. Drugs that cause vasodilation reduce peripheral resistance.

Blood Pressure

Blood pressure (BP) is a result of all of the factors that regulate cardiac output (CO) and peripheral resistance (PR). The formula for BP is:

$$BP = CO \times PR$$

Increasing any of the factors (HR, SV, or PR) will cause the blood pressure to rise, and stimulation of the sympathetic nervous system may increase all of them. In most cases of essential hypertension, there is increased activity of the sympathetic nervous system, so this factor is important in the control of blood pressure. Many of the antihypertensive drugs decrease the activity of the sympathetic nervous system, resulting in a reduction of the blood pressure and a decrease in the adverse effects of hypertensive disease.

Factors that Contribute to High Blood Pressure

A number of factors have been shown to affect BP. While these factors are not believed to be the cause of hypertension, controlling these factors can produce modest decreases in BP. These factors include sodium restriction, weight loss, elimination of smoking, regular physical exercise, and various relaxation techniques aimed at reducing stress. Successful control of these factors may eliminate the need for drug therapy or reduce the dosage and number of drugs required.

Role of Kidneys in Hypertension

With hypertension, there is increased peripheral resistance, and blood flow through the kidneys is reduced. The peripheral resistance is usually higher in the kidneys than in other vascular areas. The kidneys play an important role in maintaining sodium and water balance in the body. When renal blood flow is reduced, as it usually is when there is hypertension and increased peripheral resistance, a substance called **renin** is released by the kidneys into the bloodstream.

Through a series of chemical reactions, renin stimulates the formation of another substance, angiotensin. **Angiotensin** is an extremely potent vasoconstrictor that increases peripheral resistance and blood pressure. In addition, angiotensin stimulates the release of aldosterone from the adrenal cortex. **Aldosterone** causes the kidneys to reabsorb more sodium and consequently more water back into the blood. These actions increase blood volume and also BP. The function of the renin-angiotensin-aldosterone (RAA) system is to help maintain normal blood volume and blood pressure. It is thought that a disturbance of this system in many patients with hypertension contributes to the hypertensive condition.

A class of drugs known as the **angiotensin-converting enzyme (ACE) inhibitors** inhibits the formation of angiotensin and reduces the actions of the RAA system to increase blood volume and BP. In addition, newer drugs have recently been introduced that lower BP by blocking angiotensin receptors.

ANTIHYPERTENSIVE THERAPY

The drugs used to treat hypertension include the diuretics, sympathetic (adrenergic) blockers, vasodilators, calcium antagonists, and ACE inhibitors. In advanced cases of hypertension, these drugs are used in combination. Table 26:1 classifies the various degrees of hypertension.

Diuretic Agents

Since diuretic agents were discussed in Chapter 25, only applications related to the treatment of hypertension will be discussed here. It has been known for many years that a salt-restricted diet lowers BP. Salt-restricted diets were used to treat hypertension before the discovery of the modern drugs.

The diuretics, which decrease the level of salt in the body, were observed to produce a lowering of BP. Salt restriction and diuretic therapy are both effective measures to reduce BP.

Mechanism of Action

The thiazides and thiazide-like drugs are the preferred diuretics used to treat hypertension. The hypotensive effect of these drugs is caused in part by the loss of excess blood volume through diuresis. More importantly, the thiazides have a direct action on the walls of the arterial blood vessels. These drugs have been shown to lower sodium concentration in the blood vessel walls. This reduction in sodium appears to decrease the ability of norepinephrine, epinephrine, and other vasoconstrictors to increase BP. The result is vasodilation of the blood vessels and a reduction of BP.

Diuretics are used alone in mild hypertension. In moderate or severe hypertension, the diuretics are usually combined with other antihypertensive

TABLE 26:1	Classification of Hypertension
CLASSIFICATION	**BLOOD PRESSURE**
Normotensive	<130/85
High normal	130–139/85–89
Hypertension	
Stage 1 (mild)	140–159/90–99
Stage 2 (moderate)	160–179/100–109
Stage 3 (severe)	180–209/110–119
Stage 4 (very severe)	>210/120 (malignant hypertension)

drugs. The effects of thiazide-like diuretics (chlorthalidone and quinethazone) are identical to the effects of the thiazides. Recent studies have demonstrated that once-a-day, low-dose therapy with thiazide and thiazide-like diuretics provides effective antihypertensive treatment and patient compliance.

The organic acid diuretics, such as furosemide (*Lasix*) and bumetanide (*Bumex*), are used in patients who have reduced kidney function, where a more potent diuretic effect is required. The potassium-sparing diuretics are usually combined with the other diuretics and indicated when loss of potassium is of concern. There are many thiazide and potassium-sparing drug combination preparations available and they are frequently used in the treatment of hypertension. Several representative thiazide and thiazide-like diuretics are listed in Table 26:2.

Adverse Effects

Most of the adverse effects of the diuretics are caused by excessive loss of water, sodium, and potassium (hypokalemia), which usually results in dehydration, muscle weakness, and fatigue. The diuretics also interfere with the renal excretion of uric acid. In some patients, increased uric acid levels cause gout. In addition, diuretics interfere with the action of insulin and may cause hyperglycemia, which may be significant in diabetic patients.

Sympathetic Blocking Drugs

The sympathetic division of the autonomic nervous system has a vital function in the control of blood pressure. When sympathetic nerves are stimulated, norepinephrine is released by the nerve endings. In turn, norepinephrine stimulates alpha receptors and produces contraction (vasoconstriction) of the arterioles. In hypertension, the sympathetic nerves are functioning at a higher level of activity than normal. In addition, increased amounts of epinephrine from the adrenal gland may also be contributing to increased sympathetic activity. Thus, sympathetic blocking drugs are used to reduce the hyperactivity of the sympathetic nervous system.

Students should review the pharmacology of the alpha-blockers, beta-blockers, adrenergic neuronal blockers, and ganglionic blocking drugs in Chapters 6 and 8. Table 26:3 lists some of the sympathetic blockers used in the treatment of hypertension.

Centrally Acting Sympatholytic Drugs

There are several drugs that decrease sympathetic activity and BP by an action in the central nervous system. These drugs include clonidine (*Catapres*), guanabenz (*Wytensin*), guanfacine (*Tenex*), and methyldopa (*Aldomet*). Clonidine will be used to describe the actions of this drug class. Methyldopa was previously presented in Chapter 6.

Clonidine is a centrally acting drug used in the treatment of hypertension. The main action of

TABLE 26:2	Thiazide and Thiazide-like Diuretics Used in Treatment of Hypertension
DRUG (TRADE NAME)	**COMMON DAILY ORAL DOSAGE RANGE**
Thiazide Diuretics:	
bendroflumethiazide (*Naturetin*)	2.5–20 mg
benzthlazide (*Exna*)	50–100 mg
chlorothiazide (*Diuril*)	500–1000 mg
hydrochlorothiazide (*HydroDIURIL*)	50–100 mg
polythiazide (*Renese*)	2–4 mg
Thiazide-like Diuretics:	
chlorthalidone (*Hygroton*)	25–100 mg
quinethazone (*Hydromox*)	50–100 mg
indapamide (*Lozol*)	1.25–2.5 mg

TABLE 26:3 — Sympathetic Blocking Drugs Used in Treatment of Hypertension

DRUG (TRADE NAME)	COMMON DAILY DOSAGE RANGE	MECHANISM OF ACTION
clonidine (*Catapres*)	0.2–0.8 mg	Inhibits cardiovascular centers in the medulla
guanethidine (*Ismelin*)	25–100 mg	Interferes with release of norepinephrine from nerve endings
mecamylamine (*Inversine*)	5–25 mg	Ganglionic blocker
methyldopa (*Aldomet*)	250–2000 mg	Inhibits cardiovascular centers in the medulla
metoprolol (*Lopressor*)	100–400 mg	Blocks beta receptors in the heart
prazosin (*Minipress*)	1–20 mg	Blocks alpha receptors in vascular smooth muscle
propranolol (*Inderal*)	80–240 mg	Blocks beta receptors in the heart and arteries

clonidine is exerted on the medulla oblongata. Clonidine appears to interfere with sympathetic control of the vasomotor center in the medulla. Such interference results in a reduced level of sympathetic activity and a vasodilation of blood vessels. The adverse effects of clonidine include dry mouth, constipation, and drowsiness. If clonidine is abruptly discontinued, a withdrawal reaction may occur, with patients experiencing headache, nausea, and hypertensive crisis. To avoid withdrawal symptoms of clonidine, the dose should be reduced gradually over a 2-week period.

Beta-Adrenergic Blockers

The beta-blockers have several pharmacological actions that are of benefit in the treatment of hypertension. First, they block beta-1 receptors in the heart, lowering blood pressure by decreasing CO, especially when there is increased sympathetic activity. Second, they block the release of renin to interfere with the RAA system. There is also some evidence that propranolol, which is the most lipid-soluble beta-blocker, has a central action like clonidine and methyldopa to lower BP. The pharmacology of the beta-blockers was previously discussed in Chapter 6 and a summary of beta-blocking drugs can be found in Table 6:5.

Vasodilator Drugs

The vasodilator drugs act directly on vascular smooth muscle to cause relaxation. This results in vasodilation and a reduction in BP. Vasodilators are usually used in combination with diuretics and beta-blockers. This is necessary because vasodilators often cause fluid retention and tachycardia. The most widely used vasodilator is hydralazine.

Hydralazine (*Apresoline*)

Hydralazine is used in moderate and severe hypertension in combination with diuretics and sympathetic blockers. The main adverse effects are nausea, vomiting, headache, and reflex tachycardia. Long-term use may produce rheumatoid arthritis or a systemic lupus erythematosus-like syndrome.

Minoxidil (*Loniten*)

Minoxidil is a more potent vasodilator than is hydralazine, and it is indicated for patients who do not respond to triple therapy with other drug combinations. The usual dose is 10 to 40 mg per day. Minoxidil has the potential to produce a number of serious adverse effects, including myocardial ischemia and pericardial effusion. Minoxidil may also cause hirsutism (growth of hair); a topical preparation *Rogaine* is marketed specifically for this purpose.

Calcium Antagonists

As discussed in Chapters 23 and 24, calcium antagonists are drugs that interfere with the influx of calcium in cardiac and vascular smooth muscle. In vascular muscle, this interference causes vasodilation, which is useful in the treatment of hypertension. The calcium antagonists are usually thought of as composed of two subclasses. Verapamil and diltiazem are vasodilators with additional depressant actions on the heart. Nifedipine, nicardipine, and several newer drugs such as amlodipine (*Norvasc*), felodipine (*Plendil*), and isradipine (*DynaCirc*) produce only vasodilation. This latter group of drugs is widely used in the treatment of both hypertension and angina pectoris. Some of the calcium antagonists used to treat hypertension are presented in Table 26:4. The general pharmacology and adverse effects of the calcium antagonists were presented in Chapter 24.

Angiotensin-Converting Enzyme Inhibitors

The ACE inhibitors are an important class of drugs. The prototype of this class is captopril, which initially was used only in the treatment of severe hypertension. Captopril and newer ACE inhibitors are now widely used to treat all degrees of hypertension. When used properly, these inhibitors produce a low incidence of adverse effects and have some advantages over diuretics and beta-blockers. The ACE inhibitors are presented in Table 26:5.

Mechanism of Action

Angiotensin-converting enzyme (ACE) is necessary for the formation of angiotensin, a potent vasoconstrictor found in the blood and vasculature. Angiotensin is involved in the normal regulation of BP and blood volume. Drugs that inhibit ACE decrease angiotensin formation, produce vasodilation, and produce a lowering of BP. ACE-inhibitors usually increase renal blood flow, which is desirable. ACE inhibitors cause less interference with mental and physical performance, and many patients claim a better quality of life while taking ACE inhibitors than while taking other drug treatments.

Adverse Effects

Adverse effects associated with the ACE inhibitors are similar. Headache, dizziness, gastrointestinal (GI) disturbances, and rash are common complaints. Loss of taste sensation occurs with captopril. Less frequent is the development of a nonproductive cough or angioedema (swelling) of the face and oral cavity.

TABLE 26:4 — Calcium Antagonists Used in Treatment of Hypertension

DRUG (TRADE NAME)	COMMON DAILY DOSAGE RANGE	REMARKS
diltiazem (*Cardizem*)	180–360 mg	Vasodilation; decreases heart rate and AV conduction
nicardipine (*Cardene*)	60–120 mg	Potent vasodilator; may cause tachycardia
nifedipine (*Procardia XL*)	30–60 mg	Potent vasodilator; may cause tachycardia
verapamil (*Calan*)	240–360 mg	Vasodilation; decreases heart rate and atrioventricular (AV) conduction

TABLE 26:5 — Angiotensin-Converting Enzyme (ACE) Inhibitors

DRUG (TRADE NAME)	COMMON DAILY DOSAGE RANGE	DURATION OF ACTION
benazepril (*Lotensin*)	20–40 mg	24 hr
captopril (*Capoten*)	50–150 mg	3 hr
enalapril (*Vasotec*)	10–40 mg	24 hr
fosinopril (*Monopril*)	20–40 mg	24 hr
lisinopril (*Prinivil, Zestril*)	10–40 mg	24 hr
ramipril (*Altace*)	2.5–20 mg	24 hr
trandolapril (*Mavik*)	1–2 mg	24 hr

Angiotensin Receptor Blocking Drugs

Angiotensin receptor blockers antagonize the effects of angiotensin II by blocking the angiotensin II receptors on blood vessels and in the adrenal gland. This action blocks the vasocontriction and aldosterone secretion stimulated by angiotensin II. Consequently there is a lowering of blood pressure and less sodium and water retention. Losartan *(Cozaar)* was the first drug of this class to be approved. Candesartan *(Atacand)*, eprosartan *(Teveten)*, irbesartan *(Avapro)*, telmisartan *(Micardis)*, and valsartan *(Diovan)* are newer drugs in this class. Adverse effects of these drugs are similar to ACE inhibitors: however, these drugs usually do not cause cough and angioedema.

Treatment of Hypertensive Crisis

Hypertensive crisis is a condition in which severe hypertension suddenly develops, usually in individuals who have untreated hypertension or in response to some acute disease state. When BP is over 210/120, this condition is referred to as **malignant hypertension.** Immediate parenteral therapy is usually required to reduce BP quickly and avoid serious complications. Several vasodilator drugs produce rapid effects when administered IV. These include diazoxide and sodium nitroprusside.

Diazoxide (*Hyperstat*)

Structurally, diazoxide is similar to the thiazide diuretics. It is a very potent vasodilator, but it has no diuretic activity. It is used in hypertensive emergencies when a rapid reduction of BP is essential. Diazoxide is administered via IV injection. A 300-mg bolus is injected over a 10-minute interval. The hypotensive effects usually last 6 to 12 hours. The main adverse effects of diazoxide involve fluid retention, tachycardia, and hyperglycemia.

Sodium Nitroprusside (*Nipride*)

Sodium nitroprusside is a potent vasodilating agent used in hypertensive emergencies. Administered by slow intravenous infusion, the normal dose is approximately 3 μg per kg per minute. Since the drug becomes chemically altered when exposed to light, precautions, such as wrapping the bottle with foil, are necessary. The duration of action is short, usually 1 to 5 minutes.

Patient Education

Essential hypertension is a chronic disease. It requires lifelong treatment and medical supervision. Often, people who are told they have high BP have experienced no symptoms. However, once drug therapy begins, they may experience some drug side effects and often claim they were better off before they began treatment. Patients frequently skip doses or take only one medication of a multiple-drug regimen in order to reduce side effects or save money. Patients must understand the importance of taking all of their medications at the proper times. It is also important for hypertensive patients to have regular medical checkups to ensure that their BP is under control and that the medications are not producing any deleterious effects.

NOTE TO THE HEALTH CARE PROFESSIONAL

Patients must be aware that untreated or uncontrolled hypertension is the leading cause of death and disability in the United States. Complications include stroke, heart disease, kidney disease, and blindness. Nonpharmacological measures are important for controlling blood pressure. Dietary measures (sodium restriction), attaining normal body weight, elimination of smoking, exercise, and reducing stress can often lower blood pressure and reduce the amount of drug required.

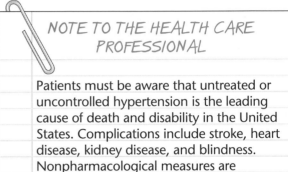

Patient Administration and Monitoring

Monitor vital signs during parenteral administration of antihypertensive drugs, especially during the treatment of hypertensive crisis.

Explain to patient the nondrug factors that can lower blood pressure and the importance of taking all medications exactly as prescribed.

Explain to patient the common side effects of the prescribed drugs (review individually).

Instruct patient to report extreme weakness, faintness, or other signs of excessive reduction of blood pressure. Also, significant changes in pulse or respiratory rate.

Instruct patient to check with the physician or pharmacist before taking over-the-counter drugs.

Explain to patient that excessive alcohol consumption may intensify the effects of blood pressure medication, and to check with the physician regarding the use of alcohol.

Chapter Review

Understanding Terminology

Match the definition in the left column with the appropriate term in the right column.

___ **1.** Measured in beats per minute.

___ **2.** Hypertension with no known cause.

___ **3.** Amount of blood pumped by the heart per minute.

___ **4.** Abnormally high blood pressure.

___ **5.** Resistance generated by the flow of blood through the arteries.

___ **6.** Blood pressure.

___ **7.** Hypertension with a known cause.

a. BP

b. CO

c. essential hypertension

d. HR

e. hypertension

f. PR

g. secondary hypertension

Answer the following questions in the spaces provided.

8. Define the following terms and explain their relationship: *CO, HR, SV.* _____
_____
_____

9. What is the relationship between *BP, CO,* and *PR?* _____
_____
_____

Acquiring Knowledge

Answer the following questions in the spaces provided.

1. List three physiological factors that determine blood pressure. _____
_____

2. List the five main classes of drugs used in the treatment of hypertension. _____
_____
_____

3. What is the mechanism of action of each of the drug classes to lower blood pressure?
_____
_____

4. When are the diuretic agents used in treating hypertension? _____
_____
_____

5. What are the three possible mechanisms of action of propranolol to lower blood pressure?
_____
_____

6. What effect do all sympathetic blocking drugs have in common? _____
_____
_____

7. Where is the site of action of clonidine? What are the adverse effects of clonidine? _____
_____
_____

8. List two adverse effects associated with each antihypertensive drug class. _____

_____

_____

9. What is hypertensive crisis? What drugs are used to treat it? _____

_____

_____

Applying Knowledge—On The Job

Use your critical thinking skills to answer the following questions in the spaces provided.

1. During a regular physical exam Mr. Johnson, who is moderately overweight and claims to smoke 10 to 15 cigarettes per day, records a blood pressure reading of 141/91. What might you tell Mr. Johnson concerning his blood pressure? Should he be put on antihypertensive medication?

_____

_____

2. Mrs. Cox is brought into the emergency room after passing out. She is sweating profusely and claims to have a pounding headache. You take her vital signs, and her blood pressure reads 215/125.

   a. What is your diagnosis? _____

_____

_____

   b. What needs to be done? _____

_____

_____

   c. What are some of the drugs that may be indicated? _____

_____

_____

3. Mrs. Goodman has stage 2 hypertension and has been prescribed chorothiazide (*Diuril*) and lisinopril (*Prinivil*) for several years. Her blood pressure reads 155/97. Upon questioning she admits that she usually only takes the diuretic and skips the other drug since it is so expensive.

   a. What should you tell Mrs. Goodman? _____

_____

   b. Is there anything that could be done to increase her drug compliance? _____

_____

_____

Internet *Connection*

Log on to the **MedicineNet** website (http://www.medicinenet.com), click on *Diseases and Conditions* heading and highlight the letter *H*. Click open *High Blood Pressure* and explore the numerous subheadings related to causes and treatments of hypertension.

Additional Reading

Dabrow-Woods, A. 2001. Improving the odds against hypertension. *Nursing 2001* 31 (8):36.

Epstein, M. 1996. Calcium channel blockers and hypertension. *Hospital Practice* 31 (12):93.

Setaro, J. F. 1995. Treatment of drug-resistant hypertension. *Hospital Medicine* 31 (4):45.

Woods, A. 2002. Patient-education guide—high blood pressure. *Nursing 2002* 32 (4):54.

27

ANTICOAGULANTS AND COAGULANTS

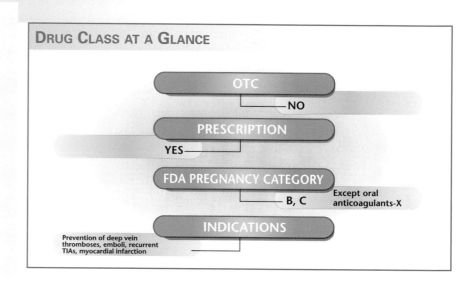

DRUG CLASS AT A GLANCE

OTC — NO

PRESCRIPTION — YES

FDA PREGNANCY CATEGORY — B, C Except oral anticoagulants-X

INDICATIONS — Prevention of deep vein thromboses, emboli, recurrent TIAs, myocardial infarction

Key Terms

agranulocytosis: condition in which the number of white blood cells, in particular the granulocytes, is less than normal.

alopecia: baldness or hair loss.

coagulation: process by which the blood changes from a liquid to a solid "plug" as a reaction to local tissue injury; normal blood clot formation.

hematuria: appearance of blood or red blood cells in the urine.

hemorrhage: loss of blood from blood vessels.

infarction: area of tissue that has died because of a sudden lack of blood supply.

mucopolysaccharide: naturally occurring substance formed by the combination of protein with carbohydrates (saccharides).

thrombocyte: cell in the blood, commonly called a platelet, that is necessary for coagulation.

thromboembolism: clots that jam a blood vessel; formed by the action of platelets and other coagulation factors in the blood.

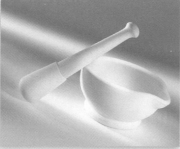

thrombophlebitis: inflammation of the walls of the veins, associated with clot formation.

thrombus: clot formed by the action of coagulation factors and circulating blood cells.

INTRODUCTION

Clot formation is essential to survival. Usually, a blood clot acts as a seal that prevents the further loss of blood, oxygen, and nutrients from a wounded area. In addition, factors present in the clot promote wound healing by signaling other cells (phagocytes) to carry off waste products and dead cells that accumulate at the site of injury. This protective mechanism (hemostasis) is always functioning to maintain homeostasis. Occasionally, the mechanism of clot formation becomes too active or the blood vessels become too narrow (atherosclerosis) to allow the clots to pass through easily. As a result, clots may become jammed in blood vessels, forming a **thromboembolism,** which prevents the normal flow of blood to other tissues. The heart, the lungs, and the brain are especially susceptible to damage caused by a loss or reduction in blood flow subsequent to thrombosis. Anticoagulants are used to prevent venous clotting in patients who have thromboembolic disorders because these drugs interfere with the ability of the blood to form stable clots.

COAGULATION

To understand how the anticoagulant drugs work, the process of normal blood clot formation **(coagulation)** must be understood. Many substances in the blood, such as platelets and clotting factors (Table 27:1), are responsible for initiating coagulation.

When an injury occurs, platelets **(thrombocytes)** immediately migrate to the damaged area. Because platelets stick to each other (aggregation) and to the vessel walls (adhesion), they form a plug around the injured tissue. Plasma clotting factors reach the platelet plug and interact with each other to form a stable blood clot. Hemostasis is the balance between clot formation and clot breakdown that occurs throughout the day. This process occurs in 4 stages.

A stable blood clot is produced in three stages:

Stage 1. A substance known as thromboplastin is produced.

Thromboplastin is produced by two different mechanisms—the intrinsic and extrinsic systems. The intrinsic system requires many clotting factors and platelets to stimulate production of thromboplastin. In contrast, the extrinsic system requires factor VII and tissue extract, a substance that is released from injured cells. Regardless of the pathway involved, once thromboplastin is produced, clotting proceeds automatically.

Stage 2. Thromboplastin converts prothrombins to thrombin.

Stage 3. Thrombin converts fibrinogen to fibrin and activates several clotting factors (V, VIII, XIII, and protein C). Fibrin is the primary element of a blood clot, and these activated factors build a fibrin mesh that holds the platelets (developing clot) together. The factors necessary for clot formation require calcium ions in order to function efficiently.

The clot is dissolved once the function has ended:

Stage 4: Plasmin is formed from the conversion of plasminogen by tissue plasminogen activator (tPA). Plasmin is an enzyme that acts upon the fibrin elements to produce a more soluble product.

ANTICOAGULANT MECHANISM OF ACTION

The clinically useful anticoagulants produce their pharmacological response by inhibiting platelet aggregation or interfering with plasma clotting factors. Antiplatelet drugs inhibit platelet aggregation, so the platelet plug does not form, or they block platelet adhesion so plug does not attach to the wall of the blood vessel and block blood flow. In general, these drugs make the platelets less sticky by directly attaching to

Anticoagulant Drug Effect on Clotting Factors

ANTICOAGULANT DRUG	CLOTTING FACTOR AFFECTED		VITAMIN K DEPENDENT
Heparins	II	Thrombin	No
	III	Thromboplastin, tissue factor	No
	X	Stuart—Prower factor	Yes
	XIII	Fibrin stabilizing factor	No
Oral anticoagulants	II	Prothrombin	Yes
	VII	Proconvertin	
	IX	Plasma thromboplastin component	
	X	Stuart—Prower factor	
	—	Protein C and S	
Antithrombin inhibitors	IIa	Thrombin	No
Chelators	IV	Calcium ions	No
Antiplatelet drugs	—	Platelet viscosity, aggregation and adhesion	No

membrane-bound receptors and by interfering with enzymes that express platelet function. Antiplatelet drugs include aspirin, dipyridamole, clopidogrel and ticlopidine.

Anticoagulants primarily inhibit plasma clotting factors. These drugs either block the formation of special proteins that are part of the coagulation cascade, or they attach to the preformed protein and disable it from performing its normal function. Heparin and the antithrombin inhibitors bind to circulating clotting factors, thromboplastin and glycoprotein IIa and prevent thrombin formation or the coagulation cascade that thrombin activates (Table 27:1). The coumarin derivatives prevent the synthesis of several clotting factors. The mechanism of anticoagulation determines the onset and duration of drug action. Heparin has a quick onset and duration of action because the anticoagulant effect occurs as soon as the thromboplastin-drug complex is formed. Coumarins have a long onset and duration of action because of the time required to clear the normal clotting factors from the circulation before an effect can be observed. Similarly, once normal protein synthesis has been interrupted, it requires days to produce fully functioning clotting factors.

Heparin and the coumarin derivatives are most frequently employed to prevent venous thrombosis, especially pulmonary embolism. These agents are used in the therapy of myocardial infarction, **thrombophlebitis** (inflammation of the walls of the veins), and stroke. The oral anticoagulants are the drugs of choice because they are relatively inexpensive, can be easily taken by patients, and are not associated with painful administration. However, standard heparin is always the preferred drug when an anticoagulant must be given to a pregnant woman. Due to its size, standard heparin does not cross the placenta and cannot affect the developing fetus. Other uses of anticoagulants include clot suppression prior to blood transfusion and during open heart surgery.

Heparins

The class of heparins is comprised of two groups: standard heparin and low molecular weight (LMW) heparins. Heparin is a naturally occurring **mucopolysaccharide** first identified in 1928. Then, as now, the main source of heparin is extraction from the lungs and intestines of cattle and pigs. Standard heparin, also called unfractionated heparin, contains the full complement of saccharides of endogenous heparin. Recently, several low-molecular-weight heparins have become available. These LMW heparins are derived from porcine heparin but only contain an active anticoagulant fraction of heparin. Compared to the molecular weight of standard heparin, 3000 daltons, the LMW heparins (ardeparin, enoxaprin, dalteparin) are smaller, ranging between 2000 and 9000 daltons. While the LMW heparins interfere with the coagulation cascade, they cannot produce the same spectrum of interference and are not interchangeable with standard heparin.

Heparins are considered peripherally acting anticoagulants because their anionic (negatively charged) character complexes with circulating clotting factors. As long as heparin is in contact with the clotting factors, coagulation is depressed and clot formation is inhibited. All heparins bind thromboplastin (factor III) and then proceed to inactivate factor X. Although the LMW heparins are more effective at binding active factor X, standard heparin is more effective at inactivating factor XIII (fibrin-stabilizing factor) and binding thrombin (active factor II). This advantage is conferred on standard heparin because the antithrombin action requires the additional chain of saccharides removed to form the LMW heparins. Unlike the LMW heparins, standard heparin also depresses platelet aggregation.

Route of Administration

All heparins cannot be administered by mouth because gastric acid would destroy the mucopolysaccharide. Standard heparin, therefore, is usually administered intravenously or subcutaneously. LMW heparins are only administered subcutaneously. Intramuscular injection should be avoided because painful hematomas can occur. The advantage of the LMW heparins is that the bioavailability is almost complete (90 percent) following subcutaneous administration compared to standard heparin (30 percent). In addition, in patients with normal renal function, the LMW heparins can be dosed based on body size without coagulation test monitoring. Standard heparin requires periodic coagulation monitoring to adjust the therapeutic dose, minimize the bleeding potential and maintaining adequate clot suppression.

The onset of action for all heparins is rapid, within 5 minutes, and the duration of action is usually 2 to 5 hours. Drugs derived from animal sources must undergo a standard biological assay to determine their purity, quality, and potency. Drugs such as heparin are administered in units of activity rather than milligrams. One hundred United States Pharmacopeia (USP) units correspond to approximately 1 mg of commercially prepared heparin. Because bioequivalence problems have been encountered with heparin products, products from different manufacturers should not be interchanged in an individual patient. Although the LMW heparins are fragments from the same parent, these drugs cannot be interchanged with standard heparin due to the variability in the anticoagulant activity. Moreover, there is no conversion that would predict a bioequivalent dosing to standard heparin.

Despite the newer heparins, standard heparin use is increasing. Standard heparin is indicated for arterial and venous thrombotic conditions.

Lipolysis

In addition to the anticoagulant action, heparin and ardeparin have the ability to clear fatty molecules from the plasma. Heparin stimulates an enzyme (lipoprotein lipase) that hydrolyzes the triglycerides in the blood. This enzyme reaction reduces large fat molecules in the plasma. This effect has no influence on heparin's anticoagulant action, and its physiological importance is not fully understood. Eventually, heparin is metabolized by the liver or excreted unchanged into the urine. Patients with renal impairment or kidney disease tend to accumulate heparin because they cannot efficiently clear it from the blood.

Adverse Effects

The major toxicity associated with the use of heparin is **hemorrhage.** At high levels, heparin causes bleeding to occur in mucous membranes (petechiae) and open wounds, such as scratches, cuts, and abrasions. If hemorrhage occurs in the gastrointestinal (GI) membranes, patients' blood pressure and hematocrit may fall even though there are no external signs of bleeding. The dose and frequency of administration should be reduced when hemorrhage is evident. Use in elderly patients requires special attention because enoxaparin elimination may be delayed. Anemia has been reported with ardeparin and enoxaparin.

Protamine sulfate is the specific antidote in heparin toxicity. Each milligram of protamine sulfate will neutralize 90 to 120 USP units of heparin, 1 mg of enoxaparin, or 100 International Units (IU) of ardeparin or dalteparin. Protamine binds to the heparin molecules and inhibits the anticoagulant action. Administration of heparin or protamine should always be accompanied by coagulation tests to determine the degree of clot suppression that is present (see "Monitoring Coagulation," page 296).

Other side effects seen with any chronic heparin use include hypersensitivity, fever, **alopecia** (hair loss), osteoporosis, and thrombocytopenia (decrease in the number of blood platelets). Thrombocytopenia occurs occasionally in patients receiving heparin who are undergoing orthopedic or cardiopulmonary by-pass surgery. The occurrence is dose-related and occurs more frequently with bovine heparin than porcine heparin. The thrombocytopenia is confirmed by a reduction in platelets by 50 percent (fewer than

50,000 mm³) within 2 weeks of initiating treatment. As the thrombocytopenia develops, the patient may have no symptoms such as bleeding that would indicate the evolving condition. The decrease in platelets appears to be mediated through an immune response; however, it is not the heparin molecule that stimulates the development of antibodies. Rather, heparin complexes with platelet factor 4 (PF-4) and binds to the platelet membrane. It is this complex that is immunogenic.

LMW heparins and heparinoids have an additional warning in the product use label which identifies a potential risk of developing epidural or spinal hematomas when these anticoagulants are administered to patients receiving epidural or spinal anesthesia. The risk of irreversible paralysis from the spinal hematoma is increased when the patient is also receiving additional anticoagulants, and nonsteroidal antiinflammatory platelet inhibitors. Although these effects have been reported, they are considered to be relatively uncommon.

Antithrombins

Thrombin inhibitors (lepirudin, argatroban, bivalirudin) reversibly bind with thrombin and reduce the thrombin-catalyzed activations of factors V, VIII, XIII, protein C and platelet aggregation. These inhibitors are highly selective for thrombin and are indicated specifically for the prophylaxis and treatment of heparin-induced thrombocytopenia. Coagulation is suppressed while heparin is withdrawn.

Thrombin inhibitors are synthetic (argatroban) or recombinant rDNA hirudin (lepirudin) that mimic the anticoagulant activity of polypeptides extracted from leech saliva. Bivalirudin is approved for use in patients with unstable angina who are undergoing percutaneous transluminal coronary angioplasty (PTCA) and concurrently taking aspirin for platelet inhibition.

Coumarin Derivatives

The coumarin derivatives include dicumarol and warfarin sodium (see Table 27:2). Dicumarol (bishydroxycoumarin) was originally discovered as a product of spoiled sweet clover. Cattle that grazed on the contaminated clover developed hemorrhagic disease. In addition, people who drank the milk from these cows developed hemorrhages because they ingested the active anticoagulant substance. The coumarins are significantly different from heparin because they can be administered orally. For this reason, these

drugs are usually referred to as the oral anticoagulants. The oral anticoagulant of choice is warfarin sodium.

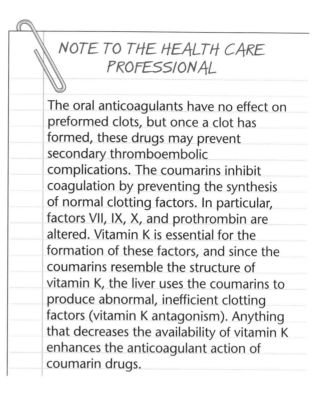

NOTE TO THE HEALTH CARE PROFESSIONAL

The oral anticoagulants have no effect on preformed clots, but once a clot has formed, these drugs may prevent secondary thromboembolic complications. The coumarins inhibit coagulation by preventing the synthesis of normal clotting factors. In particular, factors VII, IX, X, and prothrombin are altered. Vitamin K is essential for the formation of these factors, and since the coumarins resemble the structure of vitamin K, the liver uses the coumarins to produce abnormal, inefficient clotting factors (vitamin K antagonism). Anything that decreases the availability of vitamin K enhances the anticoagulant action of coumarin drugs.

The onset of anticoagulant activity with the coumarins is slow, 12 to 72 hours. Several days may be required to produce a significant amount of nonreactive clotting factors. Similarly, the duration of action is long (2 to 10 days) even after drug administration has been discontinued. The oral anticoagulants are highly bound to plasma proteins and are eventually metabolized by the liver. Both of these factors are responsible for the many drug interactions that occur with these drugs.

Adverse Effects

Hemorrhage is always the major toxicity associated with the use of an anticoagulant. **Hematuria** (blood or red blood cells in the urine), bleeding of the gums, and petechiae are common side effects that reflect local hemorrhaging. In the presence of hemorrhage, the action of the coumarins cannot be rapidly reversed by merely discontinuing the drug. The antidote for overdose includes 2.5 to 25 mg of vitamin K_1 (phytonadione) given parenterally (usually IM, SC). Because the mechanism of action involves synthetic pathways in the liver, administration of phytonadione cannot be expected to produce immediate results. The counteraction of phytonadione is evident by monitoring prothrombin time within 2 hours

Comparison of Some Commonly Employed Anticoagulant Drugs

DRUG (TRADE NAME)	DAILY MAINTENANCE DOSE	COAGULATION TEST USED TO MONITOR THE THERAPEUTIC RESPONSE
adeparin (*Normiflo*)	50 anti-Xa units/kg every 12 hr up to 14 days	Routine blood and platelet counts
anisindione (*Miradon*)	25–250 mg PO	Prothrombin time (protime, PT) or INR
clopidogrel (*Plavix*)	75 mg daily PO	Routine blood and platelet counts
dalteparin (*Fragmin*)	2500 IU/day, 1–2 hrs before surgery, up to 10 days postsurgery	Routine blood and platelet counts
dicumarol	25–200 mg PO	Prothrombin time (protime, PT) or INR
enoxaparin (*Lovenox*)	30 mg BID pre knee surgery, up to 12 days postsurgery	Routine blood and platelet counts
enoxaparin	40 mg QD for abdominal surgery	Routine blood and platelet counts
heparin sodium injection	10,000–12,000 units initially followed by 15,000–20,000 units every 12 hr SC; 5000–10,000 units every 4–6 hr IV	Whole blood clotting time; activated partial thromboplastin time (APTT)
heparin sodium lock flush solution (*Heparin Lock Flush, Hep-Lock*)	Not intended for therapeutic use; used for maintenance of indwelling IV catheters	—
ticlopidine (Ticlid)	250 mg BID PO	Routine blood and platelet counts
warfarin sodium (*Coumadin*)	2–10 mg PO	Prothrombin time (protime, PT) or INR

after the antidote is given. In severe hemorrhage, fresh whole blood or plasma may also be administered to provide a full complement of normal clotting factors.

Other side effects accompanying the use of oral anticoagulants include nausea, diarrhea, urticaria, and alopecia. To reduce gastrointestinal (GI) distress, large doses of oral anticoagulants may be administered in divided doses.

Contraindications

Anticoagulants of any type are contraindicated in patients with subacute bacterial endocarditis, ulcerative lesions (GI), visceral carcinoma, threatened abortion, severe hypertension, and recent surgery on the brain or spinal cord. Any patient with active bleeding tendencies should not receive anticoagulants. Heparins are contraindicated in patients with a hypersensitivity to individual heparins, pork products, sulfites, benzyl alcohol, or heparin-induced

thrombocytopenia. The oral anticoagulants should not be used in patients known to be vitamin K deficient.

The most important contraindication for the oral anticoagulants concerns the use of these drugs during pregnancy. The oral anticoagulants cross the placenta and may produce hemorrhaging in the fetus because the fetus is dependent on the mother for its source of vitamin K and coagulation factors. Administration of oral anticoagulants during pregnancy will result in a phenomenon known as hemorrhagic disease of the newborn (HDN). Vitamin K_1 (phytonadione) is administered to the mother (prophylaxis) or to the newborn (treatment) when HDN is anticipated. A single intramuscular dose of 0.5 to 1 mg can be administered to the newborn within 1 hour after birth. The mother may be given oral or parenteral prophylaxis 12 to 24 hours before delivery. Intramuscular injection of 1 to 5 mg or oral doses of 2 mg have been successfully used.

Intravenous administration is not recommended because severe anaphylactic-type reactions have occurred. However, if the intravenous route must be used, the phytonadione *must be injected slowly, not to exceed 1 mg per minute.*

Vitamin K Derivatives

As mentioned, natural vitamin K promotes synthesis of prothrombin (factor II), proconvertin (factor VII), plasma thromboplastin component (factor IX), and Stuart factor (X). Synthetic derivatives of vitamin K are available. Vitamin K_1 (phytonadione) and vitamin K_3 (menadione) are fat soluble, whereas vitamin K_4 (menadiol) is water soluble. Selection of the appropriate vitamin for treatment of oral anticoagulant overdose or HDN is based on the degree of activity and onset of action. Phytonadione may be the drug of choice because it has the same degree of activity as the naturally occurring vitamin and may have a better margin of safety than do the other vitamin analogs.

Indandiones

The indandiones (*anisindione*) are oral anticoagulants that produce essentially the same pharmacological actions as the coumarins. However, they have a shorter onset of action. In general, this class, which includes anisindione, produces a greater incidence of toxicity than do other available anticoagulants. The toxic reactions may include fever, rash, hepatitis, renal damage, and **agranulocytosis.** After oral administration, these drugs color the urine red-orange, which may resemble hematuria. This discoloration is of no clinical importance, but it may alarm patients if the side effect has not been explained.

Antiplatelet Drugs

The class of oral antiplatelet drugs include aspirin, dipyridamole, clopidogrel, and ticlopidine. All of these drugs are well absorbed following oral administration. Aspirin was presented in the chapter on nonsteroidal antiinflammatory drugs (NSAIDs) as a powerful inhibitor of the prostaglandins. In platelets, this enzyme pathway produces thromboxane A_2 a potent platelet aggregator and vasoconstrictor. When platelets release thromboxane A_2, it constricts blood vessels and slows blood flow so the platelets have an opportunity to stick to each other and to the wall of the blood vessel. Prostacyclin, another product of the cyclooxgenase pathway released from the blood vessel membrane, counteracts the action of thromboxane by dilating the vessels and inhibiting platelet aggregation. Normally, this balance between prostacyclin and thromboxane A_2 activity keeps the platelet plugs from significantly blocking blood flow and oxygenation of the tissues. In conditions such as arterial thrombosis, deep vein thrombosis, myocardial infarction, and stroke, platelets increase thromboxane production and demonstrate an increased sensitivity to aggregate.

Aspirin in doses from 81 mg (baby aspirin) to 325 mg (adult analgesic dose) irreversibly alters platelet cyclooxygenase. Platelets do not have a nucleus and, therefore, do not have the internal machinery to make new cyclooxygenase. Thromboxane cannot be generated until new platelets are formed. Although aspirin also blocks prostacyclin, the blood vessels are able to synthesis new cyclooxygenase within a few hours.

Clopidogrel (Plavix) and ticlopidine (Ticlid) inhibit platelet aggregation by blocking adenosine diphosophate (ADP) binding to membrane receptors and preventing ADP activation of glycoproteins IIa/IIIB in the coagulation cascade. They do not have any effect on the cyclooxygenase pathway like aspirin. These drugs irreversibly modify the receptor so the platelet cannot respond to ADP for the rest of its life span (8 to 11 days).

Dipyridamole (Persantine, Aggrenox) is a weak antiplatelet inhibitor. It reversibly interferes with platelet aggregation by increasing adenosine, an inhibitor of platelet reactivity, and inhibiting phosphodiesterase within the platelets.

Aspirin is the most inexpensive, effective antiplatelet drug recommended by physicians to reduce the incidence of clots that might injure the heart. Aspirin in doses not greater than 325 mg a day is recommended for the prevention of thrombi, stroke, and heart attack. Aspirin also prevents transient ischemic attacks (TIAs) in stroke patients but has no action on the formed clot. Aspirin is considered as effective or more effective with fewer serious adverse effects compared to the newer antiplatelet drugs. Doses of aspirin greater than 1000 mg daily are no more effective as an antithrombotic and usually increase the side effects. Clopidogrel is significantly more costly than aspirin and is used to reduce myocardial infarction, stroke, and death, especially in patients who are sensitive to the gastrointestinal bleeding induced by aspirin. Dipyridamole is only used for prevention of thromboembolism after heart valve replacement surgery. The antiplatelet drugs are used in combination to produce clinically significant reductions in reinfarction and death following myocardial infarction in men. The same clinical benefit has not been shown to occur in women post myocardial infarction.

Common less serious side effects associated with antiplatelet drugs are similar to aspirin and include headache, vomiting, rash, diarrhea, and dizziness. Ticlopidine and clopidogrel can produce severe thrombocytopenia, a dramatic reduction in platelets that does not allow the patient to clot so internal bleeding occurs.

Chelators

Several drugs inhibit coagulation by interfering with essential ions in the blood. Chelating drugs, such as edetic acid (ethylenediaminetetraacetic acid [EDTA]) and oxalic acid, bind calcium ions so that the coagulation scheme is interrupted. These agents are not routinely employed as systemic anticoagulants. However, oxalic acid in particular is present in commercially prepared test tubes to prevent the coagulation of blood taken for routine hematological tests.

Clinical Indications for Anticoagulants

The antiplatelet and anticoagulant drugs are the mainstay of clot prevention, whether given prophylactically prior to a thrombotic episode, or to reduce recurrence of thrombi in the management of peripheral vascular disease or following heart attack. Peripheral vascular disease includes deep vein thrombosis (DVT), a condition in which thrombi form within the lower extremeties usually as a result of poor circulation. Patients who are recuperating from surgery (hip and knee replacement), or have chronic inflammatory illnesses such as Crohn's disease, or vascular injury (stroke, ischemic heart disease) and women during pregnancy are more likely to develop DVT. These patients often have a period of inactivity during which the blood flow may pool or slow down creating a stasis in the circulation that encourages clotting factors and platelets to initiate coagulation. Localized coagulation is also likely to occur when additional risk factors such as smoking or hypertension are present. The localized thrombi may be associated with vascular spasms, pain, tenderness in the legs, swelling and warmth, or, in half the patients, there are no symptoms to warn of impending danger. The most significant clinical risk in DVT is that thrombi will break loose, enter the circulation within the lungs and block critical blood flow within the pulmonary system. This blockade could lead to tissue death due to stagnant blood flow and interrupted oxygenation of the tissues (ischemia). Pulmonary embolism can be a life-threatening condition.

Recently the risk of DVT has been extended to situations where people are confined or sitting motionless for long periods. "Economy Class" syndrome is a genuine condition associated with inactivity especially during long air flights, but it is not restricted to the economy section of the plane. Dehydration, through increased alcohol intake or reduced water consumption, reduces the blood volume (makes it relatively thicker) and fosters an environment of stasis and local clot formation.

Among the heparins available today, the full mucopolysaccharide referred to as heparin is approved for the broadest spectrum of use. Heparin is approved for the prophylaxis and treatment of venous thrombosis, and emboli associated with peripheral arteries and atrial fibrillation. It is also indicated for prevention of postoperative deep vein thrombosis (DVT) and pulmonary embolism in patients undergoing major abdominal surgery or who are at risk of developing thromboembolic disease. It is used to prevent clotting during cardiovascular surgery, transfusions, dialysis, and extracorporeal circulation, and in the diagnosis and treatment of disseminated intravascular coagulation.

Low-molecular-weight heparins are approved for use in prevention of DVT in selective procedures as follows: ardeparin (knee replacement), dalteparin (abdominal surgery), and enoxaparin (knee and hip replacement and abdominal surgery). For these parenteral anticoagulants the dose must be customized to the patient within recommended guidelines for time of administration (see Table 27:2).

Oral anticoagulants are approved for use in the prophylaxis and treatment of venous thrombosis, pulmonary embolism, and atrial fibrillation with embolization.

Anticoagulants and antiplatelet drugs are also indicated in coronary artery disease, to prevent heart attack, stroke, or angina. Antiplatelet drugs are routinely used in angioplasty and coronary stents to keep arteries previously obstructed by blood clots clear.

Drug Interactions

Heparin undergoes fewer drug interactions than do the oral anticoagulants. Any drugs that are known to affect platelet aggregation will probably cause increased bleeding when taken concomitantly with heparin. Such drugs include nonsteroidal antiinflammatory drugs (aspirin, ibuprofen, indomethacin, phenylbutazone), dextran, and high doses of penicillin. Digitalis and tetracyclines have been reported to counteract the anticoagulant action of heparin. The mechanism of this action is not known. Diazepam plasma levels have been reported to increase with concomitant heparin therapy.

The oral anticoagulants have the greatest potential for clinically significant interactions with other medications. These drugs are associated with three major sites where interaction may occur. Oral anticoagulants may be displaced from plasma protein binding sites, which may increase their plasma concentrations and toxicity. In addition, any drug that interferes with liver metabolism may increase or decrease the response of the oral anticoagulants. Finally, because they are taken by mouth, absorption of oral anticoagulants may be inhibited by other oral medications that bind to the anticoagulants. Several drugs, some available over the counter, such as acetaminophen, have been associated with increased bleeding from the oral anticoagulants, but the mechanism or site of action has not yet been determined.

Because it is so inexpensive and available without a prescription, aspirin is arguably one of the most frequently used medications anyone can take as needed. Cardiac prophylaxis is dependent upon aspirin's antiplatelet effect sustained by taking low doses of aspirin every day. Daily use of aspirin and ibuprofen, also available over-the-counter, can cancel the antiplatelet effects of aspirin. The reason is that ibuprofen, a COX-1 inhibitor, can occupy the same enzymatic site in the platelets but does not have the ability to alter the active site on cyclooxygenase (COX) or inhibit thromboxane production. During this time, the patient does not have the cardioprotection of altered platelets. This interaction may extend to other COX-1 inhibitors, such as naproxen and ketoprofen. Occasional ibuprofen use does not present the liability; however, another choice of NSAID may be better to take when a daily NSAID and daily aspirin prophylaxis is indicated. In general, aspirin should be taken 2 hours prior to ibuprofen so that aspirin has the opportunity to interact with the platelets first.

Table 27:3 describes numerous drug interactions that occur with anticoagulant drugs. Careful monitoring and appropriate dosage adjustments will ensure the safety of combination drug therapy in patients who receive anticoagulants.

Special Considerations

Patients receiving anticoagulant therapy should be instructed to be attentive to the appearance of bruises, bleeding gums, hematuria, or unusually heavy menstrual flow, because these are signs of an increased bleeding tendency. In addition, patients should be cautioned to avoid the concomitant use of alcohol or drugs that alter platelet function, such as over-the-counter products containing aspirin or salicylates.

Ideally, anticoagulant therapy should be administered at the same time daily. Whenever medications are added to or deleted from the regimen of patients receiving an anticoagulant, the patients' coagulation status is subject to change. Patients should therefore be carefully observed for signs of increased bleeding or hemorrhage. Fever or rash that develops during anticoagulant therapy should be regarded as an indication of potential complication. Patients must be advised to adhere strictly to the prescribed dose schedule for oral anticoagulants. Oral medication should not be discontinued unless on the specific advice of the treating physician.

Heparin is often administered by intermittent intravenous infusion. Concomitant parenteral medications should not be administered into the heparin infusion line (piggyback) to avoid potential incompatibility reactions that would inactivate the anticoagulants. The low-molecular-weight anticoagulants should not be mixed with other injects or infusions. Drug solutions known to be physically incompatible with heparin are presented in Table 27:3. When drawing blood, especially for the purpose of evaluating patients' coagulation status, samples should always be taken from the opposite arm (non-IV line) to avoid false activated partial thromboplastin time (APTT) values.

MONITORING COAGULATION

The dosage of any anticoagulant is individualized to the patient. The therapeutic dosage is established and maintained by evaluation of the patient's clotting time. Once a patient is stabilized, coagulation may be monitored every 4 to 6 weeks. To avoid the danger of hemorrhage due to too much anticoagulant, the coagulability of the blood should be measured before more drug is administered. Among the tests used to monitor coagulation status are whole blood clotting time, partial thromboplastin time (PTT), prothrombin time (PT), and the international normalized ratio (INR). The INR is being used because commercial

TABLE 27:3   Drug Interactions With Anticoagulant Drugs

Anticoagulant: Heparins

INTERACTS WITH	RESPONSE	INTERACTS WITH	RESPONSE
Aspirin cephalosporins Dextran dipyridamole ibuprofen indomethacin NSAIDs penicillin (high doses)	Increased bleeding	codeine dopamine hydrocortisone hydroxyzine meperidine methadone methylprednisolone morphine prochlorperazine promethazine vitamins (multiple)	Incompatible when mixed with these solutions for parenteral infusion
digitalis nicotine Antihistamines Tetracyclines	Decreased anticoagulant action	Oral anticoagulants platelet inhibitors (NSAIDs)	False protime values, enhances anticoagulation

Antibiotics:
  Amikacin
  Aminoglycosides
  cephaloridine
  erythromycin
  Penicillins
  Polymyxins
  Tetracyclines
	Incompatible when mixed with these solutions for parenteral infusion		

Anticoagulant: Oral Anticoagulants

INTERACTS WITH	RESPONSE	INTERACTS WITH	RESPONSE
chloral hydrate clofibrate diflusinal ethacrynic acid naldixic acid Penicillins Salicylates	Increased bleeding via protein binding displacement	amiodarone chloramphenicol cimetidine co-trimoxazole ifosfamide lovastatin methylphenidate omeprazole phenylbutazone propafenone quinidine quinine sulfinpyrazone sulfamethoxazole- trimethoprim	Increased bleeding due to decreased liver metabolism of the anticoagulants

Alteplase
Antibiotics:
  kanamycin
  neomycin
  sulfonamides
Tetracyclines
Vitamin E
	Increased bleeding time due to decreased availability of vitamin K	Aspirin
		Cephalosporins
		dipyridamole
		heparin
		phenylbutazone
		quinidine
		quinine
		Steroids
		sulfinpyrazone
			Increased bleeding due to decreased platelet aggregation, suppression of prothrombin formation, interference with other clotting mechanisms

(continued)

Drug Interactions With Anticoagulant Drugs, continued

Anticoagulant: Oral Anticoagulants, continued

INTERACTS WITH	RESPONSE	INTERACTS WITH	RESPONSE
acetaminophen Androgens Beta-blockers chlorpropamine clofibrate Corticosteroids cyclophosphamide danazol dextrothyroxine disulfiram erythromycin fluconazole Glucagon hydantoins Influenza vaccine isoniazid ketoconazole miconazole Quinolones propoxyphene propranolol ranitidine Streptokinase sulindac tamoxifen Thyroid hormone	Increased bleeding by unknown mechanism	aluminum hydroxide cholestyramine colestipol sulcralfate	Decreased anticoagulant effect via decreased oral absorption of the anticoagulant
		Oral contraceptives estrogens Vitamin K	Decreased anticoagulant effect via stimulation of clotting factor synthesis
		Adrenal corticosteroids ethacrynic acid indomethacin phenylbutazone Potassium products Salicylates	Ulcerogenic effects
Alcohol Barbiturates carbamazepine ethchlorvynol glutethimide griseofulvin nafcillin rifampin	Decreased anticoagulant effect via increased liver metabolism of the anticoagulant	ascorbic acid cholestyramine Estrogens Ethanol ethchlorvynol griseofulvin nafcillin Oral contraceptives spironolactone Thiazide diuretics Vitamin K sucralfate	Decreased anticoagulant effect of warfarin or anisindione by a variety of mechanisms

thromboplastin response to anticoagulants vary greatly between batches. The INR calibrates the commercial rabbit thromboplastins against an international human reference standard.

The effect of heparin is most frequently assessed with the whole blood clotting time and the activated partial thromboplastin time (APTT). These tests are usually performed 1 hour prior to the next scheduled dose of heparin. Generally, the PTT is maintained at twice the normal value when heparin is employed. Because of their selective inhibition of coagulation factors that are associated with the APTT monitoring reagents, the LMW drugs cannot be monitored accurately. The therapeutic effect of the LMW drugs is assessed by routine total blood and platelet counts, and urinalysis throughout therapy.

The oral anticoagulants must be monitored with the one-stage prothrombin time, or protime (PT) or the INR. Because of the long onset of action of these drugs, the initial dose cannot be changed for 3 to 5 days. It takes this long to achieve the peak anticoagulant response. During this time, periodic protime evaluation indicates the degree of clot suppression. The protime may be maintained at 1.2–1.5 times the control, which may be a 2–4 INR value. Heparin is known to interfere with accurate protime determinations when it is administered in conjunction with oral anticoagulants. When needed, oral anticoagulants should be given at least 5 hours after the last IV heparin dose or 24 hours after the last SC dose in order to achieve an accurate PT result.

THROMBOLYTIC ENZYMES

Thrombolytic enzymes are used to dissolve preformed blood clots and, therefore, are called "clotbusters." These enzymes stimulate the synthesis of fibrinolysin which breaks the clot into soluble products. This class of drugs includes urokinase (*Abbokinase*), streptokinase (*Strepase*), anistreplase (*Eminase*), alteplase (*Activase*), and reteplase (*Retevase*). Alteplase, also referred to as tissue plasminogen activator (tPA), and reteplase are thrombolytic enzymes produced through the biotechnology of recombinant DNA. Alteplase is a purified glycoprotein (527 amino acids) that binds to fibrin within the clot, stimulates conversion of plasminogen to plasmin, and initiates clot dissolution (fibrinolysis). Reteplase, derived from the alteplase glycoprotein, contains 355 of the 527 amino acids.

Thrombolytic enzymes are used to lyse pulmonary emboli and coronary artery thromboses during acute myocardial infarction. To receive maximum benefit, the enzymes must be administered as soon as possible following indications that a clot or infarct has occurred. For the treatment of acute myocardial infarction, the timing of drug administration for successful clot resolution is usually within 1 to 6 hours from the onset of symptoms. For pulmonary embolism, the time for initiation of therapy may be up to a few days. There is evidence that streptokinase is as effective as alteplase, even though the cost of alteplase therapy is tremendously more expensive than that of streptokinase. The cost of the product reflects the biotechnical development process of the drug and not necessarily a clinically significant improvement in treatment over existing products.

Dose Administration

Because thrombolytic enzymes are proteins, they are administered by parenteral infusion, usually intravenous. As proteins derived from natural sources or recombinant technology, the amount of active substance is provided as International Units (bioassay) or the milligram equivalent. Streptokinase is administered intravenously 250,000 IU over 30 minutes followed by 100,000 IU per hour up to 72 hours for the treatment of deep vein or arterial thrombosis. For the treatment of acute myocardial infarction, the available 1,500,000 IU vial diluted to 45 ml is administered as a total dose within 60 minutes. Streptokinase (and urokinase) is also used (250,000 IU per 2 ml) to clear occluded arteriovenous cannulae. Anistreplase is given as 30 units over 2 to 5 minutes, while alteplase is administered as 100 mg (58 million IU) in divided doses over a 2- to 3-hour period.

At the end of the streptokinase or urokinase infusion, treatment usually continues with heparin infusion. Heparin is begun only after the thrombin time has decreased to less than 2 times the normal control (usually 3 to 4 hours after completion of urokinase infusion). After constant intravenous infusion (4400 units per kg per hour) urokinase is cleared (within 20 minutes) by the liver. The mechanism of streptokinase elimination is not known. Alteplase is rapidly cleared from the blood within 5 to 10 minutes after the infusion is terminated.

Adverse Effects

The major adverse effect associated with the use of thrombolytic enzymes is hemorrhage. Concomitant use of heparin, oral anticoagulants, or drugs known to alter platelet function (aspirin and nonsteroidal antiinflammatory drugs) is not recommended because of the increased risk of bleeding. Since these drugs are enzymes, mild allergic reactions have occurred in patients during use. Allergic reactions include skin rash, itching, nausea, headache, fever, bronchospasm, or musculoskeletal pain. Although severe allergic reactions to enzyme therapy may require discontinuation of therapy, milder reactions are usually controlled with antihistamine or corticosteroid therapy. Contraindications to the use of thrombolytic drugs include conditions such as active internal bleeding, cerebral vascular accident (CVA) within the past 2 months, intracranial or intraspinal surgery, or intracranial tumors. Alteplase and reteplase have been associated with cardiogenic shock, arrhythmias, and recurrent ischemia among the reported adverse effects; however, these are frequent sequelae of myocardial infarction and may or may not be attributable to the drug.

Clinical Indications

Thrombolytic enzymes are approved for use in the management of acute myocardial infarction, acute ischemic stroke, and pulmonary embolism. Streptokinase is also approved for lysis of deep vein thrombi. Streptokinase and urokinase have been used for clearance of occluded arteriovenous cannulae or IV catheters obstructed by clotted blood or fibrin.

Thrombolytic enzymes are available as powders (or lyophilized powders) containing varying amounts of active substance, which must be reconstituted prior to infusion. These products are stored in powder form at room temperature (15° to 30°C) or refrigerated (2° to 8°C) prior to reconstitution.

Reconstitution should occur just before use, although urokinase solution is stable for up to 24 hours, and streptokinase may be used up to 8 hours after reconstitution. Unused solutions should be discarded after that time. Alteplase has the added requirement that it be protected from excessive exposure to light. *None of these enzyme infusion solutions should have other medications added to them.*

Coagulants/Hemostatics

There are occasions when an agent is required to decrease the incidence or severity of hemorrhage. The use of vitamin K_1 and protamine sulfate as

---

Patient Administration and Monitoring

Since many of the anticoagulants are used in a controlled hospital setting, close patient observation minimizes the risk associated with the onset of adverse reactions. In the hospital environment it is assumed that drug interactions which potentiate bleeding such as platelet inhibitors (aspirin, nonsteroidal anti-inflammatory drugs [NSAIDs]) are minimized by frequent chart review by the medical-pharmacy team. Patients certainly may continue to take oral anticoagulants on an outpatient basis for chronic prophylaxis of emboli. Therefore it becomes necessary to provide clear instruction not only to the patient, but to relatives and friends who may participate in home care of the patient. Adverse reactions with this class of drugs are potentially life-threatening and need to be communicated to the doctor immediately.

Patient Instructions

As a general safety precaution, patients taking anticoagulants should carry identification that indicates the medication, reason for use, and potential for bleeding to occur.

Patients should clearly be told that dosing is highly individual and may have to be adjusted several times to achieve the best result. For this reason patients are urged to comply with the medication schedule and follow-up appointments during which coagulation status will be monitored. Oral anticoagulants should be taken at the same time each day.

Before undergoing dental work or other surgery, the patient should confer with the physician monitoring anticoagulant therapy.

Concomitant Medications

Patients should be reminded not to discontinue other medications unless directed by the physician. Abrupt withdrawal of other medications may alter the dynamics of the oral anticoagulant.

Patients should be instructed to avoid aspirin and over-the-counter (OTC) preparations which contain products known to interfere with platelet aggregation "such as ibuprofen."

Notify the Physician

Patient and family should be instructed to report signs of bleeding to the physician immediately for evaluation. When dosage is changed or stopped for any reason, the patient should be instructed to look for signs which may indicate a change in clotting status such as bleeding gums, bruises, petechiae, nosebleeds, hematuria, hematemesis, or menses which is heavier than usual. Patients may need to change to a soft toothbrush or electric razor to avoid irritation which could predispose the patient to bleed.

Use in Pregnancy

Oral anticoagulants are designated Food and Drug Administration (FDA) Pregnancy Category X.

Any plan to become pregnant or discovery that the patient has become pregnant must be reported to the physician immediately.

Oral anticoagulants cross placental barriers resulting in hemorrhage, and possibly fetal brain and eye abnormalities, central nervous system (CNS) abnormalities among others.

Parenteral anticoagulants including thrombolytics are designated Pregnancy Category B and C. Use during pregnancy is recommended only when the potential benefit justifies the potential risk to the fetus.

---

specific antidotes for anticoagulant overdose has been discussed. A limited number of substances may be useful in arresting bleeding arising from other causes. In particular, aminocaproic acid (*Amicar*) inhibits fibrinolysin activation in situations when excessive clot dissolution is occurring. At a dose of 5 g orally or IV, aminocaproic acid promotes clotting and appears to concentrate in the newly formed **thrombus** (clot) so no dissolution can occur. The major danger with the use of aminocaproic acid is the production of a generalized thrombosis. Otherwise, the side effects include headache, diarrhea, cramps, and rash.

Thrombin (*Thrombogen, Thrombostat*), obtained from cattle, is a direct activator of fibrin formation. This plasma protein initiates clot formation when applied topically to actively oozing injuries. It is available in packages of 1000 to 10,000 units of sterile powder. Thrombin is never administered intravenously due to the potential danger of generalized thrombosis or antigenic reactions.

Hemostatic Sponges

Three popular preparations of gelatin or cellulose sponges are employed to soak up excess blood and fluids and control bleeding in procedures in which suturing is ineffective or impractical. Such procedures include oral, dental, ophthalmic, and prostatic surgery. Gelatin sponge (*Gelfoam*), gelatin film (*Gelfilm*), and oxidized cellulose (*Oxycel, Surgicel, Hemo-Pak*) expand in contact with large amounts of blood. These gauze or sponge preparations also permit clotting to occur along their surfaces when used as wound dressings and surgical packings. These agents are applied topically to control hemorrhage in situations such as amputation, resection of the internal organs, and certain neurologic surgery. Most of these packings ultimately are absorbed by the body with little or no deleterious effect. Oxidized cellulose, in particular, cannot be used as a permanent implant because it interferes with bone regeneration. It may also produce cyst formation and reduce epithelialization (healing) of surface wounds.

Chapter Review

Understanding Terminology

Match the description in the left column with the appropriate term in the right column.

_____ **1.** Several blood clots together that form a plug.

_____ **2.** Hair loss or baldness.

_____ **3.** Inflammation of the walls of the veins due to blood clots.

_____ **4.** The appearance of red blood cells or blood in the urine.

_____ **5.** A blood clot.

a. alopecia

b. hematuria

c. thromboembolism

d. thrombophlebitis

e. thrombus

Acquiring Knowledge

Answer the following questions in the spaces provided.

6. What are the major stages of coagulation? _____

_____

_____

7. Explain the action of antithrombotic drugs. _____

_____

_____

8. How does heparin differ from the oral anticoagulants? _____

_____

_____

9. What factors permit heparin to have a rapid onset of action? _____

_____

_____

10. How do the oral anticoagulants exert an antithrombotic effect? What coagulation factors are affected? Why do the oral anticoagulants have a long onset of action?

_____

_____

11. Name two specific contraindications to the use of dicumarol and warfarin sodium.

_____

_____

12. What effects does aspirin have on anticoagulant therapy?

_____

_____

13. Explain the major toxicity associated with anticoagulant therapy.

_____

_____

14. Why isn't vitamin K₁ useful in heparin overdose?

_____

_____

15. How can the effects of the oral anticoagulants or heparin be monitored prior to giving the next scheduled dose?

_____

_____

16. When is heparin preferred over the coumarins?

_____

_____

17. What are three contraindications to the use of anticoagulants?

_____

_____

Applying Knowledge—On the Job

Use your critical thinking skills to answer the following questions in the spaces provided.

18. Anticoagulants of any type are contraindicated in patients with certain health conditions. List those conditions.

_____

_____

19. Because the duration of action with warfarin is long, 2 to 10 days, hemorrhage due to toxicity requires the use of an antidote. If phytonadione is used, when would you expect to start seeing results using prothrombin time?

_____

_____

20. Because warfarin interacts with a large array of medications, patients should be advised to withhold their current medications. What should they be advised regarding additions or deletions of medications? What might they expect to happen?

_____

_____

Internet Connection

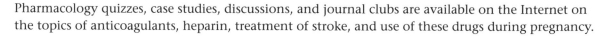

Pharmacology quizzes, case studies, discussions, and journal clubs are available on the Internet on the topics of anticoagulants, heparin, treatment of stroke, and use of these drugs during pregnancy.

a. Enter www.heartcenteronline.com and browse the broad range of information directed at educating students, patients, and health care researchers on conditions, such as stroke, heart attack, and drugs used to manage these conditions. The site provides a variety of "quizzes" to evaluate your wellness profile or calculate risk factors like diabetes, stress and immunity, heart and women's health, and cholesterol. You can browse the A to Z list, select anticoagulants, and a hyperlink will take you to a fully interactive screen. The interactive screen presents a video library on stroke factors, heart attack, and peripheral vascular disease. Some modules have a brief quiz on the material to test your understanding of the information. You can also register (free of charge) to access additional medical information.

b. Another excellent site is www.thrombosisonline.com supported by Aventis Pharmaceuticals Medical Education Division. This site presents information to patients and their families and, therefore, anticipates the viewers' need for multimedia presentation to comprehend the information. Animations about blood clot formation and deep venous thrombosis (DVT) are provided. Resource tools include a body mass index and calorie calculator, and a knowledge builder quiz.

c. The National Library of Congress supports Medlineplus at http://medlineplus.gov. At this site you can review specific prescription and over-the-counter drug information, access medical encyclopedias, or try any of the 150 interactive video tutorials.

Additional Reading

Avery, C. 1995. Improvement in heparin prophylaxis. *Nursing Times* 91 (20):11.

Harrison, M. 1997. Central venous catheters, a review of the literature. *Nursing Standards* 11 (27):43.

Herman, W. W. 1997. Current perspectives on dental patients receiving coumarin anticoagulant therapy. *Journal of the American Dental Association* 128 (3):327.

Kay, R. 1995. Low molecular weight heparin for the treatment of acute ischemic stroke. *New England Journal of Medicine* 333 (24):1588.

Normal, E. M. 1997. Low dose heparin in pediatric ivs. *American Journal of Nursing* 97:161.

Stevenson, A. L. 1997. International normalized ratio in anticoagulant therapy: Understanding the issues. *American Journal of Critical Care* 6 (2):88.

NUTRITION AND THERAPY

DRUG CLASS AT A GLANCE

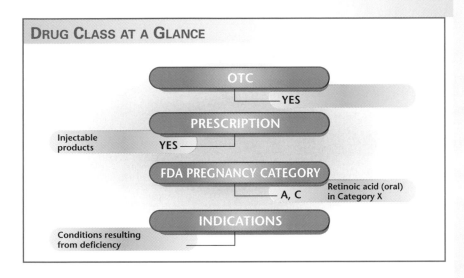

OTC
— YES

PRESCRIPTION

Injectable products
YES

FDA PREGNANCY CATEGORY
— A, C
Retinoic acid (oral) in Category X

INDICATIONS

Conditions resulting from deficiency

Key Terms

acidosis: disturbance of acid-base balance; when the pH of the blood is below 7.4.

alkalosis: disturbance of acid-base balance; when the pH of the blood is above 7.4.

anion: negatively charged ion.

cation: positively charged ion.

electrolyte: dissolved mineral that can conduct an electrical current and that exists as an ion.

essential amino acids and fatty acids: substances that are required for critical body function to sustain life and cannot be produced by the body.

hypervitaminosis: The accumulation of vitamins (fat soluble) in storage tissues that creates a deleterious condition related to the excess substance.

isotonic: normal salt concentration of most body fluids; a salt concentration of 0.9 percent.

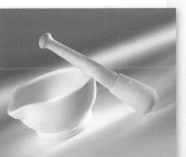

CHAPTER FOCUS

The activity of essential biochemicals and minerals is influenced by changes in body water. Therefore, it is important to explain the function of several important electrolytes and what happens when normal fluid balance is disturbed.

CHAPTER OBJECTIVES

After studying this chapter, you should be able to

- describe the difference between an energy-producing substance and minerals and list an example of each.

- describe the role of vitamins in tissue function.

- list the water-soluble vitamins and describe at least three diseases resulting from vitamin deficiency.

- list the fat-soluble vitamins and two ways deficiency can occur.

- list two main body fluid compartments and the major cation found in each compartment.

- explain the main functions of sodium, potassium, and calcium.

- describe the importance of hydrogen in relation to acidosis and alkalosis of the blood.

- list three different intravenous solutions and their main uses.

IV fluid therapy: the infusion of large amounts of fluid into a vein to increase blood volume or supply nourishment.

percent composition: common measure of solution concentration; refers to grams of solute per 100 ml of solution.

TPN: Total parenteral nutrition; a combination of nutrients that may include amino acids, carbohydrates, vitamins, and minerals (electrolytes) that is infused into patients who cannot absorb these substances from the gastrointestinal tract because of condition or disease. The combination and concentration of nutrients varies according to patient need.

NUTRIENTS

In Chapter 1 a drug was defined as a substance that alters the function of a living system. The substances covered in this chapter are traditionally not regarded as drugs even though they alter the function of living systems. In fact, these substances are required for maintaining normal function and, more importantly, they are essential for life! The body can make tissues, build and repair organs, and maintain activity and growth as long as vitamins, minerals, energy-producing substrates, and water are available. The body cannot synthesize vitamins and minerals and must therefore rely on an outside source to provide daily requirements. Energy-producing substrates, which include proteins, carbohydrates, and fats, can be synthesized by the body; however, the body relies on an outside source to provide "essential" building blocks. Nine of the 20 amino acids and two fatty acids that the body cannot produce from scratch are termed **essential amino acids and fatty acids.** These essential energy substances are presented in Table 28:1.

Diet and Disease

Even before their biochemical importance was identified, it was assumed that diet provided ample quantities of vitamins, minerals, and energy foods to sustain day-to-day activity. The content of the diet, however, varies with the culture, the ethnic group, and geographical location because eating patterns develop according to the type of food available in the region. People living at the Arctic Circle eat a different spectrum of food than those in Central America or Southeast Asia. Nevertheless, all diets must satisfy the daily demands for fuel and essential amino and fatty acids that are absorbed from plant or animal products.

It is difficult (but not impossible) to develop a deficiency to most vitamins and minerals in healthy people under the age of 70 in the United

TABLE 28:1	Essential Amino and Fatty Acids

AMINO ACIDS	FATTY ACIDS
Arginine*	Linolenic (polyunsaturated omega-3 fatty acids)
Histidine	
Isoleucine	
Leucine	Linoleic (polyunsaturated omega-6 fatty acids)
Lysine	
Methionine	
Phenylalanine	
Threonine	
Tryptophan	
Valine	

*Arginine is essential under some conditions.

States. Poorly balanced diets or poverty level diets certainly can limit the opportunity for adequate absorption of essential amino acids, vitamins, and minerals. Even in the presence of affluence and abundance, dietary composition can vary so widely that the quantities of some vitamins and minerals absorbed do not meet the level to support normal activity. In addition, decreased organ function associated with aging, medications, and disease can accelerate depletion of some elements. The value of vitamins, minerals, and substrates is easily observed in the conditions that result from deficiency, ranging from dull, brittle hair to malformed red blood cells, chronic anemias, and neuritis. Table 28:2 presents conditions that have been correlated with vitamin deficiency. Research has continually supported a relationship between diet and disease, including certain cancers.

Vitamins and Minerals: Recommended Dietary Allowances and Conditions Related to Deficiency

	RDA*	CONDITIONS RESULTING FROM DEFICIENCY	CHAPTER**
Vitamin A	1000 (800) μg	Night blindness, dry skin, decrease in epithelial cell growth	—
Vitamin C	60 (60) mg	Bleeding gums, bruising, loose teeth	—
Vitamin D	200 (200) IU	Bone loss, serum calcium	38
Vitamin E	12 (15) IU	Possible anemia	—
Vitamin K	80 (65) μg	Hemorrhage, decreased coagulation	27
Thiamine (B_1)	1.5 (1.1) mg	Anorexia, constipation, peripheral neuritis	—
Riboflavin (B_2)	1.7 (1.3) mg	Glossitis, ocular itching, vascularization	—
Niacin (B_3)	15 (19) mg	Insomnia, delusions, confusion	29
Pyridoxine (B_6)	2 (1.6) mg	Anemia, convulsions	—
Folate	200 (180) μg	Macrocytic anemia, neuropathy	30
Cyanocobalamin (B_{12})	2 (2) μg	Macrocytic anemia, muscle incoordination	30
Calcium	800 (800) mg	Bone loss	38
Iron	10 (15) mg	Microcytic anemia	30

*Recommended Dietary Allowances for 70-kg males (60-kg females) 20 to 50 years old
**Additional information presented in other chapters of this textbook

International studies have confirmed that large amounts of fat, or salt-cured or smoked meats are associated with high cancer rates for prostate, stomach, and esophageal cancers, respectively. In addition, diets that provide natural antioxidants (vitamins A, C, E) are associated with lower incidences of cancer.

Recommended Dietary Allowance and U.S.-Recommended Daily Allowance

Suggestions for the daily amount of each element needed to prevent deficiency conditions was established years ago in the U.S.-Recommended *Daily* Allowance (U.S.-RDA) and the RDA, Recommended *Dietary* Allowance. The U.S.-RDA and the RDA are not interchangeable. While both provide information, the U.S.-RDA (previously called the Minimum Daily Requirement) is used by the Food and Drug Administration to monitor the claims for quality of food processing destined for human consumption. Standards for nutrition advertising presented in product labels must meet legal requirements represented by the U.S.-RDA.

The National Research Council—National Academy of Sciences, Food and Nutrition Board publishes the Recommended *Dietary* Allowance (RDA). This is not a requirement, but a suggestion for daily intake of elements that are not produced by the body. The recommendations are derived from healthy individuals consuming a 2000-calorie daily diet balanced from the four basic food groups. Standard referenced healthy men weigh 70 kg (150 to 160 pounds), the women weigh 60 kg (130 to 148 pounds) and are between 20 and 50 years old. Diet and muscle mass of many elderly people are significantly different from younger adults; however, recommendations of dietary allowances for this population have not yet been established.

Dietary Recommendations

Except for conditions (osteoporosis, pernicious anemia, iron deficiency anemia, myelin degeneration) that result from a confirmed deficiency in vitamins or minerals, oral and parenteral supplements are not usually recommended. Conventional medical advice

Recommended Daily Food Consumption for Healthy Adults and Senior Adults

FOOD GROUPS	MINIMUM SERVINGS PER DAY	
	HEALTHY ADULTS	SENIOR ADULTS
Milk, cheese, dairy	2	3–5
Meat, poultry, fish, beans	2	2–3
Vegetable, fruit	4	3–5
Bread, cereal, whole grain, (enriched or fortified cereal)	4	4–6

suggests that adequate daily requirements of vitamins and minerals can be supplied through a healthy diet. Recommended servings for healthy adults and senior adults from a diet balanced to provide nutrition, energy, and essential vitamins and minerals is presented in Table 28:3. Specific conditions such as pregnancy, and athletic performance increase the demand for some of these elements and benefit from diet supplements. In addition, there is mounting evidence that adult vitamin supplements may be beneficial in preventing cancer (prostate, vitamin E), minimizing the toxicities of chemotherapy (vitamins A, E, C), and bone demineralization (elderly, vitamin D).

Food Guide Pyramid

A well-balanced diet is one that incorporates servings from all of the recommended food groups daily. The United States Department of Agriculture (USDA) developed a nutritional guide, called the food pyramid, (see Figure 28.1), which visually describes the relationship of the food groups required to provide the essential vitamins, minerals, and fiber each day. The foundation of the diet, and base of the pyramid, is the group of breads and grain. Ideally, 5 to 11 servings of breads and grains should be eaten daily. Three to four servings each from fruits and vegetables, and two to three servings from dairy products (milk, cheese, yogurt) and from protein such as meat, fish, poultry, and nuts are recommended daily. Individual food groups cannot be substituted for another because no single group contains the recommended full complement of vitamins, minerals, or fuel substances (carbohydrates, protein, fat). Notice the smallest group at the top of the food pyramid contains fats, oils, and sweets. Fats are an essential part of daily food consumption; however, the high number of calories and limited nutritional value associated

FIGURE 28:1

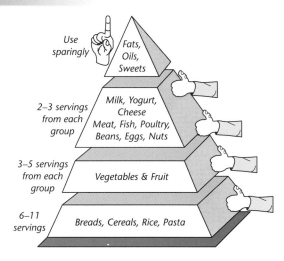

with this group warrant special attention in daily consumption.

Serving sizes vary with each food group. One serving includes:

Breads, cereals, rice, pasta, and other grains

- *1 slice of bread*
- *1/2 hamburger bun, bagel, or English muffin*
- *1 nine-inch flour tortilla*
- *1/2 cup cooked pasta, rice, or cereal*
- *1 ounce of ready-to-eat cereal*
- *2 to 4 crackers*

Fruits or vegetables

- *1/2 to 3/4 cup of raw berries or chopped fruits or vegetables*
- *3/4 cup of vegetable or fruit juice*

- *1 cup of leafy raw vegetables such as lettuce*
- *a medium apple, banana, orange, or 1/2 grapefruit*

Meat, fish, poultry, beans, eggs
- *2 to 3 ounces of cooked lean meat, poultry, or fish*
- *1 cup of cooked (dried) beans or lentils*
- *2 eggs*
- *4 tablespoons of peanut butter*

Milk, yogurt, cheese
- *1 cup milk or yogurt*
- *1–1/2 ounces natural cheese*
- *2 ounces of processed cheese*
- *1–3/4 cup of ice cream*

Finally, the amount of food eaten daily will supply calories, or fuel, for normal physiological function. Of course, the number of calories needed by each individual is dependent upon age, gender, and the level of daily activity. A moderately active person may be one who is working, including household maintenance, but doesn't perform a great deal of exercise in addition to work activities. An inactive person is one who does not exercise and engages in very little daily exertion such as walking but prefers to ride in the car or sit at home. When caloric intake from any food combination (even healthy choices) is greater than energy expenditure (burn-up), body weight will increase.

VITAMINS

Vitamins have traditionally been considered "natural substances" and food additives rather than drugs. Although vitamin K and niacin are used in doses that produce pharmacologic effects (blood clotting, cholesterol reduction), vitamins are principally associated with routine tissue activity. Vitamins act as cofactors that facilitate biochemical reactions in all tissues, yet the spectrum of their importance is still under discovery. More than 300 metabolic or enzyme reactions are known to require vitamins in order to function properly.

Vitamins are categorized as fat soluble (A, D, E, K) or water soluble (C and B vitamins). Fat-soluble vitamins characteristically are well stored in the liver and fatty tissues. They are affected by conditions that limit fat absorption such as biliary obstruction, pancreatic disease, liver cirrhosis, and absorbent resins (cholestyramine). These vitamins are absorbed in a provitamin state and metabolically converted in the intestine or kidney to the active compound that produces a specific action. Water-soluble vitamins are readily absorbed from the intestinal tract and are not influenced by biliary function. Since these vitamins are not stored in the body, they are more easily depleted through renal excretion.

FAT-SOLUBLE VITAMINS

Vitamin A

Source

Beta-carotene (provitamin A) is the most important member of a group of biologically active compounds known as vitamin A. Vitamin A_1 (retinol) is found in fish liver oils, animal liver, yellow vegetables, palm oil, parsley, spinach, and dandelion leaves. Synthetic retinol provides more consistent blood levels than do dietary sources. Vitamin A activity is expressed as retinol equivalents (RE), where one RE equals 1 μg of retinol or 6 μg of beta-carotene.

Function in the Body

Vitamin A is absolutely required for the production of the protein visual purple (rhodopsin). Dietary beta-carotene (provitamin A) is converted to retinol in the intestine. Retinol combines with a protein, opsin, to form rhodopsin. This protein enables specialized retinal cells (rods) to adapt to very low-intensity light (dark adaptation). Without beta-carotene, the rods cannot respond, resulting in "night blindness." Vitamin A is also involved in the synthesis of ribonucleic acid (RNA), cholesterol, and proteins and preserves the integrity of epithelial cells. Through these pathways, vitamin A deficiency retards cell growth and results in thickened, dry skin.

Clinical Indication

Vitamin A is administered orally as replacement therapy in deficiency conditions resulting from biliary, pancreatic, and hepatic disease, partial gastrectomy, and cystic fibrosis. Parenteral vitamin A is also available for conditions such as anorexia, malabsorption syndrome, or vomiting where oral administration is not possible.

Vitamin A is used topically for skin abrasions, minor burns, sunburn, diaper rash, and noninfected skin irritation resulting from indwelling drains as with colostomy or ileostomy.

Vitamin A acid (13-retinoic acid, *trans*-retinoic acid) is used in the management of acne vulgaris. By reducing sebum (oil) production and stimulating epithelial cell turnover, retinoic acids improve cystic acne and prevent the skin thickening (keratization) that occurs in chronic acne.

Treatment of Deficiency

The daily RDA for vitamin A is 1000 µg (RE) in men, 800 µg (RE) in women, and 800 to 1300 µg (RE) in pregnant and nursing women. Treatment of adult deficiency ranges from 100,000 to 500,000 IU per day up to 2 weeks. Treatment beyond 2 weeks may range between 10,000 to 20,000 IU daily for 2 months. Oral preparations are available over the counter (OTC) alone or in multivitamin products. Oral and injectable forms of vitamin A are also available by prescription.

Treatment of Acne

Retinoic acids (isotretinoin, trentinoin) are available as oral formulations taken twice daily for up to 20 weeks and topical gels applied once a day. The topical cream or liquid preparations will adhere to the hands and therefore necessitate thorough washing after application to avoid inappropriate exposure to other sensitive tissues; for example, the eyes.

Products

The number of available vitamin A products are numerous. Among the oral and parenteral preparations of vitamin A alone are *Aqualsol A* and *Palmitate-A 5000*. Topical OTC preparations for the skin are combinations of vitamin A with vitamin D and/or vitamin E and include *A and D, Desitin, Comfortine, Lobana Peri-Garde, Lazer Creme,* and *Aloe Grande.* Retinoic acids are available by prescription for topical application (Retin-A) and oral administration (Accutane).

Overdose

Hypervitaminosis can occur because healthy individuals should have adequate stores of vitamin A within the liver. Toxicity observed will vary with the age and condition of the person and the dose ingested. Acute toxicity may produce headache, irritability, and vertigo associated with an increase in cranial pressure. Symptoms of chronic toxicity may include lethargy; desquamation (shedding epithelial lining); dry, cracked skin; arthralgia; and cirrhotic-like liver

syndrome. Following accurate diagnosis of the condition, the vitamin A supplement should be discontinued and, if necessary, supportive treatment with prednisone begun. Liver function enzymes may be monitored until the clinical profile improves.

Overdose characteristic of hypervitaminosis A can result from overuse of the oral formulation, and from accidental oral ingestion of the topical creme or liquid formulations. Symptoms include headache, vomiting, facial flushing, dizziness, and abdominal pain. Once treatment is discontinued, the symptoms stop.

Contraindication

Oral retinoic acid (Accutane) is contraindicated in women who are pregnant or anticipating becoming pregnant. Human fetal malformations have occurred and there may be an increased risk of spontaneous abortion following treatment in women who received retinoic acid while pregnant. ***This product is classified as Food and Drug Administration (FDA) Pregnancy Category X*** because there is the potential for all exposed fetuses to be affected by maternal circulating retinoic acid. The topical formulation of retinoic acid is not associated with fetal malformation; however, use in pregnancy should be considered only when the benefit justifies the potential risk. The topical formulation is classified as FDA Pregnancy Category C.

Vitamin D (see Chapter 38 for additional information)

Source

Vitamin D is a term for a group of compounds with similar activity. Vitamin D provitamins are found in fish liver oils, egg yolks, and fortified commercial dairy products such as whole milk, butter, bread, and cereals. Following absorption of two provitamins, active forms of vitamin D are produced by metabolic conversion in the liver or by the action of ultraviolet (UV) irradiation of the skin. The liver and kidney further convert vitamin D into the more active forms of vitamin D_3, 25-hydroxydihydrotachysterol, and calcitriol. Vitamin D activity is expressed as international units (IU) of vitamin D_3.

Function in the Body

Vitamin D is essential for the metabolism of bone and cartilage. By modulating bone formation, vitamin D regulates serum calcium levels in conjunction with parathormone and calcitonin. Vitamin D deficiency produces a condition of weakened skeletal structure known as rickets in children and osteomalacia in adults. Calcitriol, the most active form of vitamin D, is responsible for intestinal calcium and phosphorus absorption. Indirectly, vitamin D affects the status of muscle contraction, nerve conduction, and blood clotting through its influence on serum calcium ions. Calcium deficiency manifests as sustained muscle contraction (tetany) or impaired nerve conduction.

Clinical Indication

Various forms of the vitamin are administered orally and parenterally in the treatment of conditions resulting from or associated with low serum calcium such as metabolic bone disease, postoperative tetany, hypoparathyroidism, and renal dialysis. It is increasingly recognized that elderly people may develop vitamin D deficiency in a number of ways. Age- or disease-related renal changes may decrease the amount of active vitamin D produced in people over 70 years old. In this age group, people may be house-bound, incapacitated, or institutionalized so that exposure to sunlight for vitamin D conversion in the skin is not a daily routine. It has been suggested that this may be complicated by the use of sunscreen products which decrease the UV activity on the skin. Finally, conditions of lactose intolerance, avoidance of dairy products because of potential constipation, or decreased appetite may contribute to an overall decrease in vitamin D absorption in older people.

As a topical cream containing vitamins A, E, and D, vitamin D is applied to the skin for the temporary relief of minor burns, chafed or dry skin, sunburn, abrasions, and noninfected irritated areas including diaper rash. Topical preparations may be applied to irritated areas resulting from ostomy connections.

Treatment of Deficiency

The daily RDA for vitamin D is 200 IU for men and women. Treatment of adult deficiency ranges between 12,000 and 500,000 IU of vitamin D activity daily. Therapy is continued with calcium supplementation until serum calcium, phosphorus, and blood urea nitrogen (BUN) indicate improvement. Ergocalciferol (D_2) and cholecalciferol (D_3) are used in the treatment and prophylaxis of vitamin D deficiency.

Other forms of vitamin D are used in the management of serum calcium disorders, tetany, hypophosphatemia, and hypoparathyroidism.

Products

Ergocalciferol (D_2) is available orally and parenterally. Oral formulations include *Calciferol Drops, Drisdol Drops, Vitamin D,* and *Deltalin Gelseals.* Cholecalciferol (D_3) is available OTC as *Delta-D* and *Vitamin D_3.* Dihydrotachysterol (*DHT, Hytakeral*), calcitriol (*Rocaltrol, Calcijex*), and calcifediol (*Calderol*) are available only by prescription.

Overdose

Hypervitaminosis can occur from administration to patients in excess of their daily needs. Acute toxicity may produce weakness, headache, nausea, vomiting, constipation, muscle or bone pain, and a metallic taste. Later changes in renal and liver function may be observed by elevations in BUN, aspartate aminotransferase (AST), alanine aminotransferase (ALT), and albumin in the urine. Finally, levels of calcium and phosphate may be elevated in the blood or urine. Bone demineralization can occur in adults, persisting after vitamin treatment has been discontinued. Death following cardiovascular or renal failure has occurred.

Drug Interactions

Patients receiving renal dialysis are predisposed to experiencing drug interactions with vitamin D preparations. Antacids containing magnesium may contribute to hypermagnesemia in combination with vitamin D therapy. Hypercalcemia resulting in atrial fibrillation has occurred with patients receiving vitamin D and verapamil or digitalis.

Vitamin E

Source

Vitamin E, alpha-tocopherol, is found in vegetable oils, eggs, cereals, milk, meat, and leafy vegetables, and is available synthetically. Like all fat-soluble vitamins, absorption depends on the availability of bile salts. Vitamin E absorption is related to ingestion of polyunsaturated fatty acids (linoleic acid). Fatty tissue, liver, and muscle store most of the alpha-tocopherol absorbed from the intestine.

Function in the Body

The mechanism of vitamin E activity is not fully known; however, it does act as an antioxidant and cofactor in metabolic reactions. As an antioxidant it prevents the formation or accumulation of toxic metabolites. In addition, vitamin E is essential to the maintenance of red blood cell (RBC) membranes.

Clinical Indication

Vitamin E is used topically for the temporary relief of minor burns, and chapped or chafed skin, especially diaper rash. Vitamin E is used in the treatment of cancer. Its antioxidant role is attributed to the ability of vitamin E to reduce the incidence of certain cancers and act as a protective agent in oxygen therapy in premature infants. Various formulations of alpha-tocopherol are available orally for the treatment of vitamin E deficiency.

Treatment of Deficiency

The daily RDA for vitamin E is 12 IU for men and 15 IU for women. Deficiency of vitamin E and the resulting anemia are rare since adequate amounts are available in foods.

Products

Vitamin E activity is expressed as IU of alpha-tocopherol. Vitamin E is available orally OTC as an individual supplement and as part of multivitamin preparations. Among the products available are *Aquasol E, E-200 I.U. Softgels, Amino-Opti-E,* and *E-Complex 600.* Topical OTC products intended for skin application only include *E-Vitamin, Vitec,* and *Vite E Creme.* Vitamin E is also available for topical use in combination with vitamins A and/or D as *Lobana-Peri Garde, Lazar Creme, Lobana Derm-Ade,* and *Aloe Grande.*

Overdose

Hypervitaminosis may produce symptoms of fatigue, headache, nausea, weakness, and diarrhea. The appropriate treatment is discontinuation of vitamin supplement until symptoms disappear.

Drug Interactions

Because vitamin E suppresses platelet aggregation, concomitant use in patients receiving oral anticoagulants may lead to episodes of increased bleeding.

Vitamin K (see Chapter 27)

Source

Vitamin K_1 (phytonadione) is found in green vegetables, cabbage, cauliflower, fish liver, eggs, milk, and meat. However, the primary source of vitamin K in humans is bacterial synthesis in the intestine.

Function in the Body

Vitamin K is required for the synthesis of blood clotting factors II, VII, IX, and X in the liver.

Interference with vitamin K synthesis or metabolism results in bleeding and hemorrhage.

Clinical Indication

Bleeding resulting from suppressed coagulation due to malformation of vitamin K-dependent clotting factors warrants vitamin K replacement therapy. Conditions that impair or eliminate bacterial vitamin K synthesis, such as antibiotic therapy, or interfere with vitamin K metabolism, are also indications for vitamin K therapy. Vitamin K is given in the prophylaxis and management of hemorrhagic disease of the newborn where the mother received oral anticoagulants, anticonvulsants, or antibiotics during pregnancy that interfered with vitamin K-dependent clotting mechanisms. ***Note: vitamin K will not reverse the bleeding associated with heparin overdose.***

Treatment of Deficiency

The RDA for vitamin K is 80 μg for men and 65 μg for women. Deficiency of vitamin K and the resulting coagulation disorder does not usually result from dietary limitations.

Replacement is achieved through oral and parenteral administration of vitamin K. Individualized doses ranging between 2.5 and 25 mg of vitamin K are taken until coagulation returns to normal or to the previous therapeutic level. Continuation of treatment is based on the protime (PT) evaluation.

Products

Vitamin K as phytonadione is available orally and parenterally by prescription as *Mephyton* and *AquaMEPHTON.*

Overdose

Hypervitaminosis is not likely to occur with oral preparations. However, patients may experience adverse reactions to parenteral vitamin K administration. Symptoms, which may include flushing, dizziness, and brief hypotension, do not necessarily obligate cessation of treatment. Pain and swelling at the injection site with repeated injections may occur. Severe allergic reactions including death, however, have occurred after intravenous administration of vitamin K.

WATER-SOLUBLE VITAMINS

Water-soluble vitamins include all the B vitamins and vitamin C. These vitamins are not stored in fatty tissues, are readily used up following absorption, and are easily excreted with water into the urine. Chronic inadequate intake of these vitamins through the diet, therefore, can lead to deficiency. Among adults the condition most commonly associated with vitamin deficiency is alcoholism. Decreased appetite, decreased food intake, and damage to digestive and metabolic systems that occur with alcoholism contribute to a deficiency state. Other conditions such as anorexia nervosa, prolonged fasting, and intravenous feeding can also precipitate vitamin deficiency. Even when diets include appropriate sources of water-soluble vitamins, overcooking and boiling food products cause the vitamins to break down (heat labile) or leach into the cooking water, making vitamin deficiency possible. Except for vitamin B_{12} and folate, it is unusual for deficiency of one vitamin to occur. As a rule, conditions that predispose an individual to vitamin deficiency will reduce the levels of multiple B vitamins concurrently.

Vitamins B_1 (Thiamine), B_2 (Riboflavin), B_3 (Niacin, Nicotinic Acid), B_5 (Calcium Pantothenate), B_6 (Pyridoxine), B_9 (Folic Acid), B_{12} (Cyanocobalamine)

Source

The family of B vitamins is available in yeast, whole grains, soybeans, liver, milk, egg yolks, leafy green vegetables, and fruit. The daily RDA for the B vitamins is presented in Table 28:2 on page 307.

Function in the Body

All of the B vitamins have coenzyme activity or are integral to cell reproduction and maturation. Thiamine combines with adenosine triphosphate (ATP) to form a coenzyme that is critical for carbohydrate metabolism. As carbohydrate intake increases in the diet, so does the requirement for thiamine. Riboflavin combines with proteins to form coenzymes in the respiratory system. Niacin forms two coenzymes in oxidation-reduction reactions. Pyridoxine forms a coenzyme in the metabolism of carbohydrates, fats, and protein. When dietary protein increases, the requirement for pyridoxine increases. Pantothenate is a precursor of coenzyme A associated with synthesis of fatty acids and steroid hormones. Cyanocobalamin and folic acid are essential for cell growth, reproduction, and hematopoiesis. A full discussion of the activity of vitamin B_{12} and folic acid is presented in Chapter 30.

Clinical Indication

Thiamine is indicated in the treatment of vitamin B_1 deficiency known as beriberi. Symptoms range from weakness, paresthesia, and hypotension to sensory and motor dysfunction. In severe cases, psychosis, ataxia, confusion (Wernicke's encephalopathy), and cardiovascular damage can occur.

Riboflavin, pantothenate, and pyridoxine are indicated for the treatment of vitamin B_2 deficiency. In the absence of riboflavin, changes occur in the cornea (vascularization) accompanied by itching, burning, and photophobia, and glossitis and seborrheic dermatitis develop.

Pantothenate deficiency induced experimentally has been shown to cause fatigue, headache, sleep disturbances, muscle cramps, and impaired coordination.

Niacin is used in the treatment and prevention of pellagra and, pharmacologically, to reduce hyperlipidemia (see Chapter 29). Pellagra is characterized by the three "Ds": diarrhea, dermatitis, and dementia.

Treatment of Deficiency

Replacement is achieved through oral and parenteral administration of thiamine (10 to 20 mg IM) until symptoms resolve. Then oral vitamin supplement is continued for a few months. In severe cases precipitated by other chronic conditions, symptoms may not fully improve.

Riboflavin deficiency is easily corrected with daily oral doses of 25 mg. While parenteral niacin is available, deficiency is usually corrected with 100 to 500 mg of niacin orally a day.

Products

Thiamine is available OTC as *Thiamilate,* and by prescription for injection as *Biamine.* Riboflavin, pantothenate, niacin, and pyridoxine are available OTC alone under the generic names, or within multivitamin supplements available under numerous labels.

Overdose

Hypervitaminosis is not likely to occur with B vitamins, although adverse reactions to individual vitamin preparations do occur. In large doses, thiamine produces a sensation of warmth, sweating, urticaria, tightness in the throat, and gastrointestinal bleeding (hemorrhage). Niacin may cause gastrointestinal distress, diarrhea, generalized flushing (vasodilation that has not been confirmed to be therapeutically useful), decreased glucose tolerance, and elevated uric acid and liver function tests.

Cautions

Parenteral administration of vitamins has caused severe hypersensitivity reactions, even death. Prior to intravenous administration of thiamine, an intradermal sensitivity test should be performed to assess potential reactivity.

Riboflavin may cause orange discoloration of the urine that is inconsequential. However, patients should be alerted to the potential for this coloration to occur.

Vitamin C (Ascorbic Acid)

Source

Vitamin C is plentiful in citrus fruits, green vegetables, tomatoes, potatoes, strawberries, and green peppers. The daily Recommended Dietary Allowance (RDA) for vitamin C is 60 mg a day for adults.

Function in the Body

Vitamin C is involved in the formation of catecholamines, steroids, and conversion reactions such as folic acid to folinic acid.

Clinical Indication

Although vitamin C has been recommended for use in a wide range of conditions from the common cold to cancer, the only clinically recognized use of ascorbic acid is in the prevention and treatment of vitamin C deficiency, or scurvy.

Treatment of Deficiency

Scurvy is characterized by degenerative changes in soft tissue and bones. Bleeding gums, loose teeth, and poor bone development have been identified with vitamin C deficiency for more than two centuries. Deficiency is readily reversed through diet as well as oral supplements in doses ranging from 70 to 500 mg daily.

Products

Ascorbic acid is available OTC alone or in combination with multivitamin supplements.

Special Consideration

There is no overdose potential with vitamin C. Doses up to 10 g daily have been used for prophylaxis of colds, as adjuncts in cancer treatment, and to improve wound healing. While these uses are still under debate, it has provided evidence that large doses of vitamin C do not produce significant adverse effects. At most, vitamin C may cause diarrhea and precipitate renal stones because it acidifies the urine. Patients prone to renal stones should not take megadoses (greater than 2 g) of vitamin C.

Prior to performing an amine-dependent stool occult blood test, ascorbic acid should not be taken for 48 to 72 hours to avoid a false-negative response.

BODY WATER

The body can tolerate acute deficiencies in food, vitamins, and minerals, but water deprivation is incompatible with life. Water is the most abundant constituent of the body, representing about 60 to 70 percent of total body weight. Many substances in the body normally exist in solution, being dissolved in water. Body water is distributed between two main compartments: the intracellular (intracellular fluid, ICF) and the extracellular (plasma and interstitial fluid, extracellular fluid [ECF]) compartments. The fluid in these compartments is normally maintained at relatively constant amounts. Loss of body water produces dehydration, whereas retention of water produces edema. In turn, the substances dissolved within the fluid compartments are directly affected by the shift or change in fluid volume.

Fluid Balance

The normal daily intake of fluids by an average-size adult is approximately 3000 ml, or about 3 quarts. This amount includes fluids from drinking, fluids in food, and water formed by body metabolism. The normal daily output of fluids is about the same as fluid intake. Fluid output is water that is normally lost in urine, sweat, feces, and through respiration. During illness, additional fluid may be lost by hemorrhage, vomiting, or diarrhea.

When a large amount of fluid is lost by the body, it must be replaced. Usually, adequate fluid intake is accomplished by drinking. In disease states or medical emergencies, fluid loss may be so great that fluid intake must be accomplished by other methods. Intravenous **(IV) fluid therapy** is commonly employed in these situations. It involves the infusion of large amounts of fluid into a vein to increase blood volume or supply nourishment.

MINERALS

Minerals, such as sodium (Na), potassium (K), and chloride (Cl), are important constituents of body composition. When dissolved in body fluids, they exist as acids, bases, and salts. These dissolved minerals are referred to as **electrolytes** because they are able to conduct an electrical current. The electrolytes form charged particles called ions. Ions that have a positive charge are known as **cations.** Ions possessing a negative charge are called **anions.**

$$NaCl \xrightarrow{dissolved} H_2O + Cl^-$$

Electrolytes are involved in many important body functions. Water is the solvent, electrolytes are the solutes, and together they form the normal salt (isotonic) concentration of the body fluids. **Isotonic** refers to a salt concentration of 0.9 percent. Alterations of water or salt levels result in fluid concentrations (hypotonic or hypertonic) that will destroy body cells (lysis or crenation). A common measure of solution concentration is **percent composition,** or grams of solute per 100 ml of solution. A 5 percent dextrose solution contains 5 g of dextrose in 100 ml of water.

Electrolytes

Sodium (Na$^+$)

Sodium, the main cation of extracellular fluid, plays a major role in maintaining normal fluid balance. The average diet is sufficient to meet body requirements for sodium. The kidneys help maintain normal levels of sodium in plasm a and other body fluids. Significant loss of sodium (vomiting and diarrhea) reduces ECF volume. Excessive use of diuretics also causes sodium depletion. Consequently, fluid moves out of the intracellular compartment in an effort to maintain blood volume. If the lost sodium and water are not replaced, blood volume and blood pressure decrease, and circulatory collapse may occur. Sodium is administered intravenously in various concentrations, as seen in Table 28:4.

TABLE 28:4	Intravenous Solutions and Their Main Uses
IV SOLUTION	**USE**
Saline:	
Sodium chloride 0.45%	Fluid and electrolyte replacement (Na, Cl)
Sodium chloride 0.9%	Fluid and electrolyte replacement (Na, Cl)
Dextrose in Saline:	
5% dextrose in 0.45% saline	Fluid and electrolyte replacement, provides carbohydrate calories
5% dextrose in 0.9% saline	
10% dextrose in 0.9% saline	
Dextrose in Water:	
5, 10, 20, and 50% dextrose in water	Fluid replacement, provides carbohydrate calories
Multiple Electrolyte Solutions:	
Ringer's solution	Fluid and electrolyte replacement (Na, Cl, K, Ca)
Lactated Ringer's solution	Same as Ringer's plus lactate, which provides buffer action in acidosis
Plasma Expanders:	
10% dextran 40 in 0.9% saline	Increases plasma volume when hypovolemia is present
Parenteral Nutrition:	
Amino acid solutions (*Aminosyn, Travasol*)	Provides protein calories
Fat emulsions 10%, 20% (*Intralipid, Liposyn*)	Provides essential fats and calories

Potassium (K$^+$)

Potassium, the main cation of intracellular fluid, is important in maintaining cell structure and function. Potassium is also vital in the regulation of muscle function, especially heart muscle. Loss of potassium can produce a loss of muscle tone, weakness, and paralysis. Excessive potassium levels can produce cardiac arrhythmias, especially heart block. The normal concentration of potassium in the serum ranges between 4.1 and 5.6 milliequivalents per liter (mEq/l). Potassium is administered IV as potassium chloride in various concentrations.

Calcium (Ca^{2+})

Calcium, another cation that is usually associated with the formation of bone, also plays a vital role in muscle contraction and blood coagulation. The normal serum concentration of calcium ranges between 4.5 and 5.7 mEq/l. A deficiency of calcium in the blood results in hyperexcitability of nerve and muscle fibers (tetany). Excess calcium produces muscle weakness and may lead to cardiac and respiratory failure. When given intravenously, calcium is usually administered in the form of calcium chloride or calcium gluconate.

Hydrogen (H$^+$)

The major source of hydrogen is from the dissociation of water.

This reaction regulates the acidity or alkalinity of body fluids. Normal pH of blood is about 7.4. When the pH of the blood falls below 7.4, a condition known as **acidosis** occurs. A pH higher than 7.4 indicates a state of **alkalosis.** The body has several buffer systems to maintain normal body pH. When these buffer systems are not able to maintain pH, acid-base disturbances occur. There are different types of acidosis and alkalosis.

Metabolic Acidosis

Metabolic acidosis occurs when there is excessive loss of bases, such as bicarbonate (HCO$_3^-$) or sodium. Such losses can occur with diarrhea, starvation, or diabetic coma. Treatment involves the administration of sodium bicarbonate along with fluids and other electrolytes, if necessary.

Respiratory Acidosis

Respiratory acidosis is associated with increased levels of carbon dioxide (CO$_2$) in the blood, occurring when there is interference with respiratory gas exchange. Carbon dioxide combines with water to form carbonic acid (H$_2$CO$_3$). Carbonic acid can dissociate into hydrogen ions, which will lower the pH of the blood (acidosis).

Metabolic Alkalosis

Metabolic alkalosis is usually associated with excessive loss of potassium (K$^+$) or chloride (Cl$^-$). This kind of loss is most often caused by severe vomiting (Cl$^-$ loss) or diarrhea (K$^+$ loss).

Respiratory Alkalosis

Respiratory alkalosis is produced by hyperventilation (salicylate poisoning or artificial respirator), which lowers the carbon dioxide (CO$_2$) levels of the blood.

The treatment of acidosis or alkalosis involves administering the appropriate electrolyte solutions so that serum electrolyte levels are returned to normal.

Intravenous Therapy

In addition to the various electrolyte solutions, a number of intravenous solutions are used as plasma expanders or to provide parenteral nutrition (Table 28:4). Patients who are unable to take fluids or food by mouth must depend on intravenous administration to ensure adequate fluid and caloric intake. Intravenous solutions usually contain some form of carbohydrate, such as dextrose, fructose, or dextran. In addition, electrolytes, vitamins, amino acids, proteins, and fat emulsions can be included. Total parenteral nutrition **(TPN)** may be used during chemotherapy in order to improve patient outcome. TPN does not influence tumor growth but may reverse the negative aspect of cancer treatment—weight loss. Its greatest value has been demonstrated in patients responding with increased white blood cell counts, improved immunocompetence, improved wound healing, and, overall, a better than expected response to chemotherapy.

Patient Administration and Monitoring

Review of the patient history should provide evidence of eating disorders, alcohol abuse, or poor dietary habits that could contribute to nutrition imbalance. Especially among elderly patients, the psychological state resulting from being socially isolated or continually worried often causes the patient to stop eating. Reassurance is the best therapy, followed by dietary adjustment and appropriate nutritional supplements. During treatment patients should be monitored for development of sensitivity reactions.

Patient Instructions

Instruct patients to take nutritional supplements with meals to avoid gastrointestinal upset.

Extended-release formulations of vitamins should not be crushed or chewed. This formulation is designed to deliver the active substance over a controlled period of time rather than all at once. Chewing will dump the vitamin into the stomach and may cause nausea or irritation depending on the vitamin; however, the patient will not experience harmful effects from the change in delivery.

Vitamin A

If being taken as an individual supplement, the recommended maximum daily dose should not be exceeded. Pregnant women should be cautioned to stay within the recommended dose range to avoid potential excess storage and adverse effects.

Vitamin D

Remind patients, especially elderly adults, that brief periodic exposure to sunlight (10 minutes a day, to 3 days each week) is beneficial to maintain a normal level of active vitamin D.

Calcium Supplements

Vitamin D and calcium are often taken together as part of a nutritional program. This may occur more frequently today due to patient anxiety about developing osteoporosis. Remind patients that calcium supplements without an adequate vitamin D level will not permit calcium to be utilized by the body. Moreover in the absence of vitamin D and estrogen, calcium supplementation (especially *Tums)* alone does not correct osteoporosis in postmenopausal women.

Niacin

Patients should be told that niacin may cause flushing and a sensation of warmth in the neck and face and tingling or itching. These effects usually subside within a few days.

Riboflavin

During treatment, patients may observe a change in urine color to deeper orange-yellow. This is not harmful and will subside when the supplement is discontinued.

Vitamin C

Daily doses in excess of 2 g may change the acidity of the urine, causing stones to develop. Patients with a history of renal stones should avoid megadose exposure of vitamin C.

Notify the Physician

Patients should be told to notify the physician if they experience weakness, headache, weight loss, vomiting, and abdominal or muscle cramps. Such symptoms may indicate an adverse reaction to the supplement or hypersensitivity.

Use in Pregnancy

Except for folic acid, pyridoxine, and thiamine (FDA Pregnancy Category A), it is suggested that vitamin supplements not exceed the recommended maximum daily amounts. Vitamins are usually found classified as FDA Pregnancy Category C. Therapy which obligates larger doses should be monitored during prenatal evaluation.

Oral retinoic acid and excessive doses of vitamin A should be avoided during pregnancy. Vitamin A is classified as FDA Pregnancy Category C because safety for use during pregnancy has not been established. **Retinoic acid, oral not topical, is classified as FDA Pregnancy Category X because of its direct deleterious actions on the developing fetus at any time during pregnancy.**

Chapter Review

Understanding Terminology

Answer the following questions in the spaces provided.

1. Explain what is meant by the term *essential amino acid.* _____
   _____
   _____

2. Why are vitamins considered essential? _____
   _____
   _____

3. What information does *RDA* convey to the reader? _____
   _____
   _____

4. Explain what *hypervitaminosis* is and which substances are potentially involved. _____
   _____
   _____

5. Explain what is meant by *percent composition* as a measure of solution concentration. _____
   _____
   _____

6. Write a short paragraph using these terms: *electrolytes, ions, cations, anions.* _____
   _____
   _____

7. What is the purpose of TPN? _____
   _____
   _____

Acquiring Knowledge

Answer the following questions in the spaces provided.

1. List the different forms of body fluids and their locations. _____
   _____
   _____

2. What are the usual sources of fluid intake and the means of fluid output? _____
   _____
   _____

3. What is the function of vitamin D? _____
   _____
   _____

4. Explain why elderly adults are more likely to experience vitamin D and calcium deficiency. ____
   _____
   _____

5. Why is it easier to develop a deficiency of the B vitamins than to develop a deficiency of vitamin A? _____

_____

_____

6. Which vitamins have a therapeutic role beyond the treatment of vitamin deficiency? _____

_____

_____

7. What are the main functions of Na^+, K^+, and Ca^{++}? _____

_____

_____

8. List the various types of acidosis and alkalosis and the common causes of each. _____

_____

_____

9. What solutions would be appropriate for the treatment of metabolic acidosis? _____

_____

_____

10. When is IV therapy indicated? _____

_____

_____

Applying Knowledge—On the Job

Use your critical thinking skills to answer the following questions in the spaces provided.

1. Accutane is contraindicated in women who are or may become pregnant. What should be included in the medication counseling when Accutane is prescribed to a female patient?

_____

_____

_____

2. What are the symptoms of vitamin D overdose? _____

_____

_____

_____

3. Pregnant women or women who are of childbearing age should take 100 to 400 mcg of folic acid daily. Why is this important? What disorder is commonly associated with folic acid deficiency? _____

_____

_____

_____

Internet Connection

A variety of websites are available that provide the most current facts to the consumer, student, and medical professional about nutrition, food contents, and/or individual vitamins and minerals. Using Yahoo as a search engine, enter www.yahoo.com to access the main menu of topics. Select *Nutrition*. Three websites are worth visiting here: **Dole5aday, Meals.com,** and **Vitamin Update.**

Dole5aday can also be entered using www.Dole5aday.com. At the home page select *Nutrition Center*. Information on fruits and vegetables from apples and pears to carambola, gooseberries, and pummelos is displayed with the FDA Nutrition Label. Facts from serving size to calories to sodium content are provided next to a color presentation of the produce item. So, go ahead, find carambola (aka star fruit). In what vitamin is its pulp richest? Then preview the separate categories of fruits and vegetables rich in vitamin A and those rich in vitamin C.

Meals.com is a website supported by Nestle at www.ut.essortment.com. Nutrition facts and ingredients from burgers, pizza, to fries and sauce are displayed. If you are advising a patient about food selections when eating out or on the run, this website details how much fat compared to protein and sodium is present in those McNuggets.

The **Vitamin Update** home page provides consumers information on the latest development in vitamins and minerals, including new natural products such as *Co-Q* enzyme and chondroitin, for example.

Additonal interactive websites that present movies, quizzes, and nutrition databases are www.nutrition.gov and www.nutrition.getschooled.com (You Are What You Eat database).

Medical World Search at www.mwsearch.com is the first search engine devoted to scanning the medical sites on the Web and search-related terms automatically. The greatest advantage is that the home page accepts "plain English terms" and quickly provides a list of online documents for review. For example, to learn more about metabolic acidosis and its impact on the body, the term *Acidosis or Metabolic acidosis* is entered at the search prompt. The articles offer a wide range of information that is convenient and reader friendly.

HYPOLIPIDEMIC DRUGS

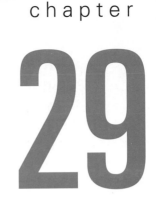

DRUG CLASS AT A GLANCE

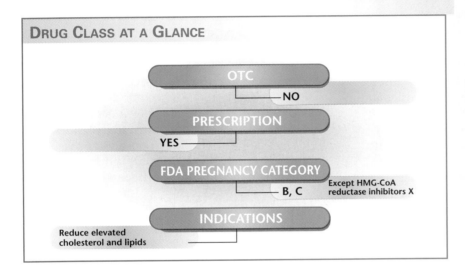

OTC — NO

PRESCRIPTION — YES

FDA PREGNANCY CATEGORY — B, C — Except HMG-CoA reductase inhibitors X

INDICATIONS — Reduce elevated cholesterol and lipids

Key Terms

cholesterol: dietary lipid normally synthesized in the body.

hyperlipidemia: abnormally high lipid levels in the plasma.

hypolipidemic drug: drug used to lower plasma lipid levels.

lipoprotein: protein found in the plasma that transports triglycerides and cholesterol.

triglyceride: dietary lipid normally used by the body.

CHAPTER FOCUS

This chapter explains how hyperlipidemia contributes to the development of several important diseases and the role that triglycerides and cholesterol play in the process. It also describes the drugs used to treat hyperlipidemia and discusses how the different hypolipidemic drugs act to lower triglyceride and cholesterol levels in the plasma.

CHAPTER OBJECTIVES

After studying this chapter, you should be able to

- describe hyperlipidemia and the importance of triglycerides and cholesterol.
- discuss the major approaches to the treatment of hyperlipidemia.
- explain the mechanism of action of four different hypolipidemic drugs and the main adverse effects each produces.

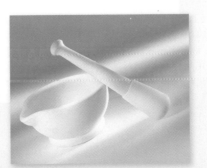

INTRODUCTION

It is often stated "you are what you eat." A balanced diet includes carbohydrates, proteins, and lipids (fats). The important dietary lipids include fatty acids, **triglycerides,** and **cholesterol.** These substances are necessary for the formation of cell membranes, nerve tissue, and plasma lipoproteins. Excess dietary lipids are stored as fat in adipose tissue, where they serve as a reserve form of energy. Cholesterol is stored in the gallbladder as a component of bile acids. The metabolism of fat, especially excess dietary fat, can contribute to other fatty deposits that line blood vessels and impede normal circulation and tissue perfusion.

LIVER METABOLISM AND LIPOPROTEINS

With a balanced nutritional diet, the body absorbs one-third of its daily cholesterol from the diet and produces two-thirds through cellular synthesis in the liver and intestines. Cholesterol is an important substrate for the body because it is the fundamental building block of steroid hormones (adrenal corticosteroids). 3-Hydroxy-3-methylglutaryl coenzyme A (HMG-CoA) is acted upon by the enzyme HMG-CoA reductase to produce mevalonic acid. After a series of reactions in the liver, mevalonic acid becomes cholesterol. The critical step that regulates cholesterol synthesis is MHG-CoA reductase. (This is important because it is a site of drug action.)

Lipoproteins

Lipoproteins, produced in the liver and intestines, transport lipids such as cholesterol and triglycerides to areas of utilization or storage. These lipoproteins differ in density and are referred to as very-low-density lipoprotein (VLDL), low-density lipoprotein (LDL), high-density lipoprotein (HDL), and chylomicrons. Each lipoprotein contains varying amounts of triglycerides and cholesterol in the core. The size of the core varies with the size of the lipoprotein. When carried as circulating lipoproteins, cholesterol is the predominate core of LDL and HDL. Low-density lipoprotein delivers cholesterol to cells for further cell-specific synthesis. By binding with LDL receptors on cell membranes, LDL is taken into the cells and the cholesterol remains in the membranes for synthesis. When cholesterol is released from LDL, HMG-CoA usually receives feedback to alter its cholesterol production.

Chylomicrons

Chylomicrons produced by the intestines transport dietary cholesterol and triglycerides. Triglycerides are the predominate core of chylomicrons and the VLDL secreted by the liver. Circulating chylomicrons become anchored to blood capillaries where catabolism occurs. During the breakdown of chylomicrons, triglycerides are hydrolyzed by the enzyme lipoprotein lipase. The resulting free fatty acids are removed from the blood. The remnants of the chylomicrons exchange triglycerides for cholesterol that can be converted to bile acids, excreted in the bile directly, or stored. These remnants also suppress internal cholesterol synthesis and downregulate the LDL receptors.

Lipoprotein Levels and Disease

There is a dynamic communication among the liver, intestines, and lipoproteins that balances the cholesterol synthesis needed day-to-day. Although lipids are essential for cell structure and function, unusually high lipid levels in the plasma have been correlated with several diseases such as diabetes mellitus, lupus erythmatosus, lipodystrophies, hypothyroidism, and premature atherosclerosis. It appears that high plasma lipid levels promote fat deposition in the walls of the arterial blood vessels. These deposits accumulate as plaque and result in the development of atherosclerosis. Cholesterol, carried by LDL, has been implicated in the formation of atherosclerotic plaque. It is thought that HMG-CoA is stimulated by macrophages after dietary cholesterol is brought into the cells. The average American diet provides large amounts of cholesterol from meat, eggs, and dairy products. Consequently, the plasma cholesterol level of many Americans can be several times higher than needed for daily metabolic balance. It is therefore not surprising that there is a significant incidence of coronary heart disease (CHD) and atherosclerosis in this culture. Atherosclerosis usually manifests itself clinically as coronary artery disease (CAD), stroke, or hypertension, each of which contributes to CHD.

Risk factors associated with the development of CHD are:

- Age (men over age 45; women over age 55)
- History of smoking, hypertension, premature menopause, obesity, antihypertension medications
- Hormone imbalance (diabetes mellitus, hypothyroidism)
- Weight (>30% overweight)
- Lipoprotein status (low HDL, high LDL)

On the other hand, cholesterol transported by HDL appears to be "protective." Individuals with high HDL-cholesterol levels are thought to be less prone to CHD because of the rapid clearance of cholesterol and triglyceride-rich lipoproteins from the circulation. When HDL is available, it can exchange its cholesterol for triglyceride through the action of lipid transfer proteins. The HDL transported lipid is readily broken down by the liver (hepatic lipase), cleared from the body, and not deposited in or on tissues. The exchanged cholesterol can then be converted to bile acids, excreted into the bile, or stored. HDL levels can be elevated through vigorous exercise, a diet that includes fish and/or diet supplementation with omega-3-polyunsaturated fatty acids (fish oils), and moderate alcohol consumption. Factors that decrease HDL include smoking, obesity, liver damage, uremia, and starvation.

The beneficial total circulating cholesterol level recommended is less than 200 mg/dl (120 to 220 mg/dl) with an HDL of 35 mg/dl or more and an LDL less than 130 mg/dl. Cholesterol values in the population range from 120 to 330 mg/dl. Circulating triglyceride values vary with age ranging from 10 to 140 mg/dl under 29 years of age to 10 to 150, 160 or 190. The upper limit of the range increases with each decade, that is, 30 to 39 years old (10 to 150 mg/dl), 40 to 49 years old (10 to 160 mg/dl), and over 50 years old (10 to 190 mg/dl). When cholesterol rises to more than 240 mg/dl associated with LDL-cholesterol of 160 mg/dl, evaluation of the lipoprotein profile will indicate the most appropriate course of therapy. Beside heredity, disease, and dietary excesses, cholesterol and triglycerides increase as a function of age. While this is probably attributable to higher fat in the diet of elderly Americans, older people are also more likely to develop cirrhosis, renal disease, and inflammation of the liver and pancreas. Even without evidence of CHD, cholesterol levels less than 200 mg/dl accompanied by two risk factors warrant evaluation of the lipoprotein profile and possibly drug treatment. Reduction in cholesterol has been demonstrated in large clinical trials to be associated with a 20 to 30 percent reduction in CAD.

MONITORING BLOOD LIPID LEVELS

Identification of circulating lipids and lipoproteins is important in monitoring patient health. Routine lipid analysis includes fasting values of total cholesterol, triglycerides, and HDL-cholesterol. Quantitative analysis of serum cholesterol is not a routine assay and must be specifically ordered. This analysis identifies the circulating levels of free cholesterol and cholesterol esters. Triglycerides and cholesterol are measured from fasting (12 to 14 hours) blood samples where the patient has not consumed alcohol for the previous 24 hours. Although the literature speaks of plasma lipid levels, or plasma lipoproteins, blood samples used for analysis are serum samples. Serum, fluid that remains after the blood has been allowed to clot, is the preferred fluid because it provides the greatest amount of (previously circulating) cholesterol and triglyceride for measurement.

Lipoprotein electrophoresis (separation of lipoproteins) is performed to characterize the lipoprotein profile. Although referred to as LDL and HDL, measurement of each lipoprotein in the blood is actually as the combination with cholesterol—that is, HDL-cholesterol. In fact, LDL-cholesterol is calculated from the values for total cholesterol (TC), HDL-cholesterol (HDL), and triglycerides (TG) as follows: LDL = TC − HDL − TG/5. From this equation it is easy to see that anything (diet, drug therapy) that lowers TC and TG and/or raises HDL promotes a reduction in LDL-cholesterol (Figure 29:1).

Correct diagnosis of primary hyperlipoproteinemia is critical because treatment of the underlying disorder often corrects the **hyperlipidemia.** The treatment of hyperlipidemia involves dietary restriction of saturated fats, cholesterol, and carbohydrates. Diet control is always the first line of defense. The American Heart Association recommends a stepped approach to diet adjustment toward a goal of 100 to 150 mg of cholesterol intake daily, and fat limited to 20 percent of the total calories. If diet does not adequately lower cholesterol, several pharmacological agents may be added to reduce plasma lipid levels. These agents are referred to as the **hypolipidemic drugs** (see Table 29:1). Use of these drugs is secondary to adequate dietary control. The drugs in this class are divided into three categories according to the site of cholesterol reduction: bile acid sequestrants, HMG-CoA reductase inhibitors, and miscellaneous alteration of cholesterol metabolism.

BILE ACID SEQUESTRANTS

Cholestyramine, Colestipol, and Colsevelam

Bile salts are synthesized from cholesterol and released into the duodenum as a part of bile. The main function of bile salts is to break down fats ingested in the diet into absorbable forms. The bile salts are recycled by intestinal absorption and storage within the gall bladder. Cholestyramine (*Questran*) is an ion-exchange resin that combines with the bile salts and cholesterol in the intestinal tract. This insoluble binding prevents the absorption of the bile salts and cholesterol. The result is an increased elimination of bile salts, cholesterol, and other fats in the feces. Low-density lipoprotein and cholesterol levels decrease during treatment. Liver synthesis of cholesterol may increase, however—the circulating cholesterol concentration decreases because cholesterol is cleared from the plasma. Changes in LDL levels may be observed within 1 week of treatment, while changes in circulating cholesterol may require 1 month. The action of colestipol (*Colestid*) is similar to that of cholestyramine. Colestipol interferes with the absorption of bile acids and cholesterol from the intestinal tract.

Dose Administration

Cholestyramine, 4 to 6 g per dose, is mixed with fruit juice and taken twice a day before meals. Cholestyramine is a powder that must be mixed with water. Noncarbonated beverages, fluid soups (broth, not cream), applesauce, or crushed pineapple may also be used to suspend the powder. The daily oral dose of colestipol tablets is 2-16 g/day given once or in divided doses. Patients are often started at 2 g once or twice daily and raised 2 g once or twice daily at 1-2 month intervals until the lipid profile is acceptable. Colestipol comes as tablets or granules.

Colesevelam (*Welchol*) is recommended to start with three tablets twice daily or six tablets once daily with a meal. Each tablet contains 625 mg of active drug so the maximum dose is more than 3 g daily.

FIGURE 29:1 Relationship of LDL-Cholesterol Values from Measured Levels of Total Cholesterol, Triglycerides, and HDL-Cholesterol

$$LDL = TC - HDL - (TG/5)$$

LDL-cholesterol	Total cholesterol	HDL-cholesterol	Triglycerides divided by 5

Before diet control	197 mg/dl	=	240 mg/dl 240	–	15 mg/dl 15	–	140 mg/dl/ 5 28

Recommended blood levels   130 mg/dl = <200 mg/dl – >35 mg/dl – [age related 10–190 mg/dl]

After diet control	117 mg/dl	=	180 mg/dl 180	–	35 mg/dl 35	–	140 mg/dl/ 5 28

Adverse Effects

Bile Acid Sequestrants—Cholestyramine is not absorbed from the gastrointestinal (GI) tract. While systemic effects do not usually occur, GI disturbances are the most common adverse effect. Constipation is the most common adverse effect, sometimes severe accompanied by fecal impacting. Existing hemorrhoids may be aggravated. Headache, dizziness, drowsiness, and anxiety have been reported to occur in some patients. Because of the large doses, nausea, vomiting, and other GI disturbances may occur. With continued use of the drug, constipation, flatulence, and nausea may disappear. The most serious adverse effect with the bile acid sequestrants is intestinal obstruction. Colestipol has produced transient elevations in aspartate aminotransferase (AST) and alanine aminotransferase (ALT) and alkaline phosphatase.

HMG-CoA REDUCTASE INHIBITORS

Statins

Lovastatin (*Mevacor*) was the first in the class of drugs that inhibit the enzyme HMG-CoA reductase. This enzyme is the rate-limiting step early in the synthesis of cholesterol. Squalene synthesis is also inhibited so that the cholesterol pathway is primarily affected while the production of essential cell growth mediators is unaffected. This inhibition reduces the circulating LDL that transports cholesterol. By reducing the plasma levels of LDL, the levels of cholesterol in the plasma are reduced; similarly, by reducing VLDL, plasma levels of triglycerides decrease. Low-density lipoprotein (LDL) can be decreased in the circulation through increased clearance from the plasma or through decreased production. At the same time, plasma levels of HDL-cholesterol are increased in the circulation.

All drugs in this class—atorvastatin (*Lipitor*), fluvastatin (*Lescol*), lovastatin (*Mevacor*), pravastatin (*Pravachol*), and simvastatin (*Zocor*)—have the same site of action and effectively reduce total cholesterol and LDL plasma levels. While the effect on circulating lipids is observable within 2 weeks of treatment, the maximum benefit requires up to 6 weeks of drug therapy. When the medication is stopped, the reduction in lipoprotein plasma levels disappears within 6 weeks. Maintenance of therapeutic benefit, therefore, requires diet adjustment and continued drug treatment.

All of these drugs are well absorbed following oral administration. However, lovastatin is better absorbed when administered with meals. Lovastatin is a prodrug (inactive) that is activated by liver metabolism. All of the other drugs in this class may be taken with or without meals without affecting the therapeutic effect. Except for pravastatin, all are highly bound (95 to 98 percent) to plasma protein. Recommended maintenance doses for HMG-CoA reductase inhibitors are presented in Table 29:1.

Lovastatin and simvastatin have been used successfully in combination with cholestyramine to lower cholesterol. Combination therapy

TABLE 29:1	Hypolipidemic Drugs	
DRUG (TRADE NAME)	**USUAL ORAL DAILY DOSE**	
Bile Acid Sequestrants		
cholestyramine (*Questran*)	8–16 g	
colestipol (*Colestid*)	2–16 g	
colesevelam (*Welchol*)	3.6 g	
HMG-CoA Enzyme Inhibitors		
atorvastatin (*Lipitor*)	10–80 mg	
fluvastatin (*Lescol*)	20–80 mg	
lovastatin (*Mevacor*)	10–80 mg/day	
pravastatin (*Pravachol*)	10–80 mg	
rosuvastatin (*Crestor*)	5–40 mg	
simvastatin (*Zocor*)	5–80 mg	
Alteration of Lipid and Lipoprotein Metabolism		
gemfibrozil (*Lopid*)	600 mg BID 30 min before meals	
fenofibrate (*Tricor*)	54–160 mg	
niacin (*Niacor*)	2 to 6 g	
Combination Drugs		
niacin and lovastatin (*Advicor*)	500–2000 mg/ 20–40 mg	
Cholesterol Absorption Inhibitor		
ezetimibe (*Zetia*)	10 mg	

dramatically reduces cholesterol and LDL-cholesterol to levels that cannot be attained by either the bile salt sequestrant or enzyme inhibitor alone. When using combination therapy, the HMG-CoA reductase inhibitor should be taken 4 to 6 hours after the bile acid sequestrant to avoid the possibility of the sequestrant binding the enzyme inhibitor while in the intestinal tract. A product is now available that combines lovastatin with niacin in a fixed dose. *Advicor* combines niacin (500, 750, or 1000 mg) with 20 mg of lovastatin.

Prior to initiation of treatment, or increase in dosage, liver function tests should be performed to confirm the status of alanine aminotransferase (ALT) and aspartate aminotransferase (AST). Because this class of drugs can elevate liver enzymes, the serum levels should be repeated every 6 to 12 weeks to avoid serious adverse effects. Persistent elevation in liver enzymes may require discontinuation of the drug.

The range of adverse effects includes headache, dizziness, alteration of taste, insomnia, diarrhea, flatulence, abdominal cramping and/or pain, and photosensitivity.

Because the HMG-CoA reductase inhibitors are absorbed and are able to affect lipid metabolism in a variety of tissues, the spectrum of adverse effects is greater than other hypolipidemic drugs. Most important is the potential for developing myalgia and muscle weakness. Transient elevations in creatine phosphokinase (CPK) may occur before and during the myalgia. Careful periodic monitoring of serum enzymes including liver function (AST, ALT) and CPK will indicate the need for dose reduction to eliminate the adverse effect. Depending on the medical profile of the patient, persistent elevation in liver function enzymes and/or CPK, the drug may require drug discontinuation.

The HMG-CoA reductase inhibitors represent a significant advance in the management of hyperlipidemias; however, they have the potential to alter muscle metabolism. Cerivastatin (*Baycol*) has recently been removed from the market due to safety concerns because of evidence of muscle breakdown in patients during chronic treatment. The incidence of this life-threatening side effect (rhabdomyolysis) was significantly higher with cerivastatin alone than with other statin drugs. Rabdomyolysis is a condition in which the contents of the skeletal muscle cells (enzymes, creatinine, myoglobin) leak into the circulation. The patient experiences muscle pain and weakness and renal failure develops when the large molecules of myoglobin obstruct normal renal flow. Patients who are taking statin drugs should be instructed to report muscle tenderness or weakness to their physician.

Accidental overdose (up to 6 g) has occurred in adults and children with these drugs. There is no specific antidote. Using general supportive measures for overdose of any medication, these patients recovered without complication.

Cholesterol Absorption Inhibitors

One of the newest drugs to reduce serum cholesterol, Ezetimibe (*Zetia*), has a mechanism of action unlike all other antihyperlipidemic drugs. Ezetimibe acts at the surface of the small intestine to block absorption of dietary cholesterol. This action reduces the amount of cholesterol delivered to the liver and facilitates clearance of cholesterol from the blood.

This drug is approved for use alone, 10 mg once a day, or in combination with HMG-CoA reductase inhibitors or bile acid sequestrants for the treatment of hypercholesterolemia. Ezetimibe can be taken together with the HMG-CoA reductase inhibitors without impeding oral absorption of ezetimibe. However, it must be taken 2 to 4 hours after bile acid sequestrant dosing to avoid an absorption interaction.

MISCELLANEOUS HYPOLIPIDEMICS

Nicotinic Acid (Niacin [*Niacor*])

Niacin is an important vitamin in the metabolism of carbohydrates. A deficiency of niacin is associated with the disease pellagra. However, in large doses, niacin (in the form of nicotinic acid) lowers plasma lipid levels. Niacin appears to reduce the level of the VLDL and LDL, lipoproteins responsible for carrying triglycerides and cholesterol in a dose-dependent manner. At the same time, fat metabolism in adipose tissue is inhibited, and lipoprotein lipase (TG breakdown) is stimulated. Consequently, the plasma lipid level is significantly reduced. These effects on lipoproteins are evident within 4 days of treatment and maximum effects occur within 3 to 5 weeks. Interestingly, the formulations of the vitamin affect circulating lipids differently. The immediate-release preparation increases HDL, while the sustained-release product reduces total cholesterol and LDL preferentially. Niacin is administered orally several times per day. Initial doses (100 mg TID) are gradually increased to 1 to 2 g three times a day. The maximum dose is usually 8 g per day. Niacin has been used in combination with colestipol and lovastatin. The triple combination is more effective in reducing LDL than dual combination of nicotinic acid with one of the others.

Common adverse effects include nausea, vomiting, diarrhea, and vasodilation. Niacin produces vasodilation that manifests as flushing of the skin. The flushing is accompanied by a sensation of warmth on the face and upper body, sometimes with tingling, itching, or headache. This effect is not harmful, but may not be well tolerated by patients who experience a persistent flushing. Patients may be advised to avoid drinking hot liquids just before and after dosing to avoid the potential for vasodilation from the liquids. Aspirin taken 30 minutes before dosing also mitigates the vasodilation in many patients.

Niacin may also increase uric acid levels in the blood (hyperuricemia). Individuals with high uric acid levels may develop symptoms of gout. The sustained release product in doses greater than 2 g per day may promote jaundice, increased bilirubin, nausea, and prolonged prothrombin time. These effects appear to be mediated by an alteration of liver function. Periodic monitoring of liver enzymes will provide adequate indication of hepatotoxicity.

Fibric Acid Derivatives

Gemfibrozil (*Lopid*) and fenofibrate (*Tricor*) are derivatives of fibric acid that decrease triglyceride and VLDL, and increase HDL. The mechanism of action is directed at triglyceride production. In addition to inhibiting the breakdown of fats into triglycerides, liver production of triglycerides is inhibited.

Both drugs are well absorbed from the intestinal tract. The oral dose of gemfibrozil is usually 600 mg BID while the dose of fenofibrate is 54–160 mg daily. These drugs are approved for use in hypertriglyceridemia patients who do not respond to diet where triglyceride levels can exceed 1000 mg/dl compared to the normal range of 10 to 190 mg/dl. They can also be used in combination with other drugs to facilitate a reduction in triglycerides that complements the cholesterol lowering action of the hypolipidemic drug.

Common adverse effects involve the GI tract and include nausea, vomiting, diarrhea, and flatulence. They may also produce dizziness and blurred vision that may interfere with the ability to perform intricate hand work or operate equipment. Since this class of drugs—fibrates—can produce muscle pain and weakness, combination with HMG-CoA reductase inhibitors potentiates the development of myopathy and significantly elevated creatine phosphokinase levels.

Gemfibrozil may increase cholesterol excretion into the bile leading to gallstone formation. The drug must be discontinued in the presence of cholelithiasis or elevated creatine phosphokinase.

CLINICAL INDICATIONS

All of the hypolipidemic drugs are indicated as adjunctive therapy for the reduction of elevated cholesterol in patients with primary hypercholesterolemia and elevated LDL who do not adequately respond to diet. This class of drugs is used to decrease mixed lipidemias of primary or secondary origin especially where high-risk patients have not responded to other treatments; for example, diabetic and nephrotic lipidemia.

3-Hydroxy-3-methylglutaryl coenzyme A (HMG-CoA) reductase inhibitors lovastatin and pravastatin are also recommended to slow the progression of coronary atherosclerosis in with CHD to reduce the risk of acute coronary episodes. Simvastatin and pravastatin are used to reduce the risk of death from coronary events, and to reduce the risk of developing acute myocardial infarction. Cholestyramine is also recommended in the management of partial biliary obstruction.

CONTRAINDICATIONS

For systemically absorbed drugs, clinical manifestations of hypersensitivity, active liver disease, or persistent elevation in liver function, enzymes are contraindications to the use or continued use of the hypolipidemic drug. 3-Hydroxy-3-methylglutaryl coenzyme A (HMG-CoA) reductase inhibitors are absolutely contraindicated during pregnancy because of their ability to inhibit essential lipid metabolism in the developing fetus. While no human data are available, skeletal malformations have occurred in animals.

Dextrothyroxine is contraindicated in patients with angina, a history of myocardial infarction, cardiac arrhythmias, congestive heart failure, hypertension, and pregnancy.

DRUG INTERACTIONS

Bile Acid Sequestrants

Cholestyramine binds with fat-soluble vitamins (A, D, and K), folic acid, and many drugs, thus reducing their GI absorption. Supplementation may be necessary to avoid vitamin deficiencies. It is recommended that any other medications be

Patient Administration and Monitoring

Compliance with drug therapy is critical to achieving the long-term benefit of cholesterol reduction, reduction of the low-density lipoproteins, and prevention of CHD. To assist patients in developing compliance habits for proper drug use, the medication, dosing schedule, and specific adverse reactions should be reviewed with the patient. A serum chemistry panel should be performed periodically during treatment to determine whether cholesterol and the LDL-HDL ratio are within the normal range. Liver function enzymes, AST, ALT, and alkaline phosphatase should be evaluated to ensure the patient is not experiencing undesirable adverse effects during treatment.

taken 1 hour before or at least 4 hours after cholestyramine to avoid interaction within the intestinal tract that would delay or inhibit absorption of the concomitant medication.

3-Hydroxy-3-methylglutaryl Coenzyme A (HMG-CoA) Reductase Inhibitors

Itraconazole increases the circulating level of HMG-CoA reductase inhibitors, predisposing the patient to developing adverse effects. The proposed mechanism is competition with hepatic enzymes. For patients who require antifungal therapy, the reductase enzyme inhibitor should be stopped until the fungal treatment is discontinued. Gemfibrozil should not be administered with HMG-CoA reductase inhibitors. Urinary excretion and protein binding of the enzyme inhibitors can decrease resulting in larger circulating drug levels. The combination predisposes patients to develop severe myopathy. Table 29:2 presents a list of specific drugs that have been shown to interact with hypolipidemic drugs.

Consideration of Formulation and Meals

Medication is usually taken before meals. Lovastatin should be taken with meals in order to absorb the maximum therapeutic amount. Niacin may be taken with meals for those patients who experience GI upset with dosing.

Powders can be mixed with beverages, soups, cereals, or pulpy fruits; however, colestipol tablets should be swallowed whole, not crushed or chewed.

Drug Interactions

Since medication may interfere with other drugs, take concomitant medications 1 hour before or 6 hours after bile acid sequestrants. 3-Hydroxy-3-methylglutaryl-coenzyme A (HMG-CoA) reductase inhibitors used as combination therapy with bile acid sequestrants should be taken 4 to 6 hours after the bile acid sequestrant.

Adverse Effects

The physician should be notified if unusual bleeding from the gums or rectum occurs. Muscle pain, tenderness, weakness, malaise, or fever while taking these medications should be reported to the doctor immediately.

With dextrothyroxine, the physician should be notified immediately if the patient experiences chest pain, sweating, palpitations, or skin rash.

Gemfibrozil may cause dizziness and blurred vision that could impair judgment in tasks requiring focused concentration or coordination. This should be reviewed with patients who need to drive or operate heavy equipment.

Patients who experience flushing (sensation of warmth on the face and upper body) with niacin treatment should avoid hot liquids immediately before and after dosing to minimize triggering of vasodilation. Patients experiencing persistent flushing may benefit from aspirin 300 mg 30 minutes before niacin dosing.

Considerations Prior to Surgery

Because of its potential to increase bleeding, dextrothyroxine should be discontinued at least 2 weeks prior to surgery. In the event the patient may be seeing another physician or oral surgeon who could schedule surgical procedures, the patient should be advised to provide full disclosure of dextrothyroxine treatment to avoid complications.

Use in Pregnancy

Hypolipidemic drugs have been designated Food and Drug Administration (FDA) Pregnancy Category B or C, except for HMG-CoA reductase inhibitors, which are designated Category X. The safety for use during pregnancy has not been clearly established through well controlled clinical trials. Therefore, use during pregnancy is only

TABLE 29:2   Drug Interactions with Hypolipidemic Drugs

HYPOLIPIDEMIC	INTERACT WITH	RESPONSE
Bile acid sequestrants	Anticoagulants (oral), aspirin, clindamycin, clofibrate, dextrothyroxine digitalis glycosides, furosemide, glipizide, imipramine, methyldopa, niacin, penicillin, phenytoin, tetracyclines, thiazides, tolbutamide, ursodiol, vitamins A, D, K, E	Decrease drug absorption
cholestyramine	HMG-CoA reductase inhibitors	Decrease bioavailability of the enzyme inhibitors when taken within 1 hour
	Anticoagulants	Increase bleeding
gemfibrozil fenofibrate	HMG-CoA reductase inhibitors	Severe myopathy
	Oral anticoagulants	Increase blood levels of anticoagulants
HMG-CoA reductase inhibitors	alcohol	Increase blood level of enzyme inhibitors
	cyclosporin, erythromycin, niacin	Increase enzyme inhibitor blood level and potential for myopathy to occur
	itraconazole	Increase enzyme inhibitor blood level by hepatic enzyme competition
	digoxin, warfarin	Increases blood levels of digoxin and warfarin
	Oral contraceptives	Increase atorvastatin blood levels
	rifampin	Decrease plasma clearance of fluvastatin
	nicotinic acid, propranolol, digoxin	Decrease fluvastatin levels
	propranolol	Decrease enzyme inhibitor hypolipidemic effect

recommended when there is clear risk from other sources to be avoided. In particular, clofibrate and gemfibrozil are Category C drugs that are not recommended for use during pregnancy. If there is a need for maintaining lowered cholesterol or triglycerides during pregnancy, bile acid sequestrants may be recommended over other systemically absorbed drugs.

3-Hydroxy-HMG-CoA reductase inhibitors **should not be taken** during pregnancy because of their ability to affect metabolism and critical growth factors in the developing fetus. Patients who may become pregnant should be advised to notify the physician immediately so that the medication can be discontinued and another appropriate treatment begun.

Chapter Review

Understanding Terminology

Match the terms in the right column with the appropriate definitions in the left column.

___ **1.** A dietary lipid normally synthesized in the body.

___ **2.** A protein in the plasma that transports triglycerides and cholesterol.

___ **3.** Abnormally high levels of lipids in the plasma.

___ **4.** A dietary lipid normally used by the body.

___ **5.** A drug used to lower plasma lipid levels.

a. cholesterol

b. hyperlipidemia

c. hypolipidemic

d. lipoprotein

e. triglyceride

Acquiring Knowledge

Answer the following questions in the spaces provided.

1. What diseases are associated with hyperlipidemia? _____

_____

2. What is the major approach to the treatment of hyperlipidemia? _____

_____

3. How does lovastatin (*Mevacor*) produce its hypolipidemic effect? _____

_____

4. List the adverse effects of niacin. _____

_____

5. How does the mechanism of action of fenofibrate (*Tricor*) differ from that of cholestyramine (*Questran*)?

_____

6. What is the primary indication for the use of gemfibrozil (*Lopid*)? _____

_____

Applying Knowledge—On The Job

Use your critical thinking skills to answer the following questions in the spaces provided.

1. The HMG-CoA reductase inhibitors may affect liver function. Liver function tests (ALT and AST) should be done at certain points during therapy using these medications. Explain when these tests should be done.

_____

_____

2. Some patients may experience persistent flushing when taking niacin. What advice might be helpful for the patients who find this to be intolerable?

_____

_____

3. What are the adverse effects listed for lovastatin? _____

_____

Internet Connection

There are a number of guidelines available online that explain the impact of serum lipids on cardiovascular function. These guidelines are prepared by a variety of professional medical and scientific organizations and made available through the National Guideline Clearinghouse (NCG) at www.guideline.gov., a public resource for evidence-based clinical practice guidelines. In the NCG search box, enter *Cholesterol* and more than 60 references will be presented that can be reviewed and printed. This site updates the index of guidelines weekly so it is always current.

The American Association of Family Practitioners at www.aafp.org provides access to current and archived volumes of the journal, *American Family Physician*. This journal presents easy-to-understand articles on topics, such as cholesterol management and prevention of heart disease. At the site, go to the left margin and select *American Family Physician Past Issues*. At the Search By Topic box, enter *Cholesterol* and all relevant articles in the journal will be provided for review.

Additional Reading

Glatter, T. R. 1991. Hyperlipidemia: What do the numbers mean? *Hospital Medicine* 27 (4):25.

Mosca, L. J. 2002. Optimal management of cholesterol levels and the prevention of coronary heart disease in women. *American Family Physician* 65 (2):217.

Safeer, R. S. 2002. Cholesterol treatment guidelines update. *American Family Physician* 65(5):871.

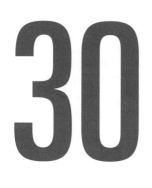

chapter

30

ANTIANEMICS

CHAPTER FOCUS

This chapter discusses the minerals and nutrients required to maintain normal function of the red blood cells (RBCs). The most critical function of the RBCs is the ability to carry oxygen to the tissues. This chapter describes how this function can be impaired, resulting in anemia, and how anemia can be treated.

CHAPTER OBJECTIVES

After studying this chapter, you should be able to

- explain the three primary ways anemia can occur.
- identify three naturally occurring substances that affect the shape of red blood cells.
- explain when it is appropriate to use iron supplements or vitamin replacement to reverse the affects of anemia.
- describe the side effects associated with iron overdose.
- explain why vitamin B_{12} and folic acid replacement are not interchangeable for the treatment of anemia.

DRUG CLASS AT A GLANCE

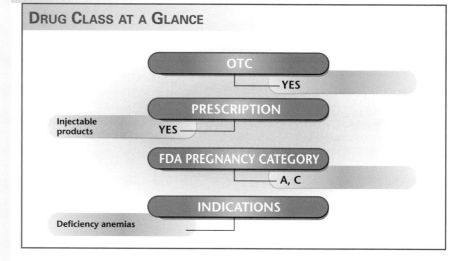

OTC — YES

PRESCRIPTION

Injectable products — YES

FDA PREGNANCY CATEGORY — A, C

INDICATIONS

Deficiency anemias

Key Terms

anemia: condition in which the oxygen-carrying function of the red blood cells to the tissues is decreased.

aplastic anemia: anemia caused by defective functioning of the blood-forming organs (bone marrow).

chelate: chemical action of a substance to bond permanently to a metal ion.

-chromic: suffix meaning color.

chronic: condition of long duration, usually months or years.

-cytic: suffix meaning cells.

enteric-coated: type of tablet or pill with a coating that enables it to pass through the stomach without being dissolved, so the stomach lining will not be irritated; the drug is then released in the intestine.

gastric lavage: flushing of the stomach.

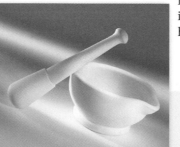

hematinic: medications containing iron compounds, used to increase hemoglobin production.

332

hemoglobin: protein in red blood cells that transports oxygen to all tissues of the body.

hypochromic: condition in which the color of red blood cells is less than the normal index.

intrinsic factor: protein necessary for intestinal absorption of vitamin B_{12}; lack of intrinsic factor leads to pernicious anemia.

malabsorption: inadequate ability to take in nutrients through the intestine.

mega-: prefix meaning large.

megaloblast: large, immature cell that cannot yet function as a mature red blood cell (RBC).

micro-: prefix meaning small.

morphology: shape or structure of a cell.

normocytic anemia: anemia in which RBCs are normal size and usually contain normal hemoglobin but are insufficient to carry adequate oxygen to the tissues; low RBC count.

pernicious: disease of severe symptoms, which could be fatal if left untreated.

RBC: red blood cell.

INTRODUCTION

Hemoglobin is a protein found in red blood cells **(RBCs).** Because the main function of hemoglobin is to transport oxygen to all tissues of the body, anything that alters the function of the RBCs or the production of hemoglobin causes a deficiency in oxygen transport, thus producing a condition known as **anemia.** In response to oxygen deficiency, the body develops the characteristic symptoms of anemia, including weakness, fatigue, irritability, and pallor.

CAUSES OF ANEMIA

Certain anemias are inherited because the synthesis of hemoglobin is genetically controlled. Cooley's anemia and sickle cell anemia are inherited diseases in which the hemoglobin is abnormal and cannot efficiently carry oxygen. Inherited anemias are **chronic** illnesses and cannot be successfully treated or cured with drug replacement therapy. Anemia may also be caused by deficiency in the amount of hemoglobin, occurring when the number of circulating red blood cells is decreased. Loss of blood (hemorrhage), increased destruction of RBCs (hemolysis), or decreased production of RBCs reduces the amount of circulating hemoglobin. The production of normal blood cells may be impaired when the bone marrow is poisoned by chemicals, such as benzene or anticancer drugs. More commonly, however, blood cell production is decreased when essential vitamins and minerals are deficient in the diet. The most commonly occurring deficiency anemias are produced by a lack of iron, cyanocobalamin (vitamin B_{12}), or folic acid. Besides decreasing RBC production, deficiency anemias may be associated with changes in the size and shape of the red and white blood cells. For this reason, deficiency anemias are also classified according to the shape, or **morphology,** and color of the blood cells.

Microcytic (**micro-** means small and **-cytic** refers to cells) anemias are characterized by unusually small RBCs. When mycrocytic anemia is associated with a hemoglobin deficiency, the RBCs appear pale (**hypochromic**—*hypo-* refers to less than normal and **-chromic** means color). Macrocyte (*macro-* means large) anemias have unusually large blood cells. When blood cell production is interrupted, large immature cells known as **megaloblasts (mega-** also means large) are released into the circulation. In megaloblastic anemias, the blood cells may appear larger, but the RBCs are normochromic (no change in color). Morphological changes associated with several different anemias are compared in Table 30:1. Unlike inherited anemias, deficiency anemias are very responsive to replacement therapy. Once the missing substance is identified and restored to the diet, the symptoms of the anemia subside. In addition, the morphology and production of blood cells return to normal.

TABLE 30:1 — Origin and Treatment of RBC Anemias

ORIGIN	CAUSE	RBC CHARACTERISTICS	TREATMENT
Excessive blood loss	Hemorrhage	Normocytic normochromic	Stop bleeding, blood transfusion
Decreased RBC production			
Deficiency anemia	Lack of iron Lack of copper Lack of folic acid	Microcytic hypochromic	Replace iron or copper in the diet Replace folic acid or cyanocobalamin in diet
	Lack of cyanocobalamin	Macrocytic (megaloblastic) normochromic	
Bone marrow failure	Chemicals Anticancer drugs Irradiation	Normocytic normochromic	Blood transfusion
Increased RBC destruction	Defective RBC metabolism Microbial toxins Drug allergy	Normocytic normochromic	Blood transfusion
Altered RBC production and destruction	Defective hemoglobin synthesis	Sickle shape microcytic	Blood transfusion
	Chronic infection Liver disease	Hypochromic Normocytic normochromic	Blood transfusion

Iron Deficiency Anemia

The amount of iron in the body is maintained at a relatively constant level between 2 and 5 g. Diets that include meat, fish, or soy products should supply an adequate amount of iron. Iron is primarily distributed in the RBCs or stored in tissues such as the bone marrow, spleen, and liver. Since the body excretes very little iron each day, iron stores are efficiently conserved. Iron deficiency occurs when the internal iron stores become depleted.

Development of Deficiency

To maintain an adequate iron balance, the National Academy of Sciences Research Council suggests that the Recommended Dietary Allowance (RDA) for iron should be between 10 and 18 mg. The RDA varies with the age, sex, and health of the individual. After age 20, healthy males require less iron intake than do females. Depletion of iron reserves in adult males does not readily occur. Most often, when it does occur, it is caused by internal bleeding or chronic disease (carcinoma or ulcers) rather than a dietary deficiency of iron.

Women, on the other hand, are always predisposed to iron deficiency, primarily as a result of the constant loss of blood during each menstrual period (in which 1 to 20 mg of iron may be lost). For this reason, iron deficiency anemia can easily develop in women, especially those who have nutritionally poor diets. Pregnancy and lactation also increase the iron requirements for women and may contribute to the development of iron deficiency.

In addition, women and young children may become iron deficient from a condition known as pica, a condition in which people eat unusual substances such as clay and laundry starch. When this continues over a long time, the clay and starch bind the dietary iron so that no iron is absorbed. Eventually, internal iron stores become depleted, and anemia results.

Chronic iron deficiency from any cause results in a microcytic hypochromic anemia. The RBCs and hemoglobin are affected because iron is essential for normal oxygen transport. Oxygen molecules are carried by the iron, which is bound to hemoglobin. In chronic iron deficiency, the function of hemoglobin is severely impaired.

TABLE 30:2   Iron Preparations*

TRADE NAME	IRON	OTHER INGREDIENTS
Femiron	63 mg ferrous fumarate	—
Feosol Spansules	159 mg ferrous sulfate exsiccated	—
Feosol Tablets	200 mg ferrous sulfate	—
Fergon Elixir	300 mg ferrous gluconate/15 ml	—
Fergon Tablets	320 mg ferrous gluconate	—
Fer-in-Sol Capsules	190 mg ferrous sulfate	—
Fer-in-Sol Drops	75 mg ferrous sulfate/0.6 ml	0.02% alcohol
Fermalox	200 mg ferrous sulfate	Magnesium hydroxide, aluminum hydroxide
Fero-Gradumet Filmtabs	525 mg ferrous sulfate	—
Ferro-Sequels	150 mg ferrous fumarate	Docusate sodium
Geritol tonic liquid	18 mg iron ammonium citrate	Niacin, thiamine, pyridoxine, choline, cyanocobalamin, methionine, 12% alcohol
Mol-Iron Tablets	195 mg ferrous sulfate	—
Mol-Iron with Vitamin C	39 mg ferrous sulfate	Ascorbic acid
Tri-Tinic Capsules	36.3 mg ferrous fumarate	Ascorbic acid, folic acid, cyanocobalamin, intrinsic factor concentrate
Vitron-C	66 mg ferrous fumarate	Ascorbic acid, tartrazine

*This is not an inclusive list of available products.

Hematinics

Anemia caused by a nutritional lack of iron is easily corrected with oral iron supplements. **Hematinics** are medications that primarily contain iron (ferrous) compounds for the purpose of increasing hemoglobin production. Hematinics are available as over-the-counter products in tablet, capsule, and liquid forms. Many iron supplements are packaged as part of a multiple vitamin preparation containing 100 percent of the RDA for iron. However, several hematinics listed in Table 30:2 contain 5 to 20 times the RDA for iron. Ferrous compounds such as fumarate, sulfate, and gluconate are equally well absorbed orally and are the agents of choice. The addition of ascorbic acid (vitamin C) appears to enhance the intestinal absorption of iron. Long-term iron-deficient patients may require 100 to 200 mg of iron TID for at least 6 months. In comparison, iron deficiency associated with pregnancy, especially in the last trimester, may be corrected with 20 to 50 mg of iron per day.

Occasionally, iron deficiency is caused by an inability to take oral medications or to absorb iron **(malabsorption).** In these situations, iron dextran (InFeD) may be administered intramuscularly or intravenously. The intravenous route is usually preferred because there is less pain at the injection site. Also, staining of the skin may occur at the injection site. The manufacturer's suggested dose is based upon the patient's weight and hemoglobin value. The parenteral use of iron dextran has resulted in anaphylactic-type reactions. Patients must be tested for sensitivity prior to administering iron dextran to avoid an anaphylactic reaction. Iron dextran should only be used in patients for whom there is a clearly established indication of lack of tolerance of oral supplements or for whom gastrointestinal (GI) absorption is impaired. Iron dextran is *incompatible* in solutions containing oxytetracycline.

Clinical Indications

Iron supplementation, including parenteral administration, is approved for the prevention and treatment of iron deficiency anemia from any source. There is no proven therapeutic value in the treatment of anemias arising from a deficiency of other vitamins or minerals.

Adverse and Toxic Effects

The most frequently occurring side effects associated with oral hematinics are gastric irritation, nausea, and constipation. Supplements are recommended to be taken on an empty stomach to optimize absorption. In sensitive patients, however, the gastric irritation may be intense. When gastric irritation occurs, the dose of the iron supplement may be reduced or taken with meals. Delayed release and **enteric-coated** iron preparations reduce the gastric irritation by releasing the iron in the lower intestine. Unfortunately, the iron in these preparations is not well absorbed, and the products usually are more expensive than are other iron supplements. Patients should be cautioned not to chew or crush these preparations prior to swallowing. Overall, the special formulations offer no significant advantage over other hematinic formulations available. Some hematinics contain a stool softener to counteract constipation, whereas others contain an antacid to alleviate the nausea.

Liquid iron preparations are recommended to be taken with juice or water to avoid staining the teeth. Patients may be advised to take such liquid preparations through a drinking straw to decrease the potential for staining.

In therapeutic doses, unabsorbed iron is excreted into the feces, causing stools to become black and tarry. This effect should not be mistaken for blood in the stool, since both iron therapy and occult bleeding produce the same fecal appearance. Iron overload (excessive iron storage) rarely occurs with oral iron therapy. However, acute iron toxicity may occur as a result of accidental overdose or poisoning. Usually, iron poisoning occurs in children who are attracted by the colored tablets and flavored liquids containing iron. In toxic doses (0.3 to 1 g), iron erodes the stomach lining, causing pain, bleeding, and vomiting. In severe cases, acidosis, hypotension, and cardiovascular collapse occur. Treatment of acute iron toxicity includes **gastric lavage** (flushing the stomach) with deferoxamine mesylate (5 to 10 g). The deferoxamine binds, or **chelates,** the iron so that none can be absorbed.

Drug Interactions

Drug interactions with hematinics are few. However, tetracyclines and antacids taken simultaneously with oral iron supplements decrease iron absorption because they chelate iron. Tetracycline absorption also decreases. Cimetidine through a different mechanism of action also decreases iron absorption. These products should not be taken within 2 hours of each other. Iron salts will decrease the absorption of penicillamine, quinolones, methyldopa, and levodopa. Allopurinol (*Zyloprim*) has been reported to increase oral iron absorption, and ascorbic acid (vitamin C—200 mg per 30 mg iron) enhances the absorption of iron from the GI tract. Coffee, tea, milk, and eggs decrease the absorption of dietary iron. The clinical effect associated with these foods and oral iron supplements is not known.

CYANOCOBALAMIN DEFICIENCY

Cyanocobalamin (vitamin B_{12}) is available in dietary products such as meats, eggs, milk, and seafood. Nursing infants receive an adequate supply of cyanocobalamin (0.3 to 2 μg) in mother's milk. The adult RDA is 3 μg.

Development of Deficiency

Deficiency of cyanocobalamin in adults due to a decreased dietary intake is difficult to produce. Cyanocobalamin is so efficiently stored in the liver that depletion of internal reserves usually takes 6 to 10 years. However, individuals who follow strict vegetarian diets may require vitamin supplementation. Pregnancy and lactation also increase the requirement for cyanocobalamin. Deficiency of this vitamin usually occurs when the absorption process is interrupted by lack of ability to synthesize **intrinsic factor,** disease, surgery, or infection. The stomach secretes a protein known as intrinsic factor, which carries cyanocobalamin to the ileum, where it is absorbed. Therefore, the intestinal absorption of cyanocobalamin is dependent upon the presence of intrinsic factor.

Some individuals lack the ability to synthesize intrinsic factor. As a result, these people are cyanocobalamin deficient and develop **pernicious** anemia. The presence of pernicious anemia implies a deficiency in cyanocobalamin absorption specifically due to lack of intrinsic factor. Pernicious anemia may occur in adults following gastrectomy (removal of the stomach) or when the secretory portions of the stomach have been damaged by gastric carcinoma or have been removed surgically. Cyanocobalamin absorption may also be decreased when there is a chronic overgrowth in intestinal bacteria or tapeworm, and the bacteria or parasites utilize the vitamin before intestinal absorption can occur.

Characteristics of Deficiency

The anemia resulting from cyanocobalamin deficiency is a megaloblastic anemia. Many tissues are affected because cyanocobalamin is essential for the normal synthesis of nucleoprotein (deoxyribonucleic acid [DNA]). In particular, DNA synthesis and cell division require cyanocobalamin and folic acid. Both of these vitamins contribute to the formation of N^{10}-methyltetrahydrofolic acid (FH_4), which is needed to synthesize nucleoprotein precursors of DNA. Cyanocobalamin (and folic acid) deficiency causes changes in all dividing cells, resulting in the production of macrocytes and megaloblasts. The blood-forming system (hematopoiesis) reflects these changes by circulating giant platelets and large red and white blood cells with short life spans.

Cyanocobalamin is essential for the formation of the myelin sheaths that surround the peripheral nerves and spinal cord. This biochemical process involves fatty acids and lipids, which are incorporated into the myelin sheath. In cyanocobalamin deficiency, the myelin sheaths are not properly formed, leading to nerve degeneration and neurological changes. Degeneration first occurs along peripheral nerves so that paresthesia (numbness, "pins and needles" feeling) is produced. Eventually portions of the spinal cord degenerate, resulting in poor muscle coordination and weakness. Optic atrophy and glossitis (smooth, sore, beefy red tongue) occur. Deficient patients may undergo mood changes ranging from nervousness to psychosis. If the deficiency of this vitamin persists for several years, the neurological changes become irreversible. Specific diagnosis of cyanocobalamin deficiency is confirmed by the Schilling test. Radioactive cyanocobalamin (0.5 μg) is given orally, and the urine is collected for 24 hours. The next day, patients receive radioactive cyanocobalamin plus intrinsic factor, and the urine is again collected. Patients with pernicious anemia do not excrete cyanocobalamin into the urine when no intrinsic factor is present.

Clinical Indications

Cyanocobalamin is approved for use in vitamin B_{12} deficiency (pernicious anemia) or to prevent deficiency where disease or physical condition increases the requirement for this vitamin. The most common medical indications for use are pregnancy, hemorrhage, malignancy, postgastrectomy, and liver or renal disease.

Preparations

Cyanocobalamin (vitamin B_{12}) is available in tablets and injectable solution. Oral preparations containing less than 50 μg are primarily supplements for nutritionally based deficiencies. Injectable solutions of cyanocobalamin are administered intramuscularly or subcutaneously 30 μg per day for up to 10 days, followed by 100 to 200 μg per month until remission occurs. Thereafter, 100 μg per month may be sufficient to maintain remission. Patients who have pernicious anemia should be advised that they will require monthly injections for the rest of their lives. Hydroxycyanocobalamin (*alpha-Redisol, Hydrobexan*) is an injectable vitamin preparation that is longer-acting than cyanocobalamin because it is highly bound to proteins. Hydroxycyanocobalamin has no significant advantage over cyanocobalamin in the treatment of pernicious anemia. For any of the parenteral formulations, intravenous administration should be avoided because it is associated with excretion of the vitamin before the therapeutic response can be achieved.

Several over-the-counter preparations, primarily multiple vitamins, contain cyanocobalamin varying from 1 to 25 μg per tablet. The trade names of some commercial preparations are listed in Table 30:3. In malnourished individuals and geriatric patients, oral supplements (1 μg per day) may be beneficial. The only recognized therapeutic value of cyanocobalamin is in the treatment of pernicious anemia or cyanocobalamin deficiency. It has not been proved to cure hepatitis, poor appetite, allergies, sterility, psychosis, and aging, for which it is often administered. There is no known toxicity to this vitamin. The kidneys excrete all of the vitamin that cannot be used.

Drug Interactions

Cyanocobalamin absorption has been reported to be decreased due to drug interactions with colchicine, neomycin, aminosalicylic acid, and timed-release potassium. Chronic heavy alcohol intake (for more than 2 weeks) may produce malabsorption of cyanocobalamin. Chloramphenicol and other drugs that suppress the bone marrow may interfere with red blood cell

TABLE 30:3 — Commercial Cyanocobalamin (Vitamin B_{12}) Preparations*

TRADE NAME	CYANOCOBALAMIN, µG		OTHER INGREDIENTS
Rubramin-PC Vitamin B_{12}	Injection	100 µg/ml	—
Crysti-12 Cyanoject Rubesol-1000 Rubramin-PC Sytobex	Injection	1000 µg/ml	—
Alpha Redisol Codroxomin Hydro-Crysti-12 Hydroxocobalamin LA-12	Hydroxocobalamin injection 1000 µg/ml		—
Enviro-Stress Tablets	Oral	25 µg	Ascorbic acid, niacin, riboflavin, thiamine
Feminins	Oral	10 µg	Ascorbic acid, folic acid, iron, niacin, pantothenic acid, pyridoxine, riboflavin, thiamine, and vitamins A, D, and E
Geritol Complete	Oral	6 µg	Ascorbic acid, iron, niacin, pantothenic acid, pyridoxine, riboflavin, thiamine, vitamin K, and assorted minerals
Geritonic Liquid	Oral	9 µg/15 ml	Iron, desiccated liver, niacin, pyridoxine, riboflavin, thiamine, yeast concentrate, assorted minerals, 20% alcohol
Golden Bounty B Complex	Oral	25 µg	Ascorbic acid, niacin, riboflavin, thiamine
Multi 75 Tablets	Oral	75 µg	Ascorbic acid, niacin, riboflavin, thiamine, and assorted minerals
One-A-Day	Oral	6 µg	Ascorbic acid, folic acid, niacin, riboflavin, thiamine, pyridoxine, and vitamins A and D
Livitamin Liquid	Oral	5 µg/15 ml	Iron, desiccated liver, niacin, pyridoxine, riboflavin, thiamine, and copper
Rogenic	Oral	25 µg	Ascorbic acid, desiccated liver, iron, and pyridoxine
Surbex-T Filmtabs	Oral	10 µg	Ascorbic acid, niacin, pantothenic acid, pyridoxine, riboflavin, thiamine

*This is not an inclusive list of commercially available products.

maturation so that vitamin B_{12} cannot function in these cells. The result may be seen in patients as an inadequate therapeutic response to vitamin B_{12}. Antiulcer drugs (H_2-receptor antagonists, cimetidine) decrease gastric acid so that vitamin B_{12} cannot combine with available gastric intrinsic factor, impairing but not totally inhibiting absorption of vitamin B_{12}.

FOLIC ACID DEFICIENCY

The RDA for folic acid (400 µg) can be satisfied by including green leafy vegetables and meat in the diet. A dietary deficiency of folic acid (folates) frequently occurs because people do not adequately supplement their diet with vegetables.

Production Pathway for Tetrahydrofolic Acid (FH₄)

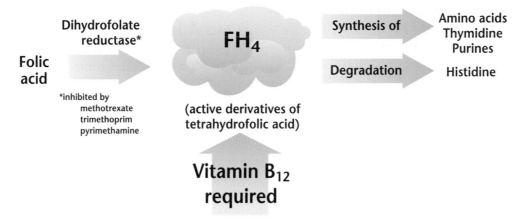

In addition, even well-balanced diets become folate deficient because the heat required for canning and cooking destroys folic acid. For this reason, folates are considered to be heat labile. Many conditions increase the requirement for folic acid. In particular, pregnancy, hemolytic anemia, rheumatoid arthritis, and hyperthyroidism are conditions associated with an increased production of blood cells that require folic acid for synthesis.

Role of Folic Acid

Folic acid is essential for cell growth and reproduction because it is necessary for protein synthesis. Folic acid is utilized in the synthesis of thymidine, an essential element in the nucleoprotein DNA. Also, synthesis of amino acids requires an activated form of folic acid known as FH₄ (see Figure 30:1). Therefore, folic acid and cyanocobalamin deficiencies produce identical anemias. Folate deficiency is associated with a macrocytic (megaloblastic) anemia. Oral preparations of folic acid in doses of 0.1 to 1 mg per day are used to treat folate deficiency. These folic acid products are available by prescription (called folic acid or *Folvite*) or as over-the-counter preparations (called folic acid). Parenteral (IM, IV, SC) formulations are available (folic acid, *Folvite*) for patients in whom the anemia is severe or gastrointestinal absorption is severely impaired. There are no known toxicities to folic acid, and allergic reactions rarely occur.

Clinical Indications

Folic acid is approved for use in megaloblastic anemia due to folate deficiency. Deficiency may arise from inadequate nutrition in infants, children,

or adults, or increased requirement due to pregnancy. Folic acid is designated Food and Drug Administration (FDA) Pregnancy Category A because of its critical role in fetal development. Folate status in pregnancy is directly related to proper neural development. Folate deficiency increases the potential for neural tube deficit (NTD).

Contraindications

Folic acid should never be given for treatment of cyanocobalamin (vitamin B₁₂) deficiency anemia. Administration of folic acid in a cyanocobalamin deficiency will reverse the production of the megaloblastic cells. Therefore, the anemia will be corrected. However, folic acid has no effect on the synthesis of myelin. Thus, folic acid cannot reverse the neurological changes associated with cyanocobalamin deficiency, and the damage may continue until it becomes irreversible. When megaloblastic anemia is present, patients must undergo tests that specifically diagnose the cause of the anemia so that proper replacement therapy can be initiated. Folic acid is not effective in the treatment of **aplastic** and **normocytic anemias.**

Drug Interactions

Drug interactions with folic acid may result in decreased absorption of folate or decreased production of FH₄. Anticonvulsants such as phenytoin (*Dilantin*), primidone (*Mysoline*), barbiturates, and oral contraceptives interfere with (decrease) the intestinal absorption of folic acid by an unknown mechanism. This decrease in folic acid absorption infrequently results in clinically significant megaloblastic anemia. However, increase in seizure frequency and decrease in serum phenytoin concentrations have been reported in patients receiving 15 to 20 mg of folic acid per day. Long-term use of aspirin, salicylamide, and caffeine has also been associated with impaired folate absorption.

Certain drugs, such as methotrexate (antineoplastic), trimethoprim (*Septra*), and pyrimethamine (antimalarial) block the formation of FH_4 because they inhibit the enzymes that convert folic acid to tetrahydrofolic acid (Figure 30:1). The treatment for anemias caused by decreased folic acid utilization (interference with the metabolic pathway that produces FH_4) is leucovorin calcium (folinic acid), a derivative of FH_4. This compound, also known as citrovorum factor, is available only by prescription and can be given orally or intramuscularly. For the treatment of megaloblastic anemia, up to 1 mg of leucovorin per day may be given IM. This compound is *contraindicated* in the treatment of pernicious anemia and other vitamin B_{12}-associated anemias because folinic acid does not influence vitamin B_{12}-dependent myelin pathways. Leucovorin also is used to prevent or treat the severe toxicity of massive methotrexate doses in the clinical management of resistant neoplasms.

ERYTHROPOIETIN

Erythropoietin is a protein normally produced by the kidneys that participates in red blood cell homeostasis. Responding to changes in tissue oxygenation, erythropoietin stimulates production of red blood cells in the bone marrow. This provides more vehicles to transport oxygen to the tissues, thus improving oxygenation. Epoetin alpha (EPO) is a synthetic glycoprotein produced through recombinant DNA technology. Its 165 amino acids mimic the activity of endogenous erythropoietin to stimulate red blood cell production, and increase hematocrit and hemoglobin in anemic patients.

Clinical Indications

Erythropoietin (*Epogen, Procrit*) is approved for use in chronic renal failure, cancer chemotherapy, or in dialysis patients where the hematocrit and hemoglobin confirm an anemic condition exists. Zidovudine related anemia in HIV patients is another indication for erythropoietin. In such cases the anemia represents a threat to patient health and/or obligates frequent transfusions to maintain adequate hematocrit and hemoglobin. The goal of therapy is to reduce the need for frequent transfusions as well as providing adequate tissue oxygenation.

Dose Administration

Erythropoietin is given either IV or SC injection, 100 to 300 mg/kg, three times a week. The dose varies according to the medical indication for treatment. Dose adjustment, based on the monitored hematocrit and hemoglobin, can be made after 8 weeks of treatment. Hematocrit values greater than 40 percent indicate a need for dose reduction to physiological hemoglobin levels of 36 percent. This is particularly important in treating patients with existing heart disease (CHF) who cannot tolerate an increased circulatory volume. Patients who do not respond to the 300 mg/kg dose are probably nonresponders to erythropoietin.

Special Considerations

Severe anemia, or anemia resulting from deficiencies in iron, folate and/or vitamin B_{12}, are not candidates for erythropoietin treatment. These anemias obligate appropriate replacement of the deficient factor until the red blood cell morphology and total count are returned to normal.

Preparations of erythropoietin cannot be frozen or vigorously shaken because the mechanical action will break (denature) the glycoprotein. In general, erythropoietin should not be added to any other drug solution; however, benzyl alcohol 0.9 percent may be added to minimize the discomfort of injection and act as a bacteriostatic.

Adverse Effects

The spectrum of adverse effects associated with erythropoietin reflects symptoms of the underlying disease and cannot always be directly attributed to erythropoietin. Among the most common effects are headache, arthralgia, nausea, hypertension (dialysis patients), and diarrhea. A significant number of patients who receive erythropoietin are on dialysis schedules. Such patients have hypertension as part of their chronic condition. Skin rashes, indicative of hypersensitivity, are mild and transient. Antibodies do not develop to erythropoietin, minimizing the potential for hypersensitivity reactions. Seizures have also occurred in some patients, making it necessary to advise ambulatory patients to avoid driving or operating heavy machinery during the treatment period.

Patient Administration and Monitoring

Compliance with diet recommendations to improve borderline deficiencies is not always successful. Thus, supplementation becomes a significant factor in treating anemias especially those not just outside the range of normal. Patients often need direction in developing a medication schedule that fosters compliance and, therefore, consistent improvement in the blood profile. The following suggestions are helpful in encouraging patients to stick with the treatment schedule.

- *Oral iron formulations may irritate the stomach lining when taken on an empty stomach. Taking the supplement with meals reduces the incidence of nausea and irritation.*

- *Sustained-released preparations should not be chewed or crushed because it will deliver more or all medication at once rather than over an extended period. This will foster GI irritation because of the larger amount of iron released.*

- *Remind patients who cannot take pill or capsule formulations to drink liquid iron formulations with a straw. This will avoid discoloration of the teeth.*

- *Review the medication history of the patient to confirm whether antacids, tetracyclines, or quinolones are being taken. These drugs should be taken at least 2 hours before iron supplements to avoid chelation.*

- *For vitamin B_{12} supplementation, make clear that treatment of pernicious anemia is for life. Monthly injection is necessary to avoid irreversible nerve damage.*

- *Caution patients taking multiple supplements that folic acid cannot substitute for vitamin B_{12}. Medication schedules must be followed as directed.*

- *Supplements used in the treatment of anemias are designated as Food and Drug Administration (FDA) Pregnancy Category C. Safety of parenteral formulations in pregnant women has not been established through controlled clinical trials. Nevertheless, when a clear benefit to the mother outweighs the risk to the fetus, these supplements are used. Folate, in particular, is designated Category A because of its absolute requirement in the fetus for normal development of the nervous system.*

Chapter Review

Understanding Terminology

Match the definition or description in the left column with the appropriate term in the right column.

___ **1.** Shape or structure of a cell.

___ **2.** A condition in which the oxygen-carrying function of the RBCs is decreased.

___ **3.** A tablet with a coating that enables it to pass through the stomach without being dissolved.

___ **4.** A disease with severe symptoms; could be fatal if left untreated.

___ **5.** Protein in RBCs that transports oxygen to all tissues of the body.

___ **6.** Large, immature RBC.

___ **7.** Medications containing iron compounds, used to increase hemoglobin production.

a. anemia

b. enteric-coated

c. hematinic

d. hemoglobin

e. megaloblast

f. morphology

g. pernicious

Match the definition in the left column with the appropriate prefix or suffix in the right column.

___ **8.** Prefix meaning large.

___ **9.** Prefix meaning small.

___ **10.** Suffix meaning cells.

___ **11.** Suffix meaning color.

a. chromic

b. cytic

c. mega

d. micro

Acquiring Knowledge

Answer the following questions in the spaces provided.

1. How are anemias produced? _____

_____

2. Describe the cell changes that may be produced in anemic individuals. _____

_____

3. What types of anemias are responsive to drug therapy? _____

_____

4. What is the most common cause of microcytic hypochromic anemia? _____

_____

5. How can the gastric irritation associated with oral hematinics be alleviated? _____

_____

6. What is the antidote for acute iron toxicity? _____

_____

7. How is cyanocobalamin absorbed? How can a deficiency be produced? _____

_____

8. Describe the anemia associated with cyanocobalamin deficiency. _____

_____

9. How can cyanocobalamin deficiency be diagnosed? _____
_____

10. When is cyanocobalamin therapy of value? _____
_____

11. How does folic acid deficiency anemia differ from cyanocobalamin deficiency? _____
_____

12. Are folic acid and cyanocobalamin interchangeable in the treatment of megaloblastic anemia? Why?
_____

13. How can a folate deficiency be produced? _____
_____

14. When is leucovorin calcium therapeutically useful? _____
_____

Applying Knowledge—On the Job

Use your critical thinking skills to answer the following questions in the spaces provided.

1. One of your jobs is to remind patients of the potential for interactions with other medications the patient is taking. Why is it recommended not to take iron supplements with tetracyclines?
_____
_____

2. Ms. Benson, who has been treated for epilepsy since 1989, has been placed on a folic acid supplement. Why do you ask whether she is still taking *Dilantin*? How can this medication affect the folate treatment?
_____
_____

3. Explain the reason for not routinely administering vitamin B_{12} for any patient presenting with chronic symptoms of anemia and a hematology profile of large immature cells consistent with vitamin B_{12} deficiency?
_____
_____

4. A patient has just received a prescription for *Procrit*. What adverse effects are associated with this medication?
_____
_____

5. Iron toxicity usually occurs with a specific group of people. Which group is most susceptible and why?
_____
_____

6. In an effort to increase patient compliance, what suggestions would you make?
_____
_____

Additional Reading

Abramson, S. D. 1999. "Common" uncommon anemias. *American Family Physician* 59 (4):851. (access online at www.aafp.org)

Cerrato, P. L. 1991. Your patient's anemic—but the problem isn't iron. *RN* 54:61.

Oral cobalamin for pernicious anemia? 1991. *Nurse's Drug Alert* 15:12.

Wimberley, T. H. 1991. Iron preparations: It's elementary, my dear. *Pediatric Nursing* 17:274.

DRUGS THAT AFFECT THE RESPIRATORY SYSTEM

Chapter 31

Antiallergic and Antihistaminic Drugs

Action of Histamine
Antiallergic Agents
Antihistaminic Agents

Chapter 32

Bronchodilator Drugs and the Treatment of Asthma

Respiratory Diseases
Role of the Autonomic Nervous
    System
Bronchodilator Drugs
Antiinflammatory Drugs
Antiallergic Agents
Mucolytics
Expectorants

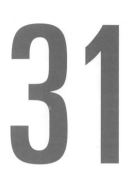

31

ANTIALLERGIC AND ANTIHISTAMINIC DRUGS

CHAPTER FOCUS

This chapter describes the drugs that reduce the symptoms produced by seasonal allergies. Many of these drugs, frequently available as over-the-counter (OTC) products, directly influence selective actions of histamine by interacting with histamine receptors (see Chapter 33 for histamine receptors in the gastrointestinal [GI] tract).

CHAPTER OBJECTIVES

After studying this chapter, you should be able to

- explain the reactions produced by histamine released in response to allergic reactions.

- describe the difference in action between an antihistaminic and a drug that is effective in the prophylactic management of asthma.

- describe two specific therapeutic uses of antihistaminics that result from an action on the central nervous system (CNS) yet are not associated with allergic responses.

- describe three side effects of antihistaminics that are extensions of their therapeutic activity.

- describe three examples of first- and second-generation antihistamines and the characteristic difference between the two groups.

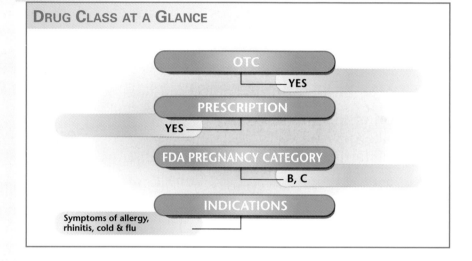

DRUG CLASS AT A GLANCE

OTC — YES

PRESCRIPTION — YES

FDA PREGNANCY CATEGORY — B, C

INDICATIONS — Symptoms of allergy, rhinitis, cold & flu

Key Terms

antiallergic: drug that prevents mast cells from releasing histamine and other vasoactive substances.

antigen: substance, usually protein or carbohydrate, that is capable of stimulating an immune response.

antihistaminic: drug that blocks the action of histamine at the target organ.

asthma: inflammation of the bronchioles associated with constriction of smooth muscle, wheezing, and edema.

dermatitis: inflammatory condition of the skin associated with itching, burning, and edematous vesicular formations.

eczematoid dermatitis: condition in which lesions on the skin ooze and develop scaly crusts.

erythema: redness of the skin, often a result of capillary dilation.

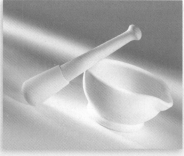

histamine: substance that interacts with tissues to produce most of the symptoms of allergy.

prophylactic: process or drug that prevents the onset of symptoms (or disease) as a result of exposure before the reactive process can take place.

sensitize: to induce or develop a reaction to naturally occurring substances (allergens) as a result of repeated exposure.

xerostomia: dryness of the oral cavity resulting from inhibition of the natural moistening action of salivary gland secretions or increased secretion of salivary mucus, rather than serous material.

INTRODUCTION

Sneezing, coughing, itching, headache, and nasal congestion often indicate that people are experiencing an allergic reaction. Severe allergic reactions can result in respiratory and cardiovascular failure (anaphylaxis). The symptoms of an allergic reaction indicate that individuals have become **sensitized** to certain antigens in the environment. **Antigens** are substances such as pollen, mold, dust, and insect venom that stimulate the production of antibodies in the blood and tissues. In certain (sensitized) people, repeated exposure to these antigens results in allergic reactions due to antigen-antibody interactions. People who suffer from **asthma,** a chronic obstructive lung disease, are highly sensitive to antigenic stimulation. Allergic reactions that occur in asthmatic people severely restrict their ability to breathe.

Once an antigen has initiated an allergic reaction, certain cells in the body (mast cells) release active substances into the blood. The most important substance released is **histamine,** which interacts with other cells to produce most of the symptoms of allergy. Drugs that block only the tissue action of histamine are known as **antihistaminics.** Such drugs alleviate the annoying discomfort that accompanies most allergic reactions.

In contrast, drugs that prevent mast cells from releasing histamine are considered **antiallergic** agents. Antiallergic drugs also block the action of other active substances (serotonin and bradykinin). Antiallergic drugs are valuable in the prophylactic therapy of asthma because they help prevent future allergic reactions.

ACTION OF HISTAMINE

Histamine is found throughout the body in the mast cells and basophilic white blood cells. The largest concentrations of mast cells are in the lungs, the gastrointestinal (GI) tract, and the skin. When an antigen comes into contact with the skin or lungs or enters the bloodstream of sensitized individuals, the mast cells and basophils immediately release histamine into the blood. Histamine then interacts with the membrane receptors in certain tissues to produce the symptoms of allergy.

Two types of receptors are associated with histamine: H_1- and H_2-receptors. Histamine interacts with the H_1-receptors, located on blood vessels, bronchiolar smooth muscle, and intestinal smooth muscle, to mediate allergic reactions. The intensity of the allergic symptoms is proportional to the amount of histamine released.

The H_2-receptors are located within the stomach, heart, blood vessels, and uterine tissue. The most important response mediated by H_2-receptors is increased secretion of gastric acid. This response is not usually associated with allergies. However, the action of H_2-receptors is clinically important in the management of GI ulcers and will be discussed in Chapter 33.

Vascular Effects

Histamine usually produces a transient drop in blood pressure because it dilates small blood vessels and capillaries. With large histamine concentrations, this drop can result in hypotension and circulatory collapse. Dilation of cerebral blood vessels stimulates pain receptors in the skull. This action explains the throbbing headache known as histaminic cephalgia. Capillary dilation in the skin results in a localized redness called **erythema.**

In addition, histamine causes fluids and proteins to leak out of the capillaries. When capillary leakage occurs in the nasal mucous membranes, nasal congestion occurs. When capillary leakage occurs in the skin, edema, wheals, or hives are produced. Itching and pain occur because histamine irritates sensory nerve endings. The erythema and edema produced by histamine in the skin are known as the Response of Lewis.

Extravascular Smooth Muscle Effects

Histamine produces contraction of the smooth muscle of the intestine and bronchioles by stimulating H_1-receptors. Contraction of intestinal smooth muscle results in disturbances of intestinal activity. Contraction of the bronchiolar smooth muscle results in bronchoconstriction, which makes breathing difficult.

Humans are more sensitive to the bronchiolar constriction produced by histamine than to the disturbances of intestinal activity. In particular, people who have pulmonary diseases (asthma and emphysema) may be unusually sensitive to the respiratory actions of histamine.

Cardiac Effects

Histamine produces several effects on the heart that are directly related to the amount of histamine present. Histamine usually produces rapid heartbeat. However, at high levels of histamine (histamine shock), cardiac conduction is impaired. Such impairment may lead to the development of arrhythmias and cardiovascular collapse. The major effects of histamine are summarized in Table 31:1.

ANTIALLERGIC AGENTS

Allergic reactions can be blocked in two ways. As shown in Figure 31:1, the mast cells can be prevented from releasing their contents or the H_1-receptors can be blocked from interacting with histamine. Cromolyn sodium (*Intal, Nasalcrom*) is the only available drug that selectively prevents the release of histamine from the mast cells. Cromolyn sodium is not a bronchodilator, a smooth muscle relaxant, or a histamine-receptor antagonist. Since this drug has no effect on histamine receptors, cromolyn sodium must be administered before histamine release has begun.

Drugs like cromolyn sodium, which prevent the onset of symptoms or disease as a result of exposure before the reactive process can take place, are called **prophylactic** drugs. Cromolyn sodium is inhaled as a fine micronized powder. The powder form allows the drug to reach the pulmonary mast cells before any antigens can induce an allergic reaction.

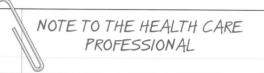

NOTE TO THE HEALTH CARE PROFESSIONAL

If a rash develops while patients are taking cromolyn sodium, the drug must be discontinued before further sensitivity occurs. Cromolyn sodium cannot be used in acute allergic or asthma attacks in which histamine has already been released.

TABLE 31:1	Physiological Responses Following Histamine Stimulation		
SYSTEM OR TISSUE	**HISTAMINE EFFECT**	**RECEPTOR**	**PHYSIOLOGICAL RESPONSE**
Blood pressure	Decreased	H_1, H_2	Hypotension
Heart rate	Increased	H_2	Rapid heartbeat
Bronchioles	Constriction	H_1	Breathing difficulty
Intestine	Contraction	H_1	Constipation/diarrhea
Skin capillaries	Redness, edema, itching	H_1	Response of Lewis
Gastric acid secretion	Increased	H_2	Nausea, heartburn

Routes of Administration

Cromolyn is available in capsule (*Spinhaler*) and solution (*Nasalcrom*) forms for inhalation use and as capsules for oral administration (*Gastrocrom*). Indications for use and dosages are presented in Table 31:2. The *Spinhaler* and *Nasamatic* devices have instructions for proper use and are readily mastered by patients of any age. The oral capsule formulation, which contains a measured dose, is opened and the powder dissolved into a glass of hot water. The full glass of liquid must be consumed to receive the proper dose. Fruit juice, milk, or food will inhibit dissolution and absorption of the drug and therefore should not be consumed until 0.5 hour after dosing.

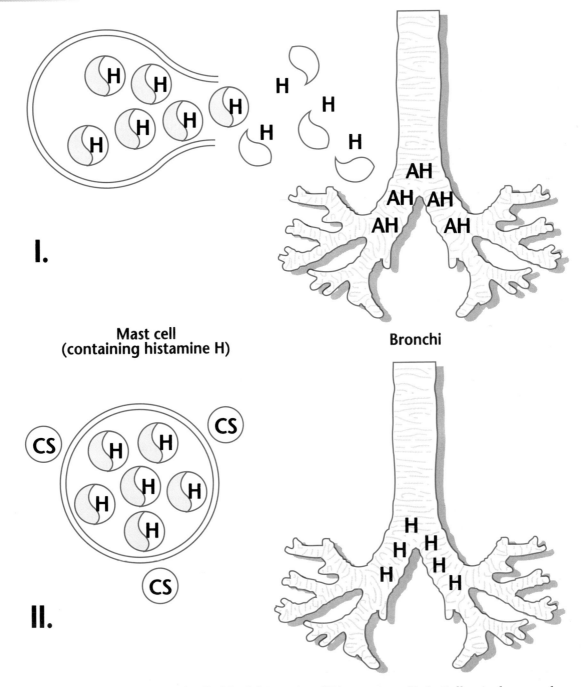

I. Antihistaminic drugs (AH) specifically block histamine (H₁) receptors. II. Antiallergic drugs such as cromolyn sodium (CS) prevent the release of histamine (H) from the mast cells.

TABLE 31:2 — Indication for Use of Cromolyn Sodium

FORMULATION	PROPHYLAXIS INDICATION	DOSE
Nebulization solution	Inhalation capsules Aerosol Severe bronchial asthma exercise-induced bronchospasm	20 mg inhaled 4 times daily at regular intervals; one 20-mg capsule or 20 mg of nebulizer solution 1 hr before exercise
Nasal solution	Allergic rhinitis	One spray in each nostril 3–6 times a day at regular intervals
Oral	Mastocytosis	200 mg 4 times a day 30 min before meals and at bedtime

Clinical Indications

Cromolyn is currently used as a prophylactic adjunct in the management of chronic bronchial asthma and allergic rhinitis to prevent bronchospasms. Pulmonary function tests must demonstrate that the patient has a bronchodilator reversible component to the airway obstruction for cromolyn to be of any benefit. Patients must be compliant with dosing at regular repeated intervals otherwise the drug cannot achieve a satisfactory response. Oral cromolyn improves diarrhea, flushing, headaches, urticaria, abdominal pain, and nausea in some patients with mastocytosis. In this condition, mast cells accumulate in organs and tissues in excessive amounts. Patients may experience symptoms associated with excessive histamine release from puritis to peptic ulcer and chronic diarrhea.

Adverse Effects and Contraindications

Adverse effects are minimal and include wheezing, nasal itching, nasal burning, nausea, drowsiness, and headache. Occasionally, bronchospasms occur because the micronized powder irritates the lung membranes. Cromolyn is contraindicated in patients who develop hypersensitivity to the drug.

ANTIHISTAMINIC AGENTS

Antihistaminic drugs are used to relieve acute reactions in which histamine has already been released. All of the antihistaminics available specifically block histamine from interfacing with its H_1-receptors. Therefore, the H_1-mediated allergic responses of histamine are prevented. Antihistaminic drugs are usually administered orally (see Table 31:3) because they are absorbed well from the intestinal tract.

A few antihistaminics are available for parenteral administration. These drugs are rapidly metabolized by the liver, necessitating repeated drug administration (usually two to four times a day) to maintain a therapeutic response. First-generation antihistamines include chlorpheniramine (*Chlor-Trimeton*), clemastine (*Tavist*), diphenhydramine (*Benadryl*), and promethazine (*Phenergan*). These agents are characterized by a nonselective interaction with peripheral and central histamine receptors. For this reason these early antihistamines produce the same spectrum of therapeutic responses, varying only in their degree of activity. These drugs can be used interchangeably and frequently cause sedation along with relief of allergy symptoms. In addition to inhibiting the actions of histamine, these drugs possess local anesthetic and anticholinergic activity. Through a local anesthetic action, antihistaminics can depress sensory nerve activity and thus relieve itching and pain. Diphenhydramine (*Benadryl*) is still considered an antihistamine of choice.

Dimenhydrinate (*Dramamine*) exerts a unique action in the brain to relieve vertigo and motion sickness and the nausea that accompanies it. Cyproheptadine (*Periactin*) and azatadine (*Optimine*) have the ability to inhibit the actions of histamine and serotonin. For this reason, these two drugs may offer a wider range of relief in highly sensitized individuals.

The second generation of antihistamines, which includes cetirizine (*Zyrtec*), fexofenadine (*Allegra*), and loratadine (*Claritin*), appears to be more selective for peripheral H_1-receptors. These agents are not sedating or drying and demonstrate equal antiallergic activity to the older drugs. The

TABLE 31:3 — Frequently Used Antihistaminic Drugs*

DRUGS**	TRADE NAME	RECOMMENDED DOSES			
		SEDATIVE DOSE	ADULT ORAL	CHILD ORAL	ADULT PARENTERAL
brompheniramine	Brovex	—	12 to 24 mg every 12 hr	0.5 mg/kg every 4–6 hr	2.5–10 mg IM, SC
cetirizine[1]	Zyrtec	—	5 or 10 mg once a day		
chlorpheniramine	Allerclor, Chlor-Trimeton[2]	—	2–4 mg every 4–6 hr	1–2 mg every 4–6 hr***	
clemastine	Tavist[2]	—	1.34–2.68 mg BID	0.67–1.34 mg BID***	—
cyproheptadine	Periactin	—	4–20 mg/day	2–4 mg BID, TID	—
dexchlorpheniramine	—	—	2 mg every 4–6 hr	0.5–1 mg every 4–6 hr***	—
desloratidine	Clarinex	—	5 mg/day	5 mg/day	—
dimenhydrinate	Dramamine	—	50–100 mg every 4–6 hr	12.5–50 mg every 6–8 hr up to 150 mg/day***	50 mg IV, IM
diphenhydramine	Benadryl[2]	50 mg at bedtime	25–50 mg every 4–6 hr	6.25–25 mg TID, QID	10–50 mg IV, IM up to a maximum of 400 mg/day
fexofenadine[1]	Allegra	—	60 mg BID or 180 mg once daily	30 mg BID	—
hydroxyzine	Atarax, Vistaril	50–100 mg before anesthesia	25 mg TID, QID	50–100 mg daily in divided doses***	
loratadine	Claritin, Alavert[2]	—	10 mg/day	5 mg/day	—
meclizine	Antivert, Bonine[2]	—	25–100 mg/day	—	—
methdilazine	Tacaryl	—	8 mg BID, QID	4 mg BID, QID	—
phenindamine	Nolahist	—	25 mg every 4–6 hr	12.5 mg every 4–6 hr (Do not exceed 75 mg in 24 hr)	—
promethazine	Phenergan	25–50 mg at bedtime	12.5 mg QID or 25 mg at bedtime	6.25–12.5 mg TID or 25 mg at bedtime	25 mg IM
pyriamine (4 mg) pheniramine (4 mg) phentoloxamine (4 mg)	Poly-Histine Elixir[2]	—	10 ml every 4 hours PO	2.5–5 ml every 4 hr PO	—
triprolidine	(Zymine)	—	—	0.3–1.25 mg every 4–6 hr	—
triprolidine (2.5 mg), pseudoephedrine (60 mg)	Actagen, Actifed[2]	—	1 dose every 4–8 hr PO up to 4 doses/day	—	—

[1]Second-generation antihistamines
[2]Available OTC and prescription; all other products prescription only
*Not an inclusive list of trade names.
**All drugs are used for actue allergy (urticaria, rhinitis, hay fever, contact dermatitis, and pruritus) except for dimenhydrinate, which is used to prevent motion sickness, and meclizine, which is used for motion sickness and vertigo. Diphenhydramine is also used as an antiemetic.
***Dose for these drugs is set for children as young as 2–6 years and 6–12 years of age. Experience younger than 2 years has not been established.

proposal that patients who were refractory to first-generation drugs would find relief with the newest antihistamines has not proven to be a significant advantage. The new antihistamines are not superior in antihistamine activity to older drugs but they are truly less sedating.

A few antihistamines have made the move from prescription to OTC status. The most recent is loratadine, under the trade name *Clarinex* as prescription, and *Alavert* as OTC preparation. The cost of OTC medications is expected to be significantly less than the equivalent prescription product. This has contributed to the interest in moving more of these drugs into the OTC market.

Clinical Indications

Antihistaminics are frequently used in acute allergic reactions including urticaria, hay fever, insect bites, rhinitis, and **dermatitis.** Because of the inherent sedation, antihistaminics may be used to induce sleep in OTC sleeping aids (for example, *Nytol*) or to relieve motion sickness (for example, *Dramamine*). Certain antihistamines—chlorpromazine, perfenazine (*Trilafon*), prochlorperazine (*Compazine*), promethazine (*Phenergan*), and triflupromazine (*Vesprin*)—are extremely effective in reducing nausea and vomiting. These drugs are used as adjunct pre- and postoperative medications to minimize anesthetic irritability and facilitate patient recovery (see Chapter 33). Antihistaminics are frequently found in cold remedies and cough syrups because of

their ability to dry nasal secretions. Many of the common OTC analgesic and cough-cold medications contain an antihistamine as an active ingredient. The most common ingredients are chlorpheniramine, brompheniramine, and doxylamine. The anticholinergic component of H_1-antagonists provides relief from symptoms associated with the common cold as well as allergic reactions such as runny nose. In addition, sedation caused by an antihistaminic in a multiingredient cold product aids recovery by promoting bed rest. Examples of over-the-counter cold and allergy products that contain antihistaminics are given in Table 31:4.

Adverse Reactions

Antihistaminics generally produce similar side effects but differ in the predominance or intensity of one side effect over another. The most common side effects produced by the antihistaminics are drowsiness and sedation. Another frequently occurring side effect is dry mouth **(xerostomia).** At any dose, most of these drugs exert an anticholinergic effect that dries the mucous linings of the mouth and nasal passages. This side effect is therapeutically useful in treating the common cold. Other adverse effects include hypotension, rapid heartbeat, anorexia, epigastric distress, and urinary retention. Within the class of antihistamines, diphenhydramine (*Benadryl*), promethazine (*Phenergan*), and hydroxyzine (*Vistaril*) reportedly cause sedation most often,

	Over-the-Counter Cold and Allergy Preparations That Contain Antihistaminics*			
TRADE NAME	**ANTIHISTAMINE**	**FORM**	**OTHER ACTIVE INGREDIENTS**	
Allerest Maximum Strength	12 mg chlorpheniramine	Tablet	Pseudoephedrine 30 mg	
Dimetane Decongestant	4 mg brompheniramine	Caplet	Phenylephrine 10 mg	
Nyquil Nighttime Cold/Flu Medicine Liquid	12.5 mg doxylamine/ml	Liquid	Alcohol 10%, acetaminophen 1000 mg, dextromethorphan 30 mg, pseudoephedrine 60 mg	
Sting-eze	diphenhydramine		benzocaine, camphor, eucalyptol, phenol	
Triaminic Nite Time	1.0 mg chlorpheniramine/5 ml	Liquid	Pseudoephedrine 15 mg, dextromethorphan 7.5 mg	
Ziradryl	1% diphenhydramine	Lotion	Alcohol, camphor, parabens, zinc oxide 2%	

TABLE 31:4

*Not an inclusive list of available products.

whereas chlorpheniramine (*Chlor-Trimeton*) and cyproheptadine (*Periactin*) are associated with little or no sedation. In unusual circumstances, patients may become nervous and unable to sleep (insomnia) while taking chlorpheniramine. In patients over 60 years of age, paradoxical stimulation rather than sedation can occur and may warrant dose reduction to eliminate this adverse experience.

Cautions and Contraindications

Because of their anticholinergic activity, antihistaminic drugs should be used with caution in patients with cardiovascular disease or hypertension or patients predisposed to developing an increase in intraocular pressure or urinary retention. Antihistaminics should not be used by patients with a known hypersensitivity to antihistaminics or patients with narrow-angle glaucoma, stenosing peptic ulcer, or prostatic hypertrophy. Antihistaminics should not be used in newborn or premature infants because these patients are more susceptible to the adverse effects. Similarly, antihistaminics should not be used by nursing mothers, since these drugs are excreted into breast milk and thus passed into the newborn. These drugs should not be given to dehydrated children because dystonias (abnormal tissue tone) may occur. Phenothiazine antihistaminics such as promethazine (*Phenergan*) are contraindicated for use in patients with CNS depression or a history of phenothiazine-induced jaundice.

Astemizole (*Hismanal*) and terfenadine (*Seldane*), both second-generation antihistamines, have been removed from the market because they produced serious cardiovascular and hepatic effects that were fatal in some patients. Especially when plasma concentrations were elevated, these drugs prolonged the QT interval. On the ECG, prolongation of the QT interval reflects a change in cardiac conduction that makes it possible for life-threatening ventricular arrhythmias to occur. The mechanism is a direct interaction with selective ion channels (K^+, Na^+, Ca^{++}) in the myocardium that interrupts normal cardiorhythm. Prolongation of the QT interval is a hot topic in drug development because of the potential for serious arrhythmias and, since astemizole and terfenadine, the vast number of drugs that have been confirmed to produce this effect.

Antihistaminics are found as active agents in many ointments, sprays, and cream preparations to be used on the skin. The prolonged indiscriminate use of topical antihistaminic preparations can lead to the development of hypersensitivity in some people. This hypersensitivity may range from rashes to **eczematoid dermatitis,** in which lesions on the skin surface ooze and develop scaly crusts. Antihistaminics may also produce drug fever, which will subside only when the drug is stopped. The mechanism of this drug-induced fever is not known. Antihistaminics are not harmless drugs, even though they may be found in many over-the-counter products (see Table 31:4). The potential for adverse effects increases when any individual takes three to five medications *or more* daily and older patients are likely to be taking multiple medications. Patients taking multiple medications, including the elderly, are more likely to experience dizziness, excessive sedation, paradoxical stimulation, or confusion with these drugs. Medications that affect the cardiovascular system or CNS may predispose patients to developing mental confusion. In addition, the availability of antihistamines in OTC preparations contributes additional seasonal exposure—that is, winter colds, and spring and fall allergies. Even with appropriate magnification in eyeglasses, it is difficult to read the fine print that identifies the contents of OTC products. Antihistamines are not recommended for use during pregnancy. Animal studies have demonstrated abnormalities in the offspring with certain antihistamines. Convulsions in newborns after exposure to antihistamines in the third trimester has been reported. Safe use during pregnancy has not been established.

Drug Interactions

In general, antihistaminics interact with many drugs. Some antibiotics, muscle relaxants (curare), and narcotic analgesics (morphine) cause the release of histamine from mast cells. If patients are taking such a drug, it is not unusual for an antihistaminic to be given to counteract the effects of histamine. Drugs that depress the activity of the CNS (sedatives, tranquilizers, and alcohol) increase the incidence of drowsiness when taken with antihistaminics. This synergistic effect is most likely to occur with OTC products (see Table 31:4) that contain an antihistaminic in addition to alcohol as an active ingredient.

Astemizole (*Hismanal*) has potentially serious interactions with a wide variety of drugs. Macrolide antibiotics, erythromycin, clarithromycin, troleandomycin, and antifungals, ketoconazole, itraconazole, and miconazole, elevate the plasma levels of these antihistamines when taken concurrently. The mechanism of interaction is inhibition of hepatic metabolism predisposing the patient to potentially life-threatening cardiotoxic effects. While these drugs significantly increase the plasma concentration of loratadine as well, this antihistamine does not appear to produce clinically significant adverse effects at higher blood levels. Table 31:5 describes potential drug interactions that can occur with antihistaminics. While some of the second-generation antihistamines undergo food interactions, only astemizole has a precautionary recommendation. Astemizole must be taken on an empty stomach. Food interacts with astemizole to inhibit absorption so that the effective dose is not achieved.

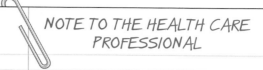

NOTE TO THE HEALTH CARE PROFESSIONAL

Because the antihistaminics can depress the CNS, patients must be warned not to operate vehicles or heavy machinery while taking these drugs.

TABLE 31:5	Drug Interactions With Antihistaminic Drugs
DRUG	**RESPONSE**
antibiotics: azithromycin, clarithromycin, erythromycin, troleandomycin	Increase plasma concentrations of loratadine through inhibition of hepatic metabolism
Anticholinergics: atropine	Increase nervousness, insomnia, and constipation
Anticoagulants: coumarins	Delay absorption of anticoagulant
Antidepressants: imipramine	Increase anticholinergic effect, urinary retention, and intraocular pressure
Antifungals: fluconazole, itraconazole, ketoconazole, miconazole	Increase plasma concentrations of loratadine through inhibition of hepatic metabolism
cimetidine	Increases the plasma concentration of loratadine
CNS depressants: alcohol, barbiturates, hypnotics, narcotic analgesics, phenothiazines, tranquilizers	Increase drowsiness, sedation, and lethargy
Corticosteroids: oral drugs	Increase risk of glaucoma in susceptible patients
MAO Inhibitors: amphetamines, tranylcypromine	Intensify the drying effects of antihistaminics and may cause hypotension with phenothiazines

Abbreviations: MAO, monoamine oxidase.

Patient Administration and Monitoring

Antihistamines provide symptomatic relief for a variety of acute and chronic conditions when used at the recommended dose and at regular, approved intervals. Because these products are widely available OTC, patients frequently assume the drugs have less potential for producing adverse effects. In all cases where the antihistamine is available OTC and prescription, the formulation of the OTC product contains the active agent, only in a lower amount. Therefore, with children, elderly, and hectic working adults, it becomes extremely easy to take multiple doses that are comparable to the prescription antihistamines. Whenever possible it is worthwhile reviewing the following facts with patients who are using antihistamines or cromolyn.

Patient Instruction

Special formulations should be reviewed with patients to ensure the product is delivering the designated amount of drug appropriately.

Sustained-release (SR) preparations should not be chewed or crushed. These capsules should not be opened to divide the dose. The pellets are coated to release the drug at a variety of time intervals that cannot be determined by the patient. Sustained-release preparations should be swallowed intact with water.

Oral capsules of cromolyn *are* designed to be opened so the powder can be dissolved in hot water. Patients should be reminded not to take the drug with fruit juice, milk, or food because it will not be absorbed.

Instructions for use of the Spinhaler and nasal inhalation are included in the package. Patients should receive instructions demonstrating the insertion of the capsule to facilitate compliance with dosing.

Dosing Schedule

The time of dosing should be provided in writing if necessary to ensure adequate drug absorption. Oral cromolyn should be taken 30 minutes before meals to avoid any delay in drug absorption.

Dosing With Meals

Oral antihistamines may cause gastric upset in some patients. Although patients may take most antihistamines with meals to minimize the irritation, astemizole must be taken on an empty stomach.

Adverse Effects

Patients should be instructed to avoid prolonged exposure to sunlight because antihistamines may produce photosensitivity.

Even with nonsedating antihistamines, patients should be reminded to avoid alcohol and CNS depressants that could potentiate adverse effects. This includes OTC preparations for relief of coughs, colds, flu, and allergy. Any product designated "elixir" contains alcohol in amounts that can interact with antihistamine effects.

Notify the Physician

Patients should notify their physician immediately if they develop involuntary muscle spasms, wheezing, or edema. These may be signs of extrapyramidal reactions or hypersensitivity respectively.

Patients should notify their physician immediately if their medical history changes or they develop signs and symptoms of glaucoma, peptic ulcer, or urinary retention.

Use in Pregnancy

Antihistamines are designated as Food and Drug Administration (FDA) Pregnancy Category B or C. They are not recommended for use in pregnancy because the safety for use in humans has not been established. The physician should be notified if the patient becomes pregnant during therapy.

Chapter Review

Understanding Terminology

Answer the following questions in the spaces provided.

1. What is the difference between an antiallergic and an antihistaminic drug? _____
   _____
   _____

2. Differentiate between erythemia and dermatitis. _____
   _____
   _____

3. Define *prophylaxis.* _____
   _____
   _____

4. Define *xerostomia.* _____
   _____
   _____

Acquiring Knowledge

Answer the following questions in the spaces provided.

1. Where is histamine located in the body? What stimulates histamine release? _____
   _____
   _____

2. What are the effects of histamine on various tissues? _____
   _____
   _____

3. How does cromolyn sodium produce its antiallergic response? When is cromolyn sodium used?
   _____
   _____

4. How do the antihistaminics prevent the action of histamine? What receptors are involved in allergic reactions?
   _____
   _____

5. What other pharmacological actions do antihistaminics produce? _____
   _____

6. Why are antihistaminics found in over-the-counter products? What are two examples?
   _____
   _____

7. What adverse effects are associated with antihistaminic use? _____
   _____
   _____

8. What drugs commonly interact with antihistaminics? _____
   _____
   _____

Applying Knowledge—On the Job

Use your critical thinking skills to answer the following questions in the spaces provided.

1. Mrs. Lewis calls the clinic where you are working. She says when she was in the clinic 2 days ago, the doctor diagnosed her with allergic rhinitis and gave her prescriptions for *Nasalcrom* and *Chlor-Trimeton*. She claims she has used *Nasalcrom* for the past 48 hours without any relief of her nasal symptoms. "My nose is running like a faucet with this pollen count so high. I didn't fill the *Chlor-Trimeton* prescription because I have to work and can't tolerate the drowsiness." What should you tell her?

    _____

    _____

2. Six months later, during cold season, Mrs. Lewis calls the office for a refill on her *Nasalcrom* prescription. She says she has a terrible cold with a runny nose and the *Nasalcrom* worked so well when she used it during hay fever season she wants to use it now. What should you do?

    _____

    _____

3. A patient has just received a prescription for *Gastrocrom*. What should be included in his instructions for proper administration?

    _____

    _____

4. What are the listed contraindications for anticholinergic antihistamines? _____

    _____

    _____

5. Can antihistamines be used safely during pregnancy? Why or why not? _____

    _____

    _____

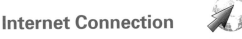

Internet Connection

The American Academy of Family Physicians maintains a website at familydoctor.org (enter without "www." prompt) for kids, teens, and parents to learn about health topics. At the home page select *Healthy Topics* to access more than 200 health and medication topics or enter a specific word or phrase at the search box.

Oral second-generation antihistamines are the treatment of choice for mild seasonal rhinitis without nasal obstruction. Information on worldwide results on antihistamine use is maintained by the World Allergy Organization at www.worldallergy.org/professional/allergyupdate/rhinitis/rhinitisglobal.shtml.

Among the best sites providing information on rhinitis, allergy, and specific medications used in the management of allergic rhinitis is www.nlm.nih.gov/medlineplus/druginformation. Topics include *Itching for Some Allergy Relief?*

Additional Reading

Cross, S. 1997. Rhinitis management. *Practical Nurse* 13 (5):262.

Mathewson, H. S. 1996. Drug capsule: Antihistamines and asthma. *Respiratory Care* 41 (3):212.

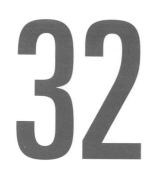

32

BRONCHODILATOR DRUGS AND THE TREATMENT OF ASTHMA

CHAPTER FOCUS

This chapter describes the common diseases that affect the respiratory system and the pharmacology of drugs used to treat these conditions. It also explains the role of the autonomic nervous system in asthma and how different bronchodilators interact with this system. In addition, it describes how corticosteroids, mucolytics, and other drugs are used to affect respiratory function.

CHAPTER OBJECTIVES

After studying this chapter, you should be able to

- describe chronic obstructive pulmonary disease (COPD) and asthma.

- list four respiratory components affected by asthma.

- list three chemical mediators involved in asthma.

- describe the mechanism of action and main pharmacological effects of the three types of bronchodilators.

- explain the role of corticosteroids, cromolyn, and mucolytics in respiratory therapy.

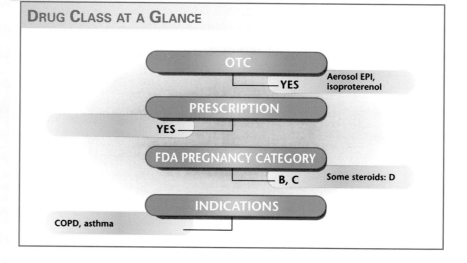

DRUG CLASS AT A GLANCE

OTC — YES Aerosol EPI, isoproterenol

PRESCRIPTION YES

FDA PREGNANCY CATEGORY — B, C Some steroids: D

INDICATIONS COPD, asthma

Key Terms

asthma: respiratory disease characterized by bronchoconstriction, shortness of breath, and wheezing.

bronchodilator: drug that relaxes bronchial smooth muscle and dilates the lower respiratory passages.

chemical mediator: substance formed by mast cells, certain blood cells, and other body cells and that is released during inflammatory and allergic reactions.

chronic bronchitis: respiratory condition caused by chronic irritation that increases secretion of mucus and causes degeneration of the respiratory lining.

COPD: chronic obstructive pulmonary disease, usually caused by emphysema and chronic bronchitis.

emphysema: disease process causing destruction of the walls of the alveolar sacs.

mucolytic: drug that liquefies bronchial secretions.

prostaglandins: series of chemical mediators that are released by most body cells and are often involved in disease processes.

SRS-A: slow-reacting substance of anaphylaxis; a prostaglandin derivative that is a potent bronchoconstrictor and mediator of asthma.

INTRODUCTION

The respiratory system plays a vital role in the exchange of the respiratory gases, oxygen (O_2) and carbon dioxide (CO_2). Functionally, the respiratory system consists of a series of anatomical tubes (trachea, bronchi, bronchioles, and alveolar ducts) that conduct air to and from the air sacs (alveoli) of the lungs. Each alveolus is surrounded by a network of capillaries. Both the alveoli and the capillaries consist of a single cell layer that allows rapid diffusion of O_2 into the blood and equally rapid diffusion of CO_2 out of the blood.

The respiratory passageways are composed of smooth muscle and cartilage (C-rings). The smooth muscle controls the size of the lumen of the respiratory passages. The autonomic nervous system regulates the contraction of the smooth muscle. Stimulation of the sympathetic nervous system, mainly through the release of epinephrine from the adrenal gland and the subsequent stimulation of beta-2 receptors, produces smooth muscle relaxation (bronchodilation). Parasympathetic stimulation (acetylcholine [ACH]) produces contraction (bronchoconstriction). Bronchodilators are drugs that relax bronchial smooth muscle and dilate respiratory passages.

RESPIRATORY DISEASES

Any disease process or condition that interferes with respiratory exchange causes serious alterations in the levels of the gases in the blood (plasma O_2 and plasma CO_2). The most common causes of respiratory difficulties are chronic obstructive pulmonary disease (COPD) and asthma.

Chronic Obstructive Pulmonary Disease (COPD)

Chronic obstructive pulmonary disease **(COPD)** is a common respiratory condition that is caused by emphysema and chronic bronchitis. Both conditions cause irreversible changes to the respiratory system. **Chronic bronchitis** is caused by chronic irritation of the respiratory tract. Cigarette smoke and other environmental pollutants increase and thicken respiratory secretions of mucus. These secretions interfere with gas exchange, resulting in eventual fibrotic changes in the respiratory lining. Chronic cough, increased susceptibility to infection, and restriction of physical activity are characteristic of this condition. Drug therapy can provide some relief, but it cannot reverse the fibrosis and other physical changes in the respiratory lining.

Emphysema

Emphysema is a disease process involving destruction of the alveolar walls. Consequently, there is an enlargement of the air spaces within the lungs. Individuals with emphysema have difficulty expelling air from the lungs. Respiratory exchange is reduced, and shortness of breath occurs. Irreversible lung damage takes place, forcing the individuals to restrict daily activities. Treatment involves respiratory exercises designed to increase the efficiency of respiration, oxygen therapy, and medications. Bronchodilators and mucolytic agents are used to dilate the bronchi and to promote expectoration of bronchial secretions.

Asthma

Asthma is a respiratory condition characterized by shortness of breath and wheezing. These effects are caused by bronchiolar constriction. Many factors can cause asthma in susceptible individuals. These factors include respiratory irritants (dust and noxious chemicals), exercise (particularly in cold weather), respiratory tract infections, aspirin and related drugs, and allergy to foreign proteins (pollen and animal dander).

In allergic asthma, individuals develop antibodies to the foreign protein (antigen). After exposure to the antigen, an antigen-antibody reaction occurs in the respiratory tract, precipitating an asthmatic attack. The immediate result is shortness of breath, wheezing, and the terrifying feeling of suffocation. Relief of asthmatic attacks involves use of drugs that relax respiratory smooth muscle (bronchodilators) and drugs that produce antiinflammatory effects on the respiratory passageways.

Asthma has several components in addition to the characteristic bronchoconstriction and wheezing. There is usually mucosal edema and increased production of bronchial mucus. Ciliary activity of the respiratory tract is usually depressed. This decrease interferes with the clearing of mucus and other debris from the lower respiratory airways. Most importantly, asthma is also an inflammatory condition of the respiratory passages.

Chemical Mediators

During an inflammatory reaction, **chemical mediators** are formed and released from injured tissue, mast cells, and leukocytes in the respiratory tract. These mediators are responsible for most of the symptoms and complications of asthma. The chemical mediators involved include histamine, eosinophilic chemotactic factor of anaphylaxis (ECF-A), and various prostaglandin derivatives (leukotrienes and the slow-reacting substance of anaphylaxis [SRS-A]). Recent advances in molecular biology have identified additional mediators that are referred to as cytokines. Tumor necrosis factor and several other cytokine mediators, known as interleukins, are currently undergoing intense investigation. The large number of chemical mediators involved in asthma presents a complicated situation both for the understanding of the disease and for its treatment.

Histamine

Whenever there is injury or insult to body tissue, histamine is rapidly released from mast cells. The pharmacology of histamine was presented in Chapter 31. In the respiratory tract, histamine causes bronchoconstriction, increased vascular permeability that contributes to mucosal edema, and infiltration of leukocytes, particularly eosinophils. Antihistamines are usually of little benefit in the treatment of asthma, and for this reason, histamine is not considered to be the most important mediator in asthma.

Eosinophilic Chemotactic Factor of Anaphylaxis (ECF-A)

Eosinophilic chemotactic factor (ECF-A) is also released by mast cells and functions to attract eosinophils to the site of cell injury or irritation. Eosinophils are part of the general inflammatory and allergic reaction that often occurs in the lining of the respiratory tract in asthma. The inflammatory and allergic reactions worsen and prolong the asthmatic process. When this occurs, antiinflammatory corticosteroid drugs are used to suppress the inflammatory process.

Prostaglandins

The **prostaglandins** are a series of chemical mediators produced by almost all body cells. When cells are irritated or injured, various prostaglandins are rapidly formed and released by the cell membranes. The prostaglandins produce numerous biological effects, including effects on smooth muscle, secretion of mucus, and the inflammatory process. In asthma, one of the most important prostaglandin mediators is the slow-reacting substance of anaphylaxis **(SRS-A).**

The leukotrienes (LT) are one type of prostaglandin that is formed in asthma. During anaphylaxis (a severe allergic reaction) and asthma, the mast cells produce and release several different leukotrienes. The most important of these are referred to as LTB, LTC, LTD, and LTE. Three of these leukotrienes (C,D,E) chemically combine to form SRS-A. Slow-reacting substance of anaphylaxis is an extremely potent bronchoconstrictor that has a long duration of action, much greater than the duration of histamine. In addition, SRS-A promotes mucosal edema, secretion of mucus, and leukocyte infiltration. Slow-reacting substance of anaphylaxis is considered to be an extremely important mediator involved in asthma. There is an intense search by drug manufacturers to discover drugs that block the production of the leukotrienes that would prevent the formation of SRS-A. New drugs that interfere with the actions of the leukotrienes have been approved.

ROLE OF THE AUTONOMIC NERVOUS SYSTEM

Bronchiolar smooth muscle tone and secretion of mucus are normally influenced by the sympathetic and parasympathetic divisions of the autonomic nervous system. Sympathetic stimulation by epinephrine (beta-2 receptor) produces bronchodilation. Parasympathetic activation, via the vagus nerve, produces bronchoconstriction and increased secretion of mucus. Noxious irritants of the respiratory tract stimulate vagal reflexes that result in parasympathetic activation. It has been suggested and often demonstrated that in asthmatics there is a predominance or hyperactivity of the parasympathetic division. This factor may be important and may contribute to the increased sensitivity and hyperreactivity of the asthmatic airway.

The general approach to the treatment of asthma is to give drugs that increase sympathetic activity or decrease parasympathetic activity (anticholinergic drugs). Research has shown that in certain cells, sympathetic activation stimulates the formation of an intracellular nucleotide called cyclic adenosine monophosphate, or AMP. Parasympathetic activation stimulates the formation of another nucleotide, cyclic guanosine monophosphate, or cyclic GMP.

Cyclic AMP appears to be responsible for mediating the effects of sympathetic stimulation to produce bronchodilation. Also during asthma, the formation and release of mediators (histamine, SRS-A, and ECF-A) from mast cells is inhibited by increased levels of cyclic AMP. Cyclic GMP appears to be responsible for mediating the effects of parasympathetic stimulation to produce bronchoconstriction, secretion of mucus, and increased release of mediators from mast cells.

In summary, the current approach to the treatment of asthma takes into account that during asthma, there may be increased parasympathetic activity, which increases intracellular levels of cyclic GMP. The high levels of cyclic GMP result in release of mast cell mediators that cause bronchoconstriction, increased secretion of mucus, mucosal edema, and leukocyte infiltration. Treatment of asthma is aimed at increasing intracellular levels of cyclic AMP with sympathomimetics and other drugs. As levels of cyclic AMP increase in bronchial smooth muscle and mast cells, there is relaxation of smooth muscle (bronchodilation) and inhibition of release of the mast cell mediators that cause inflammation. These effects give relief from the asthmatic attack and help prevent further complications. The main drugs used to treat asthma are the bronchodilators, corticosteroids, and leukotriene inhibitors.

BRONCHODILATOR DRUGS

A number of different drug classes are used in the treatment of asthma. **Bronchodilators** include beta-adrenergic drugs (sympathomimetics), theophylline, and anticholinergic drugs.

Beta-Adrenergic Drugs

Sympathetic stimulation of bronchial smooth muscle causes bronchodilation. This effect is mediated by the beta-2-adrenergic receptors. Consequently, drugs that stimulate the beta-2 receptors produce bronchodilation.

Epinephrine (which is normally released from the adrenal gland) and isoproterenol are two potent beta receptor stimulators. As discussed in Chapter 6, these drugs stimulate both beta-1 (heart) and beta-2 (smooth muscle) receptors. As a consequence, increased heart rate and other sympathetic effects occur in addition to bronchodilation. Overuse of these drugs may cause tachycardia and cardiac arrhythmias. These two drugs are available as over-the-counter (OTC) aerosols.

Adrenergic drugs that selectively stimulate the beta-2 receptors at therapeutic doses are available. These drugs are preferred over the older drugs, which stimulate both beta-1 and beta-2 receptors. However, at higher than therapeutic doses or in susceptible individuals, the selective beta-2 drugs may cause some beta-1 receptor and cardiac stimulation.

There are several other advantages of the newer, selective beta-2 drugs over older drugs such as epinephrine. The newer drugs can be administered orally, whereas the older drugs are administered only by subcutaneous injection or aerosol. Also, the duration of action of the newer drugs is much longer, and therefore provides longer protection with fewer drug administrations. However, epinephrine is still preferred in the treatment of acute asthmatic attacks, when it is usually administered by subcutaneous injection. The beta-adrenergic drugs used in the treatment of asthma are presented in Table 32:1.

Patients who experience infrequent asthmatic attacks usually carry an aerosol preparation and inhale the drug when they experience difficulty in breathing. Patients who experience more frequent asthmatic attacks usually use the aerosols or take one of the oral preparations on a regular basis.

Theophylline

Xanthine compounds—including caffeine, theophylline, and theobromine—are found naturally in tea, cocoa, and coffee. Theophylline is the only xanthine used in the treatment of asthma. Theophylline inhibits an intracellular enzyme, phosphodiesterase, which normally inactivates cyclic AMP. By inhibiting phosphodiesterase, levels of cyclic AMP increase in bronchiolar smooth muscle and in mast cells. As discussed, cyclic AMP

Sympathomimetic (Beta-Adrenergic) Bronchodilator Drugs

DRUG (TRADE NAME)	ADULT DOSE	PEAK EFFECT/DURATION OF ACTION (MINUTES)
Adrenergic Drugs:		
epinephrine injection, USP	0.2–0.5 mg (1:1000) SC or IM PRN	5–60
epinephrine mist	1 or 2 oral inhalations every 3–4 hr	5–60
isoproterenol (*Medihaler-Iso, Mistometer*)	2–3 oral inhalations every 3–4 hr	10–60
Selective Beta-2 Drugs:		
albuterol (*Proventil, Ventolin*)	2–4 mg PO TID, QID	120–480
	2 oral inhalations every 4–6 hr	30–300
bitolterol	Nebulization every 6 hr	360–480
isoetharine	Nebulization every 4 hr	15–120
metaproterenol (*Alupent*)	2–3 oral inhalations every 6 hr	30–360
pirbuterol (*Maxair*)	2 oral inhalations every 4–6 hr	360–480
terbutaline (*Brethine*)	2.5–5 mg PO TID	120–480
	0.25–0.5 mg SC	15–240
salmeterol (*Severent*)	2 oral inhalations every 12 hr	60–720

produces bronchodilation and inhibits the release of mediators from mast cells. Consequently, both beta-adrenergic drugs and theophylline increase cyclic AMP levels, which are important in the control and treatment of asthma.

Theophylline can be administered orally, rectally, or intravenously. There is significant patient variability in regard to absorption and metabolism. Therefore, the dose must be adjusted carefully. Plasma concentrations of theophylline are periodically determined to ensure that theophylline levels are in the therapeutic range (10 to 20 μg per ml).

Numerous preparations of theophylline, including extended-release tablets, are available. Aminophylline is a water-soluble preparation of theophylline that is used for intravenous administration, usually during acute asthmatic attacks. Theophylline can be administered in combination with sympathomimetics in situations where one drug is unable to control the asthmatic condition alone.

The most frequent side effects from oral administration of theophylline are nausea and vomiting. Since theophylline produces

vasodilation, some patients experience flushing, headache, and hypotension. Caution is necessary in patients with existing cardiovascular disease, since theophylline may cause excessive cardiac stimulation. Theophylline also stimulates the CNS and may cause restlessness, insomnia, tremors, and convulsions, especially when plasma levels are above the therapeutic range.

Anticholinergic Drugs

Anticholinergic drugs (atropine-like) are not widely used in the treatment of asthma. Although they do produce some bronchodilation, they tend to dry mucous membranes. However, in patients where other bronchodilators cannot be used or are not effective, administration of anticholinergic drugs by aerosol may produce bronchodilation and offer some relief. By blocking the actions of acetylcholine (which increases intracellular levels of cyclic GMP), the anticholinergic drugs decrease intracellular levels of cyclic GMP.

Ipratropium Bromide (*Atrovent*)

Ipratropium is a derivative of atropine and is the most widely used anticholinergic drug for asthma.

TABLE 32:2 — Corticosteroids Administered by Aerosol Inhalation

DRUG (TRADE NAME)	USUAL DOSE
beclomethasone (*Beclovent, Vanceril*)	1–2 inhalations (42–84 μg/inhalation) BID to QID
budesonide (*Pulmicort*)	1–3 inhalations (200–400 μg/inhalation) BID
flunisolide (*Aerobid*)	2 inhalations (250 μg/inhalation) BID
fluticasone (*Flovent*)	1–3 inhalations (44–220 μg/inhalation) BID
triamcinolone (*Azmacort*)	2 inhalations (100 μg/inhalation) TID to QID

Ipratropium is administered by oral inhalation. It has a slow onset but prolonged duration of action (6 hours). It is poorly absorbed into the systemic circulation, and therefore causes few adverse effects. Excessive drying of the mouth and upper respiratory passages may cause discomfort and is the most common side effect. The pharmacology of the anticholinergic drugs was presented in Chapter 7.

ANTIINFLAMMATORY DRUGS

Two drug classes, the corticosteroids and the leukotriene inhibitors, are used to reduce and control the inflammatory reaction that occurs in asthma. When inflammation is under control, the actions of the bronchodilator drug are more effective, and often the dosages can be reduced. Lower dosages decrease the incidence and severity of adverse drug effects.

Corticosteroids

The general pharmacology of the glucocorticoids will be detailed in Chapter 36. One of the main uses of these drugs is for treatment of inflammatory and allergic conditions such as asthma. The major effect of steroids in the treatment of asthma is to inhibit the inflammatory response that occurs in the respiratory airways. Steroids are used in acute asthmatic conditions when bronchodilators have failed to provide relief or maintain control. In addition, they are used to control bronchiolar inflammation, which is a major component of asthma. In addition, use of corticosteroids usually allows reduction of the dosages of bronchodilator drugs.

During acute asthmatic attacks, steroids are administered either parenterally or orally to achieve effective drug levels rapidly. Prednisone (*Deltasone*) is widely used in these situations. Steroids have the potential to produce a large number of adverse effects, some of which can be serious. For this reason, steroids should be used with caution and withdrawn from the treatment plan as soon as possible.

Steroids are more commonly administered by oral inhalation for the chronic control of asthma. The advantage of inhalation is that lower dosages of steroid are delivered directly into the respiratory tract. Use of this route greatly reduces systemic absorption and the adverse effects associated with steroid use. Corticosteroids available for inhalation are listed in Table 32:2.

Adverse Effects

Adverse effects associated with steroid use include fluid retention, muscle wasting, metabolic disturbances, and increased susceptibility to infection. These effects are not usually observed with aerosol therapy. However, steroids increase the incidence of oral infections (usually fungal infections) and they can cause hoarseness and other vocal chord disturbances. The incidence of these adverse effects can be reduced by rinsing the mouth with water after inhalation to minimize the amount of steroid that remains in the oral cavity.

Leukotriene Inhibitor Drugs

A major focus of asthma research has been to discover drugs that interfere with the formation of the prostaglandin derivatives known as leukotrienes. These substances cause bronchoconstriction, mucus production, and inflamation. In addition, several leukotrienes combine to form SRS-A. Recently, two new drugs that interfere with leukotriene formation were approved.

Zafirlukast (*Accolate*) and montelukast (*Singulair*) are leukotriene receptor antagonists that block the receptor that leukotrienes bind to. The drugs are administered orally, 20 mg BID and 10 mg once/day, respectively for the prophylaxis and chronic treatment of asthma. The most common adverse reactions are headache, infection, nausea, and diarrhea.

Zileuton (*Zyflo*) blocks the formation of leukotrienes by inhibiting an enzyme, 5-lipoxygenase, that is required in the synthesis of leukotrienes. Zileuton 600 mg is administered orally four times a day.

ANTIALLERGIC AGENTS

Cromolyn Sodium

Allergic conditions involve the interaction of an antigen (foreign protein) and an antibody (produced by the body). This interaction causes the release of histamine and other chemical mediators from mast cells that then trigger an asthmatic attack. Cromolyn sodium is a drug that interferes with the antigen-antibody reaction to release mast cell mediators. The drug is taken prophylactically (before allergic exposure) on a daily basis. Cromolyn is also useful in certain types of nonallergic asthma.

Administration of cromolyn is by inhalation, three to four times per day. It is available as a nasal spray (*Nasalcrom*) for allergic rhinitis, as an oral inhaler (Cromolyn Sodium Inhalation, USP) or with a special device (*Intal Inhaler*) that delivers the drug as a fine, micronized powder for the treatment of asthma. Occasionally, the powder irritates the respiratory airways and causes bronchospasm. Cromolyn is not a bronchodilator, and it has no use in the treatment of acute asthma. The therapeutic effect to prevent asthmatic attacks requires several weeks to fully develop.

The most frequent adverse effects are nasal stinging, nasal irritation, headache, and bad taste. In addition, allergic reactions have occurred involving rash, hives, cough, and angioedema.

Nedocromil (*Tilade*) is a drug similar to cromolyn in mechanism and pharmacological effect. It is administered by oral inhalation, usually two inhalations four times per day.

MUCOLYTICS

Mucolytics are chemical agents that liquefy bronchial mucus. In various conditions, such as asthma, bronchitis, and respiratory infections, the production of mucus increases. In these situations the mucus thickens and also contains glycoproteins, cellular debris, and inflammatory exudate. During respiratory infections, the mucus becomes purulent. These changes in the mucus make it difficult for the respiratory tract to remove the mucus by way of ciliary action. The upward movement of mucus by the cilia is often referred to as the mucociliary escalator system. When increased production and thickening of mucus contributes to airway obstructions and interferes with normal respiration, mucolytics are administered by aerosol to thin or liquefy the secretions. Then, the mucus and other respiratory secretions can be removed by coughing or a suction apparatus. Acetylcysteine is a widely used mucolytic. It is also important that patients be adequately hydrated, since water itself can help liquefy and mobilize secretions.

Acetylcysteine (*Mucosil*) contains a chemical group (sulfhydryl) that breaks apart the glycoproteins in bronchial secretions. This action decreases the viscosity (resistance to flow) of bronchial secretions and promotes easier mobilization and removal. Acetylcysteine is irritating and can cause bronchospasm. For this reason, a bronchodilator is added to the inhalation mixture. Administration is usually by nebulization, three or four times a day, followed by postural drainage and tracheal suction when necessary.

EXPECTORANTS

Dryness of the respiratory tract causes irritation and stimulates cough reflexes. The result is a dry, hacking, unproductive cough. Expectorants are agents that stimulate the production of respiratory secretions, which then decrease the irritation and cough caused by excessive dryness of the airways. Consequently, the main use of expectorants is to increase the output of respiratory tract secretions, which indirectly suppresses cough. The expectorants include salts (ammonium chloride and potassium citrate), ipecac syrup, and guaifenesin. Expectorants are added to many cough syrups and cold medications. After oral administration, the expectorants produce their effect by first irritating the lining of the stomach. This gastric irritation stimulates gastric reflexes that increase both gastric and respiratory tract secretions. Because of the gastric irritation, expectorants may cause nausea and vomiting. There is controversy over the use of expectorants, because the effectiveness of these agents has never really been adequately demonstrated.

Chapter Review

Understanding Terminology

Match the definition or description in the left column with the appropriate term in the right column.

___ **1.** Slow-reacting substance of anaphylaxis.

___ **2.** A disease in which patients have difficulty expelling air from the lungs; causes destruction of the walls of the alveolar sacs.

___ **3.** Characterized by shortness of breath and wheezing.

___ **4.** A drug that relaxes bronchial smooth muscle and dilates the lower respiratory passages.

___ **5.** Chronic obstructive pulmonary disease.

___ **6.** A respiratory condition caused by chronic irritation that increases secretion of mucus and causes degeneration of the respiratory lining.

___ **7.** A drug that liquifies bronchial secretions.

a. asthma

b. bronchodilator

c. chronic bronchitis

d. COPD

e. emphysema

f. mucolytic

g. SRS-A

Acquiring Knowledge

Answer the following questions in the spaces provided.

1. What are some of the factors that can precipitate an asthma attack? _____

_____

2. List four physiological changes that can occur in the respiratory tract during an asthma attack.

_____

3. What chemical mediators are released from mast cells? What effects do they produce? _____

_____

_____

4. Discuss the relationship of cyclic AMP and cyclic GMP to the autonomic nervous system. _____

_____

_____

5. What effects do increasing the level of cyclic AMP or decreasing the level of cyclic GMP have on the respiratory tract during asthma? _____

_____

_____

6. Compare the pharmacological effects of epinephrine and albuterol. What is the main indication for each? _____

_____

_____

7. Explain the mechanism of action of theophylline. _____

_____

_____

8. Discuss the indications for the use of corticosteroids. What advantage is there to using beclomethasone by inhalation? _____

_____

_____

9. Explain the mechanism of action of cromolyn. How is it administered? _____

_____

_____

10. How does acetylcysteine liquefy mucus? _____

_____

_____

Applying Knowledge—On the Job

Use your critical thinking skills to answer the following questions in the spaces provided.

1. Mrs. Willard has been prescribed *Ventolin* plus *Atrovent Inhalation Aerosol* while in the hospital to treat her chronic obstructive pulmonary disease (COPD). When you walk into her room to do your afternoon assessment, you notice she is wheezing more than on admission 3 days ago. She is due to take both inhalers within the next half hour. Which inhaler would you administer first to provide her with the quickest relief?

_____

_____

_____

_____

_____

2. Mr. Wiblin calls his physician's office complaining of a dry throat, raspy voice, and a couple of white, patchy areas in his throat. He requests a prescription for an antibiotic. You pull his chart and see that he was given new prescriptions for *Azmacort* and theophylline 1 week ago for newly diagnosed asthma. What additional questions would you ask him? Is an antibiotic appropriate for this patient? If not, why?

_____

_____

3. Following a bee sting, a young boy developed hives and had difficulty breathing. What drug is indicated for immediate treatment of this condition? How should it be administered?

_____

_____

4. Mrs. Peabody is an elderly woman who has taken theophylline for years for her asthma. Recently she has complained of trouble sleeping and she says her hands are shaking and her heart is pounding. What do you think is happening to her? What would be a logical course of action to take?

_____

_____

5. Patient compliance is an important factor in the treatment and control of asthma. Of the selective beta-2 drugs listed, assuming that each medication would be equally effective, which medication do you feel would lend itself to better patient compliance? What was the main factor in choosing this medication?

_____

_____

6. Why is it important to advise patients using corticosteroid inhalers to rinse their mouth with water after inhalation?

_____

_____

7. What is the usual dosing with Tilade inhaler?

_____

_____

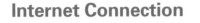

Internet Connection

Visit the **MedicineNet** website (http://www.medicinenet.com) and click on the _Diseases and Conditions_ heading. Highlight the letter _A_ and find both the _Asthma_ and _Allergic Rhinitis_ subheadings. Both provide additional background and drug information concerning these two common respiratory conditions.

Additional Reading

Blanchard, A. R. 2002. Treatment of COPD exacerbations: Pharmacologic options and modification of risk factors. _Postgraduate Medicine_ 111 (6):65

Korenblat, P. E. 2000. The role of cysteinyl leukotriene receptor antagonists in asthma therapy. _Hospital Physician_ 36 (12):50.

Toygen, D., and Brenner, P. 2001. Metered dose inhalers. _American Journal Nursing_ 101 (10):26.

PHARMACOLOGY OF THE GI TRACT

Chapter 33

Therapy of Gastrointestinal Disorders: GERD, Ulcers, and Vomiting

Digestion and Ulcer Production
Management of Ulcers
Management of Gastroesophageal
  Reflux Disease (GERD)
Antisecretory Drugs
Antacids

Sucralfate
Management of Emesis

Chapter 34

Agents That Affect Intestinal Motility

Bowel Function
Antidiarrheals
Laxatives and Cathartics

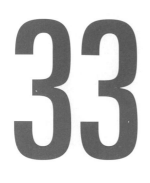

33

THERAPY OF GASTROINTESTINAL DISORDERS: GERD, ULCERS, AND VOMITING

CHAPTER FOCUS

This chapter describes drugs that limit the development of ulcers and/or prevent the recurrence of ulcers by eliminating specific bacteria that are associated with ulcer development, affecting the action of acid or the production of acid in the stomach. Drugs that inhibit vomiting are also discussed.

CHAPTER OBJECTIVES

After studying this chapter, you should be able to

- explain what stimulates the production of acid and pepsin in the GI tract.

- identify examples from the three classes of drugs that inhibit acid secretion.

- describe the differences between an antihistaminic antiulcer drug, an antacid and a proton pump inhibitor.

- explain the appropriate use of antihistaminic (H_2) drugs.

- explain the rationale for drugs used in gastroesophageal reflux disease.

- explain the action of drugs that inhibit vomiting.

- describe three side effects commonly associated with antiulcer drugs.

- describe three drug interactions associated with antisecretory antiulcer drugs.

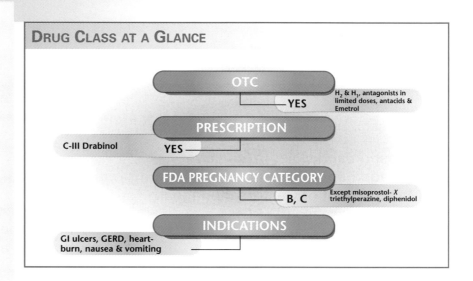

DRUG CLASS AT A GLANCE

OTC — YES — H_2 & H_1, antagonists in limited doses, antacids & Emetrol

PRESCRIPTION — C-III Drabinol — YES

FDA PREGNANCY CATEGORY — B, C — Except misoprostol- X triethylperazine, diphenidol

INDICATIONS — GI ulcers, GERD, heartburn, nausea & vomiting

Key Terms

abortifacient: substance that induces abortion.

acid rebound: effect in which a great volume of acid is secreted by the stomach in response to the reduced acid environment caused by antacid neutralization.

antacid: drug that neutralizes hydrochloric acid (HCl) secreted by the stomach.

antisecretory: substance that inhibits secretion of digestive enzymes, hormones, or acid.

GERD: gastroesophageal reflux disease.

hepatic microsomal metabolism: specific collection of enzymes in the liver (P_{450}) that metabolizes some drugs and can be increased (stimulated) by some medications or decreased (inhibited) by other medications so that therapeutic drug blood levels are altered.

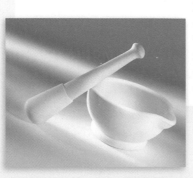

hyperacidity: abnormally high degree of acidity (for example, pH less than 1). In the gastric environment, this term usually refers to an abnormally high amount of acid secretion rather than an abnormal decrease in pH (see *hyperchlorhydria*).

hypercalcemia: elevated concentration of calcium ions in the circulating blood.

hyperchlorhydria: excess hydrochloric acid in the stomach.

hypermotility: increase in muscle tone or stimulation of muscle contractions causing faster clearance of substances through the GI tract.

hypophosphatemia: abnormally low concentrations of phosphate in the circulating blood.

parietal (oxyntic) cell: cell that produces hydrochloric acid (HCl) in the gastric mucosa.

perforation: opening in a hollow organ, such as a break in the intestinal wall.

proteolytic: action that causes the decomposition or destruction of proteins.

systemic: occurring in the general circulation, resulting in distribution to most organs.

ulcer: open sore in the mucous membranes or mucosal linings of the body.

ulcerogenic: capable of producing damage to tissues ranging from minor irritation or lesions to an integral break in the mucosal lining (ulcer).

INTRODUCTION

The organs of the upper gastrointestinal (GI) tract are concerned primarily with the digestion and absorption of nutrients. The stomach and small intestine (particularly the duodenum) secrete several enzymes that aid in the digestion of food. Secretion of these digestive juices is usually stimulated by food or increased motility of the GI muscles. Specialized cells in the stomach produce hydrochloric acid (HCl) and **proteolytic** enzymes (for example, pepsin), which break down food particles into an absorbable form.

DIGESTION AND ULCER PRODUCTION

Process of Digestion

Gastric acid secretion is stimulated when food enters the stomach. However, even the sight, smell, or thought of food stimulates acid and pepsin secretion through the vagus nerve (parasympathetic and cholinergic) as depicted in Figure 33:1. When food enters the stomach, additional acid is secreted by the action of the hormone gastrin. In addition, the food bulk may distend the gastric muscle and stimulate the vagus nerve to elicit even more acid secretion. The secretion of HCl causes the contents of the stomach to become extremely acidic (pH 1.0). This acid pH is necessary to activate the digestive enzymes such as pepsin.

NOTE TO THE HEALTH CARE PROFESSIONAL

Cigarette smoking has been shown to be closely related to ulcer recurrence and reversal of antiulcer drug effectiveness.

Eventually, the digested mass passes from the stomach into the small intestine (duodenum) where the final phase of digestion occurs, and absorption begins. When digestion is nearly complete, the duodenum secretes an inhibitory enzyme that stops gastric acid secretion. This action prevents excess secretion of HCl and pepsin, which could damage the GI tissue. Gastric acid is even produced and secreted between meals in response to appropriate stimuli. Acid secretion between meals, during the evening hours, and during sleep reduces bacterial growth in the stomach, thus minimizing the risk of infection. Normally, the cells of the GI tract are protected from the destructive action of acid and pepsin. The mucosal lining of these organs is continuously lubricated with secretions of mucus to prevent autodigestion (self-destruction). This protective mechanism is extremely important during the evening hours, when acid is secreted into an empty stomach. Anything that interferes with the protective function of the mucosal cell barrier may contribute to the production of ulcers.

Production of Ulcers

Ulcers are open sores in the mucous membranes or mucosal linings of the body. Gastrointestinal ulcers frequently occur in the stomach and duodenum, where acid and pepsin activity are

Gastrointestinal Organs Involved in Digestion. Sites of Antiulcer Drug Action

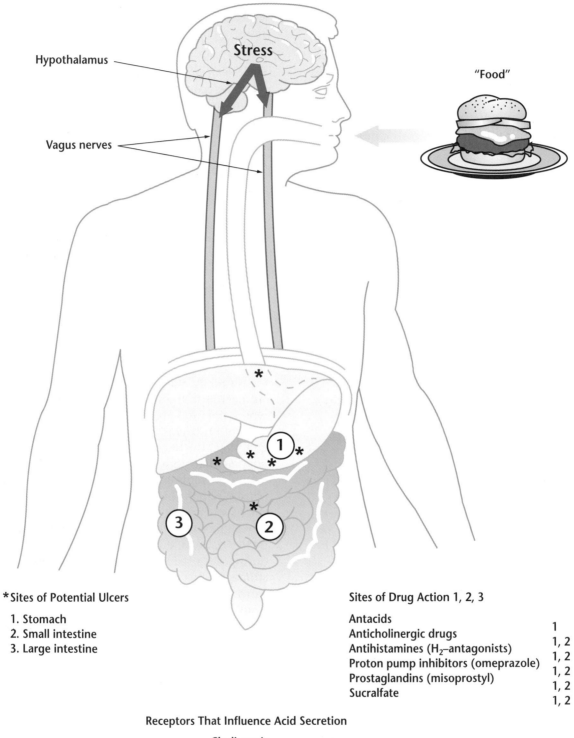

*Sites of Potential Ulcers

1. Stomach
2. Small intestine
3. Large intestine

Sites of Drug Action 1, 2, 3

Antacids   1
Anticholinergic drugs   1, 2
Antihistamines (H₂–antagonists)   1, 2
Proton pump inhibitors (omeprazole)   1, 2
Prostaglandins (misoprostyl)   1, 2
Sucralfate   1, 2

Receptors That Influence Acid Secretion

Cholinergic
Gastrins
Histamine H₂
Prostaglandin

greatest (Figure 33:1). These sites of local damage are known as peptic ulcers (digestive destruction).

There is no simple cause of ulcers. Some individuals secrete excess amounts of gastric acid (**hyperacidity** or **hyperchlorhydria**) even when food is not present in the stomach. Other individuals may not produce enough protective mucus or inhibitory enzyme to stop acid secretion. In addition, many other factors make individuals susceptible to ulcer production. For example, emotional stress, alcohol, smoking, and increased cholinergic (vagus) activity stimulate the secretion of acid. Drugs, such as the nonnarcotic analgesics and steroids, are **ulcerogenic** because they inhibit the secretion of mucus and interfere with the normal production of the mucosal lining. In addition, there is evidence that some people are genetically susceptible to ulcer formation. Usually, a combination of ulcerogenic factors is involved in the development of peptic ulcers. Whether gastric or duodenal, peptic ulcers are associated with acid-induced injury to the mucosa.

Regardless of the cause, GI ulcers may be accompanied by periodic pain, nausea, loss of appetite, and vomiting. The pain is characteristically described as a dull, gnawing, burning sensation, and it often resembles heartburn or acid indigestion. Duodenal pain is usually (but not always) relieved by food, whereas gastric pain is brought on by food. In both cases, the pain may be intense enough to awaken patients from sleep. Chronic erosion of the mucosa may produce a bleeding hole (**perforation**) in the GI wall. Such a development is suspected when blood appears in the stool or vomit. The immediate danger is that the GI perforation will lead to hemorrhage, hypotension, and shock.

MANAGEMENT OF ULCERS

Treatment of gastric and duodenal ulcers is directed toward removing the source of the irritation and pain and allowing the mucosal sores to heal. Recommended treatment of active ulcers is short term, 4 to 8 weeks. Frequently, therapy is continued (maintenance therapy) to minimize the risk of ulcer recurrence. Therefore, inhibition of gastric acid and pepsin secretion is a major part of ulcer therapy. Therapy includes avoiding situations that contribute to or augment the secretion of acid, such as emotional stress; ingestion of alcohol, spicy foods, high-protein diets; and ulcerogenic drugs. In addition to diet manipulation, several types of drugs are

therapeutically useful because they influence secretory activity by different mechanisms. Today, H_2-antagonists (antihistamines), prostaglandins, proton pump inhibitors, anticholinergic drugs, and antacids are frequently used in combination with proper diet in the management of ulcers. These drugs are not always curative. In some instances, recurrent ulcers require surgical repair to avoid further damage, pain, and hemorrhage.

Recent clinical research has confirmed that *Helicobacter pylori* (*H. pylori*) bacteria are present in 100 percent of patients with chronic active gastritis and 90 percent of patients with duodenal ulcers. The Centers for Disease Control has reported that nine out of ten cases of GI ulcer are caused by *H. pylori*. The organism promotes ulcer recurrence in patients who have received conventional antiulcer treatment. Once the organism has been eradicated, chances of reinfection is minimal and ulcer recurrence is dramatically reduced. Management of these patients requires extensive combination therapy. Antibiotics must be administered to eradicate the bacteria. Antibiotic monotherapy is not recommended because bacterial resistance develops. One of the standard regimens recommends at least two antibiotics in combination with bismuth salts. Bismuth is believed to lyse the bacterial cell wall and prevent further adhesion of the bacteria to the gastric mucosa. This provides greater opportunity for the antibiotics to eradicate the bacterial infection. Amoxicillin, tetracycline, metronidazole (*Flagyl*), and clarithromycin (*Biaxin*) are the drugs of choice because *H. pylori* is sensitive to them. A variety of regimens are in use: "dual therapy" refers to the simultaneous administration of two antibiotics; "triple therapy" includes two antibiotics plus bismuth; and "quadruple therapy" is the triple combination plus a proton pump inhibitor. The wide variety of drugs used in the treatment and management of ulcers is presented in Table 33:1.

MANAGEMENT OF GASTROESOPHAGEAL REFLUX DISEASE (GERD)

Gastroesophageal reflux disease (**GERD**) is a disorder characterized by a burning sensation behind the sternum (retrosternal pain), better known as heartburn. Patients frequently describe the symptom as an irritation and/or burning in

Antisecretory Drugs/Adult Oral Daily Doses Used in the Clinical Management of Ulcers

| DRUG (TRADE NAME) | DUODENAL ULCER | | GASTRIC ULCER | GERD | PATHOLOGICAL HYPERSECRETORY CONDITIONS |
	SHORT-TERM ACTIVE	MAINTENANCE			
Histamine H₂-Receptor Antagonists:					
cimetidine (*Tagamet*)	800 mg at bedtime or 400 mg BID or 300 mg QID	400 mg at bedtime	800 mg at bedtime or 300 mg QID	800 mg BID or 400 mg QID	300 mg QID not to exceed 2400 mg/day
cimetidine OTC (*Tagamet-HB*)	Heartburn	200 mg QD, BID no more than 2 weeks			
famotidine (*Pepcid*)	40 mg at bedtime or 20 mg BID	20 mg at bedtime	40 mg at bedtime	20 or 40 mg BID or 1 hr before eating (up to 2 tablets BID)	20 mg every 6 hr
famotidine OTC (*Pepcid-AC*)	—	Heartburn	10 mg (1 tablet) BID 1 hr before the meal causing symptoms (do not exceed 2 tablets/day)		
nizatidine (*Axid Pulvules*)	300 mg at bedtime or 150 mg BID	150 mg at bedtime	—	150 mg BID	—
OTC (*Axid AR*)	—	—	—	75–150 mg	
ranitidine (*Zantac*)	300 mg at bedtime or 150 mg BID	150 mg at bedtime	150 mg BID	150 mg BID	150 mg BID
OTC (*Zantac 75*)	—	—	—	75–150 mg	
Prostaglandins:					
misoprostol (*Cytotec*)	For patients unresponsive to H₂ antagonists 200 µg		100–200 µg QID with food for prevention of NSAID-induced gastric ulcers	—	—

(continued)

their chest or throat. While heartburn is a common complaint among otherwise healthy people, in GERD this symptom is part of a chronic disease. Heartburn occurs after meals, worsens when the patient is lying down, and involves regurgitation of digestive juices into the esophagus. In severe GERD, the patient may also have signs of chronic blood loss, ulcerative esophagitis and strictures, and fibrous tissue bands resulting from the chronic injury to the esophagus.

The normal barriers to regurgitation of acid involve contraction of the gastroesophageal sphincter, dilution of acid by swallowed saliva, peristalsis that moves digested material away from the esophagus and stomach, and, ultimately, resistance by the mucosal lining.

In GERD, the sphincter in the lower esophagus (LES) relaxes inappropriately such that gastric acid washes back (reflux) into the esophagus. When this occurs out of synchrony with peristalsis, the acid in

Antisecretory Drugs/Adult Oral Daily Doses Used in the Clinical Management of Ulcers, *continued*

DRUG (TRADE NAME)	DUODENAL ULCER		GASTRIC ULCER	GERD	PATHOLOGICAL HYPERSECRETORY CONDITIONS
	SHORT-TERM ACTIVE	MAINTENANCE			
Proton Pump Inhibitors:					
omeprazole (*Prilosec*)	20 mg daily*	—	20 mg daily	20 mg daily	60 mg once a day to 120 mg TID
lansoprazole (*Prevacid*)	15 mg QD	15 mg QD	—	30 mg/day	60 mg/day up to 120 mg
esomeprazole (*Nexium*)	—	—	—	20 or 40 mg daily	—
pantoprazole (*Protonix*)	—	—	—	40 mg daily	—
rabeprazole (*Aciphex*)	20 mg daily	—	—	20 mg daily	60 to 120 mg daily
H. pylori Combination Treatment**					
bismuth subsalicylate (525 mg) plus metronidazole 250 mg plus tetracycline (500 mg) (*Helidac*) 1 dose (4 tablets) QID					
ranitidine bismuth citrate (*Tritec*)	400 mg BID (1 tablet)	—	—	—	—
omeprazole	40 mg once a day	—	—	—	
clarithromycin	500 mg TID				
Triple therapy					
omeprazole or esomeprazole	20mg BID 40 mg daily	— —	— —	— —	
clarithromycin		500 mg BID	—	—	—
amoxicillin		1000 mg BID	—	—	—
lansoprazole	30 mg QD***	—	—	—	—
clarithromycin	500 mg BID***	—	—	—	—
amoxacillin	1 g BID***	—	—	—	—
GI Stimulants (Prokinetic drugs)					
metoclopramide (*Reglan, Maxolon*)	—	—	—	10–15 mg up to QID 30 minutes before each meal	—

*4–8 weeks.
**Not an inclusive list of *H. pylori* regimens.
***Up to 14 days.

contact with esophageal tissue remains longer. Certain foods are known to relax this sphincter (reduce lower esophageal pressure) in anticipation of digestion (see Table 33:2). In GERD, the normal barriers are not able to respond correctly to the damaging triggers. Any additional complication, such as hiatal hernia, that impedes the flow of digestive contents, or drug-induced relaxation of the sphincter, predisposes patients to prolonged acid contact and irritation, even erosion. Once the mucosa is eroded, hydrogen ions have a direct path to injure the cells.

Diet and lifestyle adjustments that have an important place in maintenance therapy usually meet with poor compliance in the routine of hectic, stress-filled days. Until recently, GERD patients received only temporary relief of heartburn with antacids. With the availability of a variety of antisecretory drugs and gastric stimulants, GERD is significantly better managed today. In the management of mild to moderate GERD, sphincter relaxation can be lessened by the use of the gastric stimulants, also known as prokinetic drugs. However, the primary therapeutic objective is suppression of normal acid production that limits esophageal contact with gastric acid. The H_2-antagonists have brought dramatic relief to many patients with mild to moderate GERD. Where ulcerative damage is present, especially in severe GERD, the proton pump inhibitors are considered the first-line therapy. In severe GERD, especially to avoid lifetime drug therapy, the patient may undergo surgery to remove damaged tissue and delay further erosion. The mechanisms of action of the drugs used in the management of GERD are presented in Table 33:3.

ANTISECRETORY DRUGS

Two primary mechanisms are involved in drug-mediated ulcer healing: reduction of gastric acidity and enhancement of mucosal barrier defenses. Antihistaminics, prostaglandins, proton pump inhibitors, and anticholinergic drugs reduce the volume and concentration of gastric acid. **Antacids,** on the other hand, neutralize the acid already present. Sucralfate (*Carafate*) is neither an antacid nor an antisecretory drug. It acts to enhance the mucosal defense by a local action at the site of the ulcer. Among the drugs used in the management of gastric and duodenal ulcers, the antihistaminics (H_2-receptor antagonists) represent a revolutionary change in therapy, especially for patients who cannot or will not tolerate the unpleasant side effects associated with the use of anticholinergic and antacid drugs.

H_2-Receptor Antagonists (Antihistamines)

The autocoid histamine is a potent stimulator of gastric secretions in humans. Histamine is in mast cells located throughout the GI mucosa. Histamine receptors are found in the gastric mucosa that mediate the secretion of gastric acid and pepsin. These receptors are designated H_2-receptors to distinguish them from the H_1-receptors involved in hypersensitivity and allergic reactions (see Chapter 31). The **parietal,** or **oxyntic, cells** located in the stomach are responsible for acid production. Evidence suggests that the receptors involved in mediating gastric secretion are located on the parietal cells. These receptors include cholinergic and histamine receptors, which facilitate acid secretion as well as sensitize the cells to gastrin stimulation. Stimulation of these receptors increases the volume and strength (decreases pH) of acid secretion. If either the cholinergic receptors or H_2-receptors are blocked, acid secretion decreases and gastrin-induced secretion is inhibited.

TABLE 33:2	Examples of Drugs and Foods Known to Lower Esophageal Sphincter Pressure

FOOD	DRUGS
Chocolate	Alcohol calcium channel blockers
Fat	Cigarettes, morphine
Onion	Dopamine
Coffee	Diazepam
Peppermint	Barbiturates
Spearmint	Prostaglandins
	Digestive hormones

Cimetidine (*Tagamet*), famotidine (*Pepcid*), nizatidine *(Axid),* and ranitidine *(Zantac)* are H_2-receptor antagonists that competitively inhibit the interaction of histamine with H_2-receptors. Blockade of these receptors significantly reduces the secretion of acid and pepsin output from the target issue. These drugs are neither anticholinergic nor antispasmodic drugs. Their antiulcer action is directed at the histamine (H_2-) receptors. These drugs act at the end organ to inhibit acid secretion **(antisecretory).** Therefore, in the presence of other acid-promoting (secretory) stimuli, gastric acid secretion is suppressed. The pharmacology of H_2-receptor antagonists is similar. These drugs differ in their potency, pharmacodynamic characteristics (bioavailability or protein binding), and ability to influence the **hepatic microsomal metabolism** of other medications. The currently available H_2-receptor antagonists are presented in Table 33:1.

Route of Administration

All of the H_2-receptor antagonists except nizatidine can be administered orally and parenterally. Following oral administration, these drugs are absorbed into the blood. Peak absorption occurs within 90 minutes for cimetidine and 2 to 3 hours for famotidine, nizatidine, and ranitidine. Overall absorption does not appear to be adversely affected by the presence of food in the GI tract. Therefore, these drugs can be taken with meals. Cimetidine absorption has been reported to be delayed by the concomitant use of antacids, but the data are not as clear for famotidine, nizatidine, and ranitidine. Antacids should be taken 1 hour after cimetidine and ranitidine administration to avoid an interaction resulting in decreased absorption of these drugs. No special precautions are associated with the oral use of other H_2-receptor antagonists and antacids. The primary route of drug elimination is the kidneys, although hepatic metabolism occurs to some extent.

Adverse Effects

The H_2-receptor antagonists are very well tolerated during short-term or chronic maintenance therapy requiring high daily doses. Adverse effects may include headache or constipation. Cimetidine has been associated with reversible central nervous system (CNS) effects, mental confusion, and disorientation, usually in severely ill patients. Liver or renal disease may contribute to elevated circulating levels of cimetidine due to

---

TABLE 33:3 Drugs Used in the Management of GERD: Mechanisms of Action

DRUG	MECHANISM OF ACTION
antacids	Increase pH of the refluxed fluid local cytoprotection
GI Stimulants/Prokinetic Drugs:	
bethanachol	Increase lower esophageal pressure through a cholinergic pathway
	Induce intestinal peristalsis
metoclopramide	Increase lower esophageal pressure, increase gastric and esophageal peristalsis, increase gastric emptying
H_2-Receptor Antagonists	
cimetidine	Decrease gastric acid secretion
famotidine nizatidine	Decrease gastric volume
Proton Pump Inhibitors:	
esomeprazole omeprazole	Inhibit gastric acid secretion
lansoprazole pantoprazole rabeprazole	Decrease gastric volume

decreased metabolism and excretion and predispose elderly patients to CNS effects. Nizatidine and ranitidine have been associated with elevations in hepatic enzyme levels, in particular, AST (aspartate aminotransferase, serum glutamic oxaloacetic transaminase [SGOT]), ALT (alanine aminotransferase, serum glutamate pyruvate transaminase [SGPT]), and alkaline phosphatase. These levels return to normal when the medication is discontinued.

A safety profile in children under 16 years of age has not been established with this class of drugs. A relatively small number of pediatric patients have required antihistaminic therapy, usually for hypersecretory conditions. Since there is little experience with these drugs in infants, and because these drugs are secreted into breast milk, female patients should be cautioned not to nurse their infants while taking H_2-receptor antagonists.

No serious adverse effects have been associated with reported overdose of these drugs. Treatment of overdose is symptomatic and supportive.

Drug Interactions

Cimetidine has been reported to increase blood levels of several drugs by altering their metabolism. The mechanisms of metabolic interference are thought to be inhibition of hepatic microsomal systems (binding to cytochrome P_{450}), as well as alteration of hepatic blood flow leading to decreased hepatic clearance of certain drugs. Although ranitidine binds to cytochrome P_{450} less than cimetidine, famotidine and nizatidine have no effect on this metabolic pathway. Since an inhibition of the hepatic microsomal metabolizing system may lead to an elevation in the drug levels of certain concomitant medications, famotidine or nizatidine may be a favored choice under these conditions. Drugs that may be affected by inhibition of the hepatic microsomal metabolizing system with cimetidine (and possibly ranitidine) use are presented in Table 33:4. Drug interactions associated with any H_2-antagonists are also presented in Table 33:4. In order to maintain therapeutic blood levels of these drugs, dosage adjustment may be necessary when concomitant H_2-receptor antagonist therapy is begun or ended. To avoid clinically significant variation in anticoagulant action, patients receiving warfarin concomitantly with cimetidine should have their prothrombin time monitored during the treatment period. Ranitidine does not affect the hepatic microsomal system to the same extent as does cimetidine. However, ranitidine has been reported to interact with some of the same types of drugs. Absorption of ranitidine, for example, appears to be decreased by concomitant use of antacids. Other drugs, such as diazepam and metoprolol, are affected by concomitant use of ranitidine (Table 33:4).

Information regarding the compatibility of mixing H_2-receptor antagonists with other drug solutions for parenteral administration is available for cimetidine. Cimetidine is incompatible when added to solutions of barbiturates, cefamandole nafate, cefazolin sodium, cephalothin sodium, and theophylline. These drugs should not be mixed in the same syringe with cimetidine because precipitation of cimetidine will occur.

Clinical Indications

H_2-receptor antagonists are recommended for the short-term treatment (up to 8 weeks) of benign gastric and duodenal ulcers. This class of agents will heal 60 to 80 percent of ulcers within 4 weeks of treatment. Although patients often take medication beyond 4 weeks, it is not necessarily associated with total cure or eradication of all lesions. In the treatment of active ulcers, the doses of these drugs may vary from a single dose taken at bedtime to BID or QID regimens. Prophylaxis or maintenance therapy may be continued with a single daily dose taken at bedtime (Table 33:1). The specific doses of the H_2-receptor antagonists vary because each drug has a different potency. However, all of these drugs are effective in alleviating the symptoms and subsequent tissue damage or complications of peptic ulcer disease to the same extent when used in the recommended regimens. At this time, cimetidine (*Tagamet-HB*), famotidine (*Pepcid-AC*), nizatidine (*Axid AR*), and ranitidine (*Zantac 75*) are available OTC in dosages per tablet which are less than those available by prescription. The dosage of *Tagamet-HB* is 100 mg per tablet compared to the prescribed dose range of 200–800 mg per dose form, while the dose of *Pepcid-AC*, which has an effect on pepcid acid control, is 10 mg per tablet compared to 20 or 40 mg. OTC nizatidine and ranitidine are available in 75-mg tablets.

H_2-receptor antagonists are used in the treatment of special hypersecretory conditions such as multiple endocrine adenomas, **systemic** mastocystis (mast cells), or Zollinger-Ellison (ZE) syndrome. Zollinger-Ellison syndrome is a disease characterized by the presence of gastrin-containing tumors (gastrinomas) and ulceration of the GI tract. In most ZE syndrome patients, gastric acid hypersecretion is present. The flood of

TABLE 33:4	Drug Interactions Associated With Antisecretory Drugs		

ANTISECRETORY DRUG	INTERACTS WITH	MECHANISM OF ACTION	RESPONSE
cimetidine or ranitidine	Antacids, sucralfate	Delay absorption	Decreased cimetidine or ranitidine availability
cimetidine	Cisapride	Accelerate GI absorption	Increase in plasma levels of cimetidine, ranitidine
cimetidine	Caffeine, calcium channel blockers, carbamazepine, chlordiazepoxide, chloroquine, diazepam, labetalol, lidocaine, meperidine, metoprolol, metronidazole, pentoxifyline, phenobarbital, phenytoin, propranolol, quinidine, quinine, sulfonylureas, tacrine, theophylline, triampterene, tricyclic antidepressants, warfarin	Cimetidine inhibits hepatic metabolic enzymes	Increased blood levels of these drugs
lansoprazole, omeprazole	Sucralfate	Delay absorption	Decrease availability of lansoprazole
metoclopramide	Alcohol, cyclosporin	Accelerate gastric emptying	Increase absorption of alcohol, cyclosporin
metoclopramide	Cimetidine	Accelerate gastric emptying	Decrease cimetidine absorption
metoclopramide	MAO Inhibitors	Release catecholamines	Increase potential hypertension
metoclopramide	Anticoagulants, narcotic analgesics		
nizatidine	Aspirin, doses greater than 3 g/day	Unknown	Increased serum salicylate levels
omeprazole	Clarithromycin	Unknown	Increase plasma levels of both omeprazole and clarithromycin
omeprazole	Diazepam, flurazepam, triazolam, phenytoin, warfarin	Interfere with metabolism	Increased blood level of these drugs
ranitidine	Diazepam, midazolam	Ranitidine alters drug absorption	Increased blood levels of midazolam; decreased blood levels of diazepam
ranitidine	Warfarin	Ranitidine may decrease warfarin clearance	Increased hypoprothrombinemia

hydrochloric acid into the intestine ultimately contributes to severe diarrhea, whereas the acid and pepsin erode the GI mucosa, producing peptic ulcers. Zollinger-Ellison syndrome patients are often resistant to other modes of therapy but have successfully responded to the H_2-receptor antagonists at doses three times the usual daily dose. Cimetidine and ranitidine have been given to ZE patients in doses of 3 to 6 g per day to control ulcers. In these patients, treatment with H_2-antagonist drugs must be continued indefinitely to avoid ulcer recurrence.

At present, most of the H$_2$-receptor antagonists are approved for the short-term management of duodenal ulcers, gastric ulcers, and pathological hypersecretory conditions. However, some of these drugs are also used clinically for the treatment of GERD, stress ulcers induced in critically ill patients (burns, intracranial lesions, trauma), and gastric irritation in susceptible patients requiring nonsteroidal antiinflammatory drugs (NSAIDs) or chronic aspirin treatment. Table 33:1 indicates the recommended doses for the approved uses of each H$_2$-receptor antagonists.

Prostaglandins

Several pathways and receptors are involved in the production and secretion of gastric acid and cytoprotective mucus. In addition to the H$_2$-histamine receptors, prostaglandins are believed to have specific receptors in the gastric mucosa. Prostaglandins are a variety of naturally occurring substances that interact with specific prostaglandin receptors. These receptors mediate bicarbonate production and secretion of mucus, and therefore they directly influence the protective environment of the stomach. Drugs that inhibit prostaglandin synthesis, such as NSAIDs, are known to induce gastric ulcers, presumably by inhibition of the prostaglandin-mediated secretions.

NOTE TO THE HEALTH CARE PROFESSIONAL

Women who are in their child-bearing years should be instructed about the effects of taking prostaglandins and urged never to give their medication to friends or relatives.

Route of Administration

At present, only one synthetic prostaglandin is approved for use in the management of NSAID- and aspirin-induced gastric ulcers. An analog of prostaglandin E$_1$, misoprostol (*Cytotec*), is available for oral administration (tablets) in doses of 100 to 200 μg QID. Misoprostol may be taken with meals to minimize any local irritation. For those patients who cannot tolerate the 200 μg dose, the recommended dose is 100 μg. Misoprostol is recommended to be taken throughout the duration of NSAID therapy in patients at high risk for developing gastric ulcers, but misoprostol does not appear to prevent duodenal ulcers in patients on chronic NSAID therapy.

Adverse Effects and Contraindications

Unlike the other antisecretory drugs, prostaglandins mediate a number of physiological effects in the body. Besides their involvement in peripheral pain pathways, prostaglandins are directly involved in the process of uterine contraction, from premenstrual cramping to induction of labor at term. Misoprostol (*Cytotec*) produces uterine contractions (**abortifacient**) and may cause miscarriage if patients become pregnant while on therapy. For this reason, misoprostol is contraindicated for use in pregnant women. If women become pregnant during treatment, the drug should be terminated immediately and the patients should be counseled about the potential hazards to the fetus. Misoprostol should not be given to women of child-bearing potential until the abortifacient risks and sequelae have been thoroughly explained and an effective contraception method begun. Other effects produced during therapy appear to be related to the effect of prostaglandin on the smooth muscle of the GI and genitourinary (GU) tract. Misoprostol has been associated with self-limiting diarrhea in men or women on therapy and, to a lesser extent, abdominal pain, headache, flatulence, nausea, and constipation may occur.

The toxic dose of prostaglandins in humans has not been determined. However, signs of overdose may include sedation, tremor, palpitations, hypotension, bradycardia, and fever.

Proton Pump Inhibitors

Gastric acid secretion may be affected by blocking receptors that mediate physiological responses (H$_2$-histamine, prostaglandin E$_1$, or cholinergic receptors) or by directly inhibiting the exchange of hydrogen (H$^+$) and potassium (K$^+$) ions within the parietal cells. This adenosine triphosphatase (ATPase)-driven exchange of hydrogen and potassium ions within the gastric parietal cells is absolutely essential for the production of HCl. Within the past few years, a new class of drugs has been studied that directly inhibits this enzyme-specific secretory system. For this reason, these compounds are referred to as proton pump inhibitors. These compounds have no effect on any other receptor-mediated activity.

Omeprazole (*Prilosec*), esomeprazole *(Nexium)*, lansoprazole *(Prevacid)*, pantoprazole *(Protonix)*, and rabeprazole *(Aciphex)*, the drugs currently available in this class, are used in the management of ulcers. The proton pump inhibitors are approved for the short-term treatment of benign gastric ulcers, active duodenal ulcers, GERD, or long-term therapy in pathological hypersecretory conditions. These drugs are part of the effective combination treatment with antibiotics to eradicate *Helicobacter pylori,* promote ulcer healing, and prevent ulcer recurrence in susceptible patients. When administered with clarithromycin and amoxicillin, the proton pump inhibitors promote ulcer healing.

Adverse Effects

Oral administration of the proton pump inhibitors is generally well tolerated. The more common side effects include headache, abdominal pain, diarrhea, nausea, and constipation. There has been no evidence that omeprazole alters human gastric cell function to predispose patients to develop malignancies. However, because of the ability of this drug to sustain an inhibition of acid production, coupled with cell changes in laboratory animals, caution is indicated in the product labeling, which recommends that the drug be used only under the conditions and dosage described.

In the event of overdose, treatment is symptomatic and supportive, since there is no specific antidote. Because omeprazole is extensively bound to circulating plasma proteins, the drug cannot be dialyzed readily from the blood.

Drug Interactions

Omeprazole *(Prilosec)* is metabolized through the hepatic microsomal system and has been reported to cause elevated blood levels of diazepam, phenytoin, and warfarin when these drugs have been taken concomitantly. Since omeprazole profoundly affects the pH of the gastric contents, it may interfere with the absorption of drugs that depend upon an acid environment for optimal absorption. At this time, however, there have been no significant interactions reported. Although lansoprazole, pantoprazole, and rabeprazole are metabolized through the hepatic microsomal system, there have been no reported clinically relevant drug interactions at this time.

Gastrointestinal Stimulants

Gastrointestinal stimulants induce contractions within the upper GI tract that prevent reflux of acid into the esophagus and promote gastric emptying. This combination of actions moves the potentially damaging digestive material away from the lower esophagus. Metoclopramide *(Reglan)* stimulates contraction of the lower esophageal sphincter by enhancing the action of endogenous acetylcholine. Metoclopramide increases tissue sensitivity to acetylcholine, while cisapride enhances the release of acetylcholine at the myenteric plexus. Neither of these drugs interacts with cholinergic receptors nor stimulates cholinergic nerves. The selectivity of action for upper GI smooth muscle makes the drugs clinically valuable for the treatment of GERD and minimizes the potential for unnecessary stimulation of gastric and biliary secretion.

Metoclopramide *(Reglan)* reduces symptoms best in daytime heartburn, especially meal induced. For this reason the recommended dose schedule is 10 to 15 mg 30 minutes prior to the meal or provocative situation. Metoclopramide is readily absorbed orally. In the treatment of GERD metoclopramide can be taken up to four times a day—that is, at each meal and before bedtime, for 8 to 12 weeks.

Metoclopramide *(Reglan)* is also available for other therapeutic uses and parenteral administration. Diabetic patients may experience delayed gastric emptying. This physiological alteration, known as diabetic gastroparesis, is usually accompanied by a persistent feeling of fullness, nausea, and heartburn. The degree of gastric stasis and intensity of the accompanying symptoms will determine whether intravenous administration is warranted to stabilize the patient. After the nausea and/or vomiting have stopped, the patient may continue on oral outpatient treatment. Metoclopramide, 10 mg prior to meals, is indicated for the relief of symptoms associated with acute and recurrent diabetic gastroparesis.

Metoclopramide *(Reglan)* is also used in the treatment of chemotherapy-induced vomiting.

Cisapride has been removed from the commercial market through a mutual decision between the FDA and the drug manufacturer over safety concerns. Cisapride has been associated with alterations in cardiac conduction, observed as a prolongation of the QT interval on the electrocardiogram. In many patients, this resulted in life-threatening arrhythmias and death. The potential for an alteration in cardiac function was raised by the concomitant use of a variety of other medications. Because there was no way to reasonably minimize the interaction of such drugs in patients, especially those with conditions such as existing ventricular arrhythmias, cisapride was voluntarily removed from the market.

Adverse Effects and Contraindications

Metoclopramide (*Reglan*) is generally well tolerated. The type of nontherapeutic effects that have been reported with GI stimulants are also observed as symptoms of GERD. Adverse effects with metoclopramide, which are transient and usually mild, include restlessness, drowsiness, diarrhea, and headache. Patients have reported hypersensitivity reactions to metoclopramide. In such situations, the drug should be stopped immediately.

Metoclopramide (*Reglan*) may produce cardiovascular effects such as palpitations and sinus tachycardia. At normal therapeutic levels, cardiovascular function is not compromised.

Metoclopramide (*Reglan*) is contraindicated in three conditions. Metoclopramide is contraindicated in patients in whom GI motility may precipitate hemorrhage or perforation. Such patients are those who have active GI hemorrhage, bowel perforation, or bowel obstruction. Patients with pheochromocytoma, tumor of the catecholamine producing adrenal tissue, may develop hypertension because GI stimulants evoke release of catecholamines from the tumor. Patients who have demonstrated sensitivity or intolerance to the drug should not receive the drug in the future.

In addition, metoclopramide is contraindicated in patients who are epileptic or are receiving drugs that are likely to cause extrapyramidal reactions. In epileptic patients, the severity and frequency of seizures may be increased. On rare occasions, metoclopramide produces a potentially irreversible, involuntary contraction of muscle known as tardive dyskinesia. Although it can affect any muscle, most often it is associated with the limbs, tongue, and facial muscles. The patient cannot control bizarre mouth gestures of grimacing and protruding tongue. The mechanism of action is related to chronic blockade of endogenous dopamine within the extrapyramidal system of the brain. Chronic blockade of dopamine in this system causes an increase in the number and sensitivity of dopamine receptors that avidly await any dopamine molecules to produce muscle contraction. In some patients the symptoms may correct months after the drug is withdrawn. Elderly female patients are most likely to develop this condition at 30 to 40 mg per day. On the other hand, children and young adults may develop extrapyramidal reactions at higher doses used to block vomiting during chemotherapy.

Anticholinergic, Antiserotonin, and Antispasmodic Drugs

The secretion of gastric acid is medicated by several substances including hormones (gastrin), neurotransmitters (acetylcholine), and histamine. There is no question that stimulation of the vagus nerve increases the secretion of gastric acid. Stimulation of the parasympathetic nerves that supply the GI tract increases intestinal motility, and this activity may also enhance gastric secretion. Drugs that inhibit cholinergic activity by blocking the autonomic ganglia or blocking muscarinic receptors directly decrease gastric acid secretion and intestinal motility. Among the anticholinergic drugs, the belladonna derivatives (atropine, hyoscyamine, and scopolamine), glycopyrrolate, isopropamide, and propantheline have been used in the management of peptic ulcers because of their pharmacological effects on acid secretion and intestinal motility (see Table 33:5). Synthetic antispasmodic drugs such as dicyclomine and oxyphencyclimine do not exhibit anticholinergic activity, but they are used for their ability to relax intestinal smooth muscle via nonspecific pathways. Drugs with an antispasmodic action may be useful in the clinical management of irritable bowel syndrome (spastic colon), GI **hypermotility** (increased muscle tone or stimulation of muscle contractions, causing faster clearance of substances through the GI tract), neurogenic colon, and other functional GI disorders. The mechanisms of action of these drugs have been discussed in previous chapters dealing with the parasympathetic nervous system and autonomic ganglia.

Many of these drugs are available as combination preparations. In general, the combination may include a sedative (barbiturate), an antianxiety drug (chlordiazepoxide, hydroxyzine, or meprobamate), or an H_2 antagonist. Examples of the available combination products include *Bellacane-SR, Bellergal-S, Butibel Elixir, Clindex, Donnatal,* and *Librax.*

Tegaserod (*Zelmac*) belongs to a new chemical class of compounds that selectively target and act on serotonin ($5\text{-}HT_4$) receptors present throughout the GI tract. These serotonin receptors are believed to potentially play a key role in pain perception and GI motility. By acting on these receptors that lie on the surface of the gastric cells, *Zelmac* may reduce abdominal pain and may normalize altered gastrointestinal function in patients with irritable bowel syndrome (IBS) who suffer from abdominal pain and constipation as their primary symptoms.

Route of Administration

Oral and parenteral preparations of these drugs are available. In the management of GI disorders, anticholinergic compounds are usually administered orally 30 minutes before meals and at bedtime (see Table 33:5). These drugs must be absorbed (systemically) in order to produce the desired pharmacological effects. Following oral administration, the synthetic anticholinergic compounds are not as readily absorbed as the belladonna derivatives.

Adverse Effects

Because the naturally occurring belladonna alkaloids are easily absorbed and readily cross the blood-brain barrier, they are associated with CNS side effects (dizziness, headache, insomnia, and drowsiness) at therapeutic doses.

Since the synthetic anticholinergic drugs are quaternary compounds (ionized) that cannot cross membranes easily, including the blood-brain barrier, the synthetic anticholinergics are not associated with CNS side effects. The synthetic anticholinergic drugs, however, may produce ganglionic blockade and neuromuscular blockade at toxic doses. Other adverse effects associated with the use of anticholinergic drugs include mydriasis, blurred vision, dry mouth, bradycardia or tachycardia, increased intraocular pressure, and urinary retention. By the nature of their effect on GI motility, these drugs frequently produce constipation. Anticholinergic drugs are eventually metabolized in the liver and are relatively short-acting. The synthetic (quaternary) derivatives have a longer duration of action than do the belladonna alkaloids.

Tegaserod (*Zelmac*), 6 mg twice daily, was found to be well tolerated. Diarrhea, the predominant adverse event, is transient and resolves with continued therapy. The most common side effects are similar to the spectrum of symptoms of the underlying gastrointestinal disorder—abdominal pain, diarrhea, nausea, flatulence, and headaches.

Special Considerations and Contraindications

Anticholinergic and antispasmotic drugs should be used with caution in patients who have glaucoma, tachyarrhythmias, or bladder obstructions. They are contraindicated in patients

---

TABLE 33:5	Selected Anticholinergic, Antiserotonin, and Antispasmodic Drugs Used in the Clinical Management of Gastrointestinal Disorders

DRUG (TRADE NAME)	USE	ADULT ORAL DOSE
Belladonna Alkaloids:		
atropine	Bradyarrhythmia	0.25–0.5 mg TID
belladonna (*Bellafoline*)	Spasm, peptic ulcer, intestinal and biliary colic	0.125–0.25 mg TID, QID
l-hyoscyamine (*Levsin*)		up to 1.5 mg
scopolamine hydrobromide	Sedation preoperative, motion sickness	0.4–1.0 mg every 1–2 hr
Synthetic Anticholinergics:		
glycopyrrolate (*Robinul*)	Peptic ulcer	1–3 mg TID
propantheline (*Pro-Banthine*)	Peptic ulcer	7.5–22.5 mg
Synthetic Antispasmodics:		
dicyclomine (*Bentyl, Dyspas*)	Irritable bowel	80–160 mg/day in four divided doses
oxyphencyclimine (*Daricon*)	Peptic ulcer	5–10 mg BID, TID
Serotonin Antagonists:		
tegaserod (*Zelmac*)	Irritable bowel syndrome	6 mg BID

who have myasthenia gravis, narrow-angle glaucoma, or obstructive bowel disease. Elderly patients may be sensitive to the effects of these drugs, as evidenced by episodes of mental confusion and excitement even at low doses. Because of the potential for interaction, these drugs should be used with caution in patients who are receiving cardiac glycosides, antihistaminics, levodopa, or other parasympathomimetic drugs.

Drug Interactions

Any pharmacological agent that has an anticholinergic component will enhance the anticholinergic activity of these drugs. Such drugs include amantidine, antihistaminics, antipsychotics, antiparkinsonism drugs, meperidine, and tricyclic antidepressants. Monoamine oxidase (MAO) inhibitors may inhibit the metabolism of these drugs, thus potentiating anticholinergic activity. Since antacids decrease the oral absorption of these drugs, anticholinergics should be given 1 or 2 hours before the antacids.

Clinical Indications

Anticholinergic drugs will affect secretion and muscle contraction within the GI system. The appropriate drug is selected according to the desired site of action. Synthetic anticholinergics are approved as adjunct treatment of peptic ulcer. Synthetic antispasmodics are approved for use in peptic ulcer (oxyphencyclimine) or irritable bowel (dicyclomine). Belladonna alkaloids are used as adjuncts to peptic ulcer treatment, in functional GI disorders (diarrhea, spasm, diverticulitis) and intestinal and biliary colic, including infant colic.

ANTACIDS

Antacids are used to relieve the pain and indigestion that accompany overeating, hyperacidity associated with heartburn, GERD, gastritis, hiatal hernia, or peptic ulcers. Antacids are usually taken orally as liquids or tablets so that they are readily distributed to the GI tissues. A phenomenal number of antacid products are available over the counter as single or combination products, too many to present in the scope of this chapter. The majority of over-the-counter (OTC) antacid products contain magnesium (Mg^{2+}), aluminum (Al^{3+}), or calcium (Ca^{2+}) ions (see Table 33:6). However, one of the oldest antacids, sodium bicarbonate (baking soda), can be found in almost every home.

Mechanism of Action

Antacids neutralize gastric acidity. These drugs react with hydrochloric acid (HCl) to form water and salts (see Table 33:6). Since the hydrogen ions are used to form water, gastric acidity decreases and the pH of the stomach juices increases. When the pH of the stomach contents reaches 4 or 5, pepsin activity is completely inhibited, and the mucosal irritation is removed.

All antacids produce a similar spectrum of effects because they directly neutralize gastric acid. Selection of an antacid may be based on the acid neutralizing capacity. Otherwise, advantages of some OTC products may not be related to their acid neutralization but to the ability of additional ingredients to produce other pharmacological actions. For example, saccharin may be added to increase the palatability (overcome the chalky taste), simethicone may be added as an antigas agent, and aspirin or acetaminophen may be included in varying amounts to ameliorate the symptoms of headache and minor muscle aches associated with tension (Table 33:7).

Classification of Antacids

Most antacid drugs are nonsystemic drugs, implying that they are not absorbed into the bloodstream. Therefore, their action is primarily exerted along the GI tract. Although small amounts

TABLE 33:6	Neutralization of Gastric Acid (HCl) by Antacids		
ANTACID	GASTRIC ACID	INSOLUBLE SALT	
$Mg(OH)_2$ magnesium hydroxide	+ 2 HCl $\longrightarrow$	$MgCl_2$ magnesium chloride	+ 2 H_2O
CaCO3 calcium carbonate	+ 2 HCl $\longrightarrow$	$Ca^{2}+$ calcium ions	+ H_2O + CO_2 gas
Al $(OH)_3$ aluminum hydroxide	+ 3 HCl $\longrightarrow$	Al $(Cl)_3$ aluminum chloride	+ 3 H_2O

of magnesium, aluminum, and calcium ions may be absorbed, these antacid components primarily remain in the GI tract. Cations (Mg^{2+}, AL^{3+}, Ca^{2+}), which are absorbed, are usually excreted by the kidneys. The nonsystemic antacids interfere with the intestinal absorption of other elements.

Constipation is a frequent adverse effect of these drugs because the absorption of water and phosphate ions is inhibited. For this reason, individuals using antacids over a long period of time may also require a laxative to improve bowel function. While constipation may occur with aluminum and calcium antacids, diarrhea is likely to develop with magnesium-containing antacids. **Hypophosphatemia** (phosphate depletion) occasionally occurs with the chronic use of antacids containing aluminum compounds.

Sodium bicarbonate is a systemic antacid that is capable of producing metabolic alkalosis as a result of sodium (Na^{2+}) and bicarbonate (HCO_3^-) ion absorption. The excess bicarbonate absorbed is eventually excreted by the kidneys, causing the urine to become more alkaline. Absorption of sodium ions promotes fluid retention, which can lead to edema or increased blood pressure. Such fluid is particularly important in patients who have renal insufficiency, congestive heart failure, or hypertension. These individuals are usually on a sodium- (salt-) restricted diet, which is counteracted by the systemic antacid.

Chronic use of systemic antacids in combination with milk or calcium may lead to the milk-alkali syndrome. Here, in addition to metabolic alkalosis, **hypercalcemia** (elevated concentration of calcium ions), nausea, headache, weakness, and mental confusion are present. These symptoms subside when the antacids are discontinued.

The use of antacids is limited by their short duration of action. When taken on an empty stomach, the duration of action is about 30 minutes. Since food acts as a buffer, most antacids are taken 1 hour after meals so that the buffering activity continues for 2 to 3 hours.

TABLE 33:7	Selected Over-the-Counter Preparations of Antacids		
TRADE NAME	**ANTACID CONTENT**	**ADDITIONAL ACTIVE INGREDIENTS**	**AVAILABLE PREPARATIONS**
Alka-Seltzer Plus	Sodium bicarbonate	Citric acid, sodium, 325 mg aspirin	Effervescent tablets
Extra Strength Alka-Seltzer	Sodium bicarbonate	Citric acid, sodium, 500 mg aspirin	Effervescent tablets
Amphojel	Aluminum hydroxide	—	Tablets, suspension
Bromo-Seltzer	Sodium bicarbonate	Citric acid, sodium, 325 mg acetaminophen	Effervescent granules
Di-Gel	Aluminum hydroxide, magnesium hydroxide	Simethicone, saccharin, sorbitol	Tablets, liquid
Gaviscon	Aluminum hydroxide, sodium bicarbonate	Alginic acid, magnesium trisilicate	Tablets, liquid
Gelusil	Aluminum hydroxide, magnesium hydroxide	Simethicone, saccharin, sorbitol	Tablets, liquid
Maalox	Aluminum hydroxide, magnesium hydroxide	Simethicone, saccharin, sorbitol	Tablets, liquid
Milk of Magnesia	Magnesium hydroxide	—	Tablets, suspension
Riopan	Hydroxymagnesium aluminate (magaldrate)	Simethicone, saccharin, sorbitol	Tablets, suspension, liquid
Rolaids	Dihydroxyaluminum, sodium carbonate	—	Tablets
Tums	Calcium carbonate	—	Tablets, liquid

Chronic use of antacids may produce a condition known as **acid rebound.** As the pH of the stomach increases in the presence of antacids, the secretory cells respond by increasing the secretion of gastric acid. This eventually counteracts the neutralization potential of the antacids.

Another consideration in the selection or long-term use of antacids involves the sodium content of the product. The sodium associated with the sodium bicarbonate component of these products may be significant for patients with hypertension, congestive heart failure, or other conditions requiring maintenance on a low-sodium diet. The contents of the product should be reviewed before selection of an antacid is made.

Drug Interactions

Antacids may alter the absorption and excretion of other drugs by forming insoluble complexes or altering the pH of the stomach or urine. Absorption of oral tetracyclines is inhibited by antacids (especially magnesium and calcium compounds) because the antacids bind the tetracyclines into a nonabsorbable form (see Table 33:8). Alteration of the urinary pH (alkaline) causes increased blood levels of drugs that are weak bases. Drugs such as quinidine, morphine, and pseudoephedrine are reabsorbed into the blood during antacid therapy. Conversely, acid drugs such as aspirin, penicillins, and isoniazid are excreted more quickly in an alkaline urine.

Clinical Indications

Antacids are approved for reduction of hyperacidity associated with peptic ulcer; relief of upset stomach associated with heartburn, GERD, and acid indigestion. Individual antacids have been formulated to be of value in replacement therapy as follows: magnesium deficiency resulting from alcoholism, restricted diet or magnesium-depleting drugs (magnesium hydroxide); treatment of hyperphosphatemia (aluminum carbonate); and calcium deficiency associated with postmenopausal osteoporosis (calcium carbonate).

SUCRALFATE

Sucralfate (*Carafate*) is a complex of aluminum hydroxide and sulfated sucrose that is used to promote healing of peptic ulcers. Similar to the antacids, sucralfate is a nonsystemic drug that exerts its effect locally in the GI tract. Unlike antacids, however, sucralfate does not alter gastric pH.

Mechanism of Action

Sucralfate acts by forming a protective barrier over damaged gastric mucosa. Sucralfate binds proteins, such as albumin and fibrinogen, that are exuded from damaged mucosal cells and are present in the ulcer crater. A coating is formed that prevents further damage by blocking contact with gastric

TABLE 33:8	Drug Interactions Associated With Antacid Drugs	
DRUGS	**INTERACTION**	**RESPONSE**
allopurinol, anticholinergics, chloroquine, chlorpromazine (phenothiazines), corticosteroids, digoxin, ethambutol, H_2 antagonists, iron, isoniazid, penicillamine, salicylates, tetracyclines, thyroid hormones	Bind with antacids to form insoluble complexes	Decreases the oral absorption of drug
Weak Acids:		
pentobarbital, salicylates	Alkaline urine produced by the antacid	Increases the renal excretion of drug (decreases blood drug level)
Weak Bases:		
morphine, pseudoephedrine, quinine, quinidine, benzodiazepines	Alkaline urine produced by the antacid (increased toxicity)	Increases renal reabsorption of drugs
dicumarol	Unknown mechanism, interacts with magnesium antacid	Increases the absorption of dicumarol (increases the anticoagulant effect)

acid and pepsin, allowing healing to occur. In addition, sucralfate inhibits pepsin activity and may absorb bile salts that can cause irritation of the gastric lining. A small amount of sucralfate is absorbed from the GI tract and eventually excreted in the urine. The most common side effect associated with the use of sucralfate is constipation.

Clinical Indications

Sucralfate is recommended for short-term treatment of duodenal ulcers. It is available only in tablet form. The usual dose is 1 g taken four times daily on an empty stomach, 1 hour before meals and at bedtime. Antacids may also be part of the combined antiulcer therapy. However, antacids should not be taken within 30 minutes before or after sucralfate administration.

Drug Interactions

Concomitant administration of sucralfate has been shown to affect the absorption of digoxin, quinolone, quinidine, ketaconazole, and warfarin resulting in decreased bioavailability of these drugs. The interaction is believed to be a direct result of sucralfate's binding to the drug, leading to a decrease in absorption from the GI tract. Sucralfate has been reported to reduce the bioavailability of phenytoin. The dose of phenytoin may need to be adjusted to maintain a therapeutic response in patients who are taking sucralfate. Oral administration of any of these drugs should be separated from sucralfate administration by at least 2 hours to avoid drug interaction. Sucralfate may interfere with the absorption of fat-soluble vitamins, possibly resulting in deficiencies with long-term use of the drug. Small amounts of aluminum absorption do occur with sucralfate. Although this is of little clinical significance in most patients, use of sucralfate in patients with chronic renal failure may lead to accumulation of aluminum because of inability to excrete these ions efficiently. In other patients, the concomitant use of sucralfate and aluminum-containing antacids may result in aluminum accumulation. However, the clinical significance in patients who are not renally compromised is not known.

MANAGEMENT OF EMESIS

Process of Emesis

Vomiting is a natural defense mechanism that may signal the presence of disease, or organ dysfunction or provide a route for removal of harmful ingested substances. Emesis may be self-induced (bulimia) or involuntary, associated with cold and flu, pregnancy, motion sickness, inner ear infection, or exposure to certain drugs. Vomiting occurs in response to a signal from the vomiting center (VC) located in the brainstem (Figure 33:2). The status of the body is monitored via afferent nerves bringing information to the chemoreceptor trigger zone (CTZ) or directly to the VC. Harmful stimuli carried in the blood to the CTZ include poisons, metabolic toxins (uremia), and electrolyte imbalances. In addition hormones (pregnancy, endocrine imbalances), radiation, and chemotherapy provoke the CTZ to stimulate the VC.

The VC may be directly triggered by afferent nerves receiving stimulation from visceral distention, increased intracranial pressure, rotation, unequal stimulation of the inner ear (labyrinth), or pain. Even sight, smell, and memory can precipitate activation of the VC. The message is received to reverse peristalsis through stimulation of the salivary glands (increased secretion), the diaphragm, and muscles of the upper GI tract.

Frequently, vomiting is self-limiting and of short duration such as viral-induced symptoms of cold and flu. Even without medication, vomiting will resolve within 2 to 3 days. Persistent vomiting, however, results in electrolyte, fluid, and acid-base imbalance. Infants and elderly are more susceptible to developing life-threatening electrolyte changes if the vomiting is not controlled. Nausea and vomiting associated with motion sickness may require pharmacological control because the labyrinthine stimulation may persist well beyond the initial trigger. Other circumstances where vomiting can be detrimental to the patient include the postoperative period where the force of emesis could tear sutures or dangerously increase pressure on the organs (eye or cranial surgery).

Emetics

Stimulation of emesis is primarily restricted to removal of noxious substances—that is, drug overdose following oral administration. Gastric lavage has replaced the use of emetics; however, ipecac syrup is still available for home use. Gastric emptying, when warranted, should occur within the first 2 hours to minimize absorption of the toxic substance. Ipecac syrup given in one or two doses acts on the gastric mucosa locally and on the CTZ centrally to induce vomiting. Oral dosing should be followed by 200 to 300 ml of water.

Vomiting Reflex: Pathway Between the Chemoreceptor Trigger Zone (CTZ) and the Vomiting Center (VC) and the Stomach

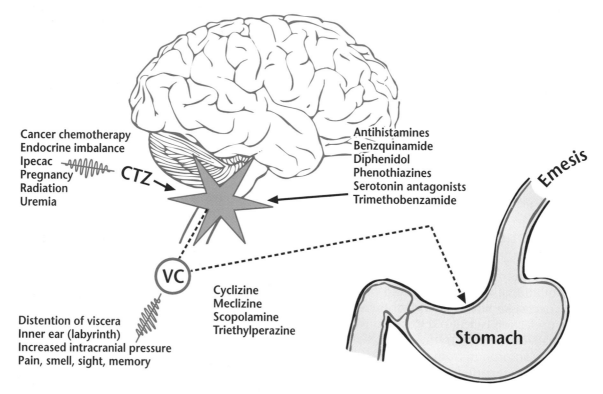

Carbonated beverages should not be given because it may enhance absorption of ipecac. Systemic absorption of ipecac is limited because vomiting removes it from the body as well. Ipecac should not be administered until contact with a trained health professional has been established (for example, emergency service, paramedics, poison control). If vomiting does not occur after 2 doses of 15 to 30 ml (infants 5 ml), the patient should be transported to a proper facility for gastric lavage.

If vomiting does not occur within 30 minutes, absorbed ipecac may produce adverse reactions from diarrhea, hypotension, arrhythmia, and bradycardia to CNS depression. In systemic doses it is cardiotoxic.

Ipecac syrup should never be administered to individuals who are unconscious, semiconscious, severely inebriated, or who are having seizures. These individuals cannot control muscle contraction, which could lead to aspiration of gastric contents and bronchospasm. Life-threatening pulmonary edema and aspiration pneumonitis can result.

Ipecac is contraindicated when the ingested substance is unknown, caustic (lye), or petroleum

based, such as kerosene or gasoline. Regurgitation of caustic substances will damage the esophagus. Vegetable oil delays the absorption of the petroleum substances.

Ipecac syrup is available OTC and by prescription. Unfortunately it is a drug currently used by bulimic women to complete the binge and purge cycle.

Antiemetics

Commonly used antiemetics, such as antihistamines (H_1-antagonists) and phenothiazines, mitigate vomiting by influencing dopaminergic or cholinergic mechanisms within the CNS. In this regard, drugs that are not phenothiazines but are antidopaminergic such as metoclopramide (*Reglan*) also inhibit the vomiting reflex. Antihistamines (H_1-antagonists) effective in relieving vomiting are H_1-antagonists that exert significant anticholinergic activity. These antihistamines are also effective in relieving the nausea and vomiting associated with motion sickness. Serotonin (5-HT) antagonists are among the newest drugs that prevent or reduce the nausea and vomiting produced by highly emetogenic cancer chemotherapy (cisplatin, carboplatin). While the specific mechanism or sites of action have not yet been identified for all these agents, many are known to act at the CTZ, the VC, or both (see Figure 33:2). The H_1-antihistamine and serotonin antagonists also influence peripheral nerves.

One product stands out in this class because it produces its effect directly on the stomach and does not affect the nervous system or receptor-mediated functions. Phosphorated carbohydrate solution (*Emetrol, Nausetrol*) is a combination of sugars (fructose, dextrose) and phosphoric acid. Because it is a hyperosmolar solution, it delays gastric emptying, and acts on the wall of the GI tract to reduce smooth muscle contraction. It is safe for use during pregnancy, especially for morning sickness during the first trimester. It is also used in infants and children.

Another noteworthy drug is Dronabinol. Dronabinol *(Marinol),* the principal psychoactive substance in *Cannabis sativa,* is indicated for the treatment of nausea and vomiting associated with cancer chemotherapy. Most often Dronabinol is only used after conventional antiemetics have failed.

Adverse Effects and Contraindications

For the most part, the adverse effects of the phenothiazines, antihistamines, and serotonin antagonists are extensions of their therapeutic activity. The spectrum of adverse effects presented in previous chapters includes dry mouth, sedation, drowsiness, diarrhea, and blurred vision. The phenothiazines, metoclopramide (*Reglan*), and ondansetron (*Zofran*) have the potential to produce extrapyramidal reactions at antiemetic doses. Diphenidol (*Vontrol*) has anticholinergic activity and has produced hallucinations, disorientaton, or confusion in patients. It is recommended that this drug be used only in a supervised setting; for example, in hospital.

Dronabinol, although used in patients who have not responded to other therapy, is considered highly abusable, and thus is designated a Schedule C-III drug. Mood changes (euphoria, confusion, depression, dizziness) can develop especially in elderly patients, and irritability, insomnia, and restlessness characteristic of withdrawal syndrome has occurred. Dronabinol may cause an increase in central sympathethic activity and therefore should be used with caution in patients who are hypertensive or manic or schizophrenic.

Contraindications to the use of these drugs, except for phosphorated carbohydrate, include hypersensitivity or pregnancy. Safety for use in pregnancy has not been established in humans.

Phosphorated carbohydrates should be used with caution in diabetic patients, and should be avoided in patients with a family history of fructose intolerance. Otherwise, the most common adverse effects associated with this product are abdominal pain and diarrhea. These effects are dose related and a direct result of hyperosmotic fluid in the intestine.

Clinical Indications

The drugs in this class provide symptomatic relief ranging from morning sickness in pregnancy to severe nausea and vomiting of cancer chemotherapy. Promethazine (*Phenergan*) is used as preanesthetic medication to prevent nausea and vomiting. Chlorpromazine (*Thorazine*) and perphenazine (*Trilafon*) also inhibit intractable hiccoughs within the antiemetic dose range. Metoclopramide (*Reglan*), ondansetron (*Zofran*), and granisetron *(Kytril)* are specifically used as prophylaxis and treatment in cancer chemotherapy. When given prior to chemotherapy, vomiting can be reduced or prevented so that the patient is able to complete chemotherapy without discomfort or interruption. This predisposes the patient to be compliant with subsequent chemotherapy sessions—that is, to complete the full protocol. Ondansetron (*Zofran*) and granisetron (*Kytril*) are also used for prevention of vomiting postoperatively and with radiotherapy; however, they are not recommended for use where the incidence of emesis is expected to be low. Dronabinol (*Marinol*), a derivative of tetrahydrocannabinol, is an alternative antiemetic when other conventional drugs have proven unsuccessful in cancer chemotherapy.

Perphenazine (*Trilafon*), prochlorperazine (*Compazine*), and triflupromazine (*Vesprin*) are drugs of choice for severe nausea and vomiting of any cause. Severe vomiting should not be treated with antiemetics alone. Because fluids and electrolytes will be affected by severe, protracted vomiting, fluid replacement is essential to stabilizing the patient. The recommended doses for the antiemetic drugs are presented in Table 33:9. Except for a few products, these drugs are available only by prescription. Cyclizine (*Marezine*), meclizine (*Antivert*), and diphenhydramine (*Benadryl*) are available in therapeutic doses OTC and by prescription, while phosphorated carbohydrate solution (*Emetrol*) is only OTC.

Drugs Used to Relieve Vomiting or Motion Sickness

DRUG (TRADE NAME)	NAUSEA AND VOMITING	MOTION SICKNESS
Antidopaminergic		
Phenothiazines:		
chlorpromazine (*Thorazine*)	10–25 mg every 4–6 hr PO	No
perphenazine (*Trilafon*)	50–100 mg every 6–8 hr rectal	No
prochlorperazine (*Compazine*)	8–16 mg daily in divided doses PO	No
	5 or 10 mg TID, QID PO, 25 mg BID rectal	No
promethazine (*Phenergan*)	12.5–25 mg every 4–6 hr PO, rectal	No
	25 mg BID initial dose 0.5–1 hr before travel	No
thiethylperazine (*Torecan*)*	10–30 mg daily PO	No
Other		
metoclopramide (*Clopra, Octamide, Reclomide, Reglan*)	1–2 mg/kg IV 30 min before cancer chemotherapy repeat every 2 hr for 2 doses, then every 3 hours for 3 doses	No
Anticholinergic		
Antihistamines (H_1-antagonists):		
cyclizine (*Marezine***)	50 mg every 4–6 hr PO, initial dose 0.5–1 hr before travel; do not exceed 200 mg daily	Yes
diphenhydramine (*Benadryl***)	25–50 mg TID, QID PO	Yes
dimenhydrinate (*Dramamine***)	50–100 mg every 4–6 hr PO; do not exceed 400 mg daily	Yes
meclizine (*Antivert, Bonine*)	25–50 mg 1 hr before travel; repeat every 24 hr as needed	Yes
Anticholinergics:		
Scopolamine (*Transderm-Scop*)	Apply behind the ear 4 hr before effect is required	Yes
trimethobenzamide (*Tigan*)	250 mg TID, QID PO, rectal	No
Serotonin Antagonists:		
ondansetron (*Zofran*)	3 doses 0.15 mg/kg of diluted solution IV 30 min before then 4 and 8 hr after chemotherapy or single 32-mg dose 30 min before; 16 mg PO 1 hr before anesthesia	No
granisetron (*Kytril*)	10 µg/kg IV 30 min before chemotherapy or 1 mg BID PO; first dose within 1 hr before chemotherapy; second dose 12 hr later	No
Miscellaneous:		
dronabinol (*C-III Marinol*)	5 mg/m² PO 1–3 hr before chemotherapy; then every 2–4 hr after up to 6 doses daily	No
carbohydrate solution (*Emetrol***)	15–30 ml every 3 hr for morning sickness	

*For severe nausea and vomiting.
**Over-the-counter preparation.

Patient Administration and Monitoring

Drugs effective in the relief of symptoms associated with acute or recurrent heartburn, nausea, esophagitis, or GI ulcers are often used by patients between physician visits. It is not uncommon for individuals to delay proper evaluation because they fear the worst diagnosis (for example, ulcer and/or need for a change in diet). Since many of these medications are available OTC, patients self-medicate rather than return for periodic reevaluation when symptoms return. With the increasing availability of drugs in this class, especially in the wide variety of formulations (tablet, liquid, suspension, suppository), and the likelihood that concurrent medications can cancel therapeutic effects, it is important that patients receive instructions on proper drug administration.

Rules for Antiulcer Medication

While the drugs in this class are extremely effective, there are two rules essential for successful therapy and patient safety. Rule number one: If symptoms persist, especially when medication has been taken for 1 to 2 weeks, notify the physician for further evaluation. Rule number two: If signs of bleeding occur such as black or tarry stools, or dark material appears in vomited fluids ("coffee grounds"), notify the physician immediately. Adequate evaluation includes changing medication until the appropriate efficacy is attained. Bleeding may herald the recurrence or onset of mucosal damage, which can lead to life-threatening hemorrhage.

Patient Instruction on Formulation

Product formulation should be explained to patients so that active drug is released at the appropriate time and in the designated amount to effectively relieve symptoms.

Chewable tablets should be chewed before swallowing, and followed with a full glass of water. These tablets are not designed to be swallowed whole and the delay in tablet dissolution will reduce or eliminate their effectiveness. Tablets not designated as chewable and capsules should not be chewed when taking medication with meals. Omeprazole must be swallowed whole, not chewed, before meals. Lansoprazole capsules, however, can be opened and contents put onto applesauce for patients having difficulty taking the medication.

Sustained-release preparations should not be crushed or chewed. This formulation releases drug over a specific period of time to maintain therapeutic blood levels of drug.

Effervescent tablets should dissolve completely before swallowing. Bubbling should have stopped before swallowing.

Hyperosmolar solutions used for nausea and vomiting should not be diluted before dosing. The product exerts its effect through the concentrated sugars. Dilution removes the product's ability to produce a response.

Transdermal patch formulations should be placed on an area of skin that is not covered with hair, sores, or cuts. For scopolamine, the patch is placed directly behind the ear. Patients must be instructed to wash hands thoroughly with soap after handling the patch. Drug that may have transferred to the hands could cause temporary dilation of the pupils or blurred vision if scopolamine comes in contact with the eyes (rubbing).

Antacid Interactions

Patients who are expected to use antacids concurrent with other GI medication should receive clear instructions on the antiulcer dosing regimen to avoid drug incompatibility. Where medications may be prescribed by other physicians (for example, gynecologist, ophthalmologist), patients should be reminded not to take antacids until they have checked with the prescribing physicians for potential interaction or incompatibility.

H_2-antagonists, especially cimetidine and ranitidine, should not be taken with antacids. Dosing should be staggered by at least 1 hour.

Sucralfate should be taken on an empty stomach 1 hour before meals. Antacids should be used 2 hours before or 2 hours after sucralfate.

Magnesium-containing antacids may act as a laxative when taken in large doses resulting in diarrhea. Aluminum- and calcium-containing antacids may cause constipation.

H. pylori Therapy

All of the combination regimens for *H. pylori* require the patient to drink large amounts of fluid during the treatment. This not only keeps the drugs adequately circulating through the system, it minimizes the potential for irritation of the lower esophagus, especially from the tetracycline component.

When tetracyclines are part of the combination therapy for eradication of *H. pylori* in women, the patient must be asked whether she uses oral contraceptives. Tetracyclines used concomitantly with oral contraceptives reduce the effectiveness of the contraceptive. Patients should be advised to use another form of contraception during the antibiotic therapy.

If metronidazole is part of the antibiotic regimen (*Helidac*), the patient must be instructed to avoid alcohol during therapy. This includes OTC alcohol-containing products. Metronidazole will produce an Antabuse-type reaction—that is, nausea and vomiting—by interfering with alcohol metabolism.

Bismuth salts produce a unique cosmetic effect. It will darken the tongue during treatment. The effect is temporary and does not harm the patient.

Antacids *can be used* while taking lansoprazole.

Common Adverse Effects

Antiemetic drugs may produce drowsiness and sedation, and impair judgment.

Patients should receive instruction to use caution when driving, operating equipment, or performing tasks which require coordination and dexterity.

Patients should be instructed to avoid alcohol or CNS depressants since the antiemetic may enhance sedation, mental confusion, and depression.

Use in Pregnancy

All of the drugs used in the treatment of ulcers or GERD are designated Food and Drug Administration (FDA) Pregnancy Category B or C except for **misoprostol,** which is designated **Category X.** In general there are no specific studies that have established the safety of these drugs for use during pregnancy. The longstanding availability and use of antacids suggest that there are no deleterious effects to the fetus with short-term therapy. A recent study that followed pregnant patients during cisapride therapy concluded that short-term exposure had no damaging effects of the fetus. The recommendation during pregnancy is that these drugs be used only when clearly needed.

Misoprostol is designated pregnancy Category X because it causes miscarriage and potentially dangerous bleeding. This drug should never be taken during pregnancy. Female patients should be advised to avoid becoming pregnant while receiving misoprostol. If the patient becomes pregnant, the physician should be notified immediately.

Except for phosphorated carbohydrate solution, antiemetic drugs are not recommended for use in pregnancy. Safety for use in pregnancy has not be established in humans.

Patients who become pregnant while receiving combnation *H. pylori* therapy should notify the physician immediately.

Chapter Review

Understanding Terminology

Match the definition or description in the left column with the appropriate term in the right column.

___ **1.** A substance that inhibits secretion of digestive enzymes, hormones, or acid.

___ **2.** A substance that causes abortion.

___ **3.** An open sore in the mucous membranes or mucosal linings.

___ **4.** Occurring in the general circulation, resulting in distribution to most organs.

___ **5.** A drug that neutralizes gastric acid.

___ **6.** A cell that produces hydrochloric acid in the gastric mucosa.

___ **7.** An opening in a hollow organ, such as a break in the intestinal wall.

___ **8.** An abnormally high amount of acid secretion.

___ **9.** An action that causes the decomposition of proteins.

___ **10.** An excess of HCl in the stomach.

___ **11.** Hydrochloric acid.

a. abortifacient

b. antacid

c. antisecretory

d. HCl

e. hyperacidity

f. hyperchorydia

g. parietal

h. perforation

i. proteolytic

j. systemic

k. ulcer

Acquiring Knowledge

Answer the following questions in the spaces provided.

1. What factors contribute to ulcer production? _____

_____

_____

2. What usually stimulates gastric secretion of digestive enzymes and acid? _____

_____

_____

3. How does the mechanism of action of an antisecretory drug differ from that of an antacid? _____

_____

_____

4. How do the H_2-receptor antagonists differ from other antiulcer drugs? _____

_____

_____

5. How do the H_2-receptor antagonists differ from each other? _____

_____

_____

6. What would predictably occur from the administration of prostaglandins to a pregnant woman?

_____

_____

7. How does the mechanism of action of proton pump inhibitors differ from that of antacids and sucralfate? _____

_____

_____

8. How do anticholinergic and antispasmodic drugs affect gastric secretions? _____

_____

_____

9. Are all antispasmodic drugs also anticholinergic? _____

_____

_____

10. How do systemic antacids differ from nonsystemic antacids? _____

_____

_____

11. Can antacids be used in conjunction with antisecretory drugs in the treatment of ulcers? _____

_____

_____

Applying Knowledge—On the Job

Use your critical thinking skills to answer the following questions in the spaces provided.

1. Assume that you work for an internist who treats numerous ulcer patients, many of whom are prescribed *Tagamet* or *Zantac*. For the following patients, decide whether *Tagamet* or *Zantac* is right for them.

   a. Patient A is taking *Toprol* for hypertension. _____

   _____

   _____

   b. Patient B is taking *Coumadin* for thrombosis. _____

   _____

   _____

   c. Patient C is taking *Valium* for anxiety. _____

   _____

   _____

   d. Patient D is taking *Donnatal* for epilepsy. _____

   _____

   _____

2. Jeri works in a hospital pharmacy, where she's responsible for checking patient charts to spot potential drug interaction problems. Yesterday, she checked the following four adult ulcer patients for whom antacids were recommended. In each case, the patient was taking another drug that could affect the bioavailability of the antacid. For each patient, decide whether the antacid dose should be increased or decreased because of the drug interaction.

   a. Patient A is taking quinidine for heart arrhythmias. _____

   _____

   _____

   b. Patient B is taking penicillin for gingivitis. _____

   _____

   _____

   c. Patient C is taking *Trinalin* for allergic rhinitis. _____

   _____

   _____

d. Patient D is taking *INH* for tuberculosis. _____

_____

_____

3. A 25-year-old female patient has been taking NSAIDs on a regular basis for a chronic inflammatory disease of the joints. Her physician has decided to initiate *Cytotec* therapy. What should this patient be advised regarding pregnancy? Why?

_____

_____

4. A woman calls inquiring about syrup of ipecac. She was told by a friend that every house that has children in it should have syrup of ipecac. What should she be told regarding the administration?

_____

_____

Internet Connection

There is a wonderful library of information available through the National Institutes of Health at www.niddk.nih.gov. The National Institute of Diabetes and Digestive and Kidney Diseases provides free literature, online articles, and general information for the consumer, patient, or student. At the home page, double-click on any of the topics or enter a specific term in the search box. Publications are available on gastritis, GERD, *H. pylori,* peptic ulcer, including a Digestive Disease Dictionary to assist the student in understanding medical terminology. NIDDK distributes publications through the National Digestive Disease Information Clearing House. All information is available in English and Spanish.

Another site maintained by the National Institutes of Health and the National Library of Medicine is *MEDLINEplus health information.* At www.nlm.nih.gov/medlineplus, select the *Health Topics* tab or *Drug Information* tab to obtain articles on specific topics, such as Nutrition Tips for Managing Nausea and Vomiting.

A path to information on ulcers and vomiting is through the Altavista search engine. Enter www.altavista.com to access the home page. At the top of the screen, type the item of interest into the search inquiry box. Try *H. pylori Ulcer Treatment.* You will be provided with more than 13,000 documents that discuss *Ulcers and Treatment.* Scroll down the first 20 titles. Notice the references *Peptic Ulcer Treatment* and *H. pylori—Introduction,* and *Acid Suppression* or *H. pylori Eradication—The Choice.* You can click on the title to read the information. To return to the list of titles at any time during your reading, click the right mouse button and select *Back.*

Using www.altavista.com, enter *Vomiting Treatment* into the search box and hit *Search.* 351,000 documents are waiting for you. Just scroll through 10 to 20 to see the range of information from vomiting control in cancer chemotherapy to gastroentritis. At the bottom of each page is a line of blue buttons numbered 1 through 20. Each button brings the next 20 documents on screen. When you are finished, click the right mouse button to select *Back* or select return to home page at the bottom of the current web page on screen.

Additional Reading

1996. Famotidine-induced deliurium in the elderly. *Nurses Drug Alert* 20 (11):81.

Blair, D. 1997. Patient characteristics and life style recommendations in the treatment of gastrointestinal reflux disease. *Journal of Family Practice* 44 (3):266.

Keller, V. E. 1995. Management of nausea and vomiting in children. *Journal of Pediatric Nursing* 10 (5):280.

Podolski, J. L. 1996. Recent advances in peptic ulcer disease. *Helicobacter pylori* infection and its treatment. *Gastroenterology Nursing* 19 (4):128.

Taha, A. S. 1996. Famotidine for the prevention of gastric and duodenal ulcers caused by NSAIDs. *New England Journal of Medicine* 334 (22):1435.

The student is referred to www.findarticles.com to obtain online current articles without the difficulty of finding medical journals. This website provides two types of information: sponsored listings, provided by companies, and published articles, authored by physicians, nurses, and scientists. The articles are usually one to two pages in length and are fully available for on-screen review.

AGENTS THAT AFFECT INTESTINAL MOTILITY

chapter

34

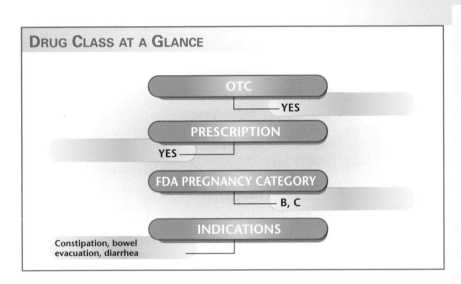

DRUG CLASS AT A GLANCE

OTC
— YES

PRESCRIPTION
YES —

FDA PREGNANCY CATEGORY
— B, C

INDICATIONS
Constipation, bowel
evacuation, diarrhea

Key Terms

adsorbent: substance that has the ability to attach other substances to its surface.

cathartic: pharmacological substance that stimulates defecation.

defecation: process of discharging the contents of the intestines, usually feces.

electrolyte: ion in solution (sodium, potassium, chloride) that permits conduction of impulses to occur.

emollient: substance that is soothing to mucous membranes or skin.

evacuation: process of removal of waste material from the bowel.

hernia: protrusion of an organ through the tissue usually containing it; for example, intestinal tissue pushing outside the abdominal cavity, or stomach pushing into the diaphragm (hiatal hernia).

hypokalemia: decrease in the normal concentration of potassium in the blood.

hyponatremia: decrease in the normal concentration of sodium in the blood.

CHAPTER FOCUS

This chapter describes drugs that have a specific action on the intestines.

CHAPTER OBJECTIVES

After studying this chapter, you should be able to

- explain three actions of laxatives to promote bowel movement.
- describe two actions of narcotics on intestinal function.
- describe the action of adsorbents as it differs from that of narcotics.
- differentiate between a simple laxative effect and bowel evacuation.
- describe the adverse effects of laxatives or antidiarrheals that are a natural extension of their therapeutic action.

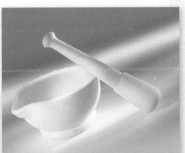

osmosis: process in which water moves across membranes following the movement of sodium ions.

peristalsis: movement characteristic of the intestines, in which circular contraction and relaxation propel the contents toward the rectum.

INTRODUCTION

The intestines are concerned primarily with the absorption of dietary nutrients and water. Rhythmic contractions known as **peristalsis** move the intestinal contents through the bowel. In the colon or large bowel, water is absorbed from digested material passing through. Eventually, the digested material that cannot be absorbed further is compacted into a fecal mass. Intestinal contraction pushes the fecal mass into the rectum, causing distention of the tissue. Rectal distention initiates a massive reflex contraction of the large bowel (colon and rectum) that expels the feces through the anus. This process is called **defecation.**

BOWEL FUNCTION

To some extent, defecation is under voluntary control. In order to initiate defecation, individuals can voluntarily increase abdominal pressure (straining) to force contraction and **evacuation** (removal of waste matter) of the bowel; however, the bowels are very sensitive to emotional stress or changes in the nervous system. Defecation can be enhanced or inhibited by stimulating the divisions of the autonomic nervous system. Stimulation of the parasympathetic fibers (cholinergic) that innervate the intestines increases intestinal motility, whereas stimulation of the sympathetic fibers (adrenergic) decreases motility.

Occasionally, intestinal motility is drastically altered, so that normal bowel function is impaired. Increased bowel motility may cause the fecal mass to move rapidly through the intestines and into the rectum. This increased activity does not permit adequate time for colonic water absorption to occur. As a result, frequent defecation of a watery stool (diarrhea) occurs. In contrast, decreased intestinal motility permits the fecal mass to remain in the colon so that excess water is absorbed. Often, the stool is firmer and more difficult to expel, and defecation is less frequent. This abnormality in bowel function is characteristic of constipation.

ANTIDIARRHEALS

Diarrhea is a symptom of increased intestinal activity. Acute diarrhea is associated with the production of loose stools in otherwise healthy individuals. Chronic diarrhea, on the other hand, is usually accompanied by weight loss, muscle weakness, and **electrolyte** imbalance. As diarrhea continues over a long time, large quantities of water, sodium, potassium, and chloride are lost or excreted in the fluid stool. This loss results in dehydration and electrolyte imbalance. Although chronic diarrhea occurs more readily in children, any individuals in poor health or with poor nutrition, especially the elderly, may develop serious effects from chronic diarrhea.

Causes of Diarrhea

Increased intestinal motility may be produced by several mechanisms (see Table 34:1). Accurate diagnosis of the underlying cause of diarrhea determines the proper drug therapy to ease the symptoms of diarrhea. For example, microorganisms (bacteria, viruses, or amoebae) may invade the gastrointestinal (GI) tissue, causing local inflammation and irritation. The bowel reacts by increasing its motility in order to evacuate the noxious organisms. Diarrhea arising from infection may be cured by administering the proper

TABLE 34:1 Factors That Promote Increased Intestinal Activity Resulting in Diarrhea

CONTRIBUTING FACTORS	TREATMENT OF CHOICE
Agents that Increase Intestinal Motility:	
a. Acute GI infections	Antibiotics
Salmonella *Shigella* *Escherichia coli* Viruses — Found in contaminated food	
Entamoeba histolitica *Giardia lamblia* — "Traveler's diarrhea" found in contaminated water	
b. Drugs	Reduce or discontinue drug use
Antacids Antibiotics Autonomic drugs Colchicine Iron Laxatives	
c. Bile salts malabsorption	Cholestyramine resin (*Cuemid*)
Increased Intestinal Motility Arising from Other Medical Problems:	
a. Chronic gastroenteritis resulting from	
Anemia Carcinoma Diabetes Neuropathies	Antidiarrheal drugs
b. Colitis, irritable colon resulting from	
Emotional stress Colon disorders	

antibiotic. Fluid and electrolyte supplements may be given (PO or IV) to correct any imbalances that develop during chronic infection.

Certain drug therapy may also produce diarrhea as a side effect. Drugs that stimulate the parasympathetic nervous system, inhibit the sympathetic nervous system, irritate the bowel directly, or disrupt the normal intestinal bacteria (broad-spectrum antibiotics) will produce diarrhea. Treatment of diarrhea in these cases is accomplished by reducing the dose of the specific drug or stopping the drug completely.

Treatment of Simple Diarrhea

Simple functional diarrhea is most frequently associated with poor dietary habits and emotional stress. The underlying cause of the increased intestinal motility may be difficult or impossible to determine. Therefore, treatment of mild diarrhea is usually symptomatic rather than curative. Drugs useful in the treatment of nonspecific diarrhea include adsorbents, anticholinergics, opiates, and a narcotic derivative (see Table 34:2). These antidiarrheal drugs either decrease intestinal motility (anticholinergics and opiates) or remove the intestinal irritant **(adsorbents.)** Adsorbents such as kaolin, pectin, and bismuth salts act in the intestine. In the intestine, adsorbents form a complex with irritating substances such as bacteria, digestive enzymes, or toxins, and carry them into the feces. Because of their mechanism of action, adsorbents also complex with vitamins, minerals, and other drugs, thereby impairing systemic absorption of these substances. Hence, adsorbents are not usually administered with meals or other medications.

Drugs Useful in the Clinical Management of Diarrhea

ACTIVE COMPONENTS (TRADE NAMES)	SCHEDULE	ADULT DOSE
Adsorbents:		
Bismuth subsalicylate (*Pepto-Bismol, Bismatrol, Pepto-Bismol Maximum Strength*)	OTC	2 tablets or 30 ml every 30 min to 1 hr up to 8 doses in 24 hr
Attapulgite (*Rheaban Maximum, Kaopectate Maximum Strength*)	OTC	2 tablets after each bowel movement up to 6 doses/day or 20 ml up to 3 doses/day
Anticholinergics:		
Belladonna alkaloids (various combination products)	OTC and prescription	Antidiarrheal products containing anticholinergics in doses greater than 0.125 mg require a prescription
Narcotic Derivatives:		
Difenoxin and atropine (*Motofen*)	IV	2 tablets, then 1 every 3 to 4 hr not to exceed 8 tablets in 24 hr
Diphenoxylate and atropine (*Logen, Lomotil, Lonox*)	V	5 mg up to QID
Loperamide (*Imodium*)	OTC and prescription	4 mg up to 8 mg/day
Opiates:		
Opium (*Opium Tincture*)	II	5 to 16 drops of liquid mixed in water up to four times a day
Paregoric (*Paregoric*)	III	5–10 ml of a solution containing 0.4 mg/ml one to four times a day

Opiates and anticholinergics decrease intestinal motility by two different mechanisms. Anticholinergic drugs inhibit the parasympathetic nerves that control digestive function. Opiates (tincture of opium, and paregoric) induce spasms (spasmogenic) that decrease the effective movement of the small and large intestines. The antidiarrheal opiates are natural products that contain a small amount of morphine as the active ingredient.

Paregoric is chemicaly called camphorated tincture of opium. **It is not the same as opium tincture,** also known as laudanum. **Paregoric and opium tincture are both indicated for the treatment of diarrhea; however, these drugs cannot be substituted for each other.** Opium tincture (10 mg morphine/ml) contains 25 times more morphine than paregoric (0.4 mg morphine/ml). The addiction liablility of paregoric is low because the concentration of morphine is very low and oral doses are small.

Health care professionals are bringing attention to the danger associated with the mistaken use of opium tincture instead of paregoric. Life-threatening conditions (respiratory depression) and death have occurred when opium tincture was taken instead of paregoric. The Food and Drug Administration has a relatively new division called the National Coordinating Council for Medication Error Reporting and Prevention that maintains a safety page on the Internet to alert health care professionals to drugs that have jeopardized the lives of adults and children from confusion in medication names. The FDA website (www.fda.gov/cder/drug/mederrors) presents a special safety paper that discusses clinical impact of the drug errors associated with opium tincture and paregoric. The antidiarrheal dose for paregoric in chidren is 0.25 to 0.5 ml per kilogram of body weight of a solution containing 0.4 mg/ml. This dose of paregoric delivers 0.2 mg of morphine to the child (0.5 ml times 0.4 mg morphine/ml in paregoric equals 0.20 mg morphine). Consider the serious problem that could occur if a child accidentally receives 0.5 ml of opium tincture instead (0.5 ml times 10 mg morphine/ml equals 5 mg morphine!) While young children are especially vulnerable to overdose due to medication errors, adult patients can also develop serious consequences. Alcohol, antihistamines, and CNS depressants may enhance sedation, drowsiness and respiratory depression when taken with the opiates. In the event of larger doses, the opium tincture may produce confusion, convulsions, fatigue, hypotension, bradycardia, and irregular breathing.

Diphenoxylate and loperamide are narcotic derivatives with spasmogenic and anticholinergic properties. Because diphenoxylate is absorbed at therapeutic doses, it can produce weak narcotic effects, including euphoria. Narcotic activity is usually seen with higher doses up to 40 to 60 mg. As an antidiarrheal, diphenoxylate is administered in combination with atropine (*Lomotil*). The atropine reduces the possibility of drug abuse and addiction to diphenoxylate. Severe diarrhea is often treated with a diphenoxylate-atropine combination or paregoric. Both of these products can be obtained only by prescription. Difenoxin is the active metabolite of diphenoxylate, which is available as a combination preparation with atropine (*Motofen*).

NOTE TO THE HEALTH CARE PROFESSIONAL

Antidiarrheals should not be used for more than a few days. These drugs should be kept out of the reach of children. Infants and children under the age of 5 are very sensitive to the action of these drugs, particularly the anticholinergic effects. Chronic misuse of these drugs can produce serious alterations in bowel function.

Diphenoxylate-atropine is a Schedule V drug. Difenoxin-atropine is Schedule IV because it is more potent than its parent. The recommended dose of loperamide is 4 mg, not to exceed 16 mg per day. Loperamide has been used in combination with trimethoprim and sulfamethoxazole to facilitate rapid relief of traveler's diarrhea.

Cautions and Contraindications

Most of the antidiarrheals are relatively nontoxic to organs other than the intestines because they are not absorbed into the general circulation. The most frequent side effect produced by antidiarrheal drugs is constipation. Since diphenoxylate is absorbed to some degree, it may produce rashes, dizziness, blurred vision, and nausea. The diphenoxylate that is absorbed is extensively metabolized by the liver to an active substance, diphenoxylic acid (difenoxine).

Ultimately, the metabolite is excreted into the urine. This drug should not be administered to patients with liver disease or severe colitis. Drugs that inhibit intestinal motility may induce toxic megacolon. Toxic doses of diphenoxylate could produce respiratory depression and coma similar to narcotic overdose.

Over-the-counter (OTC) preparations containing anticholinergics should not be used by patients who have glaucoma. Anticholinergic drugs may increase intraocular pressure by reducing anterior chamber drainage in patients with glaucoma. Otherwise, the amount of anticholinergic drug is small enough to avoid the likelihood of the adverse effects usually associated with these drugs in adults.

LAXATIVES AND CATHARTICS

Laxatives and **cathartics** are pharmacological agents that stimulate defecation. Although these terms are often used interchangeably, laxatives produce a mild, gentle stimulus for defecation, whereas cathartics produce a more intense action on the bowel. All laxatives and cathartics act directly on the intestine to alter stool formation. There are only a few valid indications for the use of laxatives. Primarily, these drugs are used to relieve constipation and to evacuate the intestine prior to surgery or diagnostic examination.

The accepted clinical use of laxatives and cathartics are:

- relief of constipation from nonorganic abnormalities, including poor hygiene, voluntary retention of feces, inadequate bulk food in the diet, and emotional disturbances,

- evacuation of the bowel contents for adjunct medication in the treatment of intestinal parasites (anthelmintics) and food or drug poisoning; and cleansing the bowel prior to radioisotopic examination, diagnostic examination, or surgery,

- to prevent straining at stool to avoid rupture of existing **hernia,** avoid rupture following a hemorrhoidectomy, and

- to prevent straining in patients with myocardial infarction.

Constipation, a symptom characterized by infrequent or difficult evacuation of the bowel, may be produced in several ways. Poorly developed toilet habits, such as ignoring the intestinal stimulus to defecate (rectal distention) or voluntary retention of feces, may result in constipation. Diets low in fiber also contribute to the development of constipation. Foods that have a low fiber content do not retain water in the intestine. When these foods are digested, they cannot produce adequate colonic distention to initiate a defecation reflex at regular intervals. Anxiety, fear, and other emotional disturbances also induce constipation by altering the parasympathetic control of the intestines. Stressful situations usually result in sympathetic stimulation that decreases intestinal motility. All of these factors may lead to the production of hard, dry stools that are difficult to pass.

Laxatives are employed to facilitate defecation without straining, stress, or pain. Their use is especially important in patients who have hemorrhoids or hernias or who have had a myocardial infarction. Resistance to defecation is usually overcome by voluntarily increasing abdominal pressure (straining). Such increases in pressure can affect the workload on the heart or rupture an existing hernia or hemorrhoids.

Mechanism of Action

Laxatives can be classified according to their mechanism of action, which includes stimulants, swelling agents, osmotic (saline) laxatives, and emollients (see Table 34:3). Stimulant laxatives directly irritate the mucosal lining of the intestine. In addition to the irritation, histamine is released, enhancing intestinal motility.

Swelling agents are natural fibers or grains that remain in the intestine, soak up water, and expand (swell). The water, which is retained, softens the stool, whereas the swelling action distends the rectum and initiates defecation. Osmotic, or saline, laxatives are a mixture of sodium and magnesium salts. These ions attract water **(osmosis),** which causes a more liquid stool to be formed. Lactulose is a combination of sugars (galactose, fructose) that promotes the same action because of the amount of sodium associated with the nonabsorbable sugar molecules. Polyethylene glycol-electrolyte solution (PEG-ES) is a nonabsorbable solution containing sodium sulfate that acts in a similar manner to promote complete, thorough bowel evacuation.

Emollients are laxatives that act on the stool to permit water to penetrate the fecal mass. The oily nature of these laxatives eases the passage of the stool through the rectum.

Route of Administration

Most laxatives are administered orally. The onset of action by this route varies from 6 to 36 hours,

> ### NOTE TO THE HEALTH CARE PROFESSIONAL
>
> Phenothalein has recently been removed from products because of safety considerations. Products will reissue with new laxative formulations. *Ex-Lax* now contains senna rather than phenothalein.
> Stimulant cathartics may produce dehydration and electrolyte changes (**hypokalemia**—a decrease in potassium—or **hyponatremia**—a decrease in sodium) if used too frequently. The senna preparations produce such an intense response that abdominal cramping (griping) or nausea may accompany their action.

except for the osmotic agents, which begin to work within 0.5 to 2 hours. Certain laxatives may be administered rectally as suppositories or as enemas (see Table 34:3). Administration of drug as an enema (traditionally, warm fluid injected rectally) usually has an onset of action from within 5 to 60 minutes. Hence, enemas are preferred to cleanse the bowel prior to surgery or diagnostic examination. Certain preparations are considered bowel evacuants because of their ability to empty the bowel quickly and thoroughly prior to procedures such as GI examination. Bowel evacuation is particularly successful if patients have fasted for 3 to 4 hours prior to receiving the laxative. Often, patients are given bowel preparations the evening before the GI examination and instructed to abstain from foods, except for clear liquids, until after the procedure has been completed.

Adverse Effects

Certain laxatives are absorbed when administered orally and therefore produce systemic effects. Such agents include the osmotic laxatives and phenolphthalein. The sodium and magnesium ions that are absorbed from osmotic laxatives are excreted through the kidneys. However, the increased sodium load may be harmful to patients who have impaired renal function, edema, or congestive heart failure. Also, in sensitive or debilitated patients, excess magnesium ions can depress central nervous system (CNS) and muscle function. The osmotic laxatives are not harmless drugs. These agents cause large amounts of water to be lost with the feces. Hence, it is possible to dehydrate patients from overuse of these drugs.

Over-the-Counter Laxatives*

CLASS	ACTIVE COMPOUND(S)	TRADE NAME	ADULT DOSE	ROUTE OF ADMINISTRATION
Bowel evacuants	Polyethylene glycol-electrolyte solution (PEG-ES)	GoLYTELY, CoLyte, OCL	4 liters prior to GI exam as 240 ml every 10 min	Oral solution
	Senna extract	X-Prep, X-Prep Bowel, Fleet Prep Kits (1–6)	As instructed	Oral, tablets, liquids, rectal suppositories
Emollients	Mineral oil	Agoral Plain, Neo-cultol, Kondremul	5–45 ml	Oral, liquid
Osmotic (saline) laxatives	Magnesium hydroxide	Phillips' Milk of Magnesia	30–60 ml	Oral, suspension
	Magnesium citrate	Citrate of Magnesia	1 glass	Oral, liquid
	Sodium biphosphate and sodium phosphate	Fleet Enema	118 ml	Rectal, liquid
	Lactulose (galactose, fructose)	Cephulac, Duphalac, Cholac	15–60 ml	Oral, syrup
	Polyethylene glycol-electrolyte solution (PEG-ES)	GoLYTELY, OCL	(see bowel evacuants)	
Stimulants	Bisacodyl	Dulcolax	5–15 mg 1× daily (10 mg) suppository 1× daily	Oral, tablets Rectal suppositories
	Castor oil	Purge, Fleet Flavored Castor Oil	45–60 ml	Oral, liquid
	Senna preparations	Fletcher's Castoria	10–15 ml	Oral, liquid
		Black Draught Lax Senna, Senokot	2 tablets	Oral, tablets
Stool softeners	Docusate sodium	Colace, Regutol	50–500 mg increase daily fluid intake	Oral, 1–4 tablets or capsules
	Docusate calcium	Surfak Liqui-Gels, Sulfalax Calcium	240 mg daily	Oral, capsules
Swelling agents	Bran, polycarbophil	FiberCon, Fiberall, Mitrolan	2 tablets (1 g) up to QID	Oral, tablets
	Prunes	—	6–12 prunes	—
	Psyllium hydrophilic	Effersyllium, Metamucil, Perdiem, Reguloid Natural, Serutan	1 tsp up to QID in 8 oz liquid	Oral, suspension
Mixtures	Mineral oil and magnesium hydroxide	Haley's MO	5–45 ml at bedtime with 8 oz water	Oral, liquid
	Carboxymethyl-cellulose and docusate sodium	Disoplex, Disolan, Forte	1–2 tablets/capsules at bedtime	Oral, tablets, capsules
	Senna concentrate and docusate sodium	Gentlax S, Senokot-S	1–2 tablets at bedtime	Oral, tablets
CO_2-releasing suppositories	Sodium bicarbonate and potassium bitartrate	CEO—two	1 at bedtime	Suppository

*Not an inclusive list of available preparations.

Cautions and Contraindications

Laxatives should be taken with clear liquids; usually a minimum 8 ounces of water is recommended. Chronic use (misuse) of laxatives may result in cathartic colon or laxative dependency. Cathartic colon is a situation in which the intestines do not respond to physiological stimulation (loss of bowel tone), necessitating daily use of cathartics to produce defecation. Although they relieve constipation, laxatives should never be used to treat constipation that occurs because of bowel obstruction (tumor).

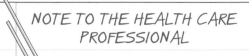

NOTE TO THE HEALTH CARE PROFESSIONAL

Laxatives and cathartics should never be used for long periods of time. Furthermore, these drugs are absolutely contraindicated in individuals with nausea, vomiting, appendicitis, or any undiagnosed abdominal pain.

Patient Administration and Monitoring

Drugs affecting the GI tract are widely available without prescription and are a cultural mainstay of self-medication among older people. It often takes a few days for the full therapeutic effect to become evident, meanwhile the patient has probably re-dosed more frequently and not taken sufficient fluid to allow the GI tract to cooperate with the medication. Proper diet incorporating fiber, fruit, and vegetables; adequate daily fluid intake, up to 10 (8 oz.) glasses; and exercise are essential for maintaining normal bowel function.

Patient Instructions

Patients should be reminded to take medication with a full glass of water or fruit juice. Juice will mask the taste of those products that taste bitter.

Discoloration of the urine is expected with the use of cascara and senna (red-brown, yellow-brown) laxatives.

Keep antidiarrheals out of the reach of children, since accidental ingestion may cause respiratory depression.

In adults, therapeutic doses may cause dizziness or drowsiness that can impair coordination and mental alertness required for operating cars or machinery.

Drug Administration

Bismuth should be avoided before GI radiologic procedures because it is radiopaque and may interfere with X-ray.

While OTC laxatives may take more than 1 day to exert an adequate effect, products recommended for bowel evacuation prior to diagnostic procedures or examination will exert their effect promptly, usually within 1 hour. Patients should be advised to take the medication so that planned activities and sleep are not interrupted.

Product Interactions

Bisacodyl-containing products should not be taken within 1 hour of antacids or milk because the enteric coating may dissolve, resulting in gastric irritation.

Docusate sodium should not be taken when mineral oil is being used because of the potential to increase the absorption of mineral oil. Mineral oil should be taken on an empty stomach.

Refrigerate magnesium citrate to retain potency and palatibility.

Notify the Physician

These drugs should not be used in the presence of nausea, vomiting, or abdominal pain. Notify the physician if rectal bleeding, muscle cramps, weakness, or dizziness occurs.

Laxatives should not be continued for more than 1 week unless under the supervision of a physician. Unrelieved constipation should be reported to the doctor for further evaluation.

Antidiarrheals should not be continued for more than 2 days if diarrhea persists; physician should be notified for evaluation.

Use in Pregnancy

The drugs in this class are designated Food and Drug Administration (FDA) Pregnancy Category B or C or NR, not rated. Castor oil should not be taken during pregnancy because of the potential for the irritant action to induce labor. Other products should only be taken during pregnancy when there is a clear indication for use and after discussion with the physician.

Chapter Review

Understanding Terminology

Answer the following questions in the spaces provided.

1. Differentiate between laxatives and cathartics. _____
   _____
   _____

2. Define *peristalsis*. _____
   _____
   _____

3. What is a hernia? _____
   _____
   _____

4. Define *adsorbents*. _____
   _____
   _____

Acquiring Knowledge

Answer the following questions in the spaces provided.

1. How do voluntary control and the autonomic nervous system affect the process of defecation?
   _____
   _____

2. What is diarrhea? What are the consequences of chronic and acute diarrhea? _____
   _____
   _____

3. How can diarrhea be produced? _____
   _____
   _____

4. What agents are used for the treatment of simple diarrhea? _____
   _____
   _____

5. How do the adsorbent antidiarrheals differ from the opiates? _____
   _____
   _____

6. What is the mechanism of action of diphenoxylate? _____
   _____
   _____

7. When are laxatives used? _____
   _____
   _____

8. What are the various types of laxatives? How do they differ? _____
   _____
   _____

9. Why are the osmotic laxatives potentially dangerous? _____
_____
_____

Applying Knowledge—On the Job

Use your critical thinking skills to answer the following questions in the spaces provided.

1. Assume that your job is physician's assistant in a county health department in a rural area. What would you recommend for each of the following patients presenting with diarrhea at the clinic where you work?

    a. Patient A thinks she ate "something spoiled." _____

    b. Patient B went deer hunting and drank water from a stream in the woods. _____

    c. Patient C is taking an antibiotic for a urinary tract infection. _____

    d. Patient D has irritable bowel syndrome. _____

2. Assume you work an eating disorders hotline. Convince the following two callers of the seriousness of their laxative abuse.

    a. Caller A is anorexic and extremely underweight. She eats very little, exercises a great deal, and takes laxatives nearly daily. She takes the laxatives because, without them, she only has a bowel movement every 2 or 3 days, and that makes her feel fat. _____
_____
_____

    b. Caller B is bulimic and of average weight. Almost every day, she binges on huge quantities of food and then purges by vomiting and taking laxatives. She takes the laxatives because she can't always induce the gag reflex after forcing herself to vomit so many times—and she can't stand the thought of all that food being turned into body fat. _____
_____
_____

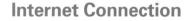

Internet Connection

There are a number of websites that support information on gastrointestinal disorders, such as www.about.com. At the home page enter *Constipation Treatment* in the search box. The site will present topics from causes of constipation in infant and elderly patients to direct web links to articles on treatment options. Or enter *Diarrhea Treatment* to access information like, "The average adult gets diarrhea four times a year. Here are some things to remember when it happens to you."

The American Gastroenterological Association provides its guideline on evaluation and treatment of constipation at www.guideline.gov/FRAMESETS/guideline.

Stimulant **laxatives** used to treat constipation or before rectal or bowel examinations or surgery are discussed at www.nlm.nih.gov/medlineplus/druginfo/medmaster/a601112.html.

Additional Reading

Arce, D. A. 2002. Evaluation of constipation. *American Family Physician* 65:2283.

Sauderlein, G. 1995. Mechanical bowel preparation in review. MEDSURG *Nursing* 4 (4):267.

Stewart, E. A. 1997. A strategy to reduce laxative use among older people. *Nursing Times* 93 (4):35.

White, T. 1995. Dealing with constipation in terminal illness. *Nursing Times* 91 (14):57.

Williams, C. M. 2002. Using medications appropriately in older adults. *American Family Physician* 66:1917.

Yuan, C. S. 2000. Treatment of constipation in chronic methadone users. *Journal of the American Medical Association* 283:367.

PHARMACOLOGY OF THE ENDOCRINE SYSTEM

Chapter 35

Introduction to the Endocrine System

Endocrine System
Uses of Hormones

Chapter 36

Adrenal Steroids

Glucocorticoids
Mineralocorticoids
Special Considerations
Drug Interactions

Chapter 37

Gonadal Hormones and the Oral Contraceptives

Female Sex Hormones
Male Sex Hormones (Androgens)
Impotence

Chapter 38

Drugs Affecting the Thyroid and Parathyroid Glands and Bone Degeneration

Thyroid Function, Pharmacology, and Disorders
Parathyroid Hormones

Chapter 39

Pancreatic Hormones and Antidiabetic Drugs

Pancreatic Endocrine Function
Diabetes Mellitus
Treatment of Diabetes

Chapter 40

Posterior Pituitary Hormones and Drugs Affecting Uterine Muscle

Diabetes Insipidus
Drugs Affecting Uterine Muscle
Tocolytics

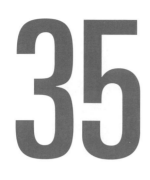

35

INTRODUCTION TO THE ENDOCRINE SYSTEM

This chapter describes organs and glands that secrete substances directly into the bloodstream to control tissue growth or repair. Hormone replacement therapy for anterior pituitary deficiency of growth hormone is also discussed.

CHAPTER OBJECTIVES

After studying this chapter, you should be able to

- describe the basic function of a hormone.
- explain how endocrine secretion differs from the secretions of neurotransmitters within synapses.
- describe the endocrine functions of the hypothalamus.
- name three groups of hormones that control endocrine function.

Key Terms

cretinism: condition in which the development of the body and brain has been inhibited.

dwarfism: condition in which individuals are particularly short (under 48 inches tall), often associated with disproportionate long bone-to-torso dimensions, but have normal mental acuity.

endocrine: glands that secrete substances directly into the blood.

gigantism: condition in which the body or any of its parts is larger than normal.

hormone: substance produced within one organ and secreted directly into the circulation to exert its effects at a distant location.

somatotropin: type of general hormone that regulates growth and maintenance of all body tissues (GH).

target organ: specific tissue where a hormone exerts its action.

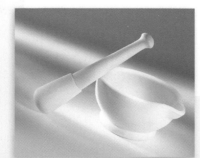

INTRODUCTION

The two main systems of the body that function to regulate the others are the nervous system and the endocrine system. The nervous system regulates activity by conducting nerve impulses to various organs. Nerve impulses travel rapidly along specific pathways to produce their effects. The response to nerve stimulation is rapid, and the duration of action is short. An example would be the contraction of skeletal muscle.

Endocrine System

The endocrine system is composed of glands located throughout the body. The **endocrine** glands are called ductless because they release chemical substances directly into the bloodstream. These chemical substances are referred to as **hormones.** Hormones stimulate various body tissues, increasing the level of activity. In contrast to stimulation of the nervous system, hormones have a slower onset and a longer duration of stimulation. Hormones travel in the blood and reach most body tissues. However, some hormones affect only certain tissues or organs. The term **target organ** is used to describe an organ that is sensitive to the effects of a particular hormone. Target organs have specific hormone receptors on their membranes. When a hormone attaches to its receptors, the effect of the hormone is produced.

Uses of Hormones

The deficiency of any hormone results in several characteristic disease states. For example, in children, the lack of growth hormone (somatotropin) results in **dwarfism,** whereas lack of thyroid hormone produces **cretinism.** There are two major therapeutic uses of hormones. In cases of hormone deficiency, the missing hormone is given as a replacement therapy to fulfill a normal physiological role. On the other hand, in certain disease states (chronic inflammation), various hormones produce beneficial effects when given in large doses. In these situations, the hormones are acting pharmacologically. The main emphasis of this chapter is the treatment of various disease states. Each endocrine gland will be discussed in the following chapters. The effects of growth hormone will be discussed in this introductory chapter.

Often referred to as the "master gland" of the endocrine system, the pituitary gland controls many of the other glands. Located in the brain and attached to the base of the hypothalamus, the pituitary gland is composed of two main lobes: the anterior lobe (adenohypophysis) and the posterior lobe (neurohypophysis). Each lobe contains a number of hormones that may be released into the general circulation.

One of the functions of the hypothalamus is to control the activity of the pituitary gland. Each lobe of the pituitary gland is controlled in a different manner. The hypothalamus and the anterior lobe of the pituitary gland are connected by small blood vessels known as the portal system. The hypothalamus produces hormones known as releasing factors, which are sent to the anterior lobe by way of the portal system. The releasing factors stimulate the release of the hormones that are produced in the anterior lobe. These hormones of the anterior lobe are known as the tropic hormones. The tropic hormones are released into the general circulation to control the activities of the other endocrine glands.

The hypothalamus also produces the hormones that are present in the posterior lobe of the pituitary gland. These hormones—oxytocin and antidiuretic hormone (ADH)—pass down nerve axons (axonal transport) to the posterior lobe, where they are stored until needed. Secretion of the posterior pituitary hormones is controlled by nerve reflexes (see Chapter 39). Figure 35:1 illustrates the relationship between the hypothalamus and the pituitary gland.

Anterior Pituitary Hormones

The main function of the anterior pituitary hormones is to regulate the activities of the other endocrine glands. With the exception of growth hormone, each of these hormones stimulates a specific endocrine gland. Table 35:1 lists the hormones of the anterior lobe of the pituitary gland and the organs that are affected.

Hormones Associated With the Pituitary Gland

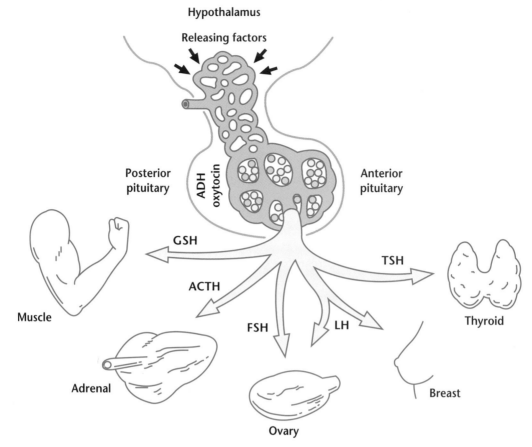

(ACTH = adrenocorticotropic hormone; ADH = antidiuretic hormone; FSH = follicle-stimulating hormone; GSH = growth-stimulating hormone; LH = luteinizing hormone; TSH = thyroid-stimulating hormone)

TABLE 35:1   Hormones of the Anterior Lobe of the Pituitary and Their Functions

ANTERIOR PITUITARY HORMONES	TARGET ORGAN	EFFECT
Growth-stimulating hormone (GSH)	All body tissues	Stimulates growth and repair
Thyroid-stimulating hormone (TSH)	Thyroid gland	Stimulates production and release of thyroxine
Adrenocorticotropic hormone (ACTH)	Adrenal cortex	Stimulates production and secretion of cortisol
Follicle-stimulating hormone (FSH)	Gonads of male and female	Stimulates development of sperm and ova
Luteinizing hormone (LH)	Gonads of male and female	Controls production of sex hormones
Prolactin	Mammary glands	Milk production

Growth hormone (**somatotropin**), or GH, is referred to as a general hormone that regulates the growth and maintenance of all body tissues. Growth hormone is associated with rises in glucose and fatty acid levels for cells' activity. Lack of growth hormone in children results in dwarfism, whereas an excess of growth hormone results in **gigantism.** The main pharmacological use of growth hormone is replacement therapy in cases of suspected dwarfism.

At first, the supply of human growth hormone was severely limited. The National Pituitary Agency controlled the procurement and dispensing of GH extracted from human cadaver tissue. Occasionally, cadaver sources were associated with the transmission of viruses to patient recipients. Fortunately, however, through DNA recombinant biotechnology, growth hormone is available as a purified polypeptide hormone now. Somatropin (*Humatrope*) is identical in amino acid sequence to the hormone produced by the human pituitary. Somatrem (*Protropin*) is another recombinant product that has one more amino acid than somatropin, but it produces the same spectrum of physiological activity.

Clinical Indication

The current indication for these products is long-term treatment of children who have growth failure because of lack of adequate endogenous growth hormone secretion. The hormone is reconstituted from a powder prior to IM or SC injection three times a week.

Adverse Effects

Adverse effects associated with the use of GH are extensions of the normal physiological action. Changes in blood sugar level (hypoglycemia or hyperglycemia) consistent with insulin fluctuations may occur. Headache, muscle weakness, and transient edema have been reported. Some patients develop antibodies to the exogenous hormone, but these antibodies do not affect the beneficial effects on growth.

Regulating Hormone Secretion

Three different groups of hormones actually control the endocrine system: the releasing factors (hypothalamus), the tropic hormones (anterior lobe), and the hormones from each of the other endocrine glands. The mechanism that controls the release of these hormones is known as negative feedback. Figure 35:2 illustrates this concept, using the thyroid gland as an example. The thyroid-

FIGURE 35:2 Negative Feedback in the Hormonal Control of the Thyroid Gland

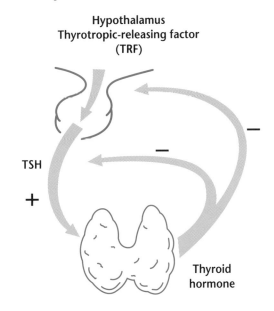

releasing factor stimulates the release of thyroid-stimulating hormone (TSH), which in turn stimulates the thyroid gland to release its hormone, thyroxine. Subsequently, the concentration of thyroxine increases in the blood. When the thyroxine concentration rises above normal, further secretion of the releasing factor and the TSH is inhibited. Consequently, normal levels of the various hormones are maintained in the blood.

Diagnostic Tests for Abnormal Anterior Pituitary Function

In order to assess the adequacy of anterior pituitary function, the serum concentration of growth hormone or TSH may be analyzed. Secretion of GH and TSH follows a diurnal pattern so that the optimal blood level of hormone is available to the tissues during the active waking state. For evaluation of pituitary and target gland function blood samples are usually taken between 6 and 8 AM. If the serum levels of the hormones are within normal levels (TSH 0–15 μIU/ml; GH 0–16 ng/ml—the maximum varies with men 3 ng/ml, women 10 ng/ml, children 16 ng/ml) the anterior pituitary and the thyroid gland are functioning normally. Serum TSH would be elevated outside the normal limits if the thyroid gland was not producing thyroxine (hormone feedback).

Since the range of normal for these hormones includes "0" or "undetectable levels," deficiency associated with anterior pituitary function must be further evaluated in conjunction with the patient's clinical profile. Further evaluation may include stimulation of the anterior pituitary to provoke secretion of growth hormone and TSH prior to obtaining an early morning blood sample. An example of a provocative test for thyroid function is the TRH Challenge Test. Thyrotropic-releasing hormone (TRH) is injected intravenously prior to drawing blood at 5, 10, 20, and 60 minutes postinjection. The TSH concentration of the blood samples is analyzed to determine whether a sudden rise in TSH occurs in response to the TRH stimulation. Observation of a spike confirms a normal functioning anterior pituitary. If the TSH level does not rise or remains undetectable, pituitary dysfunction is indicated. Note: if the patient is experiencing excess thyroid hormone secretion (thyrotoxicosis), endogenous TSH secretion should be inhibited through hormone feedback. Consequently, if TRH is injected to a patient with thyrotoxicosis, the TSH level will not rise.

Chapter Review

Understanding Terminology

Answer the following questions in the spaces provided.

1. Differentiate among dwarfism, gigantism, and cretinism. _____
   _____
   _____

2. What is a hormone? _____
   _____
   _____

3. Define *target organ*. _____
   _____
   _____

4. What is GH? _____
   _____
   _____

Acquiring Knowledge

Answer the following questions in the spaces provided.

1. What are the main uses of hormones in medical treatment? _____
   _____
   _____

2. Why is the pituitary gland referred to as the "master gland"? _____

3. What is the function of the hypothalamus in the endocrine system? _____
   _____
   _____

4. What substances are produced in the hypothalamus? _____
   _____
   _____

5. Where are the tropic hormones produced? Give two examples of a tropic hormone. _____
   _____
   _____

6. What are the functions of growth hormone? _____
   _____
   _____

7. How do the releasing factors get to the anterior pituitary gland? _____
   _____
   _____

8. What is the function of releasing factors? _____
   _____
   _____

9. Explain the concept of negative feedback in the control of hormonal secretion. _____
_____
_____

Applying Knowledge—On the Job

Use your critical thinking skills to answer the following questions in the spaces provided.

1. As a lab assistant in a hospital lab, explain to a patient why he must receive an injection before his blood is drawn to be tested for thyroid function.

_____
_____
_____
_____
_____

2. Explain why it is necessary to use a provocative challenge in order to evaluate a deficiency in pituitary function.

_____
_____
_____
_____
_____

Internet Connection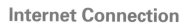

General information intended for the education of patients and their families on the endocrine system is maintained at www.endocrineweb.com. There are over 120 very detailed but easy to understand pages on endocrine disease, conditions, hormone problems, and treatment options. All pages were written by physicians who treat these diseases. The endocrine disorder home page links each endocrine gland and is a common point for all of the Endocrine Web Family of Internet Sites. It provides a quick overview of each section of this very large site.

Another excellent website is www.drkoop.com. At the home page, select Health Encyclopedia from the topics in the left column. Then select Special Topics and enter the letter E. An extensive list of clinical conditions will be provided so you can double-click on Endocrine to access excellent color illustrations and simple language explanations on the endocrine system.

Additional Readings

Cadoff, J. 1997. Your hormones. *Parents Magazine* 72 (5):39.

Kase, L. M. 1997. How hormones rule your moods. *American Health for Women* 16 (4):54.

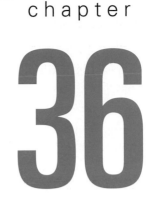

ADRENAL STEROIDS

DRUG CLASS AT A GLANCE

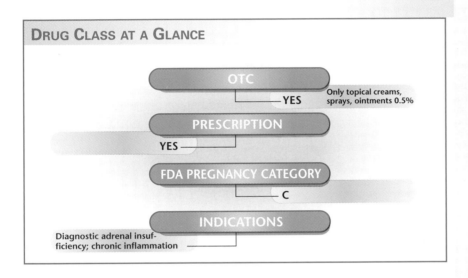

OTC
YES — Only topical creams, sprays, ointments 0.5%

PRESCRIPTION
YES

FDA PREGNANCY CATEGORY
C

INDICATIONS
Diagnostic adrenal insufficiency; chronic inflammation

Key Terms

catabolism: process in which complex compounds are broken down into simpler molecules; usually associated with energy release.

glucocorticoid: steroid produced within the adrenal cortex (or a synthetic drug) that directly influences carbohydrate metabolism and inhibits the inflammatory process.

lysosome: part of a cell that contains enzymes capable of digesting or destroying tissue/proteins.

mineralocorticoid: steroid produced within the adrenal cortex that directly influences sodium and potassium metabolism.

replacement therapy: administration of a naturally occurring substance that the body is not able to produce in adequate amounts to maintain normal function.

repository preparation: preparation of a drug, usually for intramuscular or subcutaneous injection, that is intended to leach out from the site of injection slowly so that the duration of drug action is prolonged.

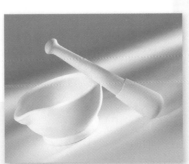

CHAPTER FOCUS

This chapter describes substances that contribute to the body's natural response to injury, particularly tissue damage. It explains how these substances produce a significant physiological effect on the kidneys to capture excreted sodium ions and on muscles to conserve glucose, which acts as fuel. Adrenal steroids are normally found in the body, but with repeated exogenous use, they are associated with a state of dependency.

CHAPTER OBJECTIVES

After studying this chapter, you should be able to

* identify the two main classes of steroids.

* describe the action of steroids on the inflammatory process.

* describe the primary action of steroids on the renal tubules.

* describe three adverse effects associated with chronic (routine) use of steroids.

steroid: member of a large family of chemical substances (hormones, drugs) containing a structure similar to cortisone (tetracyclic cyclopenta-α-phenanthrene).

tropic: having an affinity for the designated organ; for example, adrenotropic.

INTRODUCTION

The adrenal glands are located on the upper surface of each kidney. The glands consist of an inner part, known as the adrenal medulla, and an outer part, known as the adrenal cortex. The medulla, which is part of the sympathetic nervous system, secretes catecholamines during sympathetic activation. The cortex is composed of three separate tissue layers. Each layer releases one or more hormones that have important physiological functions, as shown in Table 36:1. The hormones of the adrenal cortex are divided into two main classes: the glucocorticoids and the mineralocorticoids.

The hormones of the adrenal cortex are generally referred to as corticosteroids, or just **steroids.** A deficiency in steroid production results in Addison's disease. Excess steroid production results in Cushing's disease. One of the main pharmacological uses of adrenal steroids is in the treatment of hormone deficiency conditions such as Addison's disease. This type of treatment is usually referred to as **replacement therapy.**

TABLE 36:1	Layers of the Adrenal Cortex and the Main Hormones Secreted From Each Layer	
LAYER	**HORMONES**	**MAIN FUNCTION**
Glomerulosa (outer)	Aldosterone (referred to as a mineralocorticoid)	Regulates blood levels of sodium and potassium
Fasciculata (middle)	Cortisol, cortisone (referred to as glucocorticoids)	Regulates the metabolism of carbohydrates and proteins; also has potent antiinflammatory effects
Reticularis (inner)	Minute amounts of male and female sex hormones	Normal physiological function of the sex hormones from this layer not clearly understood

GLUCOCORTICOIDS

From the standpoint of pharmacology, the most important steroids are the **glucocorticoids.** They are used frequently in the treatment of inflammatory or allergic conditions.

Regulating Cortisol Secretion

The production and secretion of cortisol are controlled by corticotropin (adrenocorticotropic hormone, ACTH) secreted by the anterior pituitary gland. The **tropic** hormones (such as corticotropin) are regulated by the releasing factors of the hypothalamus. Corticotropin subsequently stimulates the secretion of cortisol from the adrenal cortex. It is important to know which factors stimulate the hypothalamus to secrete the releasing factor for corticotropin. The main factors that influence the hypothalamus are the sleep-wake cycle (diurnal rhythm, circadian rhythm), negative feedback, and stress.

Sleep-Wake Cycle

The levels of corticotropin, and therefore of cortisol, are adjusted to each individual's sleep-wake cycle. Higher amounts of corticotropin and cortisol are secreted for availability during the waking hours, whereas lower amounts are present during sleep. The maximum secretion occurs before 8 AM while the lowest levels occur after 4 PM. During the wake period, cortisol regulates body metabolism to meet the requirements of this active period.

Negative Feedback

Releasing factor and corticotropin stimulate the release of cortisol into the bloodstream. When the level of cortisol rises above normal, further release of corticotropin and the releasing factor is inhibited. Negative feedback maintains the day-to-day levels of cortisol at relatively constant amounts.

Stress

Stress refers to a situation in which the body is subjected to increased physical or mental demands: exercise, cold weather, infections, surgery, and anxiety are all forms of stress. Stress produces an increase in corticotropin secretion, which stimulates cortisol secretion. The higher amounts of cortisol provide the body with an increased ability to cope with the demands of stress.

Effects of Glucocorticoids

The glucocorticoids regulate the metabolism of carbohydrates and proteins, particularly during stress. During periods of stress involving bodily injury (trauma or surgery), there is an increased demand for glucose. Tissues undergoing repair and wound healing use glucose almost exclusively. In addition, the brain normally uses only glucose. The main physiological effects of the glucocorticoids—producing and conserving body stores of carbohydrates (glucose)—are accomplished by two main metabolic processes: gluconeogenesis and protein **catabolism.** Both of these processes are stimulated by the glucocorticoids.

Gluconeogenesis

Gluconeogenesis is the process of making glucose. It occurs in the liver, where amino acids or glycerol are converted into glucose. The result is an increase in the production of glucose for use by injured tissue or by the brain.

Protein Catabolism

Catabolism is the breakdown of proteins into amino acids. This occurs mainly in skeletal muscle. The amino acids that are released can then be used by the liver to make glucose (gluconeogenesis).

Fluid Retention

The glucocorticoids also have some mineralocorticoid activity—that is, the ability to cause the retention of sodium by the kidneys. Wherever sodium goes, water follows; therefore, water is also retained by the body. At high concentrations, sodium and water retention may lead to the development of edema and/or hypertension.

Pharmacological Effects

The most important uses of the glucocorticoids are for replacement therapy in adrenocortical insufficiency (Addison's disease) and in the treatment of inflammatory conditions. The steroids that are available include the naturally occurring steroids and various synthetic preparations.

Replacement Therapy

The adrenal steroids are essential to life. In Addison's disease, there is a deficiency of both glucocorticoids and mineralocorticoids. The main symptoms in Addison's disease are dehydration, hypotension, and muscle weakness. Following ACTH administration, plasma cortisol and (17-hydroxycorticosteriods (17-OHCS) are measured. When the plasma levels of these steroids do not rise or cannot be detected, primary adrenal failure—that is, Addison's disease—is present. Cosyntropin is a synthetic peptide that corresponds to an active segment of ACTH. Although it provides the same therapeutic activity as ACTH with less allergenic potential, its formulation limits its use to diagnostic evaluation. Patients with Addison's disease must receive hormone replacement as chronic therapy. The naturally occurring glucocorticoids are used most frequently (see Table 36:2). Dosages administered are similar to the levels that normally exist in the

Comparison of Naturally Occurring and Synthetic Glucocorticoids

DRUG (TRADE NAME)	EQUIVALENT ANTIINFLAMMATORY DOSE (MG)	SODIUM RETENTION	DURATION OF ACTION (HOURS)
Short-Acting Steroids:			
cortisone* *(Cortone)*	25	High	12–24
hydrocortisone* *(Cortef, Hydrocortone)*	20	High	12–24
Intermediate-Acting Steroids:			
methylprednisolone* *(Depo-Medrol, Medrol, Solu-Medrol)*	4	None	24–36
prednisolone** *(Delta-Cortef, Hydeltra-TBA, Predcor 25, Predcor 50)*	5	Mild	24–36
prednisone** *(Deltasone, Meticortone, Orasone, Panasol)*	5	Mild	24–36
triamcinolone** *(Aristocort, Aristospan, Kenacort, Kenalog-40)*	4	None	36–48
Long-Acting Steroids:			
betamethasone** *(Celestone, Cel-U-Ject, Selestoject)*	0.60	None	48–72
dexamethasone** *(Decadron, Hexadrol, Decadron-LA)*	0.75	None	48–72

*Naturally occurring.
**Synthetic.

body (20 to 30 mg per day). In patients who continue to lose sodium due to a lack of aldosterone, a mineralocorticoid must also be administered along with the glucocorticoid.

Antiinflammatory Effects

Glucocorticoids are the most potent antiinflammatory agents available. Inflammation is usually considered the first step in the natural process of wound healing. However, sometimes the normal inflammatory response is too intense (acute inflammatory reaction) or is prolonged (chronic inflammatory reaction), and the inflammation itself becomes a disease process. For example, in rheumatoid arthritis, the inflammatory response can lead to permanent joint damage. Therefore, suppression of the inflammatory response becomes the most important therapeutic endpoint.

The glucocorticoids interfere with all stages of the inflammatory response, preventing edema due to capillary leakage and stabilizing cell membranes

(for example, **lysosomes**). Stabilization of the lysosomes prevents cell lysis and further cell damage. Since inflammation is also present in various allergic reactions, glucocorticoids are useful in the clinical management of allergies.

Synthetic glucocorticoids are frequently used to treat inflammatory and allergic conditions. Slight alterations in the structure of the naturally occurring glucocorticoids result in synthetic steroids with greater antiinflammatory potency. The synthetic steroids have a longer duration of action than do the naturally occurring steroids. In addition, they produce fewer undesirable mineralocorticoid effects. Features of the glucocorticoids are compared in Table 36:2.

Clinical Indications

Adrenocorticotropic hormone is primarily used for diagnostic evaluation of adrenocortical function. In established disorders, ACTH is used in the constellation of drug therapy for exacerbations of multiple sclerosis and hypercalcemia associated

TABLE 36:3	Examples of Extended-Release Injectable Steroids*
GLUCOCORTICOID	**TRADE NAMES**
Dexamethasone acetate	*Dalone LA, Decadron-LA, Decaject LA*
Hydrocortisone acetate	Generic hydrocortisone preparations
Methylprednisolone acetate	*depMedalone 40, Depo-Medrol, Depoject, D-Med 80*
Prednisolone acetate	*Articulose 50, Predalone 50*
Prednisolone tebutate	*Hydeltra-TBA, Predalone-TBA*

*These drugs are not for intravenous use; they are administered intramuscularly, intra-articularly, and intralesionally.

with cancer. Glucocorticoids are the drugs of choice in conditions where the endogenous hormone is not appropriately produced—that is, primary and secondary adrenal cortical insufficiency. Glucocorticoids are also approved for use in a wide range of inflammatory disorders where a degenerative process is out of control. These include rheumatic disorders, arthritis, collagen disease, specific ulcerative colitis, multiple sclerosis, severe allergic reaction, respiratory disease, and management of leukemias and lymphomas.

In addition to these Food and Drug Administration (FDA)-approved uses of corticosteroids, there are other uses that are medically appropriate although not specifically approved by the FDA (off-label use). Such inflammatory conditions include acute mountain sickness, bacterial meningitis, chronic obstructive pulmonary disease (COPD), Graves's ophthalmopathy, respiratory distress syndrome, septic shock, and spinal cord injury.

Administration and Dosage

Glucocorticoids may be administered orally, intramuscularly, intravenously, or topically. Intravenous administration is used in emergencies, when prompt effects are needed. Intramuscular injections are used when frequent administration is undesirable. The preparations for IM injection include **repository preparations,** in which the glucocorticoid is slowly released from the muscle, providing a longer duration of action. In general, extended-release steroids are prepared in the acetate form rather than as the sodium succinate or sodium phosphate. Examples of injectable preparations that have a slow onset and long duration of action are presented in Table 36:3. There is wide variation in the therapeutic dosages of the glucocorticoids. Doses must be adjusted to

meet the needs of individual patients. Short-term treatment with glucocorticoids absorbs scar tissue (keloids) when injected directly into the scarred skin. For exacerbations of chronically inflamed joints and soft tissue, the drugs may be injected into the specific area. For swollen joints, the edematous fluid is removed before the steroid is injected. Too frequent intra-articular administration can damage joint tissues, so patients are advised to decrease all stress on the inflamed joint to minimize the need for reinjection.

Topical use of the glucocorticoids is indicated in the treatment of inflammation and pruritic dermatosis. Topical steroids as ointments, creams, or sprays are available over-the-counter or by prescription. Over-the-counter preparations are specifically labeled for the temporary relief of minor skin irritations, itching, and rashes due to eczema, dermatitis, insect bites, poison ivy, detergents, and cosmetics, as well as itching in the genital and anal regions. Examples of over-the-counter topical steroids include *Cortaid, Bactine* hydrocortisone, and *Gynecort.* These products usually contain 0.5 percent hydrocortisone, a lesser amount of hydrocortisone than may be obtained by prescription; nevertheless, the active component is still a steroid. Misuse of these drugs may be accompanied by adverse effects similar to those described for other steroids.

Metabolism and Excretion

The glucocorticoids are metabolized by the liver and then excreted in the urine. The most common urinary metabolites are the 17-hydroxycorticosteroids (17-OHCS). These can be measured from 24-hour urine collections, and they provide an estimate of glucocorticoid secretion from the adrenal cortex. In patients with adrenocortical insufficiency, these metabolites are usually very low.

Adverse Effects

The adverse effects of the glucocorticoids usually occur in patients receiving high doses or long-term treatment. The adverse reactions, an exaggeration of the normal steroidal effects, are similar to the symptoms of Cushing's disease. The adverse effects are summarized in Table 36:4. An important adverse reaction associated with long-term use is steroid addiction, which may result in mood changes (euphoria), insomnia, personality changes, and psychological dependency. This is steroid psychosis. The incidence is usually associated with larger steroid doses. Abrupt withdrawal of the steroids may lead to severe mental depression. For this reason, discontinuation of long-term or high-dose steroids must be done under medical supervision, gradually, in small decrements to avoid precipitating withdrawal symptoms and depression.

Alternate-Day Therapy

Steroid administration is also accomplished by alternate-day therapy (ADT). Alternate-day therapy is intended to reduce or eliminate the adverse effects of prolonged steroid treatment. In ADT, a short-acting steroid is administered every other day in the morning. The effects of a single dose of a short-acting steroid will last into the next day. However, during the second day (no steroid administered), the patient's adrenal gland begins to function (that is, is released from negative feedback). On the following day (third day), the steroid is again administered and the patient's adrenal gland is once again suppressed. This therapy prevents adrenal atrophy and permanent destruction of the adrenal gland. There is also a lower incidence of other adverse effects. Doses and indication for the adrenal steroids are presented in Table 36:5.

MINERALOCORTICOIDS

The **mineralocorticoids** are hormones secreted by the outer layer of the adrenal gland. The main effect of the mineralocorticoid hormones is to regulate the fluid balance of the body. When there is a deficiency of mineralocorticoids, a condition known as hypoaldosteronism results. This condition usually is caused by adrenalectomy or by adrenal tumors. Replacement therapy is necessary because the mineralocorticoids are essential for life.

Physiological Effects

The most important mineralocorticoid is aldosterone. Its site of action is at the distal tubules of the nephrons. The main function of the nephrons is the formation of urine, during which process many essential nutrients and ions are reabsorbed through the tubules back into the

TABLE 36:4	Adverse Effects of Long-Term Steroid Therapy
METABOLIC EFFECT	**SYMPTOMS**
Glucocorticoid:	
Increased gluconeogenesis	Obesity, diabetes mellitus
Increased protein catabolism	Muscle weakness and wasting, thinning of skin (ecchymoses, striae), osteoporosis (loss of protein matrix), decreased growth (in children), decreased wound healing, increased infections (in leukopenia), peptic ulceration
Mineralocorticoid:	
Sodium and water retention	Edema, increased blood volume, hypertension
Loss of potassium	Muscle weakness and cramps
Miscellaneous Effects:	
Androgenic effects	Hirsutism, virilism, irregular menstruation
Eye complications	Glaucoma, cataract formation
Psychological changes	Euphoria, steroid addiction, depression

blood. Aldosterone increases the reabsorption of sodium ions. In exchange, potassium ions are transported into the urine. This process is usually referred to as sodium-potassium exchange. Water is also reabsorbed with sodium. Consequently, normal sodium and water levels (isotonic) are maintained in the blood and other body tissues.

Administration and Dosage

Fludrocortisone *(Florinef)* is a potent mineralocorticoid. Fludrocortisone has a greater glucocorticoid potency than does cortisone. Although fludrocortisone has dual activity, it is usually administered in conjunction with a glucocorticoid (cortisone, hydrocortisone) to achieve total replacement therapy in primary and secondary adrenocortical insufficiency. Fludrocortisone is administered orally in doses of 0.1 to 0.2 mg per day, three times per week.

Adverse Effects

Excessive use of the mineralocorticoids results in sodium and water retention and the loss of potassium. The major symptoms are edema, hypertension, and muscle weakness due to the loss of potassium. In certain patients, the edema could lead to congestive heart failure. A physician should be notified if dizziness, continuing headaches, or swelling in the lower extremities occurs. Dose adjustment usually mitigates adverse effects. Other adverse effects include increased sweating, bruising, and allergic skin rash.

SPECIAL CONSIDERATIONS

Steroids are administered for their antiinflammatory activity in patients with normal adrenal function. With continued use (as well as misuse of these drugs), patients may experience changes in appearance and behavior indicative of metabolic alterations. Since steroids universally affect metabolism, patients must be observed carefully for changes in body weight, electrolyte balance, and cardiac function. The sodium retention associated with these drugs may lead to elevated blood pressure, even hypertension, and edema. Patients should be weighed daily to monitor changes in overall body weight. Patients should be questioned

TABLE 36:5	Doses and Indications of Adrenal Steroids	
ADRENAL STEROID	**INDICATION**	**DOSE**
Corticotrophins		
ACTH *(Acthar, Corticotropin)*	Confirmation of adrenal responsiveness Multiple sclerosis	80 units single injection or 10–25 units diluted IV over 8 hr 80–120 units/day IM for 2–3 weeks
repository Corticotropin	IM, SC	40–80 units every 24–72 hr (IM, SC)
cosyntropin *(Cortrosyn)*	IM or IV	0.25–0.75 mg
Mineralocorticoids		
fludrocortisone acetate *(Florinef Acetate)*	Addison's disease	0.1 mg daily PO
Glucocorticoids		
betamethasone	Antiinflammatory	0.6–7.2 mg daily PO; up to 9 mg per day IV
budesonide *(Rhinocort)*	Allergic rhinitis	1 spray/nostril daily (64 mcg)
budesonide *(Entocort E. C.)*	Crohn's Disease	9 mg daily up to 8 weeks
cortisone *(Cortisone Acetate, Cortone)*	Antiinflammatory	25–300 mg/day PO
dexamethasone *(Decadron, Dexone, Dexameth)**	Allergic disorders Cushing's syndrome	0.75–9 mg daily PO 1 mg at 11 PM or 0.5 mg every 6 hr for 48 hr

(continued)

Doses and Indications of Adrenal Steroids, *continued*

ADRENAL STEROID	INDICATION	DOSE
Glucocorticoids, *continued*		
dexamethasone with lidocaine *(Decadron with Xylocaine)*	Soft tissue injection, bursitis	0.5–0.75 ml
fluticasone *(Flonase)*	Allergic rhinitis	2 sprays/nostril once daily (50 mcg/spray)
hydrocortisone *(Cortisol, Cortef)*	Antiinflammatory	20–240 mg/day PO
hydrocortisone sodium phosphate *(Hydrocortone Phosphate)*	Antiinflammatory	15–240 mg/day IV, IM, or SC
hydrocortisone sodium succinate *(A-hydroCort, Solu-Cortef)*	Antiinflammatory	100–500 mg every 2, 4, or 6 hr IM, IV
hydrocortisone acetate *(Hydrocortone Acetate)*	Intralesion, intra-articular *not* IV	12.5–50 mg
methylprednisolone *(Medrol)*	Antiinflammatory	4–48 mg/day PO or alternate-day therapy
methylprednisolone sodium *(A-Methapred, Solu-Medrol)*	Antiinflammatory	10–40 mg IV over several minutes
methylprednisolone acetate *(Depo-Medrol, Duralone-40, Depoject)**	Adrenalgenital syndrome Rheumatoid arthritis, dermatologic lesions Asthma, allergic rhinitis Intra-articular	40 mg IM every 2 weeks 40-120 mg IM weekly 80–120 mg IM 4–80 mg
mometasone (Nasonex)	Allergic rhinitis	2 sprays/nostril daily (50 mcg/spray)
prednisone *(Meticortin, Orasone, Panasol-S, Deltasone)**		50–60 mg/day PO
prednisolone *(Delta-Cortef, Prelone)*	Multiple sclerosis	200 mg daily PO for 7 days, then 80 mg every other day for 1 month
prednisolone acetate *(Key-Pred, Predcor, Articulose, Predaject-50)**	Intralesional, intra-articular, soft tissue	4–100 mg
	Multiple sclerosis	200 mg daily PO for 7 days, then 80 mg every other day for 1 month
triamcinolone* *(Aristocort, Atolone, Kenacort)*	Adrenal insufficiency Bronchial asthma Respiratory disease Tuberculous meningitis Acute leukemia and lymphoma Systemic lupus erythematosus	4–12 mg daily PO 8–16 mg daily PO 16–48 mg daily 32–48 mg 16–40 mg daily PO 20–32 mg daily PO
	Edema	16–20 mg PO until diuresis occurs

*Not an inclusive list of products.

about feeling fatigued or experiencing cramps and weakness in the extremities because these may be symptoms of hypokalemia. Patients with Addison's disease are often sensitive to drug effects and therefore often have an exaggerated response to drug therapy. Patients, especially those on high-dose therapy, should be monitored for changes in sleep patterns and mood, particularly depression or psychotic episodes.

Steroids should be used cautiously in patients who have gastrointestinal (GI) ulceration, renal disease, congestive heart failure, ocular herpes simplex, diabetes mellitus, emotional instability, or psychotic tendencies. In all of these conditions, steroids may exacerbate the underlying disease as a result of their pharmacological actions. Although steroids are ulcerogenic, it is not unusual that certain patients with gastrointestinal ulcer or colitis may be placed on a steroid regimen. In such cases, the risk of continuing degeneration outweighs the risk of short-term exposure to the steroid in order to obtain an immediate antiinflammatory response.

Contraindications

Steroids are contraindicated for use in patients who have systemic fungal infections and local viral (herpes) infections. Topical steroids should not be applied to the eyes or periorbital area. Ocular exposure to steroids may cause steroid-induced glaucoma and cataracts. Steroids and ACTH may reduce the patient's resistance to fight local infection. Live virus vaccinations should not be given during steroid therapy. Patients receiving high-dose steroids may not have the ability to develop antibody immunity, putting them at risk for developing infection and neurological complications. This does not apply to patients receiving physiological steroid doses as replacement therapy.

DRUG INTERACTIONS

Steroids have been reported to interact with a variety of drug classes (see Table 36:6). Since the glucocorticoids affect carbohydrate metabolism, it is not surprising that diabetics may have an increased insulin or oral hypoglycemic requirement during periods of steroid treatment. Steroids administered concomitantly with potassium-depleting diuretics, amphotericin B, or digitalis may potentiate the development of hypokalemia. Patients receiving coumarin anticoagulants may have a decreased coumarin response in the presence of steroids. Prothrombin time must be monitored to ensure that patients are adequately covered.

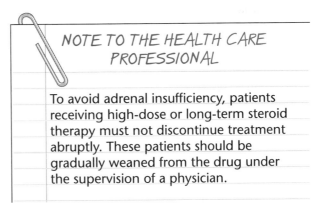

NOTE TO THE HEALTH CARE PROFESSIONAL

To avoid adrenal insufficiency, patients receiving high-dose or long-term steroid therapy must not discontinue treatment abruptly. These patients should be gradually weaned from the drug under the supervision of a physician.

TABLE 36:6 Examples of Drug Interactions Associated with Glucocorticoids

GLUCOCORTICOIDS INTERACT WITH	RESPONSE
Amphotericin B, digitalis, diuretics	Potentiate hypokalemia (possible digitalis toxicity)
Antibiotics, macrolide	Increase methylprednisolone clearance from plasma
Coumarin anticoagulants	Inhibit response to the anticoagulants
Growth hormone (*Somatrem*)	Decrease growth-promoting effect of *Somatrem*
Insulin, oral hypoglycemics	Increase requirement for insulin or oral hypoglycemics
Isoniazid	Increase requirements for isoniazid
Oral contraceptives, estrogens, ketoconazole	Increase steroid response
Phenobarbital, phenytoin, rifampin	Increase steroid requirement due to increased steroid clearance

Phenytoin, phenobarbital, and rifampin enhance the metabolism of corticosteroids, leading to reduced blood steroid levels and a decreased pharmacological response. In patients receiving these drugs chronically, the dose of corticosteroid may require adjustment.

On the other hand, oral contraceptives inhibit steroid metabolism. Concomitant use of these drugs may lead to elevated blood steroid concentrations and may potentiate steroid toxicity.

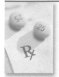

Patient Administration and Monitoring

This class of drugs has a tremendous potential for overuse and overexposure due to the availability of over-the-counter preparations. In addition, steroids may be prescribed by more than one treating physician. It is not unusual for older patients to visit orthopedists, allergists, diabetologists, ophthalmologists, and rheumatologists in addition to their family physician. Therefore, it becomes important to review steroid actions that could be misinterpreted as exacerbations of other underlying conditions.

Time of Dosing

Single steroid doses should be taken before 9 AM to allow distribution of drug to mimic diurnal levels without suppressing available adrenocortical activity. Large doses of steroids may cause GI upset. Patients may take the medication with meals or antacids to minimize the irritation.

Changes in Blood Sugar Levels

Diabetic patients should notify the prescribing (steroid) physician if changes in their monitored blood glucose levels occur. Diabetics may have an increased blood glucose concentration requiring dose adjustment in insulin or oral antidiabetic drugs. Patients should be reminded to give full disclosure of steroid use to other physicians, such as diabetologist or endocrinologist, to keep their medication history current.

Physician Notification

The physician should be notified immediately if significant fluid retention manifests as swelling of lower extremities or unusual weight gain, muscle weakness, abdominal pain, seizures, or headache occur. This may indicate the need for dose alteration or discontinuation if hypersensitivity develops. Topical steroids will more likely produce skin or ocular itching and irritation rather than the spectrum of other effects.

Elderly patients should be reminded to call if they develop signs of hypertension, hyperglycemia, and potassium loss. These include dizziness, muscle weakness, and headaches. Because of the reduced muscle mass, elderly patients are more sensitized to the effects of steroids and should be monitored in the office at least every 6 months.

For patients receiving high doses of steroids, there is a decreased resistance to fight local infection (immunosuppressive response). Patients should notify the prescribing (steroid) physician before immunizations with live vaccines are given.

Stopping Medication

Patients receiving high-dose or long-term therapy should not discontinue steroids without supervision of the prescribing physician to avoid precipitating symptoms of withdrawal.

Use in Pregnancy

Drugs in this class have been designated FDA Pregnancy Category C. Safety for use in pregnancy has not been established through adequate use or clinical trials in pregnant women. Steroids cross the placenta. Chronic maternal steroid use in the first trimester is known to produce cleft palate in newborns (about 1 percent incidence). The benefit to the mother must outweigh risk to the fetus and newborn. When clearly required, maternal steroid administration should be at the lowest effective dose for the shortest duration and the infant should be subsequently monitored for adrenal activity. Where mothers received ACTH, the newborn should be monitored for hyperadrenalism.

Chapter Review

Understanding Terminology

Answer the following questions in the spaces provided.

1. Define the term *steroid*. _____
   _____
   _____

2. Differentiate between mineralocorticoids and glucocorticoids. _____
   _____
   _____

3. Explain replacement therapy. _____
   _____
   _____

Acquiring Knowledge

Answer the following questions in the spaces provided.

1. What are the two main parts of the adrenal gland? _____
   _____
   _____

2. Which layer of the adrenal cortex secretes the mineralocorticoids? Which layer secretes the glucocorticoids? _____
   _____

3. What disease results from a deficiency of the corticosteroids? _____
   _____
   _____

4. What three factors regulate the release of cortisol? _____
   _____
   _____

5. What is the importance of higher glucocorticoid secretion during injury and wound healing?
   _____
   _____

6. List the two main therapeutic uses of the glucocorticoids. _____
   _____
   _____

7. What are the main differences between the naturally occurring steroids and the synthetic steroids?
   _____
   _____

8. List the major adverse effect of steroid therapy. What is meant by *ADT?* _____
   _____
   _____

9. What is the function of the mineralocorticoids? _____
   _____
   _____

10. What are the adverse effects of excessive administration of the mineralocorticoids?

_____

_____

Applying Knowledge—On the Job

Use your critical thinking skills to answer the following questions in the spaces provided.

1. Assume you are a pharmacy assistant in a nursing home, screening patients for contraindications and drug interactions. What is the potential drug problem—and its solution—for each of the following cases?

    a. Patient A has hypertension. He has been prescribed hydrocortisone injections for severe bursitis.

    _____

    _____

    b. Patient B is diabetic. She has been prescribed prednisolone for osteoarthritis. _____

    _____

    _____

    c. Patient C is taking coumarin anticoagulant. He has been prescribed prednisone for gout.

    _____

    _____

2. Assume you are a pharmacy intern in a university hospital. What is the potential drug problem for each of the following patients? How would you resolve the problem?

    a. A 25-year-old woman has been prescribed betamethasone for severe psoriasis. The patient is currently taking oral contraceptives.

    _____

    _____

    b. A 16-year-old boy has been prescribed dexamethasone for bronchial asthma. He is an epileptic currently taking phenobarbital for seizure control.

    _____

    _____

3. Tom is an 8-year-old who is taking 80 mg of prednisone for inflammation of the liver. He has been diagnosed with chickenpox. Would this affect his prednisone dose? Why or why not?

    _____

    _____

4. Ten-year-old Shannon has had a severe allergic reaction to poison oak. Her physician has decided to initiate prednisone therapy. The prescription reads:

    Prednisone 40 mg QS

    qd ×3d, 30 mg qd ×3d, 20 mg qd ×3d, 10 mg qd ×3d, 5 mg qd ×2d ×2d then dc. Assume the pharmacy fills this prescription with prednisone 10 mg tablets. How many tablets would the patient receive and how would you expect the label to read?

    _____

    _____

5. Why is it important for patients receiving high-dose or long-term therapy to be taken off prednisone by decreasing the dose?

    _____

    _____

Additional Reading

Anderson, B. 1991. An overview of drug therapy in chronic adult asthma. _Advances in Clinical Care_ 6:44.

O'Neil, B. J. 1991. Steroids: Drugs of a new age? _Emergency_ 23:60.

Ruholl, L. H. 1991. Your body clocks: A student guide to circadian rhythms. _Imprint_ 38:123.

37

GONADAL HORMONES AND THE ORAL CONTRACEPTIVES

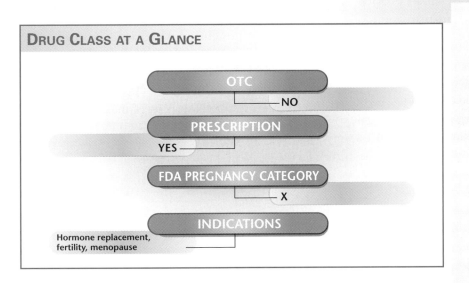

DRUG CLASS AT A GLANCE

OTC
— NO

PRESCRIPTION
YES —

FDA PREGNANCY CATEGORY
— X

INDICATIONS
Hormone replacement, fertility, menopause

Key Terms

amenorrhea: condition in which monthly menstruation (menses) no longer occurs.

anabolism: process that converts or incorporates nutritional substances into tissue; usually associated with conversion of proteins into muscle mass.

androgen: male sex hormone.

biphasic: two different amounts of estrogen hormone are released during the cycle.

buccal absorption: absorption of drug through the mucous membranes lining the oral cavity.

contraception: preventing pregnancy by preventing either conception (joining of egg and sperm) or implantation in the uterus.

diplopia: condition in which a single object is seen (perceived) as two objects; double vision.

dysmenorrhea: condition that is associated with painful and difficult menstruation.

endometrium: lining of the uterus.

CHAPTER FOCUS

This chapter describes naturally occurring substances that trigger sexual development and characteristic differences in appearance between men and women.

CHAPTER OBJECTIVES

After studying this chapter, you should be able to

- describe specific areas of the target organs affected by the male or female sex hormones.
- describe the sequence of hormone secretion during the menstrual cycle.
- discuss the pharmacological response of oral birth control pills (contraceptives) on the characteristics of the menstrual cycle.
- explain the difference between monophasic and multiphasic oral contraceptives.
- name three physiological effects that are improved during hormone replacement therapy in postmenopausal women.
- describe three adverse effects associated with chronic hormone administration in nonmenopausal women.
- name an example in which anabolic therapy is desirable.

equipotent: when drugs (substances) produce the same intensity or spectrum of activity. Usually, the absolute amount of drug (for example, 5, 10 mg) that produces the response is different for each substance, but the response generated is the same.

erythropoiesis: process through which red blood cells are produced.

fertility drug: drug that stimulates ovulation.

fibrocystic breast disease: condition in which cystic lesions form within the connective tissue of the breasts.

hirsutism: condition usually in women in which body and facial hair is excessive.

lactation: production of milk in female breasts.

menopause: condition in which menstruation no longer occurs, either because of the normal aging process in women (45 years of age and older) or because the ovaries have been surgically removed (any age); the clinical effects of menopause are a direct result of little or no estrogen secretion.

menstruation: normal periodic (every 4 weeks) physiological hemorrhage (shedding of fluid and endometrial tissue) from the uterus.

monophasic: a fixed amount (nonchanging) of estrogen is released during the cycle.

oligospermia: reduced sperm count.

osteoporosis: decrease in the amount or density of bone, usually in the elderly, which results in areas predisposed to fracture.

ovulation: release of an egg from the ovary.

perimenopause: two to 10 years before complete cessation of a menstrual period.

puberty: sequence of physiological changes associated with the expression of sexual characteristics and reproductive function that occur when a child progresses into young adulthood, usually at 12 to 14 years of age.

transdermal absorption: absorption of drug (substance) through the skin, usually associated with the application of drug-loaded patches.

triphasic: the estrogen and progestin amounts released may vary during the cycle.

virilization: development of masculine body (hair, muscle) characteristics in females.

INTRODUCTION

The sex hormones are produced and secreted by the gonads, which include the female ovaries and the male testes. The ovaries and testes are under control of the anterior pituitary gland, which releases hormones regulating the synthesis and release of the various sex hormones. Production of the sex hormones is almost entirely inhibited until the time of puberty. During **puberty,** hormone production drastically increases and is responsible for the development and maintenance of the secondary sex characteristics.

At this time, the female sex hormones have a broader spectrum of pharmacological importance than the male sex hormones. This is due to the cyclic nature of ovarian function (menstrual cycle) and its role in pregnancy and childbearing, and the evolving protective role of estrogen during the period after the childbearing years.

FEMALE SEX HORMONES

The name, female sex hormones, implies that these compounds have a singular role in female reproductive development. While this is a critical part of their physiological activity, these steroid hormones are pluripotential. This means that these hormones have a significant role in the physiology and metabolism of target tissues other than those associated with reproduction. The influence of the estrogens is becoming evident through "replacement hormone" strategies in use today. Such estrogen influence on bone and cardiovascular function and insulin sensitivity will be discussed after considering the role of the steroid sex hormones in the reproductive cycle.

Female Reproductive Cycle

Human ovaries contain roughly 400,000 eggs within undeveloped follicles at the beginning of menarche (menstruation), more than enough to accommodate reproduction needs during the next 45 years. Each month after menarche, the ovaries are stimulated to develop one dominant follicle from which one egg will be released for fertilization and hormones will be secreted to prepare the uterus to receive the fertilized embryo for continued development.

At the beginning of each monthly cycle, one of the follicles undergoes development and maturation because of the influence of follicle-stimulating hormone (FSH). Follicle-stimulating hormone enables its own receptors to flourish on the undeveloped follicles so that FSH activity is recognized; however, only one follicle will generate enough FSH receptors to continue responding even when the FSH levels decline. This is the dominant follicle for that month. As the follicle enlarges, certain cells in it begin to produce the estrogenic hormones. Among the naturally occurring estrogens are estriol, estrone, and estradiol. Estradiol is the most abundant and most active of these estrogens. The major function of the estrogens is to stimulate the development of the uterine lining (endometrium) and the mammary glands for pregnancy, should it occur.

After approximately 14 days of development, the dominant follicle ruptures and releases the egg (ovulation). The egg passes into the fallopian tube, where fertilization by a sperm cell may occur. After ovulation, the follicle, which remains in the ovary, undergoes a change. Although estrogens do not induce ovulation, they directly influence the motility of the fallopian tubes and endometrial environment for favorable ovum transport. Under the influence of luteinizing hormone (LH), the follicle is transformed into a corpus luteum. The corpus luteum continues to produce estrogen and begins to produce progesterone, the second major type of female sex hormone.

Progesterone completes the development of the uterine lining (for implantation of the fertilized egg) and the mammary duct system (for lactation). In addition, progesterone is important for maintaining the uterine lining when pregnancy does occur.

At the end of the ovarian cycle (usually day 28 ± 7 days), if fertilization of the egg has not occurred, the corpus luteum degenerates, and female hormone production ceases. The uterine lining is dependent on estrogen and progesterone for its existence. When hormone production stops, the lining sloughs off, and menstruation begins. During menstruation there is a temporary anticoagulant action within the uterine tissue and bleeding begins. The duration of menstruation is 4 days (±2 days). Menstruation stops when endometrial cells rich in thromboplastin are shed, contributing to clot formation. At this same time, a new follicle in the ovary begins to develop, and the cycle repeats itself. This monthly cycle continues throughout women's reproductive years.

A schematic representation of the rise and fall of the female sex hormones during the menstrual cycle is presented in Figure 37:1. The level of female sex hormones is constantly changing. It is low in the beginning of the cycle and high toward the end. Estrogen dominates hormone production

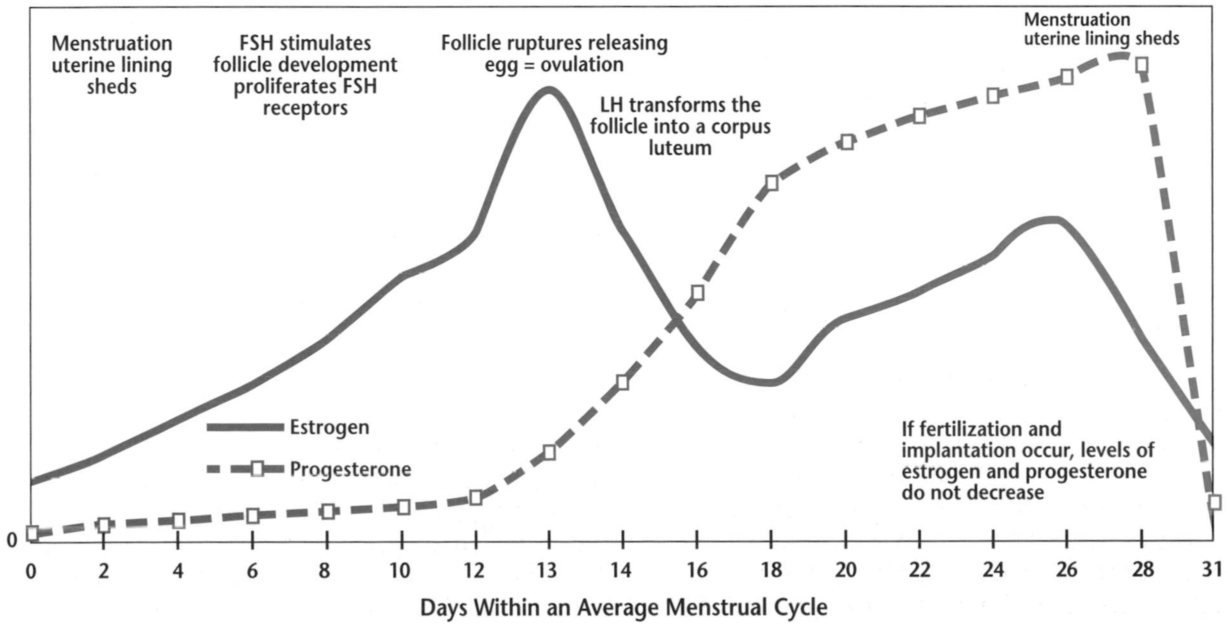

FIGURE 37:1 Female Hormone Levels During the Menstrual Cycle

during the first 2 weeks, whereas progesterone is produced during the last 2 weeks of each monthly cycle, as is estrogen. When the levels of estrogen and progesterone in the blood are high, there is inhibition of the release of FSH and LH. (This regulatory process, known as negative feedback, was discussed in Chapter 34.) Inhibition of FSH and LH prevents the subsequent development of other ovarian follicles.

If pregnancy does occur, the corpus luteum continues to produce estrogen and progesterone until the placenta is developed and can assume this function. The transition usually occurs between the second and third month of pregnancy, a critical time. If the corpus luteum degenerates before the placenta can maintain the hormone level, the uterine lining (with fetus) ruptures, hemorrhages, and sloughs off, resulting in miscarriage. During pregnancy, the levels of estrogen and progesterone are high. Such high levels continue to inhibit (negative feedback) the release of FSH. Therefore, during pregnancy, no other follicles undergo development. Similarly, oral contraceptives maintain high hormone levels in the blood, which prevent the release of FSH (such as during pregnancy). Since no follicle develops, there is no egg for fertilization.

Clinical Indications

The main uses of the female sex hormones include hormone replacement therapy (HRT), oral **contraception,** fertility enhancement, and adjunctive therapy of certain cancers (prostate and nonestrogen-dependent breast cancer). Replacement therapy is required in children who have hypogonadism, primary ovarian failure, to complete puberty and permit adequate bone growth. Replacement therapy in adults arises from removal of the ovaries during the active reproductive years (20 to 45 years of age) or cessation of ovarian activity at menopause. The clinical indication for adult HRT is management of vasomotor symptoms associated with menopause. As an outgrowth of adult HRT, estrogens are now also clinically indicated for the prevention and treatment of osteoporosis.

Route of Administration

Examples of some estrogens and progesterones and their recommended uses are presented in Table 37:1. Whether naturally occurring or synthetically produced, estrogens produce the same spectrum of activity (physiological responses and adverse effects) when **equipotent** doses are administered. Estrogens can be chemically synthesized as a specific steroid hormone, such as estradiol and estrone, or as estrogenic substances not normally produced by women—for example, ethinyl estradiol and diethylstilbestrol (DES). Conjugated estrogens, obtained from pregnant mare urine, contain a variety of estrogenic substances. Estrogen and progesterone products are available for use orally, parenterally (IM), vaginally, and topically. The active hormones are metabolized by the liver following these routes of administration and, depending on the type of conjugate formed, the metabolites are excreted into the bile or the urine.

In order to lengthen the onset and duration of estrogen action, the hormone can be administered in an oil that is more slowly absorbed from muscle tissue. Another way is to choose a route of administration that initially bypasses liver metabolism, such as transdermal administration. Estrogens are available as "drug-loaded" patches that can be applied to a clean, dry surface of the abdomen or buttocks so that the drug is absorbed through the skin **(transdermal absorption).** The skin minimally metabolizes estradiol so that the estradiol absorbed into the blood is initially greater than that following the oral route. This formulation provides an opportunity for convenient dosing of once or twice a week rather than daily.

Besides the transdermal patch, another unique delivery system is the vaginal ring. This device, also drug laden, is pressed into the vaginal canal, continuously releasing drug to the local tissue.

Vaginal inserts, creams, and long-acting "depo" formulations are designed to deliver estrogen to local site on contact or as a protracted release over a long period of time. Oral estrogen dosing is designed to mimic the physiological pattern of estrogen activity. This is especially true for the oral contraceptives. From days 0 through 21, estrogen is the dominant hormone taken daily. During the last 7 days of the monthly cycle it can be replaced by inert or iron-containing pills, progesterone, or no pill for 7 days. Oral contraceptives are considered **monophasic**— formulations that release a fixed amount of estrogen (relative to progestin) in each pill from days 0 to 21 (see Table 37:2 on page 432). With the **biphasic** and **triphasic** formulations, the pill color varies over the cycle and represents different strengths (dose ratio) of estrogens to progestin in the pill (see Table 37:3 on page 432). Clever packaging of daily medication for the 28-day cycle (one pill each day for 28 days) improves patient compliance by reducing the potential for missing doses through forgetfulness or confusion.

TABLE 37:1					

Estrogen and Progestogen Drugs*

DRUG (TRADE NAME)	FORM	DOSE FOR PROSTATIC CANCER	DOSE FOR MENOPAUSAL SYMPTOMS ATROPIC VAGINITIS	DOSE FOR REPLACEMENT THERAPY
Estrogens:				
chlorotrianisene (*TACE*)	Capsules	——————— 12–25 mg PO for 30 days ———————		
conjugated estrogens (*Premarin*)	Tablets	1.25–2.5 mg PO TID	0.3–1.25 mg/day PO	2.5–7.5 mg/day PO
estradiol (*Estrace*)	Tablets	1–2 mg PO TID	——— 1–2 mg PO cyclically ——— (21 days on drug, 7 days off drug)	
estradiol cyprionate (*Depogen, depGynogen*)	Oil, IM only	—	1–5 mg IM every 3–4 weeks	1.5–2 mg/month IM
estradiol valerate (*Delestrogen, Duragen, Estra-L-40, Gynogen*)	Oil, IM only	30 mg/week IM	——— 10–20 mg IM every 4 weeks ———	
estrone (*Aquest, Theelin*)	Aqueous suspension, IM only	2–4 mg IM two or three times/week	0.1–0.5 mg IM two or three times/week	0.1–2 mg/week
ethinyl estradiol (*Estinyl, Feminone*)	Tablets	0.15–0.2 mg/day PO	0.02–0.05 mg PO cyclically	0.05 mg PO BID, TID
quinestrol (*Estrovis*)	Tablets	—	———100 μg/day for 7 days followed——— by 100–200 μg once a week	
Progestogens:				
progesterone (*Gesterol 50, Progestaject*)	Oil, IM only	5–10 mg IM for 6–8 days	5–10 mg/day IM for 6 days	—
norethindrone (*Norlutin*)	Tablets	———5–20 mg PO on days 5–25——— of menstrual cycle		10–30 mg/day for 2 weeks
medroxyprogesterone (*Amen, Curretab, Cycrin, Provera*)	Tablets	———5–10 mg PO for 5 to 10 days———		—
Combination:				
northynodrel and mestranol (*Enovid*)	Tablets	—	20–30 mg/day	5–10 mg for 2 weeks beginning on day 5 of menstrual cycle. Increase up to 20 mg/day for 6–9 months

*Not an inclusive list of available products.

TABLE 37:2   Oral Contraceptive Preparations—Monophasic

TRADE NAME*	ESTROGEN	PROGESTIN
Demulen 1/35	Ethinyl estradiol 35 μg	Ethynodiol diacetate 1.0 mg
Demulen 1/50	Ethinyl estradiol 50 μg	Ethynodiol diacetate 1.0 mg
Desogen	Ethinyl estradiol 30 μg	Desogestrel 0.15 mg
Levlen	Ethinyl estradiol 30 μg	Levonorgestrel 0.15 mg
Loestrin Fe 1/20	Ethinyl estradiol 30 μg	Norethindrone 1.0 mg plus ferrous fumarate
Loestrin Fe 1.5/30	Ethinyl estradiol 30 μg	Ethynodiol diacetate 1.5 mg plus ferrous fumarate
Lo/Ovral	Ethinyl estradiol 30 μg	Norgestrel 0.3 mg
Micronor	—	Norethindrone 0.35 mg
Norinyl 1 + 50	Mestranol 50 μg	Norethindrone 1.0 mg
Norinyl 1 + 35	Ethinyl estradiol 35 μg	Norethindrone 1.0 mg
Nor - Q.D.	—	Norethindrone 0.35 mg
Ortho-Novum 1/35	Ethinyl estradiol 35 μg	Norethindrone 1.0 mg
Ortho-Novum 1/50	Mestranol 50 μg	Norethindrone 1.0 mg
Ovcon-35	Ethinyl estradiol 35 μg	Norethindrone 0.40 mg
Ovral	Ethinyl estradiol 50 μg	Norgestrel 0.50 mg
Ovrette	—	Norgestrel 0.075 mg

*Not an inclusive list of available products.

TABLE 37:3   Oral Contraceptive Preparations—Multiphasic

TRADE NAME	PHASE I	PHASE II	PHASE III
Progestin: Estrogen	**Norethindrone: Ethinyl Estradiol**		
Jenest 28, Nelova 10/11, Ortho-Novum 10/11	0.5 mg: 35 μg	1.0 mg: 35 μg	—
Ortho-Novum 7/7/7, Tri-Norinyl	0.5 mg: 35 μg	1.0 mg: 35 μg	0.5 mg: 35 μg
Levonorgestrel: Ethinyl Estradiol			
Tri-Levlen, Triphasil	0.05 mg: 30 μg	0.075 mg: 40 μg	0.125 mg: 30 μg
Norgestimate: Ethinyl Estradiol			
Ortho-Tri-Cyclen	0.18 mg: 35 μg	0.215 mg: 35 μg	0.25 mg: 35 μg

Doses of estrogen are significantly lower today than those pioneered 20 years ago. With these newer estrogen replacement regimens, referred to as "low-dose products," there is rarely a need to employ more than 50 μg of estrogen for effective contraception. Products range in dose from 20 to 50 μg of estrogen daily. This provides the lowest effective coverage and improves the safety profile of estrogen therapy. Although most hormone replacement regimens available contain only hormones, one product combines estrogen with an antianxiety drug, *PMB 200* (estrogen and meprobamate), for patients experiencing severe anxiety as part of the symptom complex.

Hormonal Replacement Therapy (HRT)

The most frequent causes of female hormonal deficiency are removal of the ovaries (surgical-induced menopause; premature menopause) and menopause. Menopause is an expected but not always anticipated part of the aging process.

Generations of misinformed women and health care professionals believed menopause to begin at the age of 50 and thought it to be associated with a decreased ability to enjoy life as before. At menopause, the woman was definably old and

indeed, years ago, the life expectancy of women was closer to the age of menopause. The perception of menopause has dramatically changed over the last decade, primarily as a result of the improved lifestyle of women entering menopause and because of women's increased longevity. Average life expectancy for American women who are now 65 years old is 84! It has become evident that women are entering **perimenopause,** the period leading up to menopause, as early as 40. This means that women can expect to survive 44 more years and their expectation is to be well informed about strategies that optimize their health through this time of life. More than ever before, the goal is to improve women's quality of life as they age.

Perimenopause is characterized by a significant decrease in female sex hormone production (estrogens, progestins), male hormone production (androgens are produced by the ovaries and the adrenals), frequency of ovulation, and menstruation. Initially, there is a period of physiological and emotional adjustment. During this time, individuals may experience symptoms such as fatigue, hot flashes, vasomotor spasms, nervousness, anxiety, irritability, or depression. Tissue changes in the endometrium and vagina, such as atrophy, decreased metabolism, irritation, and dryness, also take place.

Menopause, clinically defined, is the complete cessation of a menstrual period for 12 months accompanied by a circulating estrogen level less than 50 picograms/ml and an FSH blood level greater than 50 IU/ml. This transition from perimenopause to menopause is not necessarily sudden or smooth. There is such a wide variability in the decline in estrogen and progesterone production and secretion that women can be intermittently symptomatic for a number of years. Even after menopause has been clinically established, amenorrhea for one year, an estimated 60 percent of postmenopausal women will experience hot flashes or sweating years later. The hot flashes vary in intensity and duration from woman to woman. The hot flash can range from a rising warm feeling to awakening literally in a pool of sweat, referred to as night sweats. Among the other symptoms that cause women to seek treatment are insomnia, inability to concentrate, and arthritis-like aching joints. Insomnia, which contributes to depression, anxiety, myalgias, and vasomotor symptoms are effectively relieved by HRT.

Administration of estrogen reduces the severity of the symptoms and smooths the transition into this postreproductive period. The options for treatment must be considered because there is no single option that is acceptable for all women. The goal is to individualize the treatment to the particular constellation of symptoms the woman is experiencing and to establish estrogen levels within a "normal acceptable" range—that is; 50 to 150 picograms/ml. Estrogen levels that are too high for an individual woman will also produce a spectrum of adverse effects not unlike untreated menopause—that is, sweats, hot flashes, anxiety, irritability, bloating, water retention, breast tenderness, and headaches. (It is worth noting that exogenous progestin quickly relieves these symptoms.) Hormone replacement therapy options include estrogen replacement only, estrogen with cyclic progestin, and continuous estrogen and progestin. Virtually all postmenopausal women are monitored by symptoms rather than hormone blood levels, changing HRT combinations until adequate symptom relief occurs. At least 1 month is required to establish whether treatment is effective and acceptable to the patient. Annual follow-up is recommended as the treatment is continued indefinitely. Although not Food and Drug Administration (FDA) approved for this indication, it is possible that physicians may add an androgen (micronized testosterone or dehydroepiandrosterone [DHEA]) to HRT once androgen deficiency has been confirmed by the laboratory. Androgen replacement is directed at maintaining muscle mass and strength.

Recently, the Women's Health Initiative (WHI), a very large clinical study involving more than 16,000 women over 50 years old, provided results that have curbed the overwhelming enthusiasm for HRT in postmenopausal women. The study provided evidence that women taking a combination estrogen-progestin daily for at least 5 years had an increased risk of nonfatal heart attacks, thromboembolism, stroke, breast cancer and dementia including Alzheimer's disease. At the same time, the risk of colon cancer and bone fracture decreased (see Osteoporosis section). This study confirmed the coronary results of a second large study in postmenopausal women, the Heart and Estrogen/Progestin Replacement Study (HERS). Because the benefits did not outweigh the cardiovascular risks, the estrogen combination therapy part of the WHI study was stopped. The immediate reaction in the medical community has been to advise women to discuss the use of HRT with their physicians and to seek alternative therapeutic options under the direction of a physician.

HRT is still an acceptable treatment for relief of postmenopausal symptoms. It is still the most effective treatment for relief of hot flashes, sleep disturbances, and vaginal dryness. The recommendation now is to take the lowest effective dose for the shortest time (i.e., not indefinitely). As always, women are advised to have regular general medical and breast examinations with periodic mammograms during and after hormone therapy.

At the same time, drugs known as SERMs, selective estrogen receptor modulators, are in development. Drugs such as reloxifene (*Evista*) are synthetic estrogens targeted for specific estrogen receptors associated with the bones (osteoporosis) but leave other parts of the body unaffected.

For women who have not experienced age-induced menopause but become hormone deficient as a result of surgery, estrogen replacement may still be an appropriate therapy. The therapeutic goal after removal of the ovaries in women under 50 years of age is to restore the estrogen and progesterone levels to those that are more representative of endocrine support and provide adequate cyclic feedback to the hypothalamus.

Osteoporosis

Mounting evidence confirms that estrogen depletion, not specifically aging, contributes to bone loss in postmenopausal women. As estrogen declines, bone resorption begins to exceed formation, particularly in trabecular bone. This leads to a reduction in bone mass that is termed **osteoporosis.** In the presence of low calcium intake, and inadequate gravity-resisting exercise, bone fractures occur without apparent severe trauma. The incidence of fracture and osteoporosis is greater in postmenopausal women than men (6:1), but occurs asymptomatically in both. Some complain of acute pain over the fractured area or chronic lower back discomfort; however, most fractures are usually found on X-ray during medical evaluation for some other condition. These patients are not aware that the weakened skeleton has been damaged. The principal bones affected in postmenopausal women are vertebrae (crush fractures) and the distal radius. Mechanical stress or pressure, even rising from a sitting position, is enough strain to produce fractures in postmenopausal women.

Women with established osteoporosis may require a multidisciplinary approach to treatment in order to reduce or eliminate predisposing factors to fracture and to enhance elements that strengthen the body's natural defenses. Negative factors that might be eliminated include cigarette smoking, low calcium intake (recommended increase to 1500 mg daily), high caffeine and phosphate intake, sedentary lifestyle, and estrogen deficiency. Calcium can easily be consumed in the diet since one 8 oz glass of skim milk, 1 oz of cheese, and 1 cup of yogurt contain 300 to 400 mg calcium each. Otherwise calcium carbonate supplements can be taken. Weight-bearing exercises such as walking and swimming are excellent means of building the muscle support to the skeleton, thus minimizing the potential for weight-bearing fractures.

All of these recommendations are important and encouraged to begin in the perimenopausal stage of life to prevent osteoporosis. This is particularly valuable in those women who have a family history of osteoporosis, are Caucasian or Asian, have a lean body mass and short stature, and/or have premature menopause. These are among the risk factors predisposing women to osteoporosis. Whether begun earlier or not, it is expected that these positive recommendations will accompany estrogen replacement therapy in the postmenopausal woman. Because the hormone has an effect on bone metabolism, estrogen has been indicated in the treatment and prevention of osteoporosis in postmenopausal women. Estrogen reduces bone (calcium) loss and is recommended as part of the multifocal therapy of diet, calcium supplement, and exercise. In those women who have developed osteoporosis, estrogen therapy has been shown to increase bone mineral density (BMD). When estrogen treatment was discontinued or interrupted, loss of bone density was again accelerated. This beneficial action to reduce bone fracture in postmenopausal women by building bone density has been confirmed in the WHI study. However, estrogen replacement in postmenopausal women who have an intact uterus may not be the first line of treatment because the benefit to the bones may not outweigh the negative effects on the heart. Postmenopausal women who have not yet developed osteoporosis, either as a result of estrogen deficiency or senile osteoporosis, may be advised to begin calcium supplementation. Those with a family history of osteoporosis or women who begin to develop evidence of bone loss may be directed toward alternative options such as bisphosphonates (see Chapter 38). Finally, the results of the WHI study have given a new perspective on the broad recommendation of estrogens for women over 60 years old to prevent osteoporosis. Because of the increased risk of dementia reported in the WHI study, estrogen therapy may be reserved for younger women to treat the symptoms of menopause rather than long-term therapy for osteoporosis in older women. Estrogen is always a replacement therapy, it is not intended to be given to women who have functioning ovaries and normal estrogen production.

Prevention of Cardiovascular Disease

Another beneficial outgrowth of replacement therapy is the evidence that estrogen exerts a cardioprotective effect in women. The incidence of stroke and myocardial infarction in women is less than in men until age 50. At the time, the risk of cardiovascular incident is the same for men and women. Estrogen has been shown to reduce blood pressure, low-density lipoproteins (LDL-cholesterol), and serum insulin levels. At the same time, estrogen promotes high-density lipoprotein (HDL-cholesterol) levels. All of these effects were believed to directly contribute to lowering the risk of coronary heart disease and atherosclerosis. Progestins do not have the same cardioprotective effect (increase LDL).

HRT is no longer recommended as a therapy to prevent coronary heart disease in women or to protect women with preexisting coronary heart disease. The study results that led to the use of estrogen as a cardioprotective drug appear to have been done in women who, as a group, had better cholesterol levels and healthy lifestyles that favored a good environment for their heart. Therefore, the estrogen therapy alone may not have made the difference.

Alternative Estrogen Sources

There are a number of women who believe that estrogen deficiency is the natural order and do not wish to replace estrogen at all, while others at least prefer to use more natural sources of estrogen. Phytoestrogens are estrogens that are extracted from plants or absorbed from foods that contain phytoestrogens, such as spearmint. Soy products in particular are an excellent source of isoflavones, which are phytoestrogens. Soy added to the diet has been shown to decrease total cholesterol and LDL-cholesterol. The most common forms of soy are tofu, soy milk, tempeh, soy flour, and flavored soy protein powders. Such products are easily found in specialty food stores, health food stores, and stores that carry vitamin and nutritional supplements.

Oral Contraception

Combinations of estrogen and progesterone derivatives are used to prevent pregnancy. As mentioned, high hormonal levels of estrogen and progesterone inhibit the release of FSH and LH. Therefore, ovarian follicles do not undergo maturation or ovulation. In addition, changes in the endometrium and cervical mucus militate against sperm penetration as well as egg implantation. This is the most frequent method of contraception among women. If sterilization techniques for men and women are combined (tubal ligation and vasectomy), then oral contraception is second. The usual sequence is that one tablet is taken (beginning on day 5 of the menstrual cycle) for 20 to 21 consecutive days. A few days after the last tablet, bleeding (menses) occurs and the cycle is then repeated. To eliminate the need to count the days between cycles, some products are supplied with seven additional inert tablets or supplemental iron tablets. With such products, individuals take a tablet each day of the cycle. Some oral contraceptive preparations are listed in Tables 37:2 and 37:3 on page 432.

The combination (estrogen-progesterone) oral contraceptives differ in the potency of their components as well as which component exhibits predominant activity. Nevertheless, the mechanism of contraception is similar.

Oral contraceptives that contain only progesterone (progestin) are also available. The mechanism of action is not understood, but it appears that the progesterone-only contraceptives alter cervical mucus and endometrial tissue in a manner that interferes with implantation. Progestin-only contraceptives have a slightly higher failure (pregnancy) rate than do the combination products.

Most oral contraceptives are taken as individual pills each day, although quinestrol (*Estrovis*) may be taken once a week. The active drug is stored within body fat and slowly diffuses into the bloodstream over several days, where it is metabolized to the active estrogen, ethinyl estradiol. Low-dose pills, 20 to 35 μg of estrogen, are routinely used today compared to doses of 100 to 150 μg several years ago. The range of progestin dose is more flexible, going from 0.15 mg desogestrel or levonorgestrel to 1.0 mg of norethindrone or ethynodiol diacetate. (*Note:* Estrogen amounts are in microgram quantities and the progestins are always in milligram quantities.) With oral contraceptives, if one dose is missed, breakthrough spotting may occur. The potential for ovulation increases with each consecutive daily medication missed. In establishing contraception early on if the woman is sure the regimen was followed precisely yet two menstrual flow periods have not occurred, she

should be evaluated for pregnancy before continuing on hormone contraception. After several months of oral contraceptive therapy, the menstrual flow will decrease without being a signal that conception has occurred. Usually dose adjustment to a comfortable level of effectiveness is titrated against the types of unwanted effects the woman is experiencing.

Effectiveness in most cases is directly related to compliance with the daily pill schedule. Anything that facilitates user compliance decreases the chances of failure. The types of long-term contraception available today include drug delivery devices and slow-release products. Among the most recent advances in reversible contraception is the development of contraceptive implants. Levonorgestrel (*Norplant System*), a progestin enclosed within six flexible (Silastic) capsules, is implanted directly under the skin of the forearm. The unique feature of this system is that the expected life of the implanted capsules is up to 5 years. The dose of progestin (36 mg) released from each capsule is technically designed to provide adequate contraception and to ensure the progestin blood level decreases over time (years). A new set of capsules may be inserted at the end of the fifth year (as the used capsules are removed) to continue contraception. Infection or expulsion of the capsules from the site of incision (implantation) has not been a clinically significant issue among the women who have received implants. However, if a persistent infection were to develop, the capsules would be replaced. The manufacturer of *Norplant* has notified physicians and women currently using this system that this system will no longer be made available because of inconsistencies in drug availability. During the transition period, these women have to be started on another appropriate contraceptive until the implanted contraceptive is removed.

Progestasert is a T-shaped reservoir of progesterone (38 mg) that is inserted in the uterus (intrauterine). This device releases contraceptive concentrations of progesterone to the local tissue for up to 1 year. The mechanism of action is directed at interrupting pregnancy at the uterine tissue. This product does not prevent ovulation—therefore, there is a greater risk of ectopic pregnancy (ovulation and implantation outside of the uterus).

Medroxyprogesterone (*Depo-Provera*) is available for a deep IM injection that provides contraception for 3 months.

Hormone contraceptives have been used indefinitely. There is no obligatory requirement to provide a "rest period" from treatment. These contraceptives should be discontinued when a medical condition develops for which hormonal treatment is contraindicated—for example, cancer, thrombophlebitis.

The decision for women—whether to use hormone therapy even as oral contraceptives with long-term exposure—may have become more complex. It will be a few years before the results of the newest studies are fully understood.

Fertility Drugs

Anovulation

Drugs that bring about ovulation are referred to as **fertility drugs.** Currently, there are two chemical types of fertility drugs: one synthetic drug and three protein hormones extracted from human fluids. These drugs are available for patients in whom pregnancy is desired but who, for some reason, are not ovulating or releasing an egg. Anovulation can occur because the ovaries do not function (cannot respond) or do not respond to the level of endogenous anterior pituitary hormones. If the ovaries do not function, the levels of LH and FSH will be elevated due to a continuous attempt to stimulate ovulation. Elevated levels of LH and FSH are indicative of primary ovarian failure. Currently, drugs are not available that will reverse primary ovarian failure. Anovulation other than primary ovarian failure can be treated with exogenous stimulants that induce follicular growth and maturation. In these patients, fertilization and implantation may occur *in utero*. Partners therefore must engage in coitus daily during a narrow window of time after the egg has been released for fertilization to occur. Otherwise, there are a number of assisted reproductive technologies (ART), such as *in vitro* fertilization, in which ovulation may be exogenously stimulated prior to harvesting the egg for fertilization outside the body. Then implantation may be performed in the egg donor or into a surrogate uterus.

Synthetic Ovulation Stimulants

Clomiphene (*Clomid, Milophene, Serophene*) is a nonsteroidal synthetic drug that possesses some antiestrogenic activity. It is believed to stimulate the release of FSH and LH from the anterior pituitary gland. Consequently, ovarian follicle development and ovulation are stimulated. Clomiphene also binds to estrogen receptors (blocking estrogen from interacting) and through this mechanism is considered to have antiestrogenic activity. The hypothalamus and pituitary interpret the antiestrogen effect as low estrogen blood levels and respond by increasing LH and FSH secretion. This augmentation in LH, FSH, and gonadotropin secretion results in multifocal stimulation of the ovaries. Occasionally, more than one egg is produced, resulting in an increased incidence of multiple births (twinning) with the use of this drug.

Clomiphene cannot produce ovulation in patients with ovary dysfunction that will not respond to normal physiological stimulation. Frequently, this drug is used in women who are over 35 to 50 years of age, a population in whom the risk of endometrial cancer or ovulatory dysfunction is increased as a function of age. Therefore, clomiphene should not be administered without first conducting a thorough pelvic and diagnostic examination of patients.

Drug Administration

Clomiphene is readily absorbed after oral administration. The standard protocol for inducing ovulation is a 5-day treatment beginning on the fifth day of the women's menstrual cycle. One, two, or three courses of treatment may be required to achieve at least one mature follicle. If ovulation does not occur within 31 days of the first course (50 mg/day for 5 days), the second course of 100 mg/day for 5 days is given. Most women respond. However, if ovulation does not occur after the third course, the patient should be reevaluated for other underlying conditions that may be responsible for the anovulatory condition.

Polypeptide Ovulation Stimulants

Protein hormones extracted from urine are used to induce ovulation in conjunction with a polypeptide produced in placental tissue. Gonadotropin can be extracted from postmenopausal women's urine (urofollitropin, *Metrodin*) or purified (menotropins, *Pergonal, Humegon*) from the urine. These hormones acting as FSH and LH stimulate follicles to mature and rupture. After the last dose of gonadotropin, human chorionic gonadotropin (HCG, *A.P.L., Chorex-5, Gonic, Pregnyl*) is given to stimulate production of progesterone from the corpus luteum of the ruptured follicle. If implantation of a fertilized egg occurs, the placenta that develops will then supply an endogenous source of HCG. Gonadotropins are amazing polypeptides. For example, HCG has an amino acid sequence (α subunit) that is identical to endogenous FSH, LH, and TSH. While these protein hormones are primarily used in women, menotropins and HCG are also used in men to stimulate spermatogenesis. In men, HCG stimulates the Leydig cells of the testis to produce androgens, and it permits the testis to descend in certain types of prepubertal cryptorchism and hypogonadism.

Drug Administration

Urofollitropin and menotropin are administered intramuscularly in one to three courses. The first course is 75 IU/day for 7 to 12 days followed by 5000 to 10,000 U IM of HCG 1 day after the last dose of the tropins. The tropin dose represents 75 IU of LH and 75 IU of FSH. Urine is tested for estrogen concentration to determine whether multiple follicles have developed (> 150 μg in 24 hours) rather than one dominant follicle. Couples should be advised to avoid coitus when multiple follicles have developed because of the significant potential for multiple fertilization. Patient reevaluation is warranted if ovulation does not occur after three courses of treatment.

Menstrual Bleeding Disorders

In nonmenopausal women, menstrual disorders **(amenorrhea**—no menstruation—and **dysmenorrhea**—painful or difficult menstruation) or postpartum engorgement of breast tissue may also be alleviated by the use of estrogens, progesterones, or estrogen-progesterone combinations. Estrogens have been administered within 8 hours after delivery to reduce breast engorgement. However, patients often respond to analgesics and supportive therapy until tissue resorption occurs, thereby avoiding the risks of estrogen administration. Progesterone, 5 to 10 mg IM daily for 8 days, will promote bleeding in amenorrhea and spontaneous normal cycles in dysfunctional uterine bleeding.

Cancer Therapy

Certain cancers—particularly those involving the breast, uterus, and prostate gland—appear to be dependent on the presence of the sex hormones. Removal of the ovaries and testes has produced beneficial results in some cases. In other cases, use of the sex hormones appears to antagonize tumor growth, especially where the sex hormones are applied to a patient of the opposite sex. Megestrol (*Megace*) is specifically used in the treatment of advanced carcinoma of the breast, whereas medroxyprogesterone (*Depo-Provera*) is used for adjunctive and palliative treatment of inoperable cancer of the endometrium or kidney. Diethylstilbestrol is used in inoperable prostatic

cancer when patients do not have estrogen-dependent cancer or an active thromboembolic disorder.

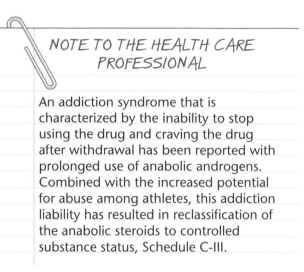

NOTE TO THE HEALTH CARE PROFESSIONAL

An addiction syndrome that is characterized by the inability to stop using the drug and craving the drug after withdrawal has been reported with prolonged use of anabolic androgens. Combined with the increased potential for abuse among athletes, this addiction liability has resulted in reclassification of the anabolic steroids to controlled substance status, Schedule C-III.

Adverse Effects of Female Hormones

Adverse effects related to estrogen or progestogen use include nausea, vomiting, headache, dizziness, irritability, depression, fluid retention, breast tenderness, and weight gain. Usually, the severity of these effects does not warrant medical intervention or can be ameliorated by reducing the dose or changing to another product. Breakthrough bleeding or amenorrhea usually resolves to a consistent menstrual pattern within 3 months of continuing treatment. However, extended hormone therapy has been associated with more serious adverse effects that require stopping the drug.

Oral contraceptives have been associated with thrombophlebitis, stroke, and myocardial infarction (see note, page 433). Recently published literature reviewing hundreds to thousands of women has provided new insight on the risks of estrogen exposure. Over the past 20 years women seem to have been carefully guided to appropriate selections of oral contraceptives based on the predisposing risk factors for cardiovascular events. Thus, women who had a family history or current evidence of hypertension, diabetes, or hypercholesterolemia were not prescribed oral contraceptives or received much lower dose regimens. As a result, the incidence of cardiovascular disorders can be evaluated in risk-free women exposed to specific estrogen doses—that is, high-dose, long-term treatment (50 to 100 μg) versus low-dose, long-term treatment (20 to 35 μg). This provides a clearer picture of the risks of estrogen exposure without complications from other underlying conditions. The results demonstrate that low-dose oral contraceptives do not increase the risk of stroke in women; however, oral contraceptives and smoking continue to increase the risk of developing hemorrhagic stroke. In addition, since estrogen reduces LDL and increases HDL-cholesterol, the risk of developing coronary heart disease is reduced 20 to 50 percent. (It is interesting that transdermal estrogen preparations that bypass the liver initially do not appear to provide cardioprotective effects.)

Women who require prolonged hormone therapy for any reason should be monitored closely. The lowest effective dose should be selected and patients should be reevaluated annually. There is no evidence that the naturally occurring hormones are safer than the synthetic drugs—the key is identifying the appropriate lowest effective dose. The dose and length of treatment are two important factors associated with the potential for adverse events after individual patient risk factors have been considered.

Fertility Drugs

Ovarian hyperstimulation syndrome is a significant adverse effect because of the potential for multiple fertilization. Virtually all physicians who engage in assisted reproductive technologies are specialists who are well acquainted with the physical risks to the mother and fetuses. Although these specialists can monitor biochemical activity, only abstinence from intercourse will ensure multiple fertilization will not occur. Other effects during the course of treatment may include bloating, stomach or pelvic pain, enlarged ovaries, ovarian cysts, blurred vision, and hypersensitivity reactions. Hot flashes, breast discomfort, headache, or nausea may be directly related to the antiestrogenic actions of clomiphene. Men may experience gynecomastia, breast pain, and mastitis.

Risks of Hormone Replacement Therapy

The serious cardiovascular events associated with oral contraceptive therapy do appear to occur in postmenopausal women who are receiving hormone replacement therapy. Recent studies have demonstrated that among postmenopausal women who took conjugated estrogens for up to 10 years, the risk of death from any cause is decreased 37 percent. This is because of the lower doses of estrogen used in postmenopausal women. Estrogen protects against osteoporosis and reduces fatality. Although physicians are encouraging women to begin estrogen therapy after menopause, it is estimated that 70 percent of the prescriptions written are never taken to the pharmacy to be filled. Why? Because the better-informed growing population of postmenopausal women (40 million) is concerned about two specific effects of long-term hormone therapy: endometrial cancer and breast cancer.

Chronic estrogen use taken unopposed (no progestin) is associated with an increased risk of developing endometrial cancer in postmenopausal women. This risk is one to six times higher than the risk for endometrial cancer in women with an intact uterus who never took endogenous estrogen. When a variety of factors is considered, the risk ranges between 2 and 13 times greater. Progestin, which is now added to estrogen replacement therapy, reduces the risk of endometrial cancer by directly downregulating estrogen receptors.

The risk for breast cancer does not have a similar story. Women with a history of early onset of menstruation and late menopause (long natural estrogen production) who are on HRT appear to have a greater incidence of breast cancer. These are women with intact ovaries at menopause. Whether this incidence is due to a synergistic estrogen action on breast tissue or better medical follow-up today is not known.

NOTE TO THE HEALTH CARE PROFESSIONAL

Patients receiving hormone therapy should be instructed to report incidences of pain or alteration in their vision (**diplopia**—double vision—or loss of vision). Pain in the legs, groin, or chest or changes in vision may be associated with thrombosis and may necessitate immediate drug discontinuation. A physician should be alerted if patients experience shortness of breath, abnormal bleeding, breast lumps, or yellowing of the skin or eyes.

Nevertheless, a positive history of breast cancer in the family or personal history mitigates against HRT in such women.

For HRT, women are faced with a complex decision: good health, improved longevity, or possible cancer. Women are anticipating a potential hormone exposure of 40-plus years (treatment for life), and the peak risk for heart disease and/or osteoporosis doesn't occur until 10 to 20 years after menopause. One school of thought is that hormone treatment need not begin until much later (60 years old) so that the long-term benefits outweigh potential risks. Meanwhile, the next significant development in this area of pharmacology is likely to be specially designed hormone molecules that do not effect endometrial and/or breast cancer.

Contraindications

Because of the potentially life-threatening adverse effects, oral contraceptives should not be used in women with a history of thrombophlebitis, liver disease, undiagnosed breast lumps, or unexplained vaginal bleeding. Persistent vaginal bleeding in women with an intact uterus should be monitored to rule out the possibility of carcinoma. Women with a history of diabetes, high blood pressure, or a seizure disorder may not be good candidates for oral contraceptives either.

Estrogens and oral contraceptives are contraindicated in women who are pregnant or have an estrogen-dependent cancer. Estrogen use during early pregnancy can affect fetal development. Congenital heart defects and limb formation defects have occurred even with localized intrauterine exposure to female hormones. Fertility drugs are also contraindicated in primary ovarian failure and during pregnancy. Birth defects have occurred in patients exposed to gonadotropins and clomiphene during pregnancy. Estrogens, progestins, and drugs used to induce ovulation are designated FDA Pregnancy Category X: The risk of use in pregnant women clearly outweighs any possible benefit.

Diethylstilbestrol (DES) has been linked to alterations in fetal development when given to pregnant women. Female fetuses exposed *in utero* to DES reportedly developed changes in vaginal and cervical tissue (vaginal adenosis and vaginal and cervical cancer) that do not become evident until the offspring reach maturity. Congenital abnormalities such as structural problems of the genitourinary tract have also occurred in males exposed *in utero* to DES. It is worth noting that DES is an effective postcoital contraceptive when taken orally within 72 hours after intercourse (25 mg BID for 5 days). At present, however, DES is considered an emergency treatment, not a routine method of birth control.

Drug Interactions

Reports of drug interactions with the use of estrogens or progestogens have been associated primarily with the use of oral contraceptives. Although numerous drugs have been indicated, evidence of a clinically significant interaction is usually not overwhelming. Nevertheless, it is probably prudent for patients taking oral contraceptives to seek an alternate form of contraception if the following drugs also are used: barbiturates, carbamazepine, griseofulvin, neomycin, penicillin, phenytoin, salicylates, tetracyclines, and rifampin. These drugs may increase the metabolism of oral contraceptives, thus reducing their effectiveness. Estrogens not necessarily associated with oral contraceptives have reduced the clearance of corticosteroids, prolonging the steroid action. It has also been hypothesized that contraceptive-induced fluid retention may precipitate seizures in epileptic patients. Although additional evidence is needed to support this proposal, an alternate form of contraception should be used in appropriate patients at risk. Estrogens interact with hydantoins used for seizure control, resulting in breakthrough bleeding, spotting, and pregnancy.

Oral contraceptives have been reported to decrease the anticoagulant response to dicumarol. The mechanism appears to involve hormone-induced stimulation of clotting factors rather than interference with the metabolism of the oral anticoagulant. Oral contraceptives increase the elimination of clofibrate and increase the clearance of benzodiazepines through enhanced metabolism. This may reduce the effectiveness of clofibrate and benzodiazepines in some patients.

Special Considerations

Women interested in using oral contraceptives must be educated about the proper use of these drugs as well as the associated risks. A combination product or progestin-only product must be taken daily as recommended by the manufacturer. Sexually active women should be aware that not taking the drug as scheduled increases the risk of becoming pregnant. If two consecutive menstrual periods are missed while a woman is taking an oral contraceptive, a physician should be consulted immediately. The physician can perform appropriate tests to establish whether conception has occurred. The risks of exposing a developing embryo or fetus to these hormones clearly warrant such caution. Women using oral contraceptives who want to become pregnant should discontinue the oral contraceptive 3 months before trying to conceive and use alternate birth control during that time.

Diabetic women who are receiving hormone therapy may experience changes in glucose tolerance. For this reason, during estrogen therapy, diabetic patients should be alerted to the potential for changes in glucose levels observed during routine glucose monitoring and the symptoms that may accompany these changes.

Women who choose to have an intrauterine device inserted should have the placement just after a menstrual flow and a confirmed negative pregnancy test to ensure fertilization has not occurred. The device should be replaced every 12 months. If the retrieval threads are not visible at any time during the year, the device should be removed by the physician and replaced.

MALE SEX HORMONES (ANDROGENS)

Male sex hormones are generally referred to as **androgens.** The main sex hormone of the male is testosterone, which is produced by the testes. The adrenal cortex of both sexes produces small amounts of other male hormones. Testosterone production is controlled by the release of LH, also known as interstitial cell-stimulating hormone (ICSH) from the anterior pituitary gland. The major function of testosterone is to stimulate the development of male sex organs (prostate, seminal vesicles, scrotum, and penis) and to maintain the secondary sex characteristics (hair distribution, vocal cord thickening, and changes in musculature) of the male. In addition, testosterone produces an anabolic effect that promotes synthesis and retention of proteins (muscle and bone) in the body.

Androgens

Deficiencies of testosterone may be caused by pituitary disorders, testicular failure, or castration. Androgens are administered as replacement therapy to maintain male sex characteristics and organ function. Testosterone is often the drug of choice over the available synthetic androgens. Testosterone is metabolized in the intestine and liver; therefore, the intramuscular route of administration is preferred to achieve adequate blood levels. Testosterone is available for injection as an aqueous or oil suspension (short acting). In addition, various depo preparations can provide adequate blood concentrations for a period of 4 weeks. There are two transdermal testosterone patch products that

are interesting because they cannot be applied in the same manner. The *Transderm* patch is applied to the scrotal region for 24 hours and changed daily for up to 8 weeks. If scrotal descent does not occur within 8 weeks, the patient must be reevaluated for another type of testosterone. The *Androderm* patch, used for the same indication as *Transderm,* cannot be applied to the scrotum. *Androderm* is applied to the back, abdomen, arms, or thighs daily until clinical results are adequate. The patch remains on the application site for 24 hours and must be rotated so that the same site is used no less than every 7 days. Some androgenic drugs are listed in Table 37:4.

Clinical Indications

Androgens are approved for use in males as replacement therapy in primary hypogonadism, hypogonadotropic hypogonadism, delayed puberty, and impotence that is the result of androgen deficiency. The hypogonadism may be congenital or acquired. In women, androgens are approved for the treatment of metastatic inoperable breast cancer and postpartum breast engorgement.

Anabolic Action

Many chronic diseases are characteristically associated with significant protein catabolism and weight loss. In some clinical situations, androgens are administered because of their ability to stimulate protein synthesis **(anabolism).** In conjunction with a diet designed to increase caloric intake, patients usually experience an increase in appetite and weight on anabolic therapy.

Androgens have been used to stimulate the production of red blood cells **(erythropoiesis)** in patients with refractory anemia, particularly those with renal disease. Anabolic steroids have been used as adjunctive drugs to improve athletic performance. Anabolic steroids do increase lean muscle mass, partly through the tissue retention of sodium and water. There is some question, however, whether this practice actually enhances physical ability and warrants exposure to the potential adverse effects of these drugs. Adverse effects associated with chronic use of these hormones may be serious and irreversible.

Androgen Use in Females

Androgen therapy has been beneficial in some cases of metastatic breast cancer. Androgen therapy has inhibited tumor growth while retaining the anabolic effects of increased protein

TABLE 37:4 Examples of Androgenic Drugs

DRUG (TRADE NAME)*	DOSE	ROUTE	USE
Short-acting Parenteral Androgens*:			
testosterone (*Histerone 100, Tesamone Testosterone Aqueous*)	25–50 mg 2–3 times/week	IM	Androgen deficiency, replacement therapy
testosterone Transdermal System (*Transderm, Androderm*)	1 patch applied to the skin for 24 hours		Transdermal
Androgen Deficiency			
testosterone (oil) (*Testosterone Propionate*)	50 mg–400 mg every 2–4 weeks	IM	Androgen deficiency, replacement therapy
	25–50 mg/day 3–4 days (40–100 mg/m^2/dose)		Hypogonadism
	50–100 mg 3 times/week	IM	Carcinoma of the breast
Long-acting Parenteral Androgens*:			
testosterone (oil) (*Andro-LA 200, Delatestryl, Depo-Testosterone, Depotest 100, 200, Duratest-100, 200, Everone 200, Testosterone Enanthate*)	50–400 mg every 2 weeks 200–400 mg every 2–4 weeks	IM IM	Deficiency, replacement therapy Carcinoma of the breast
Oral Androgens*:			
fluoxymesterone (*Halotestin*)	5–20 mg/day	PO	Replacement therapy
	5–10 mg/day for 4 to 5 days	PO	Postpartum breast engorgement
	10–40 mg/day	PO	Carcinoma of the breast
methyltestosterone (*Oreton Methyl, Android-25, Testred, Virilon*)	10–50 mg/day (5–25 mg) 80 mg/day for 3 to 5 days	PO (Buccal) PO (Buccal)	Replacement therapy Postpartum breast engorgement
	50–200 mg/day (25–100 mg) 30 mg/day	PO (Buccal)	Carcinoma of the breast Postpubertal cryptorchism
Anabolic Androgens:**			
nandrolone (*Durabolin*)	25–50 mg/week	IM	Breast cancer in women
nandrolone decanoate (*Deca-Durabolin*)	50–100 mg/week 100–200 mg/week	IM	Anemias of renal disease in women Anemias of renal disease in men
oxandrolone (*Oxandrin*)	2.5 mg BID to QID every 2–4 weeks	PO	Promote weight gain where protein breakdown is part of the underlying condition
oxymetholone (*Anadrol 50*)	1–5 mg/kg/day	PO	Anemias from deficient RBC production
stanozolol (*Winstrol*)	2 mg TID	PO	Aplastic anemia

*Not an inclusive list of available products.
**These preparations are classified as Schedule C-III.

synthesis and weight gain. Androgens have also been used to manage the symptoms (pain and swelling) associated with **fibrocystic breast disease,** but this therapy has been replaced by therapy using other agents.

Miscellaneous Use

Androgens are classified as Schedule III drugs because of their high potential for abuse and misuse. These drugs are being used by men who believe the anabolic actions maintain strength and virility after the age of 50. Between 40 and 70 years of age, men may lose 10 to 20 pounds of muscle mass, 15 percent of their bone mass resulting in a loss of 2 inches in height, and testosterone levels drop 30 percent. An estimated 15 percent of men are completely impotent by age 70. Testosterone has been shown to increase muscle mass and reduce bone loss through mineral excretion. While moods, libidos, and cholesterol levels improved, testosterone does not correct impotence. In the vast majority of cases, impotence at any age is related to vascular disease, or conditions that impair tissue perfusion such as cardiovascular disease, diabetes, smoking, and alcoholism. Testosterone has been used for years by athletes, especially body builders, to increase size, strength, and endurance. Today testosterone is available in a variety of convenient formulations, tablets, injection, and a transdermal patch. With the generation of postwar babies entering this zone (age 50 years or older), there is a great likelihood that androgen use will increase during the next 10 to 20 years. Dihydroepiandrosterone (DHEA) is naturally produced by the adrenals and promotes testosterone production. Dihydroepiandrosterone is currently not categorized as a drug but as a nutritional supplement, not requiring a prescription for purchase. Proponents of DHEA believe that oral supplements produce the desired physiological and psychological effects through testosterone production.

Adverse Effects

The main adverse effects produced by the androgens are caused by overdose. In adult males, high testosterone levels inhibit the release of FSH (anterior pituitary), which is needed for sperm production. The result is **oligospermia,** or a reduced sperm count. Adult males also may develop gynecomastia and priapism during androgen therapy. In prepubertal boys, there is a stunting of growth due to premature closure of the bone epiphyses. In females, masculinization occurs, which is characterized by **hirsutism,**

menstrual irregularities, changes in the external genitalia, acne, and a deepening of the voice. Other adverse effects include jaundice, nausea, vomiting, and diarrhea. Long-term high-dose testosterone exposure such as that seen with use in athletes has been associated with tumors, reduced HDL-cholesterol, and sterility.

Drug Interactions

Anabolic steroids have been reported to alter the pharmacological effects of such drugs as oral anticoagulants, antidiabetic drugs, and other steroids. With concomitant androgen therapy, the dose of oral anticoagulants may need to be reduced to maintain coagulation control. It has been proposed that the androgens may decrease the formation of clotting factors, which are also influenced by the oral anticoagulants. By affecting carbohydrate metabolism, androgens may decrease blood glucose levels, necessitating a reduction in insulin or oral antidiabetic dosage to maintain proper glucose levels in diabetic patients. Because androgens are steroids that facilitate the retention of sodium and water, it is not surprising that androgens given in the presence of other steroid therapy enhance the development of edema.

Special Considerations and Contraindications

Androgens are contraindicated in men with carcinoma of the breast or prostate. Androgens should never be used during pregnancy because **virilization** of the female fetus will occur. Although virilization occurs to some extent in female patients being treated for breast carcinoma, these patients should report changes to the physician to avoid irreversible virilizing effects. Androgenic steroids cause the retention of sodium, water, and calcium. In patients with carcinoma, hypercalcemia may be a signal to discontinue androgen therapy.

Since androgenic steroids are metabolized quickly following oral use, patients using buccal tablets should be instructed not to swallow the tablets, but to allow each tablet to dissolve under the tongue or in the cheek. **Buccal absorption** enables the drug to bypass intestinal and hepatic metabolism. Diabetic patients receiving androgen therapy should be monitored for alterations in glucose tolerance so that antidiabetic medications can be adjusted to meet their needs. Similarly, patients receiving oral anticoagulants should be observed for petechiae or other signs of hemorrhage. Such signs indicate the need to adjust the oral anticoagulant dose during androgen therapy.

IMPOTENCE

Impotence is the inability to perform sexual function often associated in men as dysfunctional erection or inability to achieve an erection. Impotence may result from nerve or spinal damage so that stimulatory impulses no longer reach the muscles of the penis to evoke a physical action. It is also an adverse effect of certain chronic medications (e.g., cardiovascular drugs) that apparently diminish blood flow to the penis, inhibit nerve excitability, or alter psychomotor (brain) activity, any of which eliminates or decreases the normal response during sexual stimulation. Although male hormone replacement (the subject of this chapter) is not a recommended or effective treatment for impotence, the importance of a new breakthrough therapy, sildenafil, warrants presentation here.

Sildenafil (*Viagra*) Clinical Indication

Sildenafil (*Viagra*) is an oral phosphodiesterase inhibitor specifically indicated for erectile dysfunction in men. A family of enzymes distributed throughout the body known as phosphodiesterases (PDE) catalyze reactions that influence or cause a variety of muscle and visual actions. The PDE family is differentiated by number as follows: PDE1, PDE2, . . . PDE6. . . . Amazingly, sildenafil selectively inhibits PDE5, which brokers the biochemical reaction in the blood vessels of the penis resulting in increased blood flow and penile rigidity associated with sexual stimulation. This drug does not increase or affect erection in men who are not impotent, and it does not affect erection that is not a result of sexual stimulation. The recommended effective doses are 25 to 100 mg taken within 1 hour of sexual activity, but to be taken only once a day. Since a physiological dysfunction does also occur in women, the drug is being evaluated for its potential effectiveness in women. At this time however, the drug is not approved for use in women and is designated as FDA Pregnancy Category B.

Adverse Effects

The effects most frequently reported during the investigation of sildenafil included headache, flushing of the skin, upset stomach, nasal congestion, diarrhea, and rash. Specific visual effects, color tinged vision, and sensitivity to light or blurred vision have also been reported to occur. While more investigation is required to understand these adverse effects, it is noteworthy that PDE6 is responsible for normal color vision in the retina.

Contraindications

Sildenafil should not be used in patients who are taking nitrates because a synergistic decrease in blood pressure may produce severe hypotension and/or other cardiovascular sequelae that are life-threatening. Although sildenafil increases the blood flow to the penis, it has not been associated with priapism (sustained erection often accompanied by pain). Nevertheless, this drug should be used with caution in patients who may have conditions that predispose them to priapism such as sickle cell anemia, leukemia, or predisposing anatomical conditions.

Patient Administration and Monitoring

After hormone therapy has been prescribed, patients should be contacted by phone or office visit within 4 to 12 weeks to review patient concerns, the safety profile, and potential compliance issues. Serum testosterone levels may be taken 4 weeks into treatment to confirm the dose response for male patients. Otherwise, special blood tests are not required unless there is a medical issue to be evaluated. Annually, patients should receive a full evaluation—that is, breast, abdominal, and pelvic exam for women.

Remember, once the appropriate dose is established, replacement of male or female hormones is usually associated with a positive self-image. This encourages patient compliance with the medication schedule, which is critical to the success of contraception, prophylaxis against bone and heart disease, and symptom resolution in male and female patients. The lowest effective dose is the proper choice. More is not better, especially with estrogens, testosterone, and DHEA. It should be kept in mind that the prescribing physician is not always the physician most frequently visited for physical examinations or seasonal problem—for example, flu, allergy. Women may be given hormones by a gynecologist or fertility specialist, while men today may be seen by sports medicine specialists. When interviewing and monitoring patients who are taking hormones, the information that follows should be provided to the patient.

General Information

Encourage patients to disclose all medications with all of their physicians, even if the physician is visited infrequently, so that their medication history at other health care centers is current. This counters the possibility of another medication being given that might decrease the hormone effect or produce a serious adverse effect.

Instruct patients that hormonal contraceptives do not protect against them against sexually transmitted diseases and human immunodeficiency virus (HIV). Barriers such as condoms are the only means of protection from microbial transmission during intercourse.

Patients taking clomiphene must be instructed to observe caution when driving, operating heavy machinery, or performing tasks requiring coordination or dexterity because this drug may produce dizziness, visual disturbances, and lightheadedness.

Drug Administration

Oral medications, especially contraceptives, should be taken at the same time every day. To develop compliance, the patient can be instructed to take medication with meals or at bedtime. When just starting oral contraceptive therapy, the patient should be advised to use an alternate form of birth control during the first week in addition to the oral contraceptive. This permits adequate time for the hormones to reach their effective blood levels.

If the patient experiences nausea or gastrointestinal upset when taking oral medication, the medication may be taken with meals to minimize the effect.

Buccal tablets (androgens) should not be swallowed. Instruct the patient to hold the tablet between the gum and cheek until it dissolves completely. While the tablet is in place the patient must avoid eating, drinking, and smoking.

Vaginal gels should not be used concurrently with other intravaginal treatments including douching. For patients who are using other intravaginal products, apply the hormone gel 6 hours before or after other products.

Review the appropriate application of transdermal testosterone patches with the patient. Be clear which patch system is being used (*Transderm* goes on the scrotum, *Androderm* does not go on the scrotom). The skin must be clean and dry shaved if necessary to provide adequate patch to skin contact.

Menopause

There are some changes in diet and environment that are often of help in minimizing the symptom triggers. Vasomotor symptoms may be triggered by a variety of substances such as alcohol, spicy foods, citrus, strawberries, and chocolate, as well as environmental factors, stress, and hot and humid weather. Ice water, chilled fruits, and frozen grapes often relieve the "rising hot feeling" and have minimal negative impact on weight gain. Synthetic fabrics such as polyesters or nylon do not "breathe" and, although feeling lighter in weight, actually trap perspiration against the skin. Natural fibers such as cotton are ideal for air flow. Even in winter, cotton layering is better than heavier wool or acrylic clothing. Layering (camisole, blouse, vest, cardigan) permits easy shedding of clothing for comfort as needed.

Vaginal dryness and painful intercourse may be relieved by using water-based vaginal lubricants (*Replens, Astroglide*).

Patients should be instructed that estrogens may cause photosensitivity so they should avoid prolonged exposure to sunlight. Sunscreens and protective clothing are advisable until it is evident whether the patient is experiencing photosensitivity.

Notifying the Prescribing Physician

Breakthrough bleeding or spotting that lasts for more than a few days or occurs in more than one menstrual cycle while receiving hormones should be reported to the prescribing physician immediately.

Intrauterine devices: Patients should notify the physician immediately if abnormal or excessive bleeding, severe cramping, abnormal vaginal discharge, fever or flu-like symptoms, genital lesions, or sores develop.

Diabetic patients must be instructed to be alert for changes that may occur during estrogen treatment. The prescribing physician should be notified immediately if any of the following occur:

- *pain in the calves or groin*
- *sharp chest pain*
- *shortness of breath*
- *abnormal vaginal bleeding*
- *missed menstrual period*
- *severe headache*
- *numbness in the arms or legs*
- *yellowing of the skin or eyes*
- *severe depression*

Glucose tolerance may be decreased, especially with progestins and anabolic steroids. Alert diabetic patients to the potential for fluctuations in their blood sugar levels during routine monitoring. Patients should report significant changes in glucose levels and associated symptoms to the prescribing physician.

Epileptic patients should notify the prescribing physician immediately if migraine or seizures occur during hormone therapy. Patient evaluation will determine whether the seizures are related to fluid retention associated with the hormone treatment.

Female patients receiving androgens should notify the physician if hoarseness, voice deepening, baldness, hirsutism, acne, or menstrual irregularities occur for further evaluation.

Pregnancy

Patients must be informed that all hormones are contraindicated during pregnancy. If the patient becomes pregnant, the prescribing physician should be notified immediately for appropriate discontinuation of treatment. These products are designated FDA Pregnancy Category X: the risk to the fetus outweighs any possible benefit to the mother.

Chapter Review

Understanding Terminology

Match the definition or description in the left column with the appropriate term in the right column.

___ **1.** The development of masculine characteristics, such as muscular frame and body hair, in females.

___ **2.** The lining of the uterus.

___ **3.** Reduced sperm count.

___ **4.** Absorption of a drug through the skin, such as with a patch.

___ **5.** A disease that results in a decrease in bone density, usually associated with older women.

___ **6.** A process that converts nutritional substances into tissue; usually associated with the conversion of protein into muscle mass.

___ **7.** A condition in women in which body and facial hair is excessive.

___ **8.** Male sex hormones.

___ **9.** A condition in which menstruation ceases.

___ **10.** A condition associated with painful menstruation.

___ **11.** Absorption of a drug through the mucous membranes lining the cheek.

a. amenorrhea

b. anabolism

c. androgens

d. buccal absorption

e. dysmenorrhea

f. endometrium

g. hirsutism

h. osteoporosis

i. oligospermia

j. transdermal absorption

k. virilization

Answer the following questions in the spaces provided.

12. Define *equipotent*. _____

_____

_____

13. Differentiate between conception and contraception. _____

_____

14. Write a short paragraph using the following terms: *lactation, menopause, menstruation, puberty,* and *ovulation.* _____

_____

_____

Acquiring Knowledge

Answer the following questions in the spaces provided.

1. Where are the sex hormones produced? _____

_____

2. Briefly describe the production of the estrogens and progesterone in relation to the ovarian follicle. _____

_____

_____

3. What is the mechanism of action of the oral contraceptives? _____
_____

4. List the main uses of the female sex hormones in medical treatment. _____
_____

5. What adverse effects are associated with estrogen and oral contraceptive therapy for females?
_____

6. How is the production of testosterone regulated in males? _____
_____

7. Briefly describe the main effects produced by testosterone in males. _____
_____

8. List the main uses of the androgens. _____
_____

9. What are the adverse effects of androgen therapy in females? _____
_____

Applying Knowledge—On the Job

Use your critical thinking skills to answer the following questions in the spaces provided.

1. Assume you work in an ob-gyn practice. Many of the patients are menopausal and considering estrogen replacement therapy. Which patients should be cautioned against this therapy?
_____

2. Assume you work in a family-planning clinic, where many patients consider using oral contraceptives. Which patients should be cautioned to use a different means of birth control?
_____

3. DES is contraindicated for use during pregnancy. Why? _____
_____

4. Should a patient taking oral contraceptives be warned regarding possible drug interactions with antibiotics? _____
_____

5. What should a patient being placed on oral contraceptives for the first time be told regarding sexual activity? _____
_____
_____

Internet Connection

Among the best sites providing information on hormone replacement and osteoporosis medications is www.nlm.nih.gov/medlineplus/hormonereplacementtherapy.html.

Heart and Estrogen Progestin Replacement Study (HERS) presents the risks and benefits of estrogen and progestin therapy in healthy postmenopausal women. The results of this large clinical trial are presented in the *Journal of the American Medical Association* at http://jama.ama-assn.org/issues/v288n3/ffull/joc21036.html.

At www.osteo.org, the National Institutes of Health offers current information on metabolic bone diseases such as osteoporosis and Paget's disease. The mission of this site is to educate patients and the public about metabolic bone diseases.

Data on Oral Contraceptives and Cancer Risk since these drugs first became available to American women in the early 1960s are presented at http://cis.nci.nih.gov/fact/313.htm.

Finally, www.findarticles.com is a site that allows you to enter a topic, word, or phrase such as *Androgens* or *Oral Contraceptives* to obtain relevant articles from worldwide medical information sources for online review. The articles are usually in English and are one to six pages in length. In addition to renowned journals such as the *British Medical Journal* and the *Journal of the American Medical Association,* this site provides a fair balance of information from sports medicine and news articles.

Additional Reading

Cadoff, J. 1997. Your Hormones. *Parents Magazine* 39.

Cheever, M. 1992. Cardiovascular implications of anabolic steroid abuse. *Journal of Cardiovascular Nursing* 5:19.

Gaby, A. *Preventing and Reversing Osteoporosis.* Prima Publishing, Rocklin, CA, 1994.

Gambrell, R. D. 1991. Estrogen replacement therapy and osteoporosis. *Hospital Practice Supplement* 25 (Supp. 1):30.

Petitti, D. G. 1996. Stroke in users of low-dose oral contraceptives. *New England Journal of Medicine* 335 (1):8.

38

DRUGS AFFECTING THE THYROID AND PARATHYROID GLANDS AND BONE DEGENERATION

CHAPTER FOCUS

This chapter describes substances that have a direct action on organs to promote tissue growth, particularly soft tissue and bone. It explains that these substances are produced naturally by the body but can be obtained from animal sources to replenish the body's supply in conditions associated with a deficiency.

CHAPTER OBJECTIVES

After studying this chapter, you should be able to

- describe the differences in the functions of the thyroid gland and the parathyroid glands.

- name two secretions from the thyroid that stimulate tissue growth.

- identify two effects that occur with chronic thyroid deficiency in children.

- explain why goiter occurs in adult thyroid deficiency.

- describe two sites at which antithyroid drugs reduce hyperthyroid activity.

- describe the action of calcitonin.

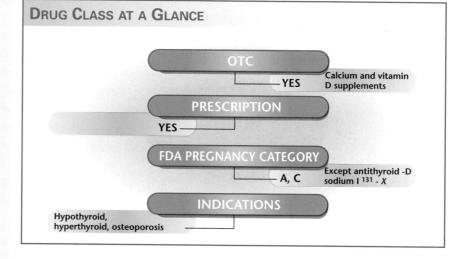

DRUG CLASS AT A GLANCE

OTC — YES — Calcium and vitamin D supplements

PRESCRIPTION — YES

FDA PREGNANCY CATEGORY — A, C — Except antithyroid -D sodium I ^{131} - X

INDICATIONS — Hypothyroid, hyperthyroid, osteoporosis

Key Terms

agranulocytosis: acute condition in which there is a reduction in the number of white blood cells (WBCs), specifically polymorphonuclear cells.

anion: ion that carries a negative (−) charge.

autoimmune disease: condition in which an individual's tissues are damaged by his or her own immune mechanisms.

cretinism: condition in which the development of the body and the brain has been inhibited.

goiter: condition in which the thyroid is enlarged, but not as a result of a tumor.

hypercalcemia: unusually high concentration of calcium in the blood.

myxedema: condition associated with a decrease in thyroid function, caused by removal of thyroid tissue or loss of tissue function because of damage to cells; also associated with subcutaneous edema and slowed metabolism.

osteoporosis: condition associated with a decrease in bone density so that the bones are thin and fracture easily.

Paget's disease: condition in older adults in which the bone density is altered so that softening and bending of the weight-bearing bones occurs.

polypeptide: substance, usually large, composed of an indefinite number of amino acids.

thyrotoxic crisis: condition caused by excessive quantities of thyroid hormone, either from a natural source of hypersecretion or exogenous administration of a drug.

INTRODUCTION

The thyroid gland produces three hormones that are essential for the growth and development of tissues. These thyroid hormones include triiodothyronine (T_3), thyroxine (T_4), and thyrocalcitonin (calcitonin, TCT). All of these hormones directly influence the activity of all peripheral tissues.

THYROID FUNCTION, PHARMACOLOGY, AND DISORDERS

The thyroid hormones triiodothyronine (T_3) and thyroxine (T_4) are concerned with tissue growth, especially muscle and nerve tissue. Thyrocalcitonin, however, primarily affects only one peripheral tissue, namely bone. The secretion of T_3 and T_4 is under the control of thyroid-stimulating hormone (TSH), which is an anterior pituitary hormone (see Figure 38:1). Once in the circulation, T_3 and T_4 stimulate protein synthesis, increase blood glucose and circulating fatty acids, and decrease serum cholesterol. These substances are essential for cell building, repair, and energy. By stimulating cell metabolism, these thyroid hormones also increase the basal metabolic rate (BMR) and heat production.

Drugs are used to influence the action of thyroid hormones in two conditions: hyposecretion of hormone (hypothyroidism) and hypersecretion of hormone (hyperthyroidism).

Hyposecretion of Hormones

Hyposecretion of thyroid hormones may occur as a result of glandular destruction. Glandular damage is produced by excessive exposure to radiation (X-ray), lack of iodine, pituitary dysfunction (lack of TSH), or surgical removal of thyroid tissue. Hypothyroidism (lack of T_3 and T_4) in infants and children produces mental and physical retardation **(cretinism).**

FIGURE 38:1   Thyroid Hormone Secretion

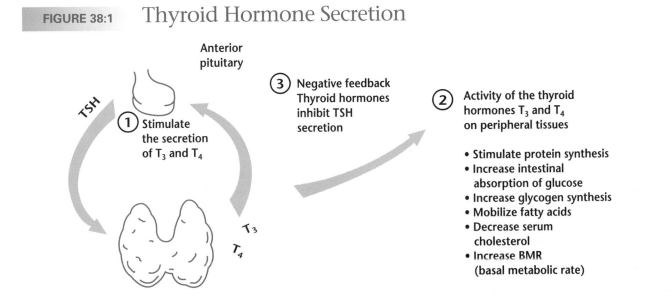

Anterior pituitary

TSH

(1) Stimulate the secretion of T_3 and T_4

(3) Negative feedback
Thyroid hormones inhibit TSH secretion

(2) Activity of the thyroid hormones T_3 and T_4 on peripheral tissues

- Stimulate protein synthesis
- Increase intestinal absorption of glucose
- Increase glycogen synthesis
- Mobilize fatty acids
- Decrease serum cholesterol
- Increase BMR (basal metabolic rate)

T_3
T_4

TABLE 38:1	Drugs Used in Hormone Replacement Therapy for Thyroid Deficiency		
DRUG (TRADE NAME)*		**ACTIVE HORMONE**	**DAILY ADULT MAINTENANCE DOSE**
levothyroxine sodium (*Levothroid, Synthroid*)		T_4	100–200 μg PO**
liothyronine sodium (*Cytomel*)		T_3	25–75 μg PO
thyroid (desiccated thyroid) (*Armour Thyroid, S-P-T, Thyrar*)		$T_3 + T_4$	60–120 mg PO

*Not an inclusive list of product names.
**Available for parenteral administration also.

Hyposecretion of T_3 and T_4 in adults results in nontoxic **goiter.** When thyroid hormone secretion is suppressed, there is no way to inhibit the secretion of TSH from the pituitary. When little or no T_3 and T_4 circulates in the blood, TSH continues to stimulate the thyroid gland to release active hormones that are not there. This constant stimulation of the thyroid results in glandular enlargement (hypertrophy). As the thyroid increases in size, it protrudes from the front of the neck, causing a swollen appearance.

Individuals who have a total absence of T_3 and T_4 develop **myxedema,** which is characterized by a round, puffy face, dry skin, hypotension, bradycardia, and an intolerance to cold temperatures. In severe cases, respiratory acidosis, electrolyte imbalance, and coma may develop (myxedema coma).

Hormone Replacement

Thyroid function is routinely evaluated by measuring serum TSH and T_4 levels. Primary hypothyroidism is associated with decreased production of total T_4, T_3, and free thyroxine index (FT_4I) but circulating TSH is increased. Secondary hypothyroidism is associated with a decrease in all three hormones. Free thyroxine index is an estimate of serum free T_4 calculated from total T_4 and thyroid hormone binding ratio. Thyroid deficiency is treated primarily by hormone replacement. To relieve the symptoms associated with thyroid deficiency, various preparations of thyroid hormones can be administered orally (see Table 38:1).

Thyroid and thyroglobulin are natural hormones that are extracted from the endocrine glands of animals. Other available thyroid hormones are prepared synthetically. Regardless of

the preparation selected, the active hormone is T_3, T_4, or a combination of the two hormones. Although these hormones produce the same spectrum of activity, T_3 and T_4 differ in potency, onset, and duration of action. Therefore, the dose of the hormone(s) must be gradually adjusted to meet patients' needs.

Once an adequate dosing schedule is established, the hormone(s) will mimic the action of normal thyroid secretion. The circulating hormone(s) will also inhibit excessive secretion of TSH (negative feedback) so that goiter production is suppressed. Hormone replacement in functionally thyroid-deficient individuals is a lifelong therapy.

Plasma Protein Binding

Thyroid hormones are usually administered orally, preferably as a single dose before breakfast. These preparations may be administered intravenously in the treatment of myxedema coma. Following absorption, T_3 and T_4 are bound to a specific plasma protein known as thyroxine-binding globulin (TBG), which transports the hormones to the various target tissues. Triiodothyronine has a quicker onset and a shorter duration of action than T_4 because T_3 is less tightly bound to TBG. Triiodothyronine is also three to five times more potent than T_4 in stimulating metabolic mechanisms. When the two hormones are given together, as in the combination preparations, T_3 acts quickly, whereas T_4 has a lag time. Eventually, both T_3 and T_4 are metabolized in the liver and excreted in the urine.

Clinical Indications

Thyroid hormones are approved for use in children and adults as replacement or supplement in hypothyroidism from any cause. Thyroid hormones are also used in the treatment of thyroid nodules because they suppress TSH and in the diagnosis of hyperthyroid conditions. Despite their ability to affect metabolism, thyroid hormones are not approved or indicated for use in the treatment of obesity. Doses necessary to effect weight reduction produce serious cardiovascular effects that can be life threatening to the patient.

Drug Administration

Thyroid hormones are usually given in the smallest doses and incrementally raised until a clinically adequate response is reached. This allows individualized dosing and minimizes the potential for adverse responses to occur. Treatment of thyroid cancer requires much larger amounts than those given for replacement therapy.

Adverse Effects

The adverse effects associated with thyroid hormone use usually result from overdose. The physiological effect of overdose is hyperthyroidism. Symptoms may include psychotic behavior, diarrhea, increased blood pressure and heart rate, fever, and angina attacks. Metabolic stimulation may result in weight loss, menstrual irregularities, and sweating. In addition, tremors, headache, nervousness, and insomnia may occur. These symptoms can be alleviated by temporarily discontinuing the drug or reducing the dose.

There is no doubt that thyroid hormones can affect the cardiovascular system. These drugs should be used with extreme caution in patients who have cardiovascular disease (hypertension, congestive heart failure, or angina) or renal disease.

Long-term use of thyroxine has been associated with osteoporosis in postmenopausal women. Bone density must be evaluated prior to therapy in order to adequately monitor the hormone's effect and adjust the dose to minimize bone demineralization.

Drug Interactions

A few drugs affect the pharmacological activity of the thyroid hormones. Cholestyramine (hypolipidemic drug) will bind the thyroid hormones when given together orally. To avoid interference with intestinal absorption of the thyroid hormones, administration of cholestyramine and the hormones should be separated by 4 or 5 hours. Long-term therapy with lithium, chlorpromazine, or imipramine has been

reported to produce hypothyroidism. The dose of T_3 and T_4 may therefore require adjustment in patients receiving these drugs chronically. Thyroid hormones (T_4 in particular) enhance the activity of oral anticoagulants, leading to increased bleeding and possible hemorrhage. Patients requiring oral anticoagulant therapy should have their thyroid dosing schedule adjusted accordingly.

Thyroid hormone therapy may cause an increase in the required dose of insulin or oral hypoglycemic drugs in diabetic patients because these hormones increase blood glucose levels. Estrogens may increase the requirement of thyroid hormone therapy if given to patients who do not have a functioning thyroid gland. Estrogens increase the binding proteins that tie up circulating thyroid hormone, thus decreasing the amount of hormone available to target tissues.

Special Considerations and Contraindications

Thyroid hormone given as replacement therapy must be taken by patients for life. Patients should not discontinue the drug without their physician's knowledge. Changes in type or brand of medication should be made only after careful examination of the product literature to ensure that the products are bioequivalent. These hormones should be taken at the same time each day to maintain constancy in the pharmacological response. Dosing is often recommended for the morning so that patients will avoid episodes of insomnia (central nervous system [CNS] stimulation).

NOTE TO THE HEALTH CARE PROFESSIONAL

Thyroid hormone therapy is contraindicated in patients with myocardial infarction or uncorrected adrenal insufficiency. Thyroid hormones should never be administered for the purpose of reducing body weight in obese individuals. These hormones should be administered to patients who have been accurately diagnosed as being hormone deficient.

Thyroid hormones must be used with extreme caution in patients who have cardiovascular disease, since the increased sympathetic and cardiotropic effects of these hormones may exacerbate the underlying disease. Patients, especially the elderly, who experience chest pain, palpitations, sweating, dyspnea (difficult or labored breathing), or tachycardia while receiving thyroid hormones should notify their physician immediately. Thyroid hormone therapy in patients who have diabetes or adrenal insufficiency may exacerbate the underlying disease, leading to an increased requirement in medications such as insulin, oral hypoglycemics, and steroids. Once the antidiabetic drug has been adjusted for patients receiving concominant thyroid therapy, the patients should not discontinue the thyroid drug without their physician's knowledge. Cessation of thyroid therapy may precipitate hypoglycemia unless the antidiabetic medication is readjusted. Thyroid replacement therapy need not be discontinued during pregnancy. Thyroid hormones administered to pregnant women do not readily cross the placental barrier to affect fetal development. These hormones are designated as Food and Drug Administration (FDA) Pregnancy Category A: adequate studies have not demonstrated a risk to the fetus in the first trimester of pregnancy and there is no evidence of risk in later trimesters.

Hypersecretion of Hormones

Hypersecretion of thyroid hormones may be produced by tumors (thyroid, pituitary, or hypothalamic malignancies), or **autoimmune disease** (Graves' disease). Graves' disease is associated with the production of a long-acting thyroid stimulator (LATS) protein. Although it is not the same as TSH, this protein produces physiological responses characteristic of chronic thyroid stimulation.

Hyperthyroidism is associated with an increased secretion and circulation of T_3 and T_4, which results in added heat production (fever and sweating), increased cell metabolism, tachycardia, muscle weakness, anxiety, and weight loss. The clinical symptoms resemble excessive stimulation of the sympathetic nervous system.

Hypersecretory conditions may be corrected with antithyroid drugs, irradiation, or surgical removal of the overactive tissue. Treatment of a hyperactive thyroid usually includes a combination of these methods.

Treating Hyperthyroidism with Antithyroid Drugs

Hypersecretory conditions of the thyroid are frequently caused by glandular tumors. Often, these overactive growths can be removed surgically.

However, the thyroid mass is frequently treated with antithyroid drugs or irradiation to reduce the tumor, inactivate the tissue, or reduce vascularity (blood flow) prior to surgery (thyroidectomy). Irradiation and drug administration in hyperthyroidism are directed toward destroying the overactive tissue or inhibiting the production and secretion of T_3 and T_4.

Route of Administration

Although small amounts of iodide are necessary for hormone synthesis, high levels of iodide inhibit the synthesis and release of thyroid hormones. In large concentrations, iodide inhibits its own uptake and binding within the thyroid gland. Iodide preparations are available in solution as potassium or sodium iodide (see Table 38:2). Strong iodine solution (*Lugol's solution*) contains 5 percent iodine and 10 percent potassium iodide. These mixtures are taken orally. The thyrotropic effects of iodide solutions are evident in 24 to 48 hours and may last several weeks when the drugs are given chronically.

Iodide suppression is not useful for long-term treatment of hyperthyroidism because the effects of iodide suppression are not permanent. Eventually, the thyroid escapes the iodide inhibition, resulting in an immediate surge in T_3 and T_4 release. As the hormones pour out of the gland (thyroid storm), an acute hyperthyroid condition develops. Presently, iodide therapy is reserved for short-term treatment (preoperative) because iodide reduces the vascularity of the gland. Lithium carbonate, when given concomitantly with iodide, may enhance the hypothyroid response.

Other, less serious side effects produced by iodide therapy include rash, headache, sore gums, hypersalivation, and pruritus.

Radioactive iodide (^{131}I) is used in the diagnosis and treatment of hyperthyroid disorders. Since radioactive iodide behaves like dietary iodide, it rapidly accumulates in the thyroid gland. However, radioactive (unstable) iodide emits two types of radiation: gamma rays and beta rays. Emission of the gamma rays (X-rays) produces a picture of the thyroid that demonstrates abnormal growth or activity. Furthermore, the beta radiation remains in the thyroid cells and destroys the overactive tissue. Thus, when ^{131}I is administered to severely hyperthyroid individuals, it reduces the thyroid mass (tumors and nodules) and destroys hormone synthesis. Radioactive iodide is used preoperatively or in the treatment of thyroid carcinoma. Occasionally, patients exposed to ^{131}I become permanently hypothyroid. In these cases,

TABLE 38:2   Antithyroid Drugs Used in Treating Hyperthyroid Conditions

DRUG (TRADE NAME)	ADULT ORAL DAILY DOSE
potassium iodide and iodine (*Lugol's solution, Thyro-Block*)	2–6 drops TID for 10 days prior to surgery
radioactive iodide (^{131}I) (*Iodotope, Sodium Iodide I 131*)	4–10 millicuries PO or IV (hyperthyroidism)
	50 millicuries PO (thyroid carcinoma)
methimazole (*Tapazole*)	15–60 mg/day (initial)*
	5–15 mg/day (maintenance)*
propylthiouracil	300–400 mg/day (initial)*
	100–150 mg/day (maintenance)*

*Given in three equal doses every 8 hours.

hormone replacement therapy must be administered for life. Because of its destructive potential, ^{131}I should never be used during pregnancy or lactation because permanent damage to the fetal thyroid can develop.

The most frequently used antithyroid drugs include propylthiouracil, methimazole, and methylthiouracil. These agents are thioamide drugs that inhibit the incorporation of iodide into tyrosine and the condensation of monoiodotyrosine and diiodotyrosine. Since these drugs have no effect on hormone release, the antithyroid action cannot be observed until the thyroid stores of T_3 and T_4 become depleted. Thereafter, no new hormones are synthesized.

Long-term treatment with the thioamide drugs usually results in remission of the hyperthyroid condition. These drugs are easily absorbed into the thyroid gland after oral use. Eventually, these drugs are metabolized and excreted in the urine.

Adverse Effects

The usual side effects of thioamide drugs include rash, fever, myalgia, jaundice, and nausea. **Agranulocytosis** also has been reported. Cross-sensitivity occurs for all thioamide drugs in sensitive individuals. Thioamide therapy frequently causes goiter formation because the negative feedback to TSH is removed. If the dose is reduced, some thyroid hormone can be synthesized. The thioamide drugs are primarily used preoperatively or as an adjunct in ^{131}I therapy.

The thioamide drugs are useful in the treatment of **thyrotoxic crisis,** which is associated with an excessive secretion of thyroid hormone. Occasionally, untreated hyperthyroid individuals undergo emotional stress or trauma that results in an intense hyperthyroid reaction. Fever, tachycardia, heart failure, and coma may result. Treatment may include thioamide drugs, iodine, and propranolol. Beta-adrenergic blockers do not affect the thyroid gland but are administered to inhibit the increased sympathetic responses that accompany hyperthyroidism.

Special Considerations and Contraindications

Antithyroid drugs will cross the placenta and inhibit fetal thyroid development, resulting in neonatal goiter and cretinism. Nevertheless, there are situations where the benefit to mother balances the potential risk to the fetus. In such cases, propylthiouracil is used because placental transfer is much lower than methimazole. Frequently hyperthyroid activity exacerbated by pregnancy diminishes during pregnancy. This allows the drug dose to be decreased or discontinued before damage to the fetus can occur. Since these drugs also appear in breast milk, they should not be administered to nursing mothers because the infant will develop hypothyroidism. Again, when necessary, propylthiouracil is the drug of choice to administer to nursing mothers. Propylthiouracil may compromise coagulation, so monitoring prothrombin time may be required for surgical patients. Propylthiouracil may cause bleeding and potentiate anticoagulants.

Patients should be evaluated for sensitivity to iodides, particularly prior to parenteral administration. Hypersensitivity reactions, which may occur immediately or several hours after administration, range from rashes to laryngeal edema. Iodide-containing medications are contraindicated in patients with pulmonary edema. Patients should be instructed to continue their iodide medications as prescribed. Sudden withdrawal of iodides may precipitate thyroid storm. Patients receiving radioactive iodide should be instructed not to expectorate and to use good toilet habits because saliva and urine may be radioactive ("hot") for 24 hours after drug exposure.

PARATHYROID HORMONES

Calcium ions, essential for neuromuscular and endocrine function, enable all muscles to contract and nerves to conduct impulses. Therefore, it is essential that all tissues receive an adequate supply of calcium through the blood. Serum calcium levels are strictly regulated by the secretion of two hormones: calcitonin and parathyroid hormone (parathormone, PTH). Calcitonin is secreted by the thyroid gland, whereas PTH is secreted by the parathyroid gland.

Calcium Homeostasis

Calcitonin and PTH are polypeptide hormones secreted in response to changes in the serum calcium level. Bone is continually formed throughout life, although the overall mass of bone peaks between age 30 and 40. Bone resorption (breakdown) is coupled to bone formation. Osteoclasts are cells that resorb bone, while osteoblasts rebuild by laying osteoid into the skeletal cavity. Mineralization of the osteoid with calcium forms new hard bone. In this metabolic balance, serum calcium rises and falls, triggering feedback to the sensing hormones, PTH and calcitonin.

Normally, serum calcium is maintained at 8 to 10 mg percent (8 to 10 mg per 100 ml serum). Low serum calcium (hypocalcemia) stimulates the secretion of PTH. Acting directly on bone cells that store calcium, PTH mobilizes calcium ions into the blood. This process is known as bone resorption. In addition, PTH increases the intestinal absorption and renal reabsorption of calcium ions. These two physiological processes require vitamin D. Overall, these effects of PTH increase the level of circulating calcium ions in response to hypocalcemia.

When the serum calcium level becomes too high (**hypercalcemia,** more than 10 mg percent), calcitonin is secreted. It lowers the serum calcium level by antagonizing the effect of PTH on bone. Calcitonin directly inhibits bone resorption so that calcium ions are retained in the bone. It does not affect intestinal and renal calcium absorption, and its action does not require vitamin D.

Treating Calcium Disorders

The major endocrine disorder that alters calcium homeostasis is hypoparathyroidism. Hypoparathyroidism is usually produced by accidental surgical removal of the glands. Since PTH is the predominant controlling factor, lack of PTH produces an imbalance in calcium regulation, and eventually hypocalcemia ensues. Hypocalcemia causes hyperexcitability of the neuromuscular system, resulting in spastic muscle contractions, convulsions, and paresthesia (a pricking, tingling, or creeping sensation). These symptoms are characteristic of tetany. Treatment of hypoparathyroidism involves the administration of calcium salts and vitamin D (cholecalciferol).

Contrary to other endocrine deficiency states, hypoparathyroidism is not usually treated by replacement of the missing hormone. The parathyroid hormone, which is available for injection, produces allergic reactions. Drug resistance usually develops within 2 weeks. Instead, hypocalcemia is usually managed by the use of oral calcium salts and vitamin D derivatives (see Table 38:3). Administration of vitamin D enhances intestinal absorption of calcium, thus increasing serum calcium levels. Through this therapy, calcium ions are immediately available to the tissues without affecting bone resorption. Any excess calcium ions are excreted by the kidneys.

However, calcium salts and vitamin D preparations are not harmless medications.

TABLE 38:3   Drugs Used in the Treatment of Calcium Disorders

DRUG (TRADE NAME)	USE	ADULT DOSE
calcitonin, salmon (*Calcimar, Miacalcin*)	Reduce hypercalcemia	4–8 IU every 12 hr SC or IM
	Paget's disease	100 IU/day IM, SC
	Postmenopausal osteoporosis	100 IU/day SC or IM; 200 IU intranasally
calcium chloride	Increase serum calcium	10–30 ml (5% solution) IV; 4–8 g/day PO
calcium gluconate	Increase serum calcium	20 ml (10% solution) IV; 15 g/day PO
calcium lactate	Increase serum calcium	0.5–2 g QID PO
alendronate (*Fosamax*)	Osteoporosis in postmenopausal women	10 mg once day, or 70 mg once a week
etidronate disodium (*Didronel*)	Paget's disease	5–10 mg/kg/day PO up to 6 months or 11–20 mg/kg/day PO up to 3 months
pamidronate (*Aredia*)	Hypercalcemia of malignancy	60–90 mg IV infusion over 24 hr
	Osteolytic bone metastases	90 mg IV infusion over 2 hr every 3–4 weeks
	Paget's disease	30 mg/day as a 4-hr infusion IV on 3 consecutive days
	Multiple myeloma	90 mg as a 4-hr infusion IV once a month
tiludronate (*Skelid*)	Paget's disease	400 mg PO with 6–8 oz of water for 3 months
risedronate (*Actonel*)	Osteoporosis in postmenopausal women	5 mg daily PO
	Paget's disease	30 mg daily for 2 months
Vitamin D:		
ergocalciferol (vitamin D$_2$)	Increase serum calcium	50,000–200,000 IU PO
dihydrotachysterol (*Hytakerol*)	Increase serum calcium	0.75–2.5 mg/day PO

Excessive use of these preparations may lead to hypercalcemia and kidney stone formation. Treatment of drug-induced hypercalcemia may involve the use of edetic acid (ethylenediamine tetraacetic acid [EDTA]), which binds (chelates) the calcium ions and removes them from the blood.

A few clinical conditions produce hypercalcemia and therefore may act synergistically with oral calcium salts. These conditions include ingestion of excess vitamin D (hypervitaminosis), neoplasia (breast or testicular carcinoma), and complications of kidney transplantation. In the United States, hypervitaminosis is not frequently encountered although it does occur.

Hypercalcemia

Although hypercalcemia may result from tumors in the parathyroid gland, this is not the most frequent cause of elevated serum calcium levels. Hypercalcemia is usually associated with certain neoplasms, multiple myeloma, and renal dysfunction. These conditions either accelerate bone resorption or impair renal excretion of calcium. The resultant hypercalcemia produces nausea, vomiting, increased secretion of gastric acid (hyperchlorhydria), headaches, and arrhythmias. Calcium may also be deposited in the cornea and kidneys, producing irreversible tissue damage.

Management of chronic hypercalcemia includes diuretics (thiazides or furosemide), which enhance the renal clearance of calcium, bisphosphonates, and calcitonin.

Degenerative Bone Disease

The two most common disorders in bone metabolism are **Paget's disease** and **osteoporosis.** In Paget's disease, bone metabolism is hyperactive in some, but not all bones, causing newly laid osteoid to be soft, calcified but fragile. The bones are characterized as thick and weak. Bones most frequently affected are the pelvis, femur, skull, and vertebrae although any bone can be affected. Microfractures seen on X-ray are usually the first indication of the chronic degenerative process. Though asymptomatic early in development, once it appears, bone pain can range from aching to severe night pain.

Osteoporosis

Osteoporosis is a condition associated with decreased bone mass. This may result from increased bone resorption, decreased mineral deposition, increased mineral excretion, or a combination of actions that remove calcium from the body. A variety of factors have been associated with the development of osteoporosis, as though predisposing certain individuals beyond the expected age-associated loss. These factors include premature menopause, leanness and short stature in women, Caucasian and oriental race, treatment with corticosteroids or phenytoin, smoking, alcoholism, and family history of osteoporosis. While osteoporosis occurs in elderly men, the incidence in women is greater, related to diminished estrogen availability. The decrease in estrogen correlates with the risk factors of premature menopause and decreased body fat (leanness) in which estrogen could be stored. In addition, calcium absorption decreases as estrogen activity decreases. Since most women are believed to have a daily dietary intake of calcium well below the Recommended Dietary Allowance (RDA 800 mg), there is concern that this further contributes to the development of osteoporosis in women.

Bone loss in osteoporosis is associated with reduction in bone density, visualized through X-ray or tomography. These tools are used to evaluate improvement in bone mineral density during therapy. While the objective is to maintain or improve bone mineral density, the goal is to prevent bone fractures. In both degenerative diseases, fractures result from stress or falls in people over 65 years old. Beyond this age, people more easily fracture vertebrae, hips, and wrists as a result of mechanical stress or pressure.

Drug Therapy of Hypercalcemia, Paget's Disease, and Osteoporosis

Calcitonin

Calcitonin, available as a synthetic polypeptide hormone, is administered to hypercalcemia patients whose thyroid and parathyroid glands function normally. In Paget's disease, bone turnover is stimulated, causing alkaline phosphatase and hydroxyproline to be excreted as markers of the abnormal bone activity. Calcitonin (*Calcimar*), injected subcutaneously or intramuscularly, inhibits the accelerated bone resorption. This hormone is available as a nasal spray (*Miacalcin*), and as an extract from salmon, is identical to human calcitonin but has a greater potency.

Calcitonin has limited clinical use because it produces allergic reactions that require termination of therapy. In addition, some patients develop drug resistance to the **polypeptide.** Drug resistance may be due to the formation of antibodies that neutralize the hormone. However, in patients who have a normal parathyroid, rebound secretion of PTH occurs when the serum calcium level falls. This effect may counteract the pharmacological activity of calcitonin. Calcitonin is usually well tolerated by patients. The usual side effects include nausea, vomiting, diarrhea, and inflammation at the injection site. The nasal preparation is associated with rhinitis, insomnia, anxiety, and headache. Overdose with 10 times the daily therapeutic dose has only produced vomiting prior to recovery.

Bisphosphonates

Alendronate (*Fosamax*), etidronate (*Didronel*), pamidronate (*Aredia*), risedronate (*Actonel*), and tiludronate (*Skelid*) inhibit normal and abnormal bone resorption and, to varying degrees, also bone formation. The mechanism of action is not completely understood but may involve dissolution of hydroxyappetite (mineralized osteoid) and a decrease in osteoclasts cells (which break down bone) and their activity.

These drugs are poorly absorbed in the gastrointestinal (GI) tract, not metabolized, and excreted in the urine. Nevertheless, enough drug is absorbed to produce a clinically significant difference in bone mineral density within 3 months of treatment. Improvement in bone density in the spine and hip did not involve demineralization of other bones. The therapeutic

Patient Administration and Monitoring

Replacement therapy is taken for life, therefore habits must be developed to assure good compliance with the dosing schedule. Patients should be alerted to a few critical items that can make lifelong therapy most convenient and safe.

Drug Administration

Hormone products cannot be interchanged. Even the same hormone cannot be substituted among different manufacturers because of the differences in bioavailability or effectiveness. Since dosing is individualized to the patient, using one product consistently maintains therapeutic efficacy with a safety profile commensurate with the dose.

Thyroid hormones may be taken as single daily dose before breakfast. More levothyroxine, however, will be absorbed if taken on an empty stomach. Patients should be instructed to be consistent in their dosing pattern—that is, with breakfast or not—so that hormone absorption does not fluctuate.

Iodine solution can be diluted with water to make it more palatable.

Calcitonin nasal preparations require demonstration and practice to ensure the patient understands how to prime the pump for initial dosing. Priming is not required again after the initial spray has discharged. The pump and the head should be held upright when spraying the dose into the nostril. Bisphosphonates, alendronate, etidronate, and tiludronate should be taken on an empty stomach or before meals to ensure that adequate absorption occurs.

Medication should never be discontinued by the patient unless supervised by the prescribing physician.

Patients should be encouraged to disclose a full medication history to all other physicians and medical professionals routinely seen by the patient. Since these drugs can produce cardiovascular changes, or symptoms resembling postmenopausal sweating and flushing, patients must alert other medical personnel that they are taking medication that could produce signs and symptoms that differ from their previous examination.

Notification of Adverse Effects

Thyroid Hormones

Patients should receive clear instruction to call the physician if nervousness, diarrhea, excess sweating, heat intolerance, chest pain, or palpitations occur. These symptoms may warrant thyroid hormone dose adjustment after evaluation by the prescribing physician.

Antithyroid Drugs

Patients should call the physician if fever, sore throat, bleeding or bruising, headache, rash, vomiting, or yellowing of the skin develops while on antithyroid medication. These symptoms may signal the need for dose interruption and further evaluation by the prescribing physician.

Iodine

Patients should call the physician if fever, skin rash, metallic taste, swelling of the throat, burning in the mouth and throat, sore gums and teeth, severe intestinal distress, or enlargement of the thyroid occurs. These signs warrant discontinuation of the drug and further evaluation by the prescribing physician.

Use in Pregnancy

Drugs that inhibit thyroid function are designated FDA Pregnancy Category D: evidence of risk to the human fetus has been demonstrated; however, the benefit of use in pregnancy may make the potential risk to the fetus acceptable. Patients who may become pregnant during therapy should notify the physician immediately for further evaluation and/or dose adjustment.

Drugs that destroy thyroid tissue, such as radioisotope ^{131}I, are designated FDA Pregnancy Category X: the risk to the woman and/or the fetus clearly outweighs any possible benefit. Women who are or may become pregnant should not be treated with ^{131}I.

Bisphosphates have been designated FDA Pregnancy Category B and C: animal studies indicate abnormalities occur that have not been evaluated in humans. The safe use of these drugs in pregnant women has not been established through appropriate controlled clinical trials. Use in postmenopausal women does not represent a health risk; however, use in women of childbearing age who may become pregnant requires clear evidence that the benefit clearly outweighs potential risk to the fetus.

effect is presumably conferred to all bones in the management of Paget's disease and osteoporosis. In the treatment of hypercalcemia due to malignancy, serum calcium levels are dramatically reduced within 24 hours, accompanied by an increase in calcium excretion.

Drug Interactions

Ranitidine and indomethacin increase the bioavailability of alendronate and tiludronate without deleterious effect. Since the absolute absorption of the administered dose is low, it is advisable not to take the bisphosphonates with calcium supplements or antacids. These drugs complex or at least interfere with bisphosphonate absorption when taken within 1 hour of the bisphosphonate. While alendronate increases the GI irritation of aspirin, aspirin taken within 2 hours after tiludronate decreases the bisphosphonate absorption. Food does interfere with drug absorption. Alendronate, etidronate, and tiludronate should be taken on an empty stomach or before meals to assure adequate absorption occurs.

Adverse Effects

The bisphosphonates are well tolerated. The most common adverse effects are flatulence, gastritis, headache, dry mouth, and musculoskeletal pain. The incidence of adverse effects is associated with the highest doses.

Estrogen

Treatment of osteoporosis had previously been limited to calcitonin and vitamin D supplementation. While still indicated for use in postmenopausal osteoporosis, calcitonin has its primary action on bone resorption, not on bone formation. The bisphosphonates combined with calcium has improved the treatment of osteoporosis, showing a prevention of related fracture incidence after 6 months of therapy. However, the most significant treatment for osteoporosis in postmenopausal women is estrogen replenishment. It has been demonstrated that estrogen receptors are located within bone cells and that estrogen not only increases bone mineral density, it reduces the incidence of osteoporotic fracture. Estrogen combined with daily calcium supplementation of 1000 to 1500 mg stimulates bone mineralization even when started up to 10 years after menopause. Estrogen therapy is promoted as a lifelong adjunct to good diet and exercise. The critical factor in achieving patient commitment to estrogen therapy is the concern women voice about the long-term effects of estrogen exposure. Of particular concern is the potential to develop breast cancer. While the data remain to be collected to answer this concern, the doses of estrogen used today are significantly lower than those in oral contraceptives over the past 25 years, which had been associated with clotting disorders and breast cancer. Additional information on the effects of estrogen as a pharmacologic agent is presented in Chapter 37.

Chapter Review

Understanding Terminology

Match the definition or description in the left column with the appropriate term in the right column.

___ **1.** A condition in which there is a significant reduction in the number of WBCs.

___ **2.** A condition characterized by a low level of physical and mental development.

___ **3.** A negative ion.

___ **4.** An enlargement of the thyroid that is not a result of a tumor.

___ **5.** A condition in which an individual's tissues are damaged by his or her own immune system.

___ **6.** A condition caused by excessive quantities of thyroid hormone.

a. agranulocytosis

b. anion

c. autoimmune disease

d. cretinism

e. goiter

f. thyrotoxic crisis

Acquiring Knowledge

Answer the following questions in the spaces provided.

1. What physiological effects are produced by the thyroid hormones T_3 and T_4? _____

_____

_____

2. What clinical symptoms reflect the metabolic changes associated with hypothyroidism?

_____

_____

3. What is the rationale for the treatment of hypothyroidism? _____

_____

_____

4. What methods are available for treating hyperthyroidism? _____

_____

_____

5. How does the action of the antithyroid drugs differ from the action of radioactive iodide?

_____

_____

6. What side effects are associated with the use of antithyroid drugs? _____

_____

_____

7. What hormones control calcium metabolism? How do these hormones differ? _____

_____

_____

8. What are the side effects of hypoparathyroid therapy? Why? _____

_____

_____

9. When is calcitonin used? _____

_____

_____

10. What drugs might influence thyroid function in normal individuals? _____

_____

_____

Applying Knowledge—On the Job

Use your critical thinking skills to answer the following questions in the spaces provided.

1. Assume that you work in the endocrinology clinic of a university hospital. Four patients treated at the clinic today had thyroid conditions. What thyroid condition do you think each of the following patients has? How should it be treated?

   a. Patient A is a 44-year-old male presenting with a round, puffy face, dry skin and hair, hypotension, anemia, drowsiness, and intolerance to cold.

_____

_____

   b. Patient B is an 18-month-old female presenting with growth failure, delayed motor and mental development, delayed tooth eruption, and intolerance to cold.

_____

_____

   c. Patient C is a 25-year-old male presenting with anxiety, weight loss, muscle weakness, tachycardia, and intolerance to heat.

_____

_____

   d. Patient D is a 65-year-old female presenting with nausea, vomiting, headaches, and heart arrhythmia.

_____

_____

2. The endocrinologist you work for has prescribed thyroid hormones to each of the following adult patients. What is the potential problem in prescribing thyroid hormones to each patient? What should be done to prevent the problem in each case?

   a. Patient A is taking the drug *Questran* for high serum cholesterol. _____

_____

_____

   b. Patient B is on long-term *Thorazine* therapy for manic-depressive illness. _____

_____

_____

   c. Patient C is an insulin-dependent diabetic. _____

_____

_____

   d. Patient D takes oral contraceptives. _____

_____

_____

   e. Patient E had a heart attack 6 months ago. _____

_____

_____

3. Is thyroid replacement contraindicated during pregnancy? Why or why not? _____

_____

4. What are the usual side effects with calcitonin? _____

_____

5. Joy has been taking synthetic thyroid replacement medications for 15 years. Her physician has decided to initiate cholestyramine therapy for her high cholesterol. What, if anything, should she be told regarding these two medications?

_____

_____

Internet Connection

Among the best sites providing information on osteoporosis and medications used in the management of osteoporosis is www.nlm.nih.gov/medlineplus/osteoporosis.html. In addition to text information, this site has a slideshow with a narrator who takes the viewer through each slide. The narrator even explains how to begin the slide show; then the viewer can select topics from how osteoporosis develops to prevention and treatment strategies. This is a tutorial setup for easy access directed at the level of the consumer, patient, or student. At the end, the viewer is presented a selection of "true or false" questions based on the material covered. The narrator, in addition to the visual graphic presentation, gives the correct answers.

At www.osteo.org, the National Institutes of Health offers current information on metabolic bone diseases such as osteoporosis and Paget's disease. The mission of this site is to educate patients and the public about metabolic bone diseases.

Facts about vitamin D and its relationship to bone development can be found at www.cc.nih.gov/ccc/supplements/vitd.html. Information intended for the education of patients and their families is maintained at "the largest website for Thyroid, Parathyroid, Adrenal, and Pancreas disorders, including Diabetes and Osteoporosis" at www.endocrineweb.com. This site adds pages weekly and now includes a large amount of information on endocrine disease, conditions, hormone problems, and treatment options. It also displays calcium requirements for maintenance of adult bones.

Finally, www.findarticles.com is a site that allows you to enter a topic, word, or phrase such as *Thyroid disorders* or *Bone density* to obtain relevant articles from worldwide medical information sources for online review. The articles are usually in English and are one to six pages in length. In addition to renowned journals such as the *British Medical Journal* or the *Journal of the American Medical Association,* this site provides a fair balance of information from sports medicine and news articles.

Additional Readings

Schroeder, B. M. 2002. ACOG practice bulletin on thyroid disease in pregnancy. *American Family Physician* 65 (10):851. (access online at www.aafp.org)

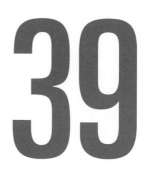

chapter

39

PANCREATIC HORMONES AND ANTIDIABETIC DRUGS

CHAPTER FOCUS

This chapter describes two naturally occurring substances that directly control the ability of cells to use glucose.

CHAPTER OBJECTIVES

After studying this chapter, you should be able to

- describe the difference in action between insulin and glucagon.

- identify the symptoms associated with insulin deficiency.

- explain the difference between the two types of insulin preparations (lente versus regular insulin).

- identify three drugs used therapeutically to release the body's available insulin.

- identify the natural extension of insulin's action that is an adverse effect of overdose.

- explain three different mechanisms of action through which drugs control blood sugar in diabetics.

DRUG CLASS AT A GLANCE

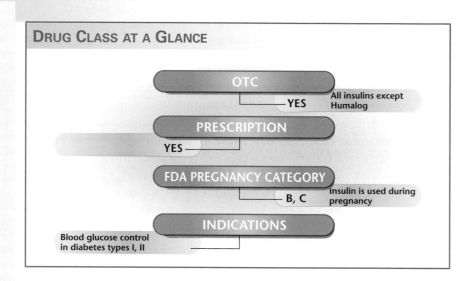

OTC — YES — All insulins except Humalog

PRESCRIPTION — YES

FDA PREGNANCY CATEGORY — B, C — Insulin is used during pregnancy

INDICATIONS — Blood glucose control in diabetes types I, II

Key Terms

acetate: compound that contains acetic acid.

adipose tissue: fat.

gluconeogenesis: conversion of amino acids to glucose.

glycosuria: presence of glucose in the urine.

hyperglycemia: higher than normal level of glucose in the blood.

ketosis: condition associated with an increased production of ketone bodies as a result of fat metabolism.

lipodystrophy: defective metabolism of fat.

neuropathy: numbness of hands and feet.

phosphate: acid solution containing molecules of combined hydrogen, phosphorous, and oxygen (H_3PO_4).

polydipsia: excessive thirst.

polyphagia: excessive eating.

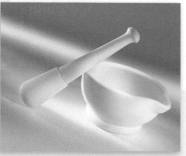

polyuria: excessive production of urine.

suspension: preparation in which undissolved solids (drugs) are dispersed within a liquid.

INTRODUCTION

The pancreas secretes two polypeptide hormones, insulin and glucagon, which regulate protein, fat, and carbohydrate metabolism. Although any of these nutrients can be used for tissue fuel, most cells use glucose, which is produced during carbohydrate digestion, as a primary source of energy. Therefore, it is essential to maintain a circulating pool of glucose for the cells and to promote efficient transport of glucose into the cells.

PANCREATIC ENDOCRINE FUNCTION

Insulin and glucagon enable cells to receive an adequate supply of fuel by regulating the blood glucose level. Insulin promotes cell use of glucose and carbohydrate storage (glycogen synthesis). As a result, the blood glucose level decreases **(hypoglycemia)**. Glucagon, however, increases circulating glucose levels **(hyperglycemia)** by stimulating glycogen breakdown (glycogenolysis). Thus, the actions of these two hormones produce opposite effects on the blood glucose level; therefore, insulin and glucagon are often referred to as mutual antagonists.

Insulin Secretion

Insulin is constantly secreted by the beta cells of the pancreas in response to changes in the blood glucose level. As the blood glucose level increases, insulin secretion increases. This effect is important because glucose cannot enter certain tissues without the presence of insulin. Skeletal muscle, heart, and **adipose tissue** (fat) are insulin-sensitive tissues.

These tissues possess insulin receptors, which interact with circulating insulin molecules to form a hormone-receptor complex. Through this complex, insulin stimulates membrane transport systems that carry glucose into the cells. The primary function of insulin is to promote glucose utilization by peripheral tissue. In addition, insulin stimulates glycogen synthesis by enhancing the conversion of glucose to glycogen in the liver. Fat and protein metabolism are also affected by insulin. It inhibits their breakdown and stimulates the synthesis and storage of fat and protein.

Glucagon Secretion

As glucose is taken up by the cells, the blood glucose level falls. This hypoglycemia stimulates the secretion of glucagon, the alpha cells of the pancreas. By stimulating glycogenolysis in the liver, glucagon enables glucose to enter the circulation. Glucagon also enhances the conversion of amino acids (found in proteins) to glucose. This process is called **gluconeogenesis.** As a result, protein synthesis decreases but glucose formation increases, leading to hyperglycemia. Consequently, as the blood glucose level increases, insulin secretion is stimulated, and the metabolic cycle begins again. Throughout the day, glucagon and insulin cooperatively maintain an adequate blood glucose level. Average blood glucose levels between meals are 80 to 100 mg per 100 ml of plasma.

DIABETES MELLITUS

Diabetes mellitus is a common disorder of pancreatic endocrine function that results from a defect in beta cell functioning. It is primarily associated with a deficiency in insulin production and secretion. In diabetic patients, the hormone deficiency may be absolute (no insulin production) or relative (insufficient secretion). Type I diabetes (insulin dependent) is characterized by a total lack of insulin production and secretion. Type I diabetes usually occurs before the age of 20, when growth is still evident. Therefore, this form of diabetes is also known as juvenile diabetes or growth-onset diabetes. Type II (maturity-onset, or adult, diabetes) usually occurs in individuals over the age of 40. Frequently, these diabetics are also overweight. Type II diabetes is characterized by a relative insulin deficiency. Either insulin production is low or secretion by the beta cells is inefficient in meeting the needs of individuals. The exact cause of diabetes mellitus is not known. In Type I diabetes, a genetic abnormality seems the most logical explanation for beta cell malfunction. However, Type II diabetes may be the result of aging, improper diet, or genetic factors.

Symptoms

The common symptoms of diabetes mellitus reflect an imbalance in carbohydrate metabolism due to insulin deficiency (see Table 39:1). The most outstanding feature of diabetes is the persistently high level of blood glucose, which leads to an increase in urine glucose **(glycosuria).** Since glucose cannot enter the cells in the absence of insulin, it becomes trapped in the circulation. Eventually, the excess glucose is filtered through the kidneys for excretion. However, as the glucose level rises in the renal tubules, it creates an osmotic effect (it attracts water). Water is pulled out of the cells and excreted into the urine with the glucose. As a result, the volume of urine increases **(polyuria),** and patients lose large amounts of water and become dehydrated. Since dehydration stimulates thirst, the patients usually drink large quantities of fluids **(polydipsia).**

Diabetics often demonstrate **polyphagia** (excessive eating). Although the blood is loaded with sugar, some cells are "starving." Therefore, diabetic patients may increase food consumption in order to avoid fatigue and hunger. Unfortunately, the absorption of dietary glucose only worsens the hyperglycemia.

Ultimately, the cells begin to use protein and fat as sources of fuel. The breakdown of fat produces an increase in ketone bodies in the blood. This condition is called **ketosis.** As the ketone level increases, metabolic acidosis (ketoacidosis) occurs. Ketoacidosis may enhance the loss of electrolytes (sodium, potassium, and chloride) and produce central nervous system (CNS) depression, resulting in diabetic coma and death. In general, Type I diabetics are prone to ketoacidosis, whereas Type II diabetics are usually resistant. Since patients with either type can develop hypoglycemia leading to a comatose state, ketoacidosis may be differentiated from severe hypoglycemia by acetone in the urine.

Complications

The symptoms of diabetes are directly related to the decreased utilization of glucose and increased catabolism of fat. However, diabetes is also associated with degenerative tissue damage. In particular, diabetics frequently develop atherosclerosis, retinal hemorrhages, blindness, renal dysfunction, and **neuropathy** (numbness of hands and feet). Diabetics are also prone to recurrent skin infections, which are often resistant to antibiotic therapy.

TREATMENT OF DIABETES

The immediate objective of therapy is to correct the metabolic imbalance and to restore lost fluid and electrolytes. Insulin administration rapidly

TABLE 39:1	Characteristics of Diabetes Mellitus	
TYPE I (ABSOLUTE INSULIN DEFICIENCY)	SYMPTOMS	TYPE II (RELATIVE INSULIN DEFICIENCY)
X	Hyperglycemia	X
X	Glucosuria (glycosuria)	X
X	Ketoacidosis	—
X	Polyphagia	X
X	Polyuria	X
X	Polydipsia	X
X	Dry skin	X
X	Dry mouth	X
Juvenile onset common	Onset age	40 years or older
X	Elevated body temperature	X
X	Persistent infections	X

reduces hyperglycemia and its complications and suppresses ketosis. Maintenance therapy of diabetes is directed at regulating the blood glucose level through diet control and consistent exercise and drug administration. In both forms of diabetes, patients' diets are adjusted to limit the intake of carbohydrates. In this way, blood glucose levels can be balanced with insulin administration.

Drugs used in the treatment of diabetes mellitus fall into five categories:

- Insulins
- Secretagogues (sulfonylureas and nonsulfonylureas)
- Glucose absorption inhibitors (alpha-glucosidase inhibitors)
- Biguanides
- Insulin sensitizers (thiazolidinediones)

The insulins and secretagogues are hypoglycemics—that is, they decrease normal or elevated blood glucose levels. As the mechanism implies, the third group of antidiabetic drugs delay dietary glucose absorption or inhibit glucose production in the liver without producing hypoglycemia. During the past few years, drugs useful in the management of diabetes have focused on improving delivery of insulin to target tissues through genetically engineered manipulation of human insulin. The oral antidiabetic drugs have also undergone a dramatic change. The confirmation of specific sites of drug action facilitated the development of new classes of oral medications such as the "insulin sensitizers."

Because of the nature of the disorder, Type I diabetics must receive insulin for life and adjust their diets accordingly. On the other hand, since Type II diabetics secrete a limited amount of insulin from the pancreas, strict diet control may balance the insulin insufficiency. Unfortunately, however, many diabetics do not adhere to the dietary limitations or cannot use diet alone to control their diabetes. In these instances, therapy of Type II diabetics may include insulin or antidiabetic drugs.

Regardless of the regimen selected, only the symptoms associated with hyperglycemia and ketosis can be controlled. Insulin use is not a cure for diabetes. Although insulin and diet may not prevent vascular or neural damage, they may greatly reduce the severity of the effects.

Insulin Therapy

Several types of insulin are available for subcutaneous or intramuscular injection. Intravenous use is reserved for emergencies, ketosis-prone Type I diabetics, or severely ill patients when an immediate onset of action is required.

Source of Insulin

In the past, the only active polypeptide hormone was extracted from pork and beef organs. Today, human insulin can now be synthesized by recombinant DNA technology. Human insulin produced by recombinant DNA is identical to the protein secreted by the human pancreas. Recombinant human insulin is also commercially available as an analog in which two amino acid positions have been switched (*Lispro; Humalog*), making it a "different molecule" but fully functional.

The commercial insulin preparations produce similar metabolic effects but vary in their onset and duration of action (see Table 39:2). The insulins can be divided into short-, intermediate-, and long-acting preparations. The duration of action varies with the size of the insulin crystal, the pH of the buffer, and the amount of protein present.

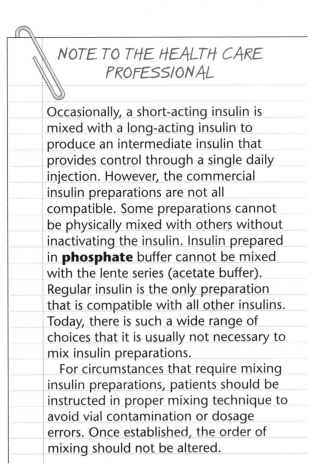

NOTE TO THE HEALTH CARE PROFESSIONAL

Occasionally, a short-acting insulin is mixed with a long-acting insulin to produce an intermediate insulin that provides control through a single daily injection. However, the commercial insulin preparations are not all compatible. Some preparations cannot be physically mixed with others without inactivating the insulin. Insulin prepared in **phosphate** buffer cannot be mixed with the lente series (acetate buffer). Regular insulin is the only preparation that is compatible with all other insulins. Today, there is such a wide range of choices that it is usually not necessary to mix insulin preparations.

For circumstances that require mixing insulin preparations, patients should be instructed in proper mixing technique to avoid vial contamination or dosage errors. Once established, the order of mixing should not be altered.

Characteristics of Commercially Available Insulin Preparations

DRUG (TRADE NAME*)	TYPE	ONSET OF ACTION (HOURS)	DURATION OF ACTION (HOURS)	REMARKS
regular insulin, crystalline zinc insulin, insulin injection (*Humulin R***, *Regular Iletin I and II*, *Novolin R Penfill*)	Short-acting	0.5–1	6–8	Can be mixed (compatible) with any other insulin preparation
Lispro insulin		0.25 hr	6–8	Can be mixed with ultralente or NPH
isophane insulin zinc suspension (*Humulin N***, *NPH Iletin I, NPH Iletin II, Novolin-N*)	Intermediate	1–2	18–24	Incompatible with the lente insulins
protamine zinc insulin suspension (*Protamine, Zinc, and Iletin I*)	Long	4–8	36	Incompatible with the lente insulins
prompt insulin zinc suspension (*Semilente Iletin I, Semilente Insulin, Semitard*)	Short	0.5–1	12–16	Incompatible with the phosphate insulin preparations
insulin zinc suspension (*Lente Iletin I, Lente-L, Humulin-L, Novolin-L*)	Intermediate	1–2.5	18–24	Incompatible with the phosphate insulin preparations
extended insulin zinc suspension (*Humulin-U Ultralente*)	Long	4–8	>36	Incompatible with the phosphate insulin preparations
insulin glargine (*Lantus*)	Long	1–2	24	Incompatible with *any* insulin preparation

*Not an inclusive list of product names.
**Recombinant DNA origin.

Regular insulin (crystalline zinc insulin), the first purified insulin available for clinical use, is a short-acting preparation that is a combination of zinc ions and insulin crystals. In order to increase the duration of action, different amounts of protein (protamine) were added to the regular insulin preparation. This addition resulted in the production of isophane insulin zinc suspension (intermediate) and protamine zinc insulin (long). Isophane insulin zinc suspension is also known as neutral protamine Hagedorn (NPH) insulin. These preparations are a **suspension** (undissolved substance dispersed within a liquid) of insulin and protamine in phosphate buffer. The amount of protein that binds to the insulin reduces the rate of absorption from the injection site.

A preparation of isophane insulin (70 percent) and regular insulin injection (30 percent) provides a rapid onset of action and a prolonged effect (up to 24 hours). This premixture is also available in a 50:50 combination of isophane and regular insulin.

The lente series includes three preparations of insulin suspended in **acetate** buffer. In the presence of acetate buffer, the size of the insulin crystals vary (small and large). The small crystals (semilente) are rapidly absorbed (short-acting), whereas the large crystals (ultralente) are slowly absorbed (long-acting). The intermediate lente preparation is actually a mixture of semilente (30 percent) and ultralente (70 percent) insulin.

All of the preparations available today have been refined to produce a single peak in glucose blood levels that can be timed to coincide with the individual's daily activity. The increased purity has contributed to less potential for allergic or adverse reaction to the protein.

Among the newer recombinant human DNA insulins, one has been developed that delivers a consistent concentration of insulin over 24 hours after a single subcutaneous injection. Insulin glargine (*Lantus*) is recommended for patients with Type 1 diabetes, or those with Type 2 diabetes who require basal control of blood glucose levels. The unique characteristic of this insulin is that a "peak" insulin blood level does not occur. Insulin is released from the injection site at a consistent rate; therefore, blood glucose levels should not rise and fall in response to changing insulin levels. Because the drug is administered at bedtime, the patient will have controlled insulin release during the next day. Although its onset of action is short, insulin glargine cannot be substituted for short-acting insulin preparations. It is not short-acting; once injected, its action lasts 24 hours. In certain patients, this is an advantage over intermediate insulins that require multiple injections to achieve 24-hour glucose control. Insulin glargine is a clear solution that cannot be diluted or mixed with any other insulin preparation.

Dosage

The potency of insulin is expressed in standard United States Pharmacopeia (USP) units. Approximately 25 USP units are contained in 1 mg of insulin. Every preparation of insulin is clearly labeled with the number of units per milliliter and the equivalent potency. There is no routine dose for insulin. Initially, 5 to 10 units of any regular insulin may be given to reduce hyperglycemia. However, the selection of the preparation and the dose must be designed to maintain an adequate blood glucose level. Adequate blood glucose levels vary with individual diabetics and their dietary and exercise (or lack of exercise) patterns. The insulin preparation is usually selected so that the peak effect coincides with patients' peak blood glucose concentrations. All insulin preparations are available in vials of 100 USP units per ml. Today, the 100 USP unit per ml strength is used most often because of the convenience in measurement.

Insulin is administered with specifically calibrated syringes that correspond to the bottle concentration. For example, a U-100 syringe delivers 100 units of insulin when filled with a U-100 preparation. If an insulin syringe is not available, a regular (tuberculin) syringe can be used. However, the dose of insulin must be converted from units to minims per cubic centimeter (16 minims = 1 cc). It is interesting that in most states, all the insulins except for *Humalog* are over-the-counter (OTC)—that is, no prescription is required. This facilitates diabetic patients obtaining an emergency source of medication; for example, when they are on vacation or out of town for any reason. A prescription may be required to obtain the syringes or for verification for insurance coverage but not necessarily for the insulin.

Usually insulin doses range between 20 and 60 units per day. Some patients who develop resistance to insulin may require 300 to 500 units to achieve adequate glucose control. Specifically indicated for such patients, concentrated insulin (*Regular Iletin II pork*), available in vials of 500 units per ml, is administered by tuberculin syringe.

Insulins are usually injected 30 to 60 minutes before meals except for lispro insulin, which is recommended to be injected 15 minutes before meals.

Changing Insulin Requirements

Once a successful dosing schedule of insulin has been established, fluctuations in the blood glucose level may still occur periodically. Many factors increase the level of cell activity and therefore the insulin requirement. Such factors as colds, fevers, infections, illness, surgery, and stress increase the blood glucose level so that higher doses of insulin are required.

Other factors may require reducing the insulin dose. For example, heavy exercise burns up excess glucose and lowers the need for insulin. This is why children, who are often very active, are especially prone to insulin reactions. Certain drugs also alter the blood glucose level and insulin requirement in diabetic individuals.

Occasionally, patients require much more than 200 units of insulin per day. Such individuals are considered to be insulin resistant. Resistance to the pharmacological effects of insulin may be due to the development of antibodies that inhibit insulin activity, or it may be associated with complications of concomitant disease, such as infection or cirrhosis of the liver. Changing the insulin preparation or putting patients on strict diet control may alleviate the resistance to hormone therapy but it may not work for all patients.

An alternate therapy is concentrated insulin (*Regular Iletin II*). Concentrated insulin can be given intramuscularly or subcutaneously in doses that are titrated to patients' needs. Accurate measurement of the dose is still important because concentrated insulin may produce a response up to 24 hours after injection. In addition, overdose may cause irreversible insulin shock. The intravenous route is not recommended for administration of concentrated insulin because of possible hypoglycemic reactions.

Refrigeration between uses is preferable, but, like other insulins, the vials should never be frozen. Avoid using (discard) discolored or turbid solutions.

Clinical Indications

Insulins are indicated and Food and Drug Administration (FDA) approved for use in the treatment of Type I diabetes mellitus, and Type II diabetes mellitus that cannot properly be controlled by diet and exercise. Insulins are also approved to reduce hyperkalemia because the protein naturally provokes a shift of potassium into cells, lowering circulating potassium levels. Of course, compensation with glucose coadministration circumvents possible hypoglycemia. Insulin is the choice for reversing severe ketoacidosis diabetic coma.

Adverse Effects

Insulin is usually well tolerated by diabetics. However, since the hormone is a polypeptide that is frequently combined with a protein (antigen), it is not unusual for diabetics to develop an allergic reaction. Allergic reactions may include itching, urticarial swelling, or anaphylaxis. Usually, patients can be switched to another species of insulin to avoid the reaction. Insulin obtained from pigs (porcine) is less antigenic than is beef insulin. In addition, regular or lente insulins are preferred because these preparations do not contain protein complexes (protamine or globin).

Some diabetics develop lipodystrophy, hypertrophy, or abscesses at the site of injection. **Lipodystrophy** is a disappearance of subcutaneous fat at the site of insulin injection. As a result, the skin becomes pitted and concave. Diabetics usually inject the insulin SC into the arms, abdomen, or thighs. To avoid atrophy of the subcutaneous tissue in these regions, a record of injection sites should be kept so that sites can be rotated.

The most common adverse effects of insulin therapy are blurred vision and hypoglycemia. During the initial period of insulin therapy, changes in the lens result in blurred vision. This effect usually subsides within 1 or 2 weeks. However, hypoglycemia is a result of insulin overdose (insulin shock). When the blood glucose level is depressed, patients often experience hunger, headache, blurred vision, fatigue, anxiety, nervousness, confusion, and paresthesia. In severe cases, fainting or convulsions may occur. Usually, candy bars, ginger ale, or fruit juices will supply an adequate amount of glucose to correct the hypoglycemia. In severe cases (diabetic coma), glucagon may be administered (0.5 to 1 mg) intravenously. Glucagon produces a rapid rise in blood glucose that lasts about 1 hour. Once patients' symptoms are controlled, dextrose can be given intravenously.

Special Considerations

Before withdrawing any solution, insulin vials should always be rotated gently in the palm of the hand to avoid foaming. Suspension preparations are not uniformly dissolved, so some crystals fall to the bottom of the bottle. This gentle rotation permits a better dispersion of the insulin in the buffer so that the proper amount can be administered on schedule. Regular insulin should appear as a clear solution.

If not exposed to strong sunlight, insulin is stable at room temperature for extended periods. Nevertheless, it is preferable to refrigerate (do not freeze) vials between uses to maintain the activity of the polypeptide. Prior to injection, it is recommended that the solution be warmed to room temperature to reduce the likelihood of producing a reaction at the site of injection. The expiration date should always be checked before administering the medication. Regular insulin that has passed the expiration date, that appears cloudy or discolored, or that has evidence of clumping should be discarded.

When preparing and administering insulin, sterile techniques should be followed. Hands should be washed prior to preparing the drug for administration. The septum of the insulin bottle should be swabbed with alcohol before the needle is inserted. Air should be injected into the bottle in order for insulin to flow easily into the syringe. The amount of air injected should be equal to the patient's insulin dose (that is, the same volume as the number of units to be given). Once air has been injected, the bottle should be turned upside down with the needle well into the insulin and the desired volume of drug withdrawn. Always check for air bubbles. Although the air is harmless, it is important to remove large bubbles because they reduce the amount of insulin injected. Always double-check the dose to be given prior to injection.

The timing of insulin administration and meals is very important for diabetic patients. The blood glucose level is delicately maintained by manipulating the carbohydrate intake. Therefore, insulin must be taken at the same time each day.

Insulin is usually administered 15 to 30 minutes before meals, although longer-acting preparations are given before breakfast. Variation in an established dosing schedule or diet will result in unstable blood glucose levels. Patients should always be observed (and they should be alert) for signals of insulin shock after receiving an injection. Patients should become aware of the onset and time of peak action of the particular insulin they use. Juice or sugar should be available to ease predictable hypoglycemic symptoms. With the long-acting insulin preparations, hypoglycemia may occur during the night, as evidenced by restless sleep and sweating. It is important to remember that the insulin requirement may change when patients become ill and experience episodes of vomiting or fever.

Regular insulin may be administered intravenously in emergencies or in severely ill patients. Plastic IV infusion sets adsorb insulin, so patients receive less insulin than prescribed. There is no way to predict the amount lost through adsorption. Therefore, following intravenous administration with an infusion setup, patients must be monitored carefully to titrate the insulin dose to the desired response.

Patients who are unconscious or severely hypoglycemic cannot offer accurate information about their medical history and therapy. Always examine patients for identification (tags, bracelets, or cards) that might disclose any insulin allergies. Never administer insulin until a positive diagnosis of insulin deficiency has been established. It is always safe to give sugar first to see if the symptoms subside. Insulin overdose is more critical than the added hyperglycemia resulting from fruit juice or candy.

Drug Interactions

Several drugs affect the action of insulin in diabetic patients (see Table 39:3 on page 472). Many have a direct effect on glucose metabolism. Salicylates, beta-blockers, adrenergic neuronal blockers, and monoamine oxidase (MAO) inhibitors reduce circulating blood glucose levels; therefore, these drugs potentiate the hypoglycemic action of insulin. In contrast, glucagon, epinephrine, diazoxide, chlorpromazine, and sympathomimetics counteract insulin's action by inhibiting glucose utilization. Insulin also can produce a shift in potassium from extracellular to intracellular sites, and this shift effectively reduces the serum potassium concentrations. When insulin is administered concomitantly with cardiac glycosides, patients should be monitored for indications of drug antagonism.

Oral Hypoglycemic Drugs (Secretagogues)

Secretagogues are the class of oral hypoglycemic drugs that describes the mechanism of action and impact on blood glucose concentration. The drugs in this class include sulfonylureas and nonsulfonylureas (also called meglitinides). These drugs are useful in the treatment of Type II diabetes, alone or in combination with other antidiabetic drugs. The term "secretagogue" is applied to a substance that induces or causes the secretion of another substance.

These antidiabetic drugs enter the beta cells of the pancreas and cause the release of insulin. These drugs bind to the potassium channel of the beta cells and allow an influx of calcium ions across the membrane that triggers insulin release from the cell. Consequently, the secreted insulin alters the blood glucose level. These drugs do not have any insulin-like activity. The hypoglycemic activity of the secretagogues is due to insulin released from the pancreas. Therefore, the secretagogues have no value in the treatment of Type I diabetes, in which there is no insulin in the beta cells.

Physiological Factors and Drugs That Alter the Actions of Insulin

FACTORS THAT INCREASE THE INSULIN REQUIREMENT (ANTAGONIZE INSULIN)	RESPONSE
Catecholamine secretion—epinephrine	
Colds, infections, illness	
Drugs: acetazolamide, AIDS antivirals, chlorpromazine, diazoxide, diltiazem, niacin, nicotine, oral contraceptives, rifampin, sympathomimetics, thiazide diuretics	These factors or agents *increase* blood glucose concentrations by:
Hormones: corticotropin, estrogens, glucagon, glucocorticoids, growth hormone, progestogens, thyroid hormones	• increasing cell activity
Obesity	• increasing gluconeogenesis
Pregnancy	• inhibiting insulin release
Smoking	• stimulating liver glycogenolysis
Stress	• stimulating the sympathetic nervous system
Surgery	

FACTORS THAT DECREASE THE INSULIN REQUIREMENT (POTENTIATE INSULIN)	RESPONSE
Alcohol	
ACE inhibitors	These factors or agents *decrease* blood glucose concentrations by:
Adrenergic neuronal blockers	
Anabolic steroids	• interfering with glucose metabolism
Anticoagulants, oral	• inhibiting the sympathetic nervous system
Beta-blockers, propranolol	
Chloroquine	
Clofibrate	
Diazoxide	
Fenfluramine	
Lithium carbonate	
MAO inhibitors	
Metoprolol	
Pentamidine	
Pyridoxine	
Salicylates	
Sulfinpyrazone	
Tetracyclines	

Abbreviations: ACE, angiotensin-converting enzyme; AIDS, acquired immunodeficiency syndrome; MAO, monoamine oxidase.

Characteristics

Four first-generation oral hypoglycemic drugs are available in the United States: acetohexamide, chlorpropamide, tolazamide, and tolbutamide (see Table 39:4). Newer, second-generation oral hypoglycemic drugs include glipizide, glimepiride, and glyburide. All of these drugs produce the same action on the pancreas. However, the onset and duration of action vary because the absorption and metabolism of these drugs differ. There is a delay in the onset of action because the drugs must be absorbed from the intestine and then transported to the pancreas.

Except for tolazamide, the oral hypoglycemics are rapidly absorbed from the intestines. Since time is required to induce insulin release from the pancreas, the onset of action varies between 1 and 4 hours. Metabolism by the liver quickly inactivates tolbutamide; therefore, tolbutamide is a relatively short-acting drug. Glyburide and glipizide are more slowly metabolized in the liver to inactive metabolites. Tolazamide and acetohexamide are metabolized to active hypoglycemic compounds so that the effective duration of action is much longer (24 hours). Since chlorpropamide is not metabolized at all, it continues to stimulate insulin release until it is excreted by the kidneys. As a result, the duration of chlorpropamide's action may be up to 60 hours. Chlorpropamide elimination is influenced by changes in the urine pH. Urine alkalinization (pH greater than 6) promotes chlorpropamide excretion.

The nonsulfonylureas are represented by repaglinide (*Prandin*) and nateglinide (*Starlix*). The mechanism of action stimulates insulin secretion out of the beta cells. These drugs, however, are more rapidly absorbed than are the secretagogues. The onset of action is 20 to 30 minutes, with peak insulin levels occurring within 60 minutes and returning to the lower, predrug level before the next meal. For this reason, these drugs must be taken within 1 to 30 minutes before each meal (dose and frequency are based on the patient's glucose-lowering requirement).

Clinical Indications

The secretagogue drugs are approved for use as an adjunct to diet to lower the blood glucose in Type II diabetes patients. These drugs have no value in the treatment of Type I diabetes or severe diabetes that occurs in the elderly. The advantage of the secretagogues over insulin is that the trauma and complications of injection, such as lipodystrophy, are avoided. However, the secretagogues are not a substitute for insulin, since these drugs have no effect on the ketosis that often accompanies diabetes. Elderly severe diabetics may undergo ketosis. Any diabetic who develops ketosis must be given insulin.

Adverse Effects

Oral hypoglycemics produce hypoglycemia as the most common side effect. This effect may be severe in elderly, debilitated, or malnourished patients. Due to the variation in the onset and duration of action, it is easy for patients to become hypoglycemic if meals are not strictly timed and well balanced. The usual treatment is to administer carbohydrates as soon as possible. Subsequent adjustment in dose or meal patterns may be necessary. Because of prolonged action, patients who become hypoglycemic on chlorpropamide must be closely observed for several (3 to 5) days. Hospitalization may be required in profound hypoglycemic episodes. In situations requiring hospitalization, dextrose may be administered by intravenous infusion to maintain an adequate blood glucose concentration.

In the absence of hypoglycemia, the secretagogues occasionally produce gastrointestinal (GI) irritation, nausea, diarrhea, weakness, fatigue, and dizziness. Reported hypersensitivity reactions include photosensitivity, rashes, jaundice, and elevation of liver enzymes. Since there is no cross-sensitivity, patients can usually be placed on another secretagogue to avoid these reactions. Some individuals receiving secretagogue therapy have reportedly developed hemolytic anemia, leukopenia, thrombocytopenia, and aplastic anemia. Leukopenia, thrombocytopenia, and mild anemia return to normal when the drug is discontinued. Oral hypoglycemic drugs have been associated with an increased rate of cardiovascular mortality, compared to treatment with diet alone or diet plus insulin.

Contraindications

Oral hypoglycemic drugs are contraindicated in patients with known hypersensitivity to secretagogues, Type I diabetes, or a diabetic

Dose and Duration of Action of Oral Antidiabetic Drugs

DRUG (TRADE NAME)	MAXIMAL EFFECTIVE DOSE	DAILY DOSE RANGE	ONSET OF ACTION (HOURS)	DURATION ACTION (HOURS)
Oral Sulfonylureas Hypoglycemics (Secretagogues)				
acetohexamide (*Dymelor*)	1.5 g	0.25–1.5 g	1	12–24
chlorpropamide (*Diabinese*)	750 mg	100–250 mg	1	60
glimepiride (*Amaryl*)	8 mg	1–4 mg	1	24
glipizide (*Glucotrol*)	40 mg	5–15 mg	1–1.5	10–16
glyburide (*DiaBeta, Micronase*)	20 mg	1.25–20 mg	2–4	24
glyburide micronase (*Glynase*)	12 mg	0.75–12 mg	1	12–24
tolazamide (*Tolinase*)	1 g	100–500 mg	4–6	12–24
tolbutamide (*Orinase*)	3 g	0.25–2 g	1	6–12
Nonsulfonylureas (Meglitinides)				
repaglinide (*Prandin*)	16 mg	0.5–4 mg QID	30 min	4
nateglinide (*Starlix*)	360 mg	60–120 mg TID	20 min	2
Glucose Absorption Inhibitors (Alpha Glucosidase Inhibitors)				
acarbose (*Precose*)	100 mg	25–100 mg TID	—	—
miglitol (*Glyset*)	100 mg	25–100 mg TID	—	—
Antihyperglycemic Drugs				
metformin (*Glucophage*)	2500 mg	500–850 mg TID	—	—
(*Glucophage XR*)	2000 mg	1500–2000 mg	—	—
Insulin Sensitizers (Thiaxolidinediones)				
rosiglitazone (*Avandia*)	8 mg	2–8 mg		
pioglitazone (*Actos*)	45 mg	15–45 mg	1–2	24

condition complicated by fever, ketoacidosis, or coma. Secretagogues are not recommended for use in patients who have moderate to severe liver or renal disease. Impairment of liver and renal function decreases the clearance of these drugs and their metabolites from the blood. The nonsulfonylurea drugs may be used with caution and careful observation in patients with mild liver or renal disease.

Special Considerations

Occasionally diabetic patients experience trauma or physiological stress from fever, concomitant disease, or a condition that increases the difficulty in maintaining glucose control. In such situations, insulin may be substituted or added to the drug regimen to stabilize glucose control. Insulin is recommended over the secretagogues during pregnancy. Insulin is also used instead of the secretagogues prior to and during surgical procedures. The insulin level is much easier to control, since the stress of surgery may cause frequent fluctuations in the blood glucose level. Secretagogues should never be used in patients with peptic ulcers or ketosis.

NOTE TO THE HEALTH CARE PROFESSIONAL

Elderly patients are particularly responsive to the pharmacological effects of oral hypoglycemic drugs. It may be necessary to lower the initial dose to one-half the adult recommended dose in geriatric patients.

When transferring patients from one oral hypoglycemic drug to another, a transitional period of dose adjustment is usually not necessary. With chlorpropamide, however, the prolonged duration of action may potentiate the hypoglycemic effect of the alternate medication. Patients must be observed carefully during the transition from chlorpropamide to another oral hypoglycemic drug. When transferring patients from insulin to an oral secretagogue, the urine can be tested easily for glucose and ketones to monitor blood glucose fluctuation.

Drug Interactions

Oral hypoglycemics are bound to plasma proteins and metabolized in the liver. Therefore, these drugs are involved in several drug interactions. Drugs that inhibit liver enzymes, displace sulfonylureas from protein-binding sites, or inhibit glucose metabolism will potentiate the hypoglycemic actions of the sulfonylureas. Repaglinide should not be started in patients who are on gemfibrozil and itraconazole because prolonged glucose lowering may occur. This is a result of inhibited metabolism of repaglinide. Table 39:5 on page 476 lists specific drugs that are known to interact with the oral hypoglycemics. Alcohol may produce a disulfiram reaction due to the accumulation of acetic acid in the blood. (See Chapter 10 for discussion of disulfiram.)

Oral hypoglycemic drugs stimulate the hepatic microsomal system and may reduce circulating blood digitoxin levels in patients receiving concomitant cardiac glycoside therapy. Rifampin has been reported to stimulate the metabolism of chlorpropamide and tolbutamide, thus reducing their hypoglycemic activity.

Other Antidiabetic Drugs

These antidiabetic drugs include three groups that have mechanisms of action that are different from those of the insulins or oral hypoglycemic secretagogues. None of these drugs is a hypoglycemic. They do not decrease blood sugar levels nor do they effect insulin release. One group influences dietary glucose absorption to maintain lower glucose blood levels; one group decreases glucose output from the liver; and one group acts directly on fat, skeletal muscle, and the liver to sensitize the action of insulin on its target tissues and enhance glucose utilization.

Glucose Absorption Inhibitors (Alpha-Glucosidase Inhibitors)

Miglitol (*Glyset*) and acarbose (*Precose*) interfere with dietary carbohydrate digestion. Ingested oligosaccharides and disaccharides are broken down to glucose through the enzymes glycoside hydrolase and alpha-amylase. In the membrane of the small intestine, miglitol and acarbose inhibit glycoside hydrolase so that glucose absorption is delayed not eliminated. Acarbose is itself an oligosaccharide and also reversibly ties up alpha-amylase (Figure 39:1 on page 477). What results is a delay in glucose absorption so that the blood glucose level after meals (postprandial) does not immediately peak. This eliminates postprandial hyperglycemia. This mechanism of action is additive to the oral hypoglycemics and insulin.

These drugs are ingested with each meal—that is three times a day—so carbohydrate metabolism can be affected. Acarbose is metabolized within the intestine by enzymes and bacteria. Miglitol is absorbed and excreted through the kidneys unmetabolized. Neither drug affects the liver and can be used in patients with liver impairment. Dosing may begin with 25 mg and range from 25 to 100 mg TID for both drugs. Dose adjustment is made at 4- to 8-week intervals after glucose monitoring confirms the drug's effectiveness 1 hour after meals.

Adverse Effects

The principal adverse effects are GI flatulence, diarrhea, and abdominal pain, which subside over continued drug use. Even in cases of overdose, only GI symptoms developed. Patients may require periodic evaluation for glycosylated

Drug Interactions With Oral Antidiabetic Drugs

DRUGS THAT POTENTIATE ORAL HYPOGLYCEMIC DRUGS	REASON
Adrenergic neuronal blocking drugs, guanethidine diazoxide fenfluramine Insulin MAO inhibitors ranitidine Salicylates Sympatholytics	Inhibit glucose metabolism or glucose utilization
alcohol Anticoagulants, oral (coumarins) chloramphenicol cimetidine gemfibrozil MAO inhibitors itraconazole	Inhibit hepatic enzymes, sulfonylurea and repaglinide metabolism
clofibrate ethacrynic acid probenecid Sulfonamide antibiotics	Displace the sulfonylureas from plasma protein-binding sites

DRUGS THAT ANTAGONIZE ORAL HYPOGLYCEMIC DRUGS OR ACARBOSE	REASON
Beta-blockers Calcium channel blockers Hormones (estrogen, glucagon, growth hormone, progestogens, thyroid hormones) isoniazid Steroids Stress Sympathomimetics	Alter carbohydrate metabolism, causing increased blood glucose concentrations; loss of blood sugar control
Alcohol, chronic Phenothiazines, chlorpromazine phenobarbital phenytoin rifampin	Increase hepatic metabolism, reducing oral hypoglycemic drug concentration in the blood

DRUGS THAT ANTAGONIZE CARBOHYDRATE ABSORPTION INHIBITORS	REASON
Digestive enzymes: amylase, pancreatin Charcoal	Decrease effect of miglitol and acarbose

hemoglobin (miglitol) and serum transaminases (acarbose) because such changes were reported in a small number of patients participating in clinical trials during drug development.

These drugs do not cause hypoglycemia when used alone. If used in combination with secretagogues or insulin, hypoglycemia may occur.

In this event, patients need to be given glucose (not sucrose) because the alpha-glucosidase inhibitors interfere with sucrose metabolism.

Contraindications to drug use include diabetic ketoacidosis, bowel disorders, or diseases that are associated with impaired absorption and hypersensitivity to the drug.

Glucose Absorption: Sites of Reversible Enzyme Inhibition

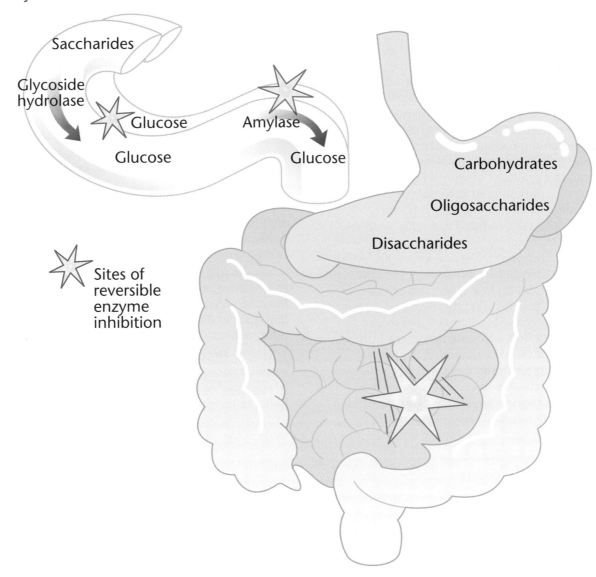

Sites of reversible enzyme inhibition.

Drug Interactions

Acarbose and miglitol are limited to interactions with products that affect GI digestion. Concurrent ingestion of digestive enzymes such as amylase, pancreatin, or charcoal would inhibit the ability of these drugs to act on carbohydrates within the intestine, thereby decreasing their efficacy.

Antihyperglycemic Biguanide

An antihyperglycemic drug keeps the glucose blood level from rising too fast or too high after meals but does not necessarily "lower" blood glucose. Metformin (*Glucophage*) chemically is a

biguanide drug that lowers postprandial glucose levels by decreasing liver glucose production and intestinal glucose absorption. It also appears to enhance glucose utilization by other tissues. Overall, this contributes to a smaller rise in postprandial glucose and smoother distribution to tissues. Unlike the secretagogues, metformin is not a hypoglycemic because it does not drive blood sugar levels down in normal or diabetic patients. It has no direct influence on insulin secretion.

The usual dose is 500 mg BID up to a maximum of 2500 mg per day. Metformin is absorbed from the GI tract and excreted unchanged by the kidneys. Elderly patients who have age-related

Patient Administration and Monitoring

This is another group of drugs that demands patient compliance not only with the medication schedule but with diet adjustment. Timing of the dose is critical to circumvent great swings in blood sugar and hypoglycemic episodes that send the patient into sweats, disorientation, pallor, immediate fatigue, and loss of consciousness. Diabetes patients require a significant amount of support to obtain encouragement and maintain a commitment to stick with the program. Fortunately, such support is readily available through community and hospital outreach education programs and the American Diabetes Association. In addition, patients need confirmation that questions can be directed to the treating physician and staff no matter how many times they need to ask. Patients can find adequate treatment from a variety of physicians ranging from family practitioners to endocrinologists or diabetologists. It is not unusual for elderly patients to change physicians because of guilt arising from not achieving the standard of control the physician has set or because they perceive they are not getting sufficient individualized attention. Therefore, diabetes patients need to receive clear, attentive, repetitive instruction in the administration of medication and the formation of new behavior patterns that will make for successful therapy.

In the Event of an Accident or Diabetes Complications

Patients must carry adequate identification that describes their medical condition and clearly identifies which antidiabetic medication they are taking. If possible, the time of usual dosing should be indicated to help medical professionals ascertain the scope of the problem. This is particularly important if the patient is taking metformin where lactic acidosis can develop.

Patients should be encouraged to disclose their medication to all other physicians who may be evaluating and/or treating the patient.

Patients should be routinely monitoring blood glucose and/or urine ketones to keep their insulin dose at the lowest effective dose.

Patients taking combination therapy should alert family members of the possibility that hypoglycemia could occur so that dextrose or oral glucose is readily available (for example, in the car, in the handbag, on the job). Anxiety, restlessness, and clammy skin often are the first signs that the patient is experiencing low blood sugar. Family members need to be well informed.

Special Note: All sugars are not alike. Table sugar is sucrose and tablets for treating hypoglycemia are dextrose or glucose. Patients taking miglitol or acarbose who experience hypoglycemia *cannot* be given table sugar or sugar cubes because the sucrose is metabolized to glucose by the enzyme that these drugs inhibit. Therefore, the patient would not have rapid absorption of glucose.

Patients and their families must be fully and clearly informed about the possibility of lactic acidosis if the patient is to receive metformin. Symptoms of acidosis need to be understood so that the patient or a relative can notify the physician as soon as symptoms become evident.

---

diminution of renal function show decreased plasma clearance of metformin. It is recommended that elderly patients not be titrated to the maximum dose because of increased plasma concentration.

Adverse Effects

The GI effects of diarrhea, nausea, vomiting, and flatulence are usually tolerable and dissipate with continued use of the drug. Sometime dose reduction will also ameliorate the adverse effect.

There is one adverse effect, although rare, that can be life-threatening—lactic acidosis. Lactic acid accumulates in the blood and contributes to lowering the pH, which directly contributes to electrolyte imbalances. This can lead to respiratory and cardiovascular distress. Patients may present with signs of lactic acidosis but no ketoacidosis. Patients often develop symptoms of fatigue, myalgia, and respiratory or abdominal distress, which should be reported to the physician immediately. Since the GI symptoms associated

Dose Administration

Remind the patient to consistently use the same brand of insulin and same type of syringe to avoid errors in medication. If more than one insulin is being administered in the same syringe, remind the patient *not to interchange* the order of mixing and not to reinject solution in the syringe into the insulin vial.

Older patients cannot easily distinguish the dose markings on transparent syringes. Recommend the use of syringes with a colored background or magnifiers that attach to the syringe to make the fluid level easier to see.

If insulin is stored in the refrigerator, remind patients to bring it to room temperature before injecting to reduce irritation at the injection site.

Patients taking glucose absorption inhibitors must take the medication at the beginning (with the first bite) of each meal—that means three meals and medication three times a day.

If the patient experiences GI upset when taking the sulfonylureas, advise the dose be taken with food.

Notify the Prescribing Physician

Patients should call the physician *whenever* they develop fever, sore throat, bruising, unusual bleeding, colds, or flu that could alter their medication requirements. Remind the patient to have the last home-monitored glucose values available for the doctor to review.

Call the physician if fatigue, profuse sweating, numbness of the extremities, excessive hunger (hypoglycemia) or excessive thirst, urination, elevation in urine glucose or ketones occurs (hyperglycemia). Evaluation and/or dose adjustment may be indicated.

Remind patients to avoid alcohol during sulfonylurea treatment because it may produce intense nausea by a disulfiram reaction.

Patients need to be advised to avoid excessive alcohol use during metformin treatment because of its potential to induce metformin lactic acidosis.

Use in Pregnancy

Antidiabetic drugs are designated Food and Drug Administration (FDA) Pregnancy Category B and C. Overall the safety for use in pregnant women has not been established through controlled clinical trials although historically women have been exposed to some of these drugs during pregnancy. Animal studies suggest that the oral antidiabetic drugs can cause birth defects so the potential risk to the patient and fetus must be seriously considered before continuing drug therapy during pregnancy. Because abnormal glucose levels during pregnancy have accompanied congenital abnormalities, blood glucose control during pregnancy is imperative in the best interests of the mother and fetus. The universal recommendation is that insulin is the treatment of choice during pregnancy. Patients should be advised to notify the prescribing physician, which is usually not the gynecologist/obstetrician, if they become pregnant while on antidiabetic drugs. Prompt evaluation will determine whether adjustment in dose and/or medication is warranted.

with initial therapy abate over time and the dose is stable, any GI distress that develops later should be considered a potential metabolic imbalance. Lactic acidosis is a medical emergency that requires patient hospitalization for treatment and observation. Hemodialysis is used to clear metformin from the system. The risk of lactic acidosis increases with renal or liver impairment and age.

Contraindications

Metformin is contraindicated for use in patients who have metabolic acidosis, including diabetic ketoacidosis, renal disease or abnormal creatinine clearance. Because iodine contrast dyes used in radiologic evaluation may cause acute renal failure, metformin should be discontinued at least 48 hours before and after such procedures to avoid the possibility of lactic acidosis.

Alcohol potentiates the action of metformin on lactic acid metabolism. Patients need to be advised to avoid excessive alcohol use during metformin treatment.

Antihyperglycemic Thiazolidinedione

Among the new classes of oral antidiabetic drugs are the "insulin sensitizers." Troglitazone

(*Rezulin*), pioglitazone (*Actos*), and rosiglitazone (*Avandia*) enhance peripheral cell response to insulin, allowing glucose to be utilized more efficiently. Although they do not stimulate insulin secretion, these drugs do decrease insulin resistance and increase insulin sensitivity of fat, skeletal muscle, and liver cells by activating receptors inside the cells (nuclear receptors) that regulate insulin activity. Both of these actions contribute to a removal of glucose from the circulation into the target cells. This requires insulin to be present in order to effect a change in glucose distribution. For this reason, they are recommended in the treatment of Type I diabetes mellitus where there is a deficiency in insulin production. However, if used in Type I patients receiving insulin, these drugs will provide the conditions for hypoglycemia due to increased insulin sensitivity.

These drugs are rapidly absorbed after oral administration and most of the drugs are excreted unchanged in the feces. Therefore, renal impairment does not affect drug blood levels. The adverse effect profile includes diarrhea and nausea.

This is a new drug class that has not been exposed to the same patient experience as other antidiabetic drugs. Troglitazone has been withdrawn from the market due to safety concerns associated with the increased incidence of liver failure and death in patients taking the drug. The two other drugs in this class have not been associated with a similar severity risk, and, therefore, are still commercially available for the management of diabetes. Reversible elevations in serum liver enzymes have occurred with pioglitazone and rosiglitazone, prompting the recommendation that evaluation of liver function such as serum enzyme profiles should be performed prior to initiating therapy with this class of drugs. Periodically, patients' enzymes should be monitored to confirm that liver injury has not developed during treatment. Other common adverse effects in this class include fluid retention and weight gain. The fluid retention (edema) can exacerbate conditions of heart failure and, therefore, do not make these the drugs of choice for patients with congestive heart failure. Otherwise, the adverse effects are headache, fatigue, and diarrhea.

Clinical Indications

All of the antidiabetic drugs are indicated for the management of diabetes mellitus Type II in combination with diet control and/or secretagogues.

This class is approved for Type II diabetics currently on insulin therapy in whom hyperglycemia is inadequately controlled.

Chapter Review

Understanding Terminology

Match the definitions or descriptions in the left column with the appropriate term in the right column.

___ **1.** Numbness of hands and feet.

___ **2.** A higher than normal level of glucose in the blood.

___ **3.** A preparation in which solid particles of an undissolved drug are dispersed within a liquid.

___ **4.** Excessive thirst.

___ **5.** Fat.

___ **6.** Excessive production of urine.

___ **7.** Excessive eating.

___ **8.** The presence of glucose in the urine.

a. adipose tissue

b. glycosuria

c. hyperglycemia

d. neuropathy

e. polydipsia

f. polyphagia

g. polyuria

h. suspension

Acquiring Knowledge

Answer the following questions in the spaces provided.

1. What is the primary deficiency in diabetes? _____

_____

2. What is the difference between Type I and Type II diabetes? _____

_____

3. What are the common symptoms of diabetes? _____

_____

4. How does insulin control the symptoms of diabetes? _____

_____

5. What role does glucagon play in diabetes? _____

_____

6. How do the commercial insulin preparations differ? _____

_____

7. Why are some insulins shorter acting than others? _____

_____

8. Why do the insulins occasionally produce allergic reactions? _____

_____

9. How do the oral hypoglycemic drugs differ from the commercial insulins? _____

_____

10. When are the oral hypoglycemics used? _____

_____

11. What factors potentiate the hypoglycemic actions of insulin and the oral hypoglycemics?

_____

_____

12. What factors antagonize the actions of insulin and the oral hypoglycemics? _____

_____

_____

Applying Knowledge—On the Job

Use your critical thinking skills to answer the following questions in the spaces provided.

1. Assume you work in a hospital preparing medications for injection. For each of the following situations, identify the error that has been made in using insulin.

   a. Your coworker on the early shift removed a vial of insulin from the freezer and left it on the counter to thaw so it would be ready for you to use when your shift starts. _____

_____

_____

   b. A vial of lente insulin in your medication refrigerator looks cloudy. You assume that it has gone bad and discard it. _____

_____

_____

   c. Your first order of the day calls for a mixture of *Semilente* insulin and isophane insulin zinc suspension. Your next order calls for *Iletin II* insulin prepared for intravenous injection.

_____

_____

2. Assume you work in an endocrinology clinic where you screen patients for potential drug interactions. What potential problem(s) do you see in each of the following cases? Should the insulin dose be increased or decreased as a result?

   a. Patient A takes oral contraceptives and is overweight. _____

_____

_____

   b. Patient B is taking *Achromycin* for a strep infection. _____

_____

_____

   c. Patient C takes *Diamox* for glaucoma. _____

_____

_____

   d. Patient D is taking *Lopressor* for hypertension. _____

_____

_____

3. Renal impairment is not uncommon in diabetics as the disease progresses. Judy has been taking *Micronase* for 10 years. Her diabetes has been fairly well controlled with diet and medication. She has just been diagnosed with moderate renal impairment due to her diabetic condition. Would you expect to see changes in her medication? Why? _____

_____

_____

4. Hal, a diabetic, has been taking *Precose* 75 mg three times daily with meals. His diabetes has been well controlled. He has just been diagnosed with liver impairment. Would you expect to see changes in his medication? Why? _____

_____

_____

5. Patients taking *Glucophage* should be cautioned to avoid excessive alcohol use during metformin therapy. Why? _____

_____

_____

Internet Connection

Healthfinder is a website maintained by the U.S. government to provide consumers and medical personnel with access to current accurate information on a variety of diseases. Through this site you can find publications, help groups, government agencies, and other organizations that provide reliable information to the public. Go onto this website by selecting http://www.healthfinder.gov. At the home page you will be provided a user-friendly menu of items. At the search box enter *Diabetes Dictionary*. This site is maintained by the NIDDK. The *Diabetes Dictionary* allows you to select any letter and you will be provided with symptoms, definitions, and conditions that are relevant to diabetes. Next, enter *Diabetes Risk Test*. This program asks you to enter information about yourself that is computed into a value indicating your likelihood for developing diabetes. Additional web pages of immediate interest for diabetes education include: www.niddk.nih.gov (National Institute of Diabetes and Digestive Disease and Kidney Disease) and www.diabetes.org (American Diabetes Association). These sites provide a review of anatomy, physiology, and pharmacology written at an easy-to-understand level and contact numbers for receiving additional information. The Diabetes Center and Endocrine Disease of the Pancreas present well-illustrated medical information directed at the education of patients and their families about diabetes and pancreatic hormones at www.endocrineweb.com. This site adds pages weekly and includes a large amount of information on endocrine disease, conditions, hormone problems, and treatment options.

Finally, www.findarticles.com is a site that allows you to enter a topic, word, or phrase such as *Type 2 diabetes* or *Insulin Sensitizer* to obtain relevant articles from worldwide medical and new-information sources for online review.

Additional Reading

Florence, J. A. 1999. Treatment of type 2 diabetes mellitus. *American Family Physician* 59 (10): 835. (access online at www.aafp.org)

Henry, R. R. 1996. Glucose and insulin resistance in non-insulin dependent diabetes mellitus. *Annals of Internal Medicine,* 124 (part 2):97.

Schumann, D. 1990. Postoperative hyperglycemia: Clinical benefits of insulin therapy. *Heart Lung* 18:165.

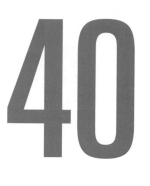

40

POSTERIOR PITUITARY HORMONES AND DRUGS AFFECTING UTERINE MUSCLE

CHAPTER FOCUS

This chapter describes two naturally occurring substances that are secreted within the brain. It explains how these two substances, antidiuretic hormone (ADH) and oxytocin, directly influence the function of the renal tubules and uterus.

CHAPTER OBJECTIVES

After studying this chapter, you should be able to

- describe how the actions of oxytocin and antidiuretic hormone differ.

- explain the clinical use for oxytocin.

- describe the natural extensions of oxytocin's action and the adverse effects such extensions produce.

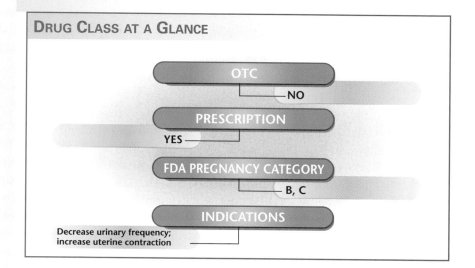

DRUG CLASS AT A GLANCE

OTC
— NO

PRESCRIPTION
YES —

FDA PREGNANCY CATEGORY
— B, C

INDICATIONS
Decrease urinary frequency; increase uterine contraction —

Key Terms

antidiuretic hormone (ADH): polypeptide substance released within the brain that regulates water balance in the body.

diabetes insipidus: chronic condition caused by inadequate secretion of antidiuretic hormone, in which individuals are extremely thirsty and produce very large amounts of pale urine.

endogenous: originating within the body.

exogenous: originating outside the body, or administered into the body from outside.

oxytocin: polypeptide substance released within the brain that has specific functions during and after pregnancy, specifically relating to the uterus and the mammary glands.

polypeptide: substance composed of an indefinite number of amino acids.

postpartum: after childbirth.

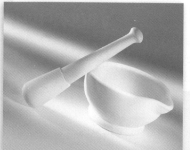

pressor: tending to increase blood pressure.

tetany: condition resulting in intermittent tonic muscle contractions.

vasopressin: another name for antidiuretic hormone because at higher doses the hormone increases blood pressure.

INTRODUCTION

The pituitary gland is located at the base of the hypothalamus and has two main lobes: the anterior lobe (adenohypophysis) and the posterior lobe (neurohypophysis). The posterior lobe stores and releases two hormones: antidiuretic hormone (ADH) and oxytocin.

Antidiuretic hormone (ADH) is a **polypeptide** substance that regulates water balance in the body. When ADH is released, it travels in the blood to the kidneys. In the kidneys, ADH increases the reabsorption of water to the blood. This action promotes conservation of body fluids. Individuals who lack ADH have a condition known as **diabetes insipidus.** This condition is characterized by the loss of large volumes of body water via the urine. To clarify names, the **endogenous** compound is generally called antidiuretic hormone, or ADH. The **exogenously** administered drug product is often called **vasopressin,** although both names refer to the same substance. The main clinical use of vasopressin and related substances is in the treatment of diabetes insipidus. In larger doses, vasopressin produces a **pressor** effect on blood vessels (vaso), from which the name vasopressin was developed.

The polypeptide **oxytocin** functions primarily during and after pregnancy. Oxytocin causes contractions of the uterus and is therefore believed to play a role during labor. Commercial preparations of oxytocin and related substances are used to induce labor, to control postpartum bleeding, and to induce therapeutic abortions. Drugs that produce contractions of the uterus are referred to as oxytocics.

Oxytocin also plays an important role during breast-feeding. Release of oxytocin is stimulated by suckling. After being released, oxytocin travels in the blood to the myoepithelial cells of the mammary glands, where it causes the ejection of milk.

DIABETES INSIPIDUS

Diabetes insipidus results from a deficiency of ADH. Individuals with diabetes insipidus excrete large volumes of dilute urine and are unable to maintain fluid balance.

Treatment mainly involves replacement therapy with vasopressin obtained from animal or synthetic sources.

Posterior Pituitary Powder

This preparation, obtained from the posterior pituitary glands of animals (cattle and swine), contains both ADH and oxytocin. The powder is inhaled several times per day in doses ranging from 5 to 20 mg. The main disadvantages of this preparation are nasal irritation and the development of allergy.

Vasopressin Injection (*Pitressin synthetic*)

Vasopressin (8-arginine vasopressin), obtained from animal sources, contains ADH and oxytocin in a ratio of 20:1. Synthetic vasopressin contains the vital sequence of amino acids that mimics endogenous hormone activity. It is injected SC or IM in the early treatment of diabetes insipidus to stabilize patients' fluid balance. The duration of action of vasopressin injection, 5 to 10 units, is approximately 2 to 8 hours. It is metabolized and excreted by the liver and kidneys.

Lypressin (*Diapid*)

Lypressin (8-lysine-vasopressin) is a synthetic compound administered by nasal spray. Lypressin produces an effective ADH action with little or no vasopressor response. Drug is administered by the patient as one or two sprays in one or both nostrils. The appropriate dose for the patient is achieved by repeated trial. If the patient requires more drug, the dosing strategy is to increase the frequency of dosing, not the number of sprays. More than two sprays in both nostrils results in excess drug, which is swallowed into the gastrointestinal (GI) tract and inactivated. Increasing the frequency of dose achieves more dose exposure for the patient. The duration of action is approximately 3 to 8 hours. Lypressin is most effective in mild cases of diabetes insipidus.

Desmopressin Acetate (*DDAVP*)

Desmopressin (1-deamino-8-*D*-arginine-vasopressin) is also chemically related to vasopressin. It is administered intranasally usually in two doses, which allows a distribution similar to the normal diurnal response. It has a duration of action of 10 to 20 hours, much longer than the natural vasopressin. Desmopressin is approved for use in conditions other than diabetes insipidus. It is proven effective in the treatment of nocturnal enuresis when administered prior to bedtime. It is also used to prevent or relieve abdominal distention associated with surgical procedures.

Adverse Effects

The most frequent side effects of vasopressin and related substances include nausea, GI cramping, and diarrhea. Tremor, vertigo, and sweating that are transient and usually not serious have also been reported with desmopressin. The physician should be notified if the patient experiences shortness of breath, nasal congestion, or nasal irritation. In higher doses, the pressor effect produces cutaneous vasoconstriction (pallor) and an increase in blood pressure. Caution must be observed with individuals who have coronary artery disease. The natural preparations (animal source) may produce hypersensitivity and allergic reactions. Because these hormones affect water balance, seizures have occurred in some patients. Careful consideration before use is necessary when patients with epilepsy require treatment.

DRUGS AFFECTING UTERINE MUSCLE

Oxytocics

Oxytocics are drugs that cause contraction of the uterus and facilitate delivery. The various preparations are usually classified according to their clinical usages.

Labor Induction

Oxytocics are used to induce labor when it does not begin spontaneously. The major problem with the use of oxytocics is the development of violent uterine contractions, which must be avoided because they result in forceful expulsion of the fetus through the undilated birth canal. Naturally occurring oxytocin is no longer available; it has been replaced by synthetic oxytocin. Oxytocin injection (*Pitocin*) is administered by IV infusion, which is carefully adjusted so that birth follows the normal sequence. The major adverse effect of oxytocin is caused by excessive administration, resulting in uterine **tetany,** or rupture, and subsequent fetal distress, injury, or death.

Postpartum Bleeding

Oxytocics are used after delivery of the placenta **(postpartum)** to cause firm uterine contractions. In this manner, oxytocics decrease uterine bleeding and reduce the possibility of serious hemorrhage. Oxytocin injection can be used as can the ergot alkaloids: ergonovine (*Ergotrate*) and methylergonovine (*Methergine*). The onset of action for these drugs, which can be administered orally or parenterally, is rapid.

The duration of their action (IM) is approximately 6 hours.

Common adverse effects include nausea and vomiting. The ergot drugs also cause constriction of blood vessels, which can produce varying degrees of hypertension. This vascular response combined with contraction of uterine muscle decreases the potential for postpartum hemorrhage and prevents muscle atony. With excessive administration, the pressor effect may be intense and may restrict blood flow to the extremities (fingers and toes). This effect can result in tissue anoxia and the development of gangrene. The ergot alkaloids should never be used to induce labor or abortions.

Therapeutic Abortions

Vigorous contraction of the uterus at any time during pregnancy will dislodge tissues, resulting in abortion. When therapeutic abortion is required, oxytocin may be administered during the first trimester and even up to the 19th week of pregnancy. However, relatively large amounts are required and, in some cases, the drug must be repeatedly administered until the abortion is complete.

The present drug of choice to induce abortion during the second trimester is a prostaglandin. Carboprost tromethamine (*Hemabate*) is a derivative of dinoprost, an $F_{2\alpha}$ prostaglandin, which is administered by deep IM injection. Dinoprostone (*Prostin E₂*), another prostaglandin, is administered by vaginal suppository.

Adverse effects of the oxytocics are usually limited after vaginal suppository or gel application. Nausea, vomiting, and diarrhea are common. Other adverse effects include fever, flushing, headache, and dizziness. Constriction of bronchial smooth muscle has been reported and, consequently, these drugs are contraindicated in patients with asthma.

TOCOLYTICS

Premature Rupture of Obstetrical Membranes

Many women develop premature contractions of the uterus early in the pregnancy that jeopardize their ability to carry the fetus to term. Intense contractions may result in premature rupture of obstetrical membranes (PROM), which could lead to premature birth. No single factor is responsible for inducing PROM so there is no specific preventative medicine. When contractions are persistent and strong, the woman is usually confined to bed. Delivery prior to 30 weeks of gestation is associated with significantly underdeveloped fetal organ systems, especially respiratory and neural functions. Premature

infants today often have the availability of "high-tech" neonatal intensive care units where ventilation and cardiovascular support are continually provided. Even though surfactants are now available that can minimize or eliminate time spent on ventilators, there is no substitute for the benefit of having the fetus come to full term *in utero*.

Ritodrine Administration

Ritodrine (*Yutopar*) is a beta-receptor agonist that has a selectivity for beta-receptors located in uterine muscle. Stimulation of these receptors sets a biochemical process in motion that affects cellular calcium and induces smooth muscle relaxation. A controlled IV infusion is continued until the contractions become less threatening or cease. Other beta-receptor agonist drugs (terbutaline IV, oral) are given as an off-label application, but only ritodrine is Food and Drug Administration (FDA) approved for the management of preterm labor in the United States.

Ritodrine does cross the placenta and is designated FDA Pregnancy Category B, which means that safe use in pregnancy has not been absolutely established through controlled clinical trials. Nevertheless, pregnant women have been exposed to the drug after 20 weeks and the children studied up to 2 years of age without showing any ill effects in growth or maturation (see Table 40:1 on page 488).

Patient Administration and Monitoring

Since this group of drugs has especially restricted use, patients will not have opportunity to misuse these drugs. Nevertheless, patients require clear instructions on the use of nasal sprays to obtain the optimum therapeutic effect.

Drug Administration

Uniform intranasal dosing is achieved when the bottle and the patient's head are held upright. Desmopressin acetate is provided as a 2.5- or 5-ml bottle containing 25 or 50 doses, respectively. Residual contents should never be mixed into another drug bottle. When the total doses have been sprayed, the residual should be discarded to avoid administering an incomplete dose.

Notify the Physician

Patients taking carbamazepine or chlorpropamide may experience an exaggerated response to ADH.

Patients with epilepsy, migraine, asthma, or heart failure may experience exacerbations of these conditions because of an increase in extracellular water with the vasopressins. Patients who experience shortness of breath, nasal congestion, irritation, or severe headache should notify the physician immediately for further evaluation.

Patients who develop skin pallor or abdominal cramping with vasopressin may eliminate the effect if one or two glasses of water are taken with the dose.

TABLE 40:1 Indications and Doses for Posterior Pituitary Hormones and Drugs Affecting Uterine Contractions

DRUG (TRADE NAME)	INDICATION	DOSE
Urination Inhibition		
vasopressin (*Pitressin*)	Diabetes insipidus postoperative abdominal distention	5–10 units IM or SC every 3 or 4 hr; intranasal 1–2 sprays in one or both nostrils
lypressin (*Diapid*)	Diabetes insipidus	1–2 sprays in one or both nostrils
desmopressin (*DDAVP, Stimate*)	Diabetes insipidus	0.1–0.4 ml daily intranasally or 0.1–1.2 mg PO BID, TID
desmopressin (*DDAVP*)	Enuresis	10–20 µg intranasally at bedtime
Uterine Contraction		
carboprost tromethamine (*Hemabate*)	Abortafacient	250–500 µg deep IM injection
dinoprostone (*Prostin E$_2$*)	Abortafacient	1 vaginal suppository up to 2 days
	Cervical ripening prior to labor	10 mg vaginal insert or gel application to the cervix
oxytocin (*Pitocin, Syntocinon*)	Medical induction of labor antepartum	1–2 mU/min (0.001–0.002 U/min) IV drip at 15- to 30-min intervals
	Postpartum contraction	Diluted 10–40 units in 1000 ml diluent
	Milk letdown	One spray in one or both nostrils 2–3 minutes before nursing or pumping
ergonovine (*Ergotrate Maleate*)	Postpartum hemorrhage	0.2 mg/ml IM, IV
methylergonovine (*Methergine*)	Postpartum hemorrhage	0.2 mg/ml IM or 0.2 mg PO TID, QID
Uterine Relaxation		
ritodrine (*Yutopar*)	Premature contractions	0.05 mg/min IV
terbutaline (*Brethine*)	Premature contractions	10–80 mg/min IV; 2.5 mg PO every 4–6 hr until term

Adverse Effects

Consistent with beta-receptor-mediated activity, fetal tachycardia, increased maternal blood pressure, and increased blood glucose and fatty acids can occur. This is usually dose related and abates on discontinuation of the drug. Nausea, vomiting, headache, anxiety, restlessness, and arrhythmia are among the other adverse effects reported to occur. Ritodrine is contraindicated for use in women who have existing conditions that would be exacerbated by beta-receptor stimulation.

Chapter Review

Understanding Terminology

Answer the following questions in the spaces provided.

1. Explain the difference between endogenous and exogenous. _____

2. What is ADH? _____

3. Define *postpartum*. _____

4. What is oxytocin? _____

5. What is vasopressin? _____

Acquiring Knowledge

Answer the following questions in the spaces provided.

1. What hormones are released from the posterior pituitary gland? _____

2. Describe the main functions of ADH and oxytocin. _____

3. What condition is associated with a lack of ADH? _____

4. List some of the preparations that are used to treat diabetes insipidus. _____

5. List the adverse effects of the drugs used to treat diabetes insipidus. _____

6. What are the drugs of choice to induce labor? _____

7. What are the drugs of choice after delivery to prevent excessive uterine bleeding? _____

8. What is an example of a drug administered to induce therapeutic abortion? _____

Applying Knowledge—On the Job

Use your critical thinking skills to answer the following questions in the spaces provided.

1. Mr. Jones has just been diagnosed with diabetes insipidus by the physician you work for.
   a. Describe the signs and symptoms Mr. Jones presented with.

   _____

   b. What drug should Mr. Jones be prescribed?

   _____

    c. Use the *Physicians' Desk Reference* (*PDR*) to advise Mr. Jones about precautions and adverse reactions when taking this drug.

_____

_____

2. Mrs. Smith has been in labor for 12 hours. Her contractions are frequent and regular but not strong enough to advance the birth process. Mrs. Smith is becoming extremely fatigued. Her doctor has recommended oxytocin.

    a. How should the oxytocin be administered?

_____

    b. What drugs would you look for in Mrs. Smith's chart to see if there might be drug interactions with the oxytocin?

_____

    c. What signs and symptoms would you look for in Mrs. Smith as you monitor her for adverse reactions?

_____

    d. What signs of adverse reactions would you look for in the newborn?

_____

3. Lila has called with an inquiry. Several weeks ago, her physician gave her a prescription for *Diapid* nasal spray. The directions on the label read "Use 1 to 2 sprays in each nostril 3 times a day." Her physician told her that she could increase her dose every week if she needed to, depending on her symptoms. She started using only one spray in each nostril; after a week she used two sprays in each nostril in the morning and at night and only one spray in the afternoon. After one week she increased it to two sprays in each nostril morning, noon, and night. Now it's been a week and she needs to increase the dose again, but she can't remember how the doctor told her to do it. She wants to know the correct way to increase it. Should she increase it by one or two sprays each dose? What is the most sprays she should use at a time?

_____

_____

4. Insipidus diabetes can be treated with DDAVP. This is also approved for other indications. What are these indications?

_____

_____

5. A patient calls. She thinks she may be experiencing a drug allergy. She was given *Methergine* after her miscarriage. After several doses, her fingers and toes are tingling as if they were falling asleep, and they are cold to the touch. Her bleeding is minimal and she wants to know if she should stop taking the medication and start taking *Benadryl*. She has some at home from when she had an allergic reaction last year.

_____

_____

Internet Connection

Healthfinder is a website maintained by the U.S. government to provide consumers and medical personnel with current accurate information on diseases such as diabetes insipidus. Go to www.healthfinder.gov and enter *Diabetes Insipidus.* The healthfinder presents the link that describes the types of diabetes insipidus, including central, nephrogenic, dipsogenic, and gestational. It also differentiates between diabetes insipidus and diabetes mellitus. This link is supported by the National Institutes of Health.

The Hershey Medical Center at www.hmc.psu.edu/healthinfo/no/nephrogenicdiabetes.htm also supports a Health and Disease Information forum.

The Nephrogenic Diabetes Foundation, formed to support education, research, and treatment for nephrogenic diabetes insipidus, is available at www.ndif.org.

At www.medlineplus.gov, information on specific drugs can be found. For example, enter *Ritodrine* or *Vasopressin* to access information from medical encyclopedias to publications on labor induction or enuresis. A separate folder titled *News* presents worldwide news articles relevant to the topic.

Additional Reading

Levy, D. B. 1990. A last resort for postpartum hemorrhage. *Emergency* 22:16.

Long, P. 1991. Bleeding and the third stage of labor. *NAACOGS: Clinical Issues Perinatology Women's Health Nursing* 2:385.

PHARMACOLOGY OF INFECTIOUS DISEASES

Chapter 41

Antibacterial Agents

Morphology of Bacteria
Chemotherapy
Penicillins
Cephalosporins
Aminoglycosides
Tetracyclines
Sulfonamides
Macrolide Antibiotics
Fluroquinolone Antimicrobials
Miscellaneous Antimicrobial Drugs
Drugs Used to Treat Tuberculosis
Chemoprophylaxis

Chapter 42

Antifungal and Antiviral (AIDS) Drugs

Antifungal Drugs
Viral Diseases and Antiviral Drugs
Antiviral Drugs
Drug Interactions

Chapter 43

Antiprotozoal and Anthelmintic Drugs

Protozoal Infections
Malaria
Dysentery
Other Protozoal Infections
Anthelmintic Drugs

Chapter 44

Antiseptics and Disinfectants

Mechanism of Action

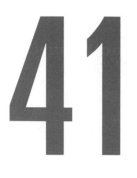

chapter

41

ANTIBACTERIAL AGENTS

CHAPTER FOCUS

This chapter describes the pharmacology of drugs used to treat bacterial infections. It explains the basic classification and identification procedures pertaining to bacteria. It also discusses the major classes of antibiotic drugs, mechanisms of antibacterial action, clinical indications, and main pharmacological and adverse effects produced by these drugs.

CHAPTER OBJECTIVES

After studying this chapter, you should be able to

- explain the use of the gram stain in bacterial identification.
- explain the mechanism of antibacterial action for each of the major drug classes: penicillins, cephalosporins, aminoglycosides, tetracyclines, sulfonamides, macrolides, fluroquinolones, and the drugs used to treat tuberculosis.
- list one drug from each major drug class and two characteristic adverse effects from each drug class.

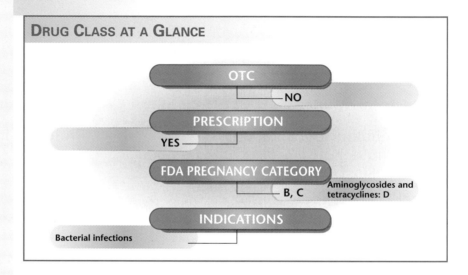

DRUG CLASS AT A GLANCE

OTC — NO

PRESCRIPTION — YES

FDA PREGNANCY CATEGORY — B, C   Aminoglycosides and tetracyclines: D

INDICATIONS — Bacterial infections

Key Terms

antibacterial spectrum: bacteria that are susceptible to the antibacterial actions of a particular drug.

antibiotic: antibacterial drug obtained from other microorganisms.

antibiotic susceptibility: identification of the antibiotics, by bacterial culture and sensitivity testing, that will be effective against specific bacteria.

antimicrobial: antibacterial drugs obtained by chemical synthesis and not from other microorganisms.

bacteria: single-celled microorganisms, some of which cause disease.

bacterial resistance: ability of some bacteria to resist the actions of antibiotics.

bactericidal: antibiotic that kills bacteria.

bacteriostatic: antibiotic that inhibits the growth of, but does not kill, bacteria.

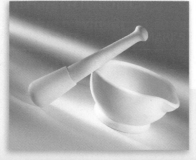

beta-lactamases: bacterial enzymes that inactivate penicillin and cephalosporin antibiotics.

broad-spectrum: drug that is effective against a wide variety of both gram-positive and gram-negative pathogenic bacteria.

cephalosporinases: bacterial enzymes that inactivate cephalosporin antibiotics.

chemoprophylaxis: use of antibiotics to prevent infection, usually before a surgical procedure or in patients at risk for infection.

chemotherapy: use of drugs to kill or inhibit the growth of infectious organisms or cancer cells.

gram negative: bacteria that retain only the red stain in a gram stain.

gram positive: bacteria that retain only the blue stain in a gram stain.

gram stain: method of staining and identifying bacteria using crystal violet (blue) and safranin (red) stains.

pathogenic: type of bacteria that cause disease.

penicillinase: bacterial enzymes that inactivate penicillin antibiotics.

INTRODUCTION

Microbiology is the study of microscopic organisms of either animal (bacteria and protozoa) or plant (fungi and molds) origin. **Bacteria** are single-cell organisms that are found virtually everywhere. Bacteria that cause disease are called **pathogenic** and those that do not are nonpathogenic.

There are no bacteria in the internal environment of the body. However, there are many different types of bacteria, including pathogens, in the externally exposed areas, such as the mouth, gastrointestinal (GI) tract, nose, upper respiratory passages, and skin. Therefore, the potential for bacterial invasion always exists. However, even when bacteria enter the body, the normal body defense mechanisms (skin, leukocytes, immune system) function to protect and prevent the development of infection. When the skin or other body tissues break down, bacteria penetrate into the internal body tissues and set up areas of infection. Bacteria produce toxins that cause inflammation, tissue damage, fever, and other symptoms associated with infection.

MORPHOLOGY OF BACTERIA

There are thousands of different types of bacteria. Bacteria are generally classified by shape and arrangement. The basic bacterial shapes are spherical (cocci), rod-like (bacilli), and curved rods (spirilla). Some of the bacterial arrangements are in pairs (diplo), chains (strepto), or clusters (staphylo). Table 41:1 illustrates some of the more common bacterial arrangements.

It is necessary to stain bacteria in order to visualize and identify them. One of the most important bacteriological stains is the **gram stain,** which contains two dyes: crystal violet (blue) and safranin (red). Bacteria that retain only the blue stain are classified as **gram positive,** whereas bacteria that retain only the red stain are **gram negative.** It is important to distinguish gram-positive from gram-negative organisms. The response to antibiotic therapy varies with the type of bacteria involved. Gram stains aid the accurate diagnosis and proper treatment of bacterial infections.

The normal procedure for bacterial identification involves taking some material from the infected area (throat swab, sputum, or urine) and growing the bacteria in a culture medium. After 24 to 48 hours the bacteria are stained. Identification is based on morphology and biochemical procedures. Newer biochemical diagnostic techniques are available for the immediate identification of some organisms.

In addition to identification, it is frequently important to determine which chemotherapeutic drugs will be most effective against the specific bacteria that are causing the infection. Identification of the antibiotics that are effective against specific bacteria is referred to as **antibiotic susceptibility.** Two of the simplest

TABLE 41:1 Bacterial Morphology and Some Common Bacterial Arrangements

BACTERIAL FORM	BACTERIAL ARRANGEMENT	CLASSIFICATION
Cocci		
Pairs		Diplococci
Chains		Streptococci
Clusters		Staphylococci
Bacilli		
Straight		Bacilli
Short curved		Vibrio
Spirillum		
Twisted		Spirilla
Twisted		Borrelia
Twisted		Treponema

methods to determine antibiotic susceptibility are the disk test and serial dilution. In each case, the bacteria are cultured in media that contain various antibacterial drugs. The drug with the greatest sensitivity will produce the greatest inhibition of bacterial growth. This screening method indicates which drug should produce the best clinical results in eradicating the infection. Bacterial identification and determination of antibiotic susceptibility are commonly referred to as culture and sensitivity testing.

CHEMOTHERAPY

Chemotherapy refers to the use of drugs to kill or to inhibit the growth of infectious organisms or cancerous cells. Chemotherapy is indicated when normal body defense mechanisms are inadequate to control infection.

Antibacterial agents are divided into two main types: bactericidal and bacteriostatic. **Bactericidal** drugs are lethal; that is, they actually kill the bacteria. **Bacteriostatic** drugs inhibit the reproduction (growth) of bacteria. With bacteriostatic drugs, elimination of the pathogenic bacteria depends upon phagocytosis by host leukocytes and macrophages, and other actions of the immune system.

Sources of Antibacterial Drugs

Antibacterial drugs are obtained from two major sources: soil microorganisms and chemical synthesis. Bacteria and other microorganisms naturally produce substances that inhibit the growth of other bacteria. In nature, these substances help protect specific types of bacteria from the harmful chemical substances released by other bacteria. These chemical substances obtained from microorganisms and used in chemotherapy are referred to as **antibiotics.** For example, the mold *Penicillium notatum* produces a substance that inhibits the growth of many gram-positive, pathogenic bacteria. This substance, known as penicillin, is the parent compound of some of the most widely used antibiotic drugs. Some antibacterial drugs, such as the sulfonamides, are produced by chemical synthesis. Antibacterial drugs that are obtained by chemical synthesis and not from other microorganisms are referred to generally as **antimicrobial** drugs.

Antibacterial Spectrum

Very few, if any, antibacterial drugs inhibit the growth of all pathogenic bacteria. Each antibacterial drug is generally effective for only a limited number of pathogenic bacteria. These susceptible bacteria make up the **antibacterial**

spectrum for that particular drug. Some drugs are effective against a limited number of bacteria, for example, only some gram-positive or only some gram-negative bacteria. These drugs are characterized as having a narrow antibacterial spectrum. Other drugs are effective against a wide spectrum of both gram-positive and gram-negative bacteria. These drugs are referred to as **broad-spectrum** or extended spectrum antibiotics.

Drug Resistance

During chemotherapy, an antibiotic may occasionally lose its effectiveness. This usually occurs when the bacteria undergo some structural or metabolic alteration or mutation that allows the bacteria to survive the actions of the antibiotic. The ability of bacteria to resist the actions of antibiotics is referred to as **bacterial resistance.** One cause of bacterial resistance involves the ability of bacteria to alter the outer cell wall so that antibiotics can no longer penetrate the bacteria. In addition, some bacteria produce enzymes that inactivate the antibiotic (see below). When resistance occurs, the bacteria are able to survive and reproduce in the presence of the drug. A common finding is that a few resistant bacteria are already present within the infection. As the nonresistant bacteria are eliminated by the antibiotic, the resistant bacteria begin to multiply rapidly and are then responsible for continuation of the infection. When drug resistance occurs, another antibacterial drug that the bacteria are sensitive to must be substituted.

Bacterial Beta-Lactamase Enzymes

Certain bacteria have the ability to produce enzymes that inactivate penicillin and cephalosporin antibiotics. These enzymes are referred to generally as **beta-lactamases** (β-lactamases). Beta-lactamases that inactivate penicillins are referred to as **penicillinases.** Beta-lactamases that inactivate cephalosporins are referred to as **cephalosporinases.** Other types of bacterial enzymes are also produced that can inactivate other antibiotics.

PENICILLINS

Penicillin is an antibiotic obtained from various species of *Penicillium* mold. Alteration of the basic structure and the addition of various salts have provided numerous penicillin preparations. The main differences between the various preparations involve differences in acid stability (in the stomach),

resistance to enzymatic destruction by penicillinase, and antibacterial spectrum. The different penicillin preparations are listed in Table 41:2.

Mechanism of Action

The penicillins are bactericidal to susceptible bacteria that are in the process of reproducing. Penicillin interferes with synthesis of the bacterial cell wall. With a defective cell wall, the bacteria cannot maintain the necessary osmotic concentration with the surrounding body fluids. Consequently, the bacterial cells gain water, swell, and burst apart (lysis).

Antibacterial Spectrum

The penicillins are divided into several different groups based on their spectrum of activity. The current classification system divides the penicillins into four generations.

First-Generation Penicillins

This group includes penicillin G and penicillin V, which have a narrow antibacterial spectrum. They are effective against common gram-positive organisms (streptococci and pneumococci) that are often responsible for causing ear and throat infections, and organisms that cause the common venereal diseases such as gonorrhea and syphilis. They are not effective against most gram-negative bacilli (rods) or organisms that produce penicillinase. These drugs are listed in Table 41:2 under first-generation penicillins.

Another subgroup of first-generation penicillins is resistant to penicillinase and is indicated primarily for the treatment of resistant staphylococcal (staph) infections. Staph infections, caused mainly by *Staphylococcus aureus,* cause abscesses and other serious infections (endocarditis and pneumonia). Staph infections are often difficult to treat because there is a high incidence of bacterial resistance due to penicillinase production among staph bacteria. These drugs are listed in Table 41:2 as penicillinase resistant.

Second-Generation Penicillins

The second-generation penicillins include ampicillin, amoxicillin, and similar drugs that are considered to have an extended, or broad, spectrum. The second-generation drugs are effective against the same organisms as penicillin G plus a number of common gram-negative organisms. These include *Escherichia coli, Proteus mirabilis,* and *Haemophilus influenzae,* which are responsible for common urinary, respiratory, and

Penicillin Antibiotics

DRUG (TRADE NAME)	ROUTE	REMARKS
First Generation:		
penicillin G (Na, K salts)	IM, IV	Produces high plasma levels, has a short duration of action
penicillin G benzathine (*Bicillin*)	IM	Penicillin G is slowly released from injection site over 28 days, provides low plasma levels
penicillin G procaine (*Wycillin*)	IM	Penicillin G is slowly released from injection site over 12–24 hr
penicillin V potassium K (*Pen-Vee K, V-Cillin K*)	PO	Resists acid destruction in stomach; used to treat minor throat and ear infections
Penicillinase Resistant:		
cloxacillin sodium (*Tegopen*)	PO	Resistance to the destructive actions of penicillinase; used to treat infections only when penicillinase-producing organisms are causing the infection
dicloxacillin sodium (*Dynapen*)	PO	
methicillin sodium (*Staphcillin*)	IM, IV	
nafcillin sodium (*Unipen*)	IM, IV	
oxacillin sodium (*Prostaphlin*)	PO, IM, IV	
Second Generation:		
amoxicillin (*Amoxil*)	PO	Broader spectrum than first-generation drugs; amoxicillin provides higher plasma levels
ampicillin sodium (*Omnipen*)	PO, IM, IV	
Third Generation:		
carbenicillin indanyl (*Geocillin*)	PO	For the treatment of urinary tract infections
ticarcillin disodium (*Ticar*)	IM, IV	Broad spectrum, generally reserved for pseudomonal and other serious gram-negative infections
Fourth Generation:		
mezlocillin sodium (*Mezlin*)	IM, IV	Increased effectiveness compared to third-generation drugs; indicated for serious gram-negative infections
piperacillin (*Pipracil*)	IM, IV	

ear infections. All second-generation penicillins can be taken orally, which is an important advantage in the treatment of a variety of common gram-positive and gram-negative infections. Amoxicillin is widely used because it is well absorbed from the GI tract and produces higher plasma drug levels than does ampicillin.

Second-generation penicillins are not effective against penicillinase-producing organisms, and in recent years, greater numbers and percentages of organisms produce penicillinase, which inactivates the penicillin molecule.

Third-Generation Penicillins

The third-generation penicillins include carbenicillin and ticarcillin, which have a broader spectrum than do the second-generation drugs. The main indication for these penicillins is in the treatment of more serious urinary, respiratory, and bacteremic infections caused by gram-negative *Pseudomonas aeruginosa* and *Proteus vulgaris*. These infections are often difficult to treat and may require combination therapy with the aminoglycoside antibiotics. Carbenicillin indanyl (*Geocillin*) is administered orally and is only indicated for the treatment of urinary tract infections. Ticarcillin (*Ticar*) is administered parenterally (IM, IV) for the treatment of systemic infections. These drugs are not resistant to penicillinase-producing organisms.

Fourth-Generation Penicillins

These drugs have been more recently introduced and generally have a wider antibacterial spectrum than do third-generation penicillins, are more effective (potent), and are administered in the form of monosodium salts. This form reduces the amount of sodium ingested compared to some other penicillins that are disodium salts. This may be important for individuals with hypertension or congestive heart failure who are usually on sodium-restricted diets.

The fourth-generation drugs are mainly indicated for serious infections caused by *Pseudomonas aeruginosa*, *Proteus vulgaris*, *Klebsiella pneumoniae*, and *Bacteroides fragilis* (anaerobe). These infections can also be difficult to treat and may require combination therapy. The fourth-generation penicillins are not resistant to penicillinase-producing organisms, and they require parenteral administration.

Beta-Lactamase Inhibitors

There still is not a single penicillin that combines all of the following: can be taken orally, has a broad spectrum, and is resistant to penicillinase. However, several drugs, known as beta-lactamase inhibitors, can be administered along with the various penicillins. These drugs inhibit the penicillinase enzymes and allow the penicillin drug to remain effective. These inhibitors include clavulanic acid, sulbactam, and tazobactam. Combinations of the various penicillins plus inhibitor are marketed together. Amoxicillin plus clavulanic acid is marketed as *Augmentin,* ampicillin is combined with sulbactam in *Unasyn,* and piperacillin is combined with tazobactam in *Zosyn.* These antibiotic combinations are indicated when bacterial resistance is suspected.

Adverse Effects

As a group, the penicillins are relatively nontoxic. Minor adverse effects, such as nausea or rashes, may occur in some patients. Diarrhea is more common with oral administration. When used in very high doses, the penicillins can cause central nervous system (CNS) disturbances, including convulsions.

The most serious adverse effect involves individuals who develop an allergy to penicillin. As a drug class, the penicillins cause the highest incidence of drug allergy. Common allergic symptoms include rashes, fever, and inflammatory conditions. The most serious allergic reaction involves anaphylaxis or anaphylactic shock. All patients must be questioned about the possibility of penicillin allergy. In cases of suspected allergy, skin sensitivity testing can be performed to determine whether patients are allergic to penicillin. Patients allergic to one penicillin are considered allergic to all of the penicillin drugs.

Antibiotics Related to the Penicillins

Imipenem (*Primaxin*) and aztreonam (*Azactam*) are two bactericidal drugs that are structurally related to penicillins and have the same mechanism of action. Imipenem is effective against both gram-positive and gram-negative bacteria, including bacteria that are resistant to penicillins. Imipenem is administered parenterally. Nausea, vomiting, seizures, and allergic reactions are adverse effects associated with imipenem.

Aztreonam is also highly resistant to penicillinase and is mainly used intravenously for resistant gram-negative infections. It can usually be used in individuals who are allergic to penicillin. Gastrointestinal disturbances and rash are common adverse reactions.

CEPHALOSPORINS

The cephalosporins are bactericidal antibiotics that have chemical structures similar to those of the penicillins. The mechanism of action of the cephalosporins is the same as that of the penicillins. The cephalosporins are considered to be broad-spectrum drugs. Their two main uses are as substitutes for penicillins in cases of allergy or bacterial resistance and in the treatment of certain gram-negative infections.

Bacterial Resistance to Cephalosporins

Some organisms, usually gram negative, can produce cephalosporinase. The cephalosporins are ineffective against organisms that produce these enzymes. The cephalosporins are also classified into four generations and are listed in Table 41:3.

First-Generation Cephalosporins

These antibiotics are considered to be the older cephalosporins. They all have a similar antibacterial spectrum, which includes both some gram-positive and some gram-negative organisms. The cephalosporins are the drugs of choice for treating infections caused by gram-negative *Klebsiella pneumoniae.* Of this group, cefazolin (*Kefzol*) is among the most widely used because of the higher plasma levels that it produces. These drugs are useful for most of the common gram-positive and gram-negative infections that cause ear, throat, and urinary tract infections.

Second-Generation Cephalosporins

These cephalosporins have a broader spectrum than the first-generation drugs and are generally more potent. They are indicated when first-generation drugs are ineffective. Cefoxitin (*Mefoxin*) is especially useful in treating infections caused by *Bacteroides fragilis* and *Serratia*

TABLE 41:3   Cephalosporin Antibiotics

DRUG (TRADE NAME)	ROUTE	REMARKS
First Generation:		
cefadroxil (*Duricef*)	PO	Used to treat common gram-positive and gram-negative infections, including *Klebsiella pneumoniae*
cefazolin (*Kefzol*)	IM, IV	
cephalexin (*Keflex*)	PO	
cephradine (*Velosef*)	PO, IV	
Second Generation:		
cefaclor (*Ceclor*)	PO	Indicated for gram-negative infections; are more resistant to the actions of penicillinase and cephalosporinase
cefoxitin (*Mefoxin*)	IM, IV	
cefonicid (*Monocid*)	IM, IV	
cefotetan (*Cefotan*)	IM, IV	
Third Generation:		
cefixime (*Suprax*)	PO	Indicated for serious gram-negative infections that are resistant to other cephalosporins; they have longer durations of action and are more potent without producing any additional toxicities compared to the first- and second-generation cephalosporins
cefoperazone (*Cefobid*)	IM, IV	
cefotaxime (*Claforan*)	IM, IV	
ceftazidime (*Fortaz*)	IM, IV	
ceftriaxone (*Rocephin*)	IM, IV	
Fourth Generation:		
cefepime (*Maxipime*)	IM, IV	Similar to third generation, but greater resistance to β-lactamase inactivating enzymes

marcescens. Also, these drugs are often effective in treating respiratory and other infections caused by *Haemophilus influenzae* and *Neisseria gonorrhoeae,* including organisms that produce penicillinase and that are often resistant to penicillins.

Third-Generation Cephalosporins

These drugs have a broader spectrum than do the second-generation drugs. They are more potent antibiotics, and they have longer durations of action than do the other cephalosporins. The third-generation cephalosporins are mainly indicated for the treatment of serious gram-negative infections that are not susceptible to second-generation drugs. These drugs are also more lipid soluble and cross the blood-brain barrier more readily than most other penicillins and cephalosporins. Consequently, they are often used for both gram-positive and gram-negative infections involving the brain (meningitis).

Fourth-Generation Cephalosporins

Cefepime (*Maxipime*), has been classified as the first drug of the fourth generation of cephalosporins. It is similar in spectrum to the third-generation drugs; the main feature is greater resistance to β-lactamase inactivating enzymes. It should be used when the lower generations of cephalosporins are ineffective.

Adverse Effects

Oral cephalosporins may cause GI disturbances, especially diarrhea and rashes. Intramuscular injections with the cephalosporins are usually painful and may cause local inflammation. Intravenous administration may cause phlebitis at the infusion site. The first-generation cephalosporins may cause nephrotoxicity, especially in patients with renal impairment or in patients who are dehydrated. In comparison, the newer cephalosporins are associated with a lower incidence of nephrotoxicity.

Cephalosporins that possess the *N*-methylthiotetrazone side chain (cefamandole, cefoperazone, cefotetan, others) may interfere with blood coagulation and cause bleeding problems. In addition, these same drugs can cause a disulfiram reaction when combined with alcohol (see Chapter 12).

TABLE 41:4	Aminoglycoside Antibiotics
DRUG (TRADE NAME)	**REMARKS**
amikacin (*Amikin*)	Reserved for treatment of serious gram-negative infections, especially with bacteria resistant to tobramycin or gentamicin
gentamicin (*Garamycin*)	Reserved for the treatment of serious gram-negative infections; produces a significant incidence of ototoxicity
kanamycin (*Kantrex*)	Used in the treatment of gram-negative infections and before intestinal surgery; also used in the treatment of tuberculosis
neomycin (*Neobiotic*)	Produces a significant degree of ototoxicity and is usually used only as a topical antibiotic (*Myciguent*) in the treatment of skin and ocular infections
streptomycin	Used in the treatment of tuberculosis, plague, and tularemia
tobramycin (*Nebcin*)	Reserved for the treatment of serious gram-negative infections, particularly *Pseudomonas aeruginosa*

Cephalosporins do cause allergic reactions, but the incidence of allergy with cephalosporins is lower than that with the penicillins. Some individuals are allergic to both penicillins and cephalosporins. Usually, cephalosporins can be used in patients who are allergic to penicillins. The guiding principle is that cephalosporins are not administered to penicillin-allergic individuals who have previously experienced the immediate type of penicillin allergic reaction (hives, anaphylaxis).

AMINOGLYCOSIDES

The aminoglycosides are a group of bactericidal antibiotics whose antibacterial spectrum mainly includes gram-negative bacilli. The mechanism of action of the aminoglycosides is that the drug passes into the bacterium, where it attaches irreversibly to the ribosomes to cause an irreversible inhibition of bacterial protein synthesis. The bacteria can no longer produce the enzymes and proteins necessary for survival and reproduction.

Pharmacokinetics

The aminoglycosides are poorly absorbed from the GI tract, and this effect is used to advantage before intestinal surgery. Large doses are given orally before abdominal surgery to reduce the number of intestinal bacteria and "sterilize the bowel." The usual route of administration for systemic effects is either IM or IV. These drugs are effective against most gram-negative organisms and generally reserved for the treatment of serious gram-negative infections in

hospitalized patients. The aminoglycosides are not significantly metabolized and are excreted mostly unchanged in the urine. Consequently, high urinary concentrations are attained, contributing to the effectiveness of the aminoglycosides in the treatment of resistant urinary tract infections. The most frequently used aminoglycosides are listed in Table 41:4.

Adverse Effects

When taken orally, the aminoglycosides may cause nausea, vomiting, and diarrhea. When administered parenterally, the two most serious adverse effects are nephrotoxicity (renal toxicity) and ototoxicity. Because of the high urinary levels, the aminoglycosides may interfere with normal renal function. Increased casts, albuminuria (protein in the urine), and oliguria (reduced urine output) may occur. The aminoglycosides interfere with the function of the auditory nerve (cranial nerve VIII). The earliest symptoms are tinnitus (ringing in the ears) and temporary impairment of hearing; this is generally referred to as ototoxicity. In some cases, in which the aminoglycosides were taken for extended periods, irreversible damage and permanent hearing loss has occurred.

Cautions and Contraindications

Pregnancy

Aminoglycosides are designated Food and Drug Administration (FDA) Pregnancy Category D and should not be used during pregnancy. The aminioglycosides have been shown to cause fetal harm; in particular, hearing loss and deafness.

Drug Interactions

The aminoglycosides possess some peripheral neuromuscular blocking activity. Administration during surgery or other procedures in which general anesthetics or other neuromuscular blockers are also being used may produce excessive degrees of muscular blockade. The most serious effect would be respiratory arrest due to paralysis of the diaphragm and the other muscles of respiration.

The ototoxic effect of the aminoglycosides is increased when other ototoxic drugs, such as some diuretics (ethacrynic acid and furosemide), are administered at the same time. Combination therapy of other nephrotoxic drugs with cephalosporins may increase nephrotoxicity.

TETRACYCLINES

The tetracyclines—a group of broad-spectrum antibiotics—are clinically useful in both gram-positive and gram-negative infections. The first tetracycline developed was chlortetracycline (*Aureomycin*). Other members of this group produce effects similar to those of chlortetracycline. Tetracyclines interfere with bacterial protein synthesis to produce a bacteriostatic effect.

Administration

The tetracyclines are usually administered orally, but IM and IV injection may be used if necessary. Foods, especially those containing calcium (milk) and substances such as antacids and mineral supplements, interfere with the GI absorption of the tetracyclines. Since tetracyclines bind calcium molecules (chelate) and form insoluble compounds, tetracycline should be taken 1 hour before meals or several hours after meals.

Doxycycline and minocycline are more completely absorbed from the GI tract than are the other tetracyclines and are least affected by calcium and other mineral-containing substances. The tetracyclines are listed in Table 41:5.

Clinical Indications

The tetracyclines are occasional alternatives to the penicillins for many of the common gram-positive and gram-negative infections. However, the most important indications for the tetracyclines are for infections caused by *Rickettsiae* (Rocky Mountain spotted fever, typhus), *Mycoplasma pneumoniae*, *Vibrio cholerae* (cholera), *Chlamydia trachomatis* (urethritis), and *Borrelia burgdorferi* (Lyme disease). In addition, the tetracyclines are sometimes used to treat lower respiratory infections that often contribute to chronic bronchitis.

Adverse Effects

The most common side effects associated with the tetracyclines are nausea, vomiting, and diarrhea. Suppression of normal intestinal bacteria may result in overgrowth of nonsusceptible organisms (superinfection), especially fungi (*Candida albicans*). These conditions usually produce diarrhea and various skin rashes. The tetracyclines also produce photosensitivity in some individuals. After ingestion of the tetracyclines and exposure to sunlight, an exaggerated sunburn may occur. The use of outdated tetracycline products may produce a particular type of reaction known as the Fanconi syndrome. The main effects of this syndrome involve the kidneys, where polyuria, proteinuria, and acidosis are most frequently observed.

Cautions and Contraindications

Pregnancy

The tetracyclines bind to calcium and therefore should not be administered to children below the age of 8 and to women who are pregnant or

TABLE 41:5	Tetracycline Antibiotics
DRUG (TRADE NAME)	**USUAL ADULT ORAL DOSE**
demeclocycline (*Declomycin*)	150 mg every 6 hr or 300 mg BID
doxycycline (*Vibramycin*)	100 mg once per day
minocycline (*Minocin*)	100 mg every 12 hr
oxytetracycline (*Terramycin*)	250–500 mg every 6 hr
tetracycline (*Sumycin*)	250–500 mg every 6 hr

nursing. These drugs are deposited in growing bones and teeth, producing a yellow discoloration and possible depression of bone growth. Tetracyclines are designated Food and Drug Administration (FDA) Pregnancy Category D and have been shown to cause growth retardation in relation to infant skeletal development.

SULFONAMIDES

The sulfonamides are a group of synthetic drugs that were discovered in 1935 as a by-product of the dye industry. The first sulfonamide was sulfanilamide. Alteration of its basic structure produced many other compounds having similar activities. The sulfonamides were initially effective against many gram-positive and gram-negative organisms. Unfortunately, early widespread use of the sulfonamides led to the development of bacterial resistance. After introduction of the penicillins (early 1940s), use of the sulfonamides rapidly declined. Today, the sulfonamides have limited uses in selected infections. Some of the sulfonamides are used topically, especially in burn cases to prevent and treat infection. Other sulfonamides are used primarily for the treatment of urinary and GI tract infections.

Mechanism of Action

Bacteria have an essential requirement for *para*-aminobenzoic acid, which is used in the synthesis of folic acid. The sulfonamides are competitive antagonists of *para*-aminobenzoic acid. The sulfonamides block the synthesis of folic acid, which subsequently inhibits bacterial growth, producing a bacteriostatic effect.

Administration

The most common route of administration is oral, although a parenteral route may be used. The main pathway of elimination is renal, and the sulfonamides tend to be concentrated in the urine. The various sulfonamides have different durations of action and generally are classified as short, intermediate, and long acting. In addition, because of their poor oral absorption, some sulfonamides are used to reduce intestinal bacteria before intestinal surgery. The sulfonamides are listed in Table 41:6.

Adverse Effects

Oral administration frequently causes nausea, vomiting, and diarrhea. One of the more serious adverse effects is crystalluria. In the presence of dehydration and acidic urine, the sulfonamides have a tendency to crystallize in the renal tubules, causing cell damage, blood in the urine, and reduced urine output. Therefore, patients must receive adequate fluid intake, and urine should be made alkaline if it is highly acidic.

The sulfonamides also may produce allergic reactions, which usually are limited to the skin and mucous membranes. The most common reactions include rashes, pruritis, and photosensitivity. A very serious type of skin

TABLE 41:6	Sulfonamide Antimicrobial Drugs	
DRUG (TRADE NAME)	**MAIN USES**	**COMMENT**
mafenide (*Sulfamylon*)	In burn cases to prevent infection	Topical
phthalylsulfathiazole	Before surgery, ulcerative colitis	Poorly absorbed
silver sulfadiazine	In burn cases to prevent infection	Topical
sulfacetamide (*Sulamyd*)	Ocular infections	Topical
sulfameter (*Sulla*)	Chronic urinary infections	Long acting
sulfamethizole (*Thiosulfil*)	Urinary tract infections	Short acting
sulfamethoxazole (*Gantanol*)	Urinary tract infections	Intermediate acting
sulfasalazine (*Azulfidine*)	Ulcerative colitis	Long acting
sulfisoxazole (*Gantrisin*)	Urinary tract infections	Short acting

condition, the Stevens-Johnson syndrome, produces a skin reaction that can be fatal. Patients who develop any rash after ingestion of the sulfonamides must receive medical evaluation.

Blood disorders, including anemia, leukopenia, and thrombocytopenia, may develop with sulfonamide therapy. Patients with existing deficiency of glucose-6-phosphate dehydrogenase (G6PD) are particularly susceptible to the development of hemolytic anemia.

Drug Interactions

The sulfonamides may produce a number of drug interactions because of their ability to displace other drugs from inactive plasma protein-binding sites. The most frequent drug interactions involve the coumarin anticoagulants (increased anticoagulant effect) and the oral hypoglycemic drugs (hypoglycemia). Patients receiving sulfonamides and any of these drugs should be closely monitored for bleeding tendencies or hypoglycemic effects.

Trimethoprim-Sulfamethoxazole

This combination, marketed under the trade names of *Septra* and *Bactrim,* has broad-spectrum antimicrobial actions. It is a combination of one of the sulfonamides, sulfamethoxazole, and the drug trimethoprim. Trimethoprim inhibits the enzyme dihydrofolate reductase, which interferes with the further synthesis of folic acid to its activated form. Together, these two drugs exert a synergistic effect to inhibit folic acid production in bacteria that is very effective. Administration is either oral or parenteral in varying concentrations.

Clinical Indications

The sulfamethoxazole-trimethoprim combination is effective against a broad spectrum of gram-positive and gram-negative bacteria. It is often used as an alternative to the penicillins and cephalosporins for respiratory, urinary, GI, and other systemic infections. It is frequently the drug of choice for treatment of *Pneumocystis carinii* pneumonial infections, and ear, sinus, and pneumonial infections caused by *Haemophilus influenzae.*

The adverse effects of trimethoprim are generally similar to the sulfonamides; however, trimethoprim does not usually cause crystalluria.

MACROLIDE ANTIBIOTICS

The term *macrolide* refers to the large chemical ring structure that is characteristic of these antibiotics. These antibiotics inhibit bacterial protein synthesis and are considered bacteriostatic. The macrolides include erythromycin and several newer derivatives that cause less gastric irritation and have a wider antibacterial spectrum than erythromycin. The newer derivatives include azithromycin, clarithromycin, and dirithromycin. The most common adverse effect of these drugs is gastrointestinal irritation.

Erythromycin (*Erythrocin, E-Mycin*)

Erythromycin is a macrolide antibiotic with an antibacterial spectrum similar to that of penicillin G, but with the addition of a few other organisms. The main uses of erythromycin are as a penicillin substitute, in the treatment of *Legionella pneumophilia* (Legionnaire's disease), *Mycoplasma pneumoniae,* and genital infections caused by *Chlamydia trachomatis.* The usual oral dose is 250–500 mg 2–4 times per day. Gastrointestinal disturbances such as nausea, vomiting, diarrhea, and minor skin rashes are usually the common adverse effects associated with erythromycin and the other macrolide drugs.

Azithromycin (*Zithromax*)

Azithromycin is administered orally, its longer half-life of 65 to 70 hours allows once a day dosing. The drug is eliminated in mostly an unmetabolized state via the biliary-intestinal route. Azithromycin has greater activity against gram-negative and anaerobic organisms than does erythromycin. It is particularly useful in ear and respiratory infections caused by *Haemophilus influenzae.*

Clarithromycin (*Biaxin*)

Clarithromycin is well absorbed after oral administration. The drug forms an active metabolite during first-pass liver metabolism. Clarithromycin has the same antibacterial spectrum as erythromycin, but it is a more potent drug. The main uses are infections caused by *Haemophilus influenzae, Legionella pneumophilia, Chlamydia trachomatis,* and *Borrelia burgdorferi* (Lyme disease).

Dirithromycin (*Dynabac*)

Dirithromycin is a prodrug that is rapidly converted into an active metabolite that is responsible for the antibacterial effect. Oral absorption is increased by food, and administration with meals is recommended. The main indications for dirithromycin are common staphlococcal and streptococcal infections, and gram-negative infections caused by *Mycoplasma pneumoniae, Legionella pneumophilia,* and *Moraxella catarrhalis.*

FLUROQUINOLONE ANTIMICROBIALS

The fluroquinolones are synthetic antimicrobial agents that have a broad spectrum of antibacterial activity, especially against gram-negative organisms. One of their advantages, over some of the other broad-spectrum antibiotics, is that they are well absorbed after oral administration. The prototype of this drug class is ciprofloxacin. Other fluroquinolones are listed in Table 41:7.

Ciprofloxacin (*Cipro*)

The mechanism of action of ciprofloxacin and the other fluroquinolones is to inhibit an enzyme, deoxyribonucleic acid (DNA) gyrase, that is essential to the function of DNA and bacterial replication. These drugs are bactericidal against a wide variety of gram-positive and gram-negative organisms.

Ciprofloxacin is used in the treatment of a wide variety of urinary, GI, respiratory, bone and joint, and soft tissue infections; especially those resistant to other antibacterial drugs.

The most common adverse reactions include headache, dizziness, GI disturbances, and rash. Some rashes are related to photosensitivity reactions. The fluroquinolones are not recommended for children or pregnant women. There is evidence of cartilage defects in animal studies, and arthralgias and joint swelling in humans.

MISCELLANEOUS ANTIMICROBIAL DRUGS

Chloramphenicol (*Chloromycetin*)

Chloramphenicol is a broad-spectrum antibiotic that is reserved for serious and life-threatening infections. Two of the main indications for chloramphenicol are the treatment of typhoid fever and certain types of meningitis. The mechanism of action of chloramphenicol is to inhibit bacterial protein synthesis, which produces a bacteriostatic effect. Absorption of chloramphenicol from the GI tract is excellent. The oral dose is 250 to 500 mg every 6 hours. Chloramphenicol is also used topically in the treatment of ocular infections.

Adverse and Toxic Effects

Common side effects usually involve nausea, vomiting, and diarrhea. Chloramphenicol is potentially a very toxic drug. One of the most serious effects is bone marrow depression, which usually produces anemia or other blood disorders. In most cases, the effects are reversible. However, in some patients the adverse effects are irreversible and may include aplastic anemia. Frequent blood cell counts should be taken while

TABLE 41:7	Fluroquinolone Antimicrobial Drugs
DRUG (TRADE NAME)	**MAIN USES**
ciprofloxacin (*Cipro*)	Used for wide variety of infections
enoxacin (*Penetrex*)	Urinary tract infections and gonorrhea
lomefloxacin (*Maxaquin*)	Respiratory and urinary tract infections
norfloxacin (*Noroxin*)	Urinary tract infections
ofloxacin (*Floxin*)	Respiratory, urinary tract, and gonorrhea
grepafloxacin (*Raxar*)	Respiratory and urinary tract infections
levofloxacin (*Levaquin*)	Respiratory and urinary tract infections
moxifloxacin (*Avelox*)	Bacterial sinusitis, bronchitis, pneumonia
sparfloxacin (*Zagam*)	Respiratory tract infections

patients are receiving chloramphenicol. As with all broad-spectrum antibiotics, suppression of normal intestinal bacterial may result in superinfections.

Cautions and Contraindications

Chloramphenicol should not be administered to infants less than 2 weeks old. Infant livers are unable to metabolize chloramphenicol and accumulation leads to toxic blood levels, resulting in a condition known as the gray baby syndrome, which is characterized by abdominal distention, circulatory collapse, and respiratory failure.

Clindamycin (*Cleocin*)

Clindamycin is a bacteriostatic antibiotic that inhibits bacterial protein synthesis. The drug is effective against most of the common gram-positive organisms and especially against anaerobic organisms, which is its major indication. The most common adverse effects involve the GI tract, usually diarrhea. Occasionally, clindamycin allows the overgrowth of another intestinal organism, *Clostridium difficile*. This can cause a condition known as pseudomembranous colitis, which causes severe diarrhea, abdominal cramps, and can be fatal if untreated.

Vancomycin (*Vancocin*)

Vancomycin is a bactericidal antibiotic that interferes with cell wall synthesis. The drug is mainly used to treat resistant staphococcal infections and pseudomembranous colitis caused by *Clostridium difficile*. Vancomycin may produce some serious adverse effects that include ototoxicity (deafness), nephrotoxicity (kidney), and a flushing redness of the neck and trunk caused by histamine release. This condition is known as "red man syndrome" and occurs when parenteral administration is too rapid.

Treatment of Vancomycin-Resistant Infections

Within the last several years there has been an increase in the number of gram-positive bacteria that are resistant to vancomycin, especially staphylococcal and enterococcal bacteria. Several new anti-infective drugs have been discovered and are now available for treatment of infections caused by these bacteria.

Quinupristin-dalfopristin (*Synercid*) is a combination of two drugs. It must be administered parenterally and is rapidly bactericidal for most resistant gram-positive organisms. The drug causes pain at the infusion site and an arthralgia-myalgia syndrome.

Linezolid (*Zyvox*) is effective against many gram-positive and some gram-negative bacteria. The drug is administered parenterally and is bacteriostatic against most bacteria. It is indicated for treatment of infections caused by vancomycin-resistant organisms. Adverse effects include gastrointestinal disturbances, headache, and a decrease in platelets and RBCs.

DRUGS USED TO TREAT TUBERCULOSIS

Tuberculosis is an infection caused by *Mycobacterium tuberculosis*. The infection usually involves the lung, but can spread to other body organs, including the brain. The infecting organism can lie dormant within the body, only to reemerge and cause infection years later. Reemergence of the organism often occurs when body resistance to infection is lowered. Infection with human immunodeficiency virus (acquired immunodeficiency syndrome [AIDS]) has been one of the factors that accounts for the increased incidence of tuberculosis in recent years. One of the biggest problems in treating tuberculosis has been the dramatic increase in bacterial resistance to drug therapy. Drug therapy usually involves administration of three or four different drugs for prolonged periods of time, often a year or more. The most important drugs for treating tuberculosis are isoniazid, rifampin, ethambutol, pyrazinamide, and streptomycin. Streptomycin is one of the aminoglycosides; it is sometimes used in initial therapy for the first few weeks. The major disadvantage is that it requires parenteral administration.

Isoniazid (*INH*)

Isoniazid is a synthetic drug that is bactericidal for reproducing organisms. The drug inhibits the production of mycolic acid, which is essential for bacterial cell wall synthesis. Isoniazid is well absorbed orally and metabolized by acetylation. This reaction is highly variable among individuals—some are "fast acetylators" while others are "slow acetylators." Slow acetylators usually experience better antibacterial results, but also experience more adverse effects of the drug.

The two most important adverse effects of isoniazid are peripheral neuritis and hepatitis.

Peripheral neuritis can usually be prevented by taking pyridoxine (vitamin B_6) supplementation. Hepatitis is more common in individuals over the age of 35 and those who drink alcohol on a regular basis. Other adverse effects include fever, rash, and central nervous system (CNS) disturbances.

Rifampin (*Rifadin*)

Rifampin is an antibiotic that has a wider antibacterial spectrum than isoniazid. The drug inhibits a bacterial enzyme required for ribonucleic acid (RNA) synthesis. Rifampin is taken orally, undergoes enterohepatic cycling, and induces drug-metabolizing enzymes. This leads to a decrease in the duration of action of both itself and other drugs and may require an increase in drug dosage.

Adverse effects include GI disturbances, hepatotoxicity, rash, and headache. A flu-like syndrome, usually fatigue and muscle ache, may occur when the drug is not taken on a regular basis. Rifampin also stains urine, tears (contact lens), and other body fluids orange-red.

Ethambutol (*Myambutol*)

Ethambutol is a synthetic compound that produces a bacteriostatic effect. The drug is believed to inhibit the incorporation of mycolic acid into the bacterial cell wall. Ethambutol is generally only used in combination with other drugs. The drug is usually well tolerated; fever, rash, and GI disturbances are common side effects. The most serious concern is the loss of visual acuity due to optic neuritis. It is recommended that visual eye tests be performed before and during therapy to prevent any permanent loss of vision.

Pyrazinamide

Pyrazinamide is a derivative of nicotinamide. Its antibactericidal effects are increased by acidic conditions. The drug is mainly used in initial therapy for the first few months. Its mechanism of action is not well understood. The most serious adverse effect is development of hepatotoxicity. In addition, some patients develop hyperuricemia and symptoms of gout.

CHEMOPROPHYLAXIS

Chemoprophylaxis refers to the use of antibiotics before bacterial infection has occurred in order to prevent infection. Chemoprophylaxis is indicated before certain surgeries that carry a high risk for infection—for example, abdominal surgery, especially after gunshot wounds where the intestines may be ruptured. In addition, individuals who are susceptible to certain infections that may be life-threatening often take antibiotics on a regular basis to prevent infection. Individuals who have had rheumatic fever, heart valve replacement, knee and hip replacement, and other conditions are particularly susceptible to infections that can cause endocarditis and heart valve damage. These individuals should receive chemoprophylaxis before dental, respiratory, urinary, and other invasive medical procedures. In addition, individuals exposed to patients with tuberculosis, meningitis, and other contagious infections are often given chemoprophylaxis to prevent infection. The selection and timing of antibiotic administration depends on the type of infection that is anticipated, patient characteristics, and other considerations related to the specific clinical situation.

Chapter Review

Understanding Terminology

Answer the following questions in the spaces provided.

1. Differentiate between the terms *bactericidal* and *bacteriostatic*. _____
   _____
   _____

2. Define the terms *antibacterial spectrum* and *broad-spectrum* drugs. _____
   _____
   _____

3. Define the terms *gram stain, gram positive,* and *gram negative*. _____
   _____
   _____

4. What is the difference between nonpathogenic bacteria and pathogenic bacteria? _____
   _____
   _____

Acquiring Knowledge

Answer the following questions in the spaces provided.

1. What are the major sources of antibacterial drugs? _____
   _____
   _____

2. Why are gram stains important? _____
   _____
   _____

3. Explain the mechanism of action of the penicillin and cephalosporin antibiotics. _____
   _____
   _____

4. What are the main advantages of the third- and fourth-generation penicillins? Third-generation cephalosporins?
   _____
   _____

5. What are the main uses, adverse effects, and drug interactions associated with the aminoglycosides?
   _____
   _____

6. Explain how the sulfonamides produce their antibacterial effect. What advantages does trimethoprim-sulfamethoxazole offer?
   _____
   _____

7. Explain the mechanisms of action of the tetracyclines, choramphenicol, and fluroquinolones.
   _____
   _____

8. What are the contraindications to the use of the tetracyclines? Chloramphenicol? _____

_____

_____

9. List some of the drugs used in the treatment of tuberculosis (TB). _____

_____

_____

10. Explain the mechanisms of action of isoniazid and rifampin. What are the major toxicities of these drugs?

_____

_____

Applying Knowledge—On the Job

Use your critical thinking skills to answer the following questions in the spaces provided.

1. Mrs. Randazzo is an elderly woman admitted to the hospital from a nursing home with a diagnosis of sepsis secondary to a urinary tract infection (UTI). She has been receiving piperacillin (*Pipracil*) for 24 hours and her temperature chart is showing a downward trend. The lab calls you with the initial results of the blood culture and states that gram-negative rods grew in two of three culture tubes. Do you need to call the attending physician for a change in antibiotic? Why or why not?

_____

_____

2. Mr. Porter is admitted to the hospital with an empiric diagnosis of pneumonia. The emergency room physician prescribed erythromycin IV—piggyback every 6 hours. In the patient's admission history, the patient states he has a penicillin allergy. Is it necessary to call the attending physician for a change in antibiotic because of the penicillin allergy? Why or why not?

_____

_____

3. Mr. Smith has just been diagnosed with a respiratory infection caused by *Pseudomonas aeruginosa*. Which penicillin antibiotic would be appropriate therapy? How is this drug administered?

_____

_____

4. John is a 22-year-old college student who is taking one of the cephalosporins for a throat infection. Last night at a fraternity party he got violently ill after a few beers. What happened?

_____

_____

5. Mrs. Evans is a 45-year-old woman who is on a four-drug regimen for treatment of her tuberculosis. At her recent checkup, her liver enzymes were increased and there were signs of jaundice. Which antitubercular drugs could be causing this condition? What other factors may make her more susceptible to this toxicity?

_____

_____

6. Mrs. Urban was prescribed clindamycin for a minor gram-positive throat infection. After 3 days she was experiencing severe diarrhea and dehydration. The next day she collapsed and was rushed to the hospital. The diagnosis was pseudomembranous colitis. Can you explain how this happened? What drug is indicated for treatment of this condition?

_____

_____

7. A woman has just presented a prescription at the pharmacy for *Velosef* 500 mg QID ×10d. Upon questioning, she states that she had a severe allergic reaction to penicillin: her throat swelled and she had a hard time breathing. Would you expect the pharmacist to call the physician to change the antibiotic? Why or why not?

_____

_____

_____

8. A man has just received a prescription for *Bactrim* DS 1 BID ×5d. He told you earlier that he was allergic to *Azulfidine.* Would you ask the patient to wait until you have spoken with the physician about this allergy? Why or why not?

_____

_____

9. A woman has just received *Zithromax* 250 mg – 2 today, then 1 QD ×4d. While talking with the patient, she tells you that she is allergic to erythromycin. When she took it previously, she had stomach cramps, was nauseated, and sometimes vomited. Should the physician be contacted to change the medication? Why or why not?

_____

_____

_____

Internet Connection

Visit the **MedicineNet** website (http://www.medicinenet.com) and click on the *Diseases and Treatments* heading. Highlight the first letter of the following topics to acquire additional background and clinical information on these antibiotic-related articles: *Diarrhea, Antibiotic Induced, Gonorrhea, Infection, Urinary, Neutropenia, Pneumonia, Pseudomembranous Colitis.* Incorporate this information with the use of the antibiotics presented in this chapter. Perhaps you and some of your classmates could each take a topic and give a brief presentation to the class.

Additional Reading

Aminoglycosides: Is once a day good enough? 1997. *Emergency Medicine* 29 (2):83.

Azithromycin versus doxycycline for Chlamydia. 1996. *Emergency Medicine* 28 (9):100.

Double trouble from the deer tick. 1997. *Emergency Medicine* 29 (3):44.

McNeil, S. A., Mody, L., and Bradley, S. F. 2002. Infectious disease: methicillin-resistant Staphylococcus aureu. *Geriatrics* 57 (6):16.

O'Donnell, J. A. and Hofman, M. T. 2002. Infectious disease: urinary tract infection. *Geriatrics* 57 (5):45.

Sheff, B. 2001. Taking aim at antibiotic-resistant bacteria. *Nursing 2001* 31 (11):62.

Tjaden, J. A., Lazarus, A. A., and Martin, G. J. 2002. Bacteria as agents of warfare. *Postgraduate Medicine* 112 (2):57.

ANTIFUNGAL AND ANTIVIRAL (AIDS) DRUGS

42

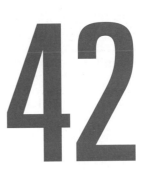

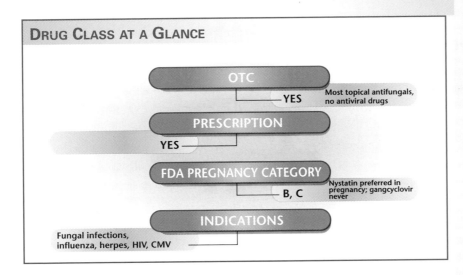

DRUG CLASS AT A GLANCE

OTC

YES — Most topical antifungals, no antiviral drugs

PRESCRIPTION

YES

FDA PREGNANCY CATEGORY

B, C — Nystatin preferred in pregnancy; gangcyclovir never

INDICATIONS

Fungal infections, influenza, herpes, HIV, CMV

CHAPTER FOCUS

This chapter describes drugs that inhibit the growth of a variety of fungi and viruses that cause infection.

CHAPTER OBJECTIVES

After studying this chapter, you should be able to

- describe two drugs that are effective against systemic fungal infections.

- describe the mechanism of action of drugs effective against viral infections, especially drugs used in the treatment of acquired immunodeficiency syndrome (AIDS).

- explain how the treatment of viral infection is different from treatment that kills microorganisms such as fungi or bacteria.

- list three side effects associated with antifungal drugs.

- describe how pathogenic fungi gain access to the human host.

Key Terms

acquired immunity: protection from viral reinfection in the form of antibodies.

acquired immunodeficiency syndrome (AIDS): viral-induced disease characterized by multiple opportunistic infections as a result of depleted lymphocytes involved in the cell-mediated immune process.

antigenic drift and antigenic shift: the ability of viruses to change the composition or structure of their surface proteins (viral coat) that are responsible for producing disease (pathogenicity).

candidiasis: infection caused by the yeast *Candida;* also known as moniliasis.

dermatophytic: infection of the skin, hair, or nails caused by a fungus.

fungicidal: substance, chemical solution, or drug that kills fungi.

HIV: human immunodeficiency virus, responsible for producing AIDS.

immunity: condition that causes individuals to resist acquiring or developing a disease or infection.

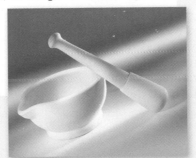

immunosuppressed: having inhibition of the body's immune response (ability to fight infection), usually induced by drugs or viruses.

keratinized: composed of a protein substance largely found in hair and nails.

mycosis: any disease caused by a fungus.

nucleoside: molecule that contains purine or pyrimidine bases in combination with sugar.

opportunistic organism: microorganism capable of causing disease only when the resistance (immunocompetence) of the host is impaired.

porphyria (acute): disease associated with excessive liver production of delta-aminolevulonic acid and characterized by intermittent hypertension, abdominal cramps, and psychosis.

Reye's syndrome: a potentially fatal illness characterized by vomiting, an enlarged liver, convulsions, and coma, in children and adolescents; linked to the use of salicylates in the management of influenza, usually type B, or chickenpox.

thrush: term used for *Candida* infection in the mucous membranes of the mouth and pharynx.

INTRODUCTION

Fungi (yeasts and molds) are plant-like microorganisms that often produce annoying symptoms in humans. Fungi that affect humans can be found in the soil, air, and contaminated food. Certain fungal infections **(mycoses)** occur throughout the body (systemic). These infections usually go undiagnosed and untreated for many months while the fungi infest several tissues (lungs, bones, and meninges). Systemic fungal infections are potentially dangerous in patients who are chronically ill (diabetes mellitus) or immunosuppressed (cancer, leukemia, acquired immunodeficiency syndrome [AIDS]) because resistance to infection is low and recurrence of infections complicates the treatment. The most common mycotic infections that occur in humans involve the hair, skin, nails **(dermatophytic),** and vagina (see Table 42:1). Dermatophytic and vaginal fungal infections are more annoying than serious, producing symptoms such as intense itching, discolored scaling patches on the skin, inflammation of the scalp, loss of hair, blisters, and broken skin between the toes. The two most common dermatophytic fungal infections are athlete's foot and ringworm of the body, scalp, and nails. The fungal culprit is in the genus *Tinea*. Table 42:1 identifies the spectrum of ringworm infections commonly encountered. Vaginal fungal infections are very common and result from an overgrowth of yeast (*Candida albicans).* Candida infections called **thrush** also can occur in esophageal and oral tissues. These sites are considered superficial fungal infections because the fungus invades dead tissue of the mucous membranes, scalp, foot, and nails.

ANTIFUNGAL DRUGS

Many drugs are available for the treatment of mycotic infections. The route of administration, doses, and accepted uses of some antifungal drugs are presented in Table 42:2 on pages 514–15. Antifungal drugs produce a selective spectrum of activity and site of action. As a rule, these drugs have no antibacterial activity and affect only certain pathogenic fungi. For example, amphotericin B is the drug of choice in the treatment of systemic fungal infections. However, amphotericin B and nystatin are also useful in the treatment of **candidiasis** (an infection caused by *Candida*) when used topically. Topical antifungal agents used primarily for dermatophytic infections may also be used for the treatment of cutaneous or vaginal candidiasis (miconazole nitrate, ciclopirox olamine, clotrimazole, gentian violet).

On the other hand, griseofulvin is effective primarily against fungal infections of **keratinized** tissues (hair, skin, or nails) and has

TABLE 42:1   Human Fungal Infections

TYPE	SITE	EXAMPLE	DRUG OF CHOICE
Systemic infections	Blood, bones, lungs	Aspergillosis, blastomycosis, histoplasmosis, candidiasis, coccidioidomycosis, cryptococcosis, paracoccidio domycosis	amphotericin B and itraconazole; Fluconazole and ketoconazole; Fluconazole, amphotericin B or itraconazole; amphotericin B plus flucytosine
Dermatophytic infections	Hair, nails, skin	Athlete's foot (*Tinea pedis*), ringworm hair (*Tinea capitis*), body (*Tinea corporis*), nails (*Tinea unguium*), jock itch (*Tinea cruris*)	griseofulvin haloprogin tolnaftate zinc undecylenate
Candida albicans	Skin, mucous membranes	Vaginal yeast infection, Candidiasis, deep mucocutaneous, oropharyngeal infections Miscellaneous subcutaneous infections, Sporotrichosis, chromomycosis, leishmaniasis	amphotericin B fluconazole, ketoconazole miconazole nystatin amphotericin B and itraconazole

no antifungal action against *Candida.* Many of the agents used in dermatophytic infections (tolnaftate, haloprogin, and undecylenic acid) have no value in the treatment of other fungal infections, particularly systemic infections. Treatment may vary according to the chronic nature of the infection. Acute superficial infections may require 1 to 2 weeks of treatment while chronic recurring infections, especially those in nail beds, may take up to 6 months of drug treatment.

In addition to amphotericin B, treatments for severe systemic fungal infections include flucytosine, and the imidazole/triazole drugs, fluconazole, ketoconazole, miconazole IV, and itraconazole. The dose of miconazole varies according to the organisms being treated, ranging from 200 to 3600 mg daily, divided over three infusions. This therapy should continue from 1 to 20 weeks in order to prevent relapse or reinfection. Table 42:2 on pages 514–15 presents the recommended doses and treatment schedules for the antifungal drugs. In the management of fungal infections in immunosuppressed patients, where resistance to infection is low and recurrence is inevitable, treatment may continue indefinitely. Selection of the appropriate drug to reduce or eliminate the infection will depend on characteristics other than excellent activity against pathogenic fungi. For example, ketoconazole is valuable because it can eliminate infections that are not responsive to other antifungal agents; however, it cannot be used for the treatment of fungal meningitis because it does not penetrate spinal fluid to reach infected meninges.

NOTE TO THE HEALTH CARE PROFESSIONAL

Corticosteroids alone are contraindicated for the treatment of acute superficial herpes simplex keratitis (ocular herpes) because of the potential to exacerbate the infection and produce cataract and/or glaucoma.

Clinical Indications

Drugs effective against fungal infections are approved for use in patients with severe fungal infections that are resistant to treatment, chronic in recurrence, and/or life-threatening. Amphotericin B is indicated for use in invasive fungal infections including *Aspergillus, Candida, Cryptococcus, Histoplasmosis,* and *Blastomycosis.*

Drugs Effective in the Treatment of Fungal Infections

DRUG (TRADE NAME)	USE*	ADULT DOSE
amphotericin B (*Fungizone, Abelcet, Amphotec*)	Severe progressive fungal infections Systemic infections Severe coccidioidomycosis Cryptococcosis	Adjusted according to the severity of the disease, test dose 1 mg/2 ml dextose solution IV over 20–30 min. Then 0.25–0.35 mg/kg slow IV infusion over 6 hr, total dose of 1.5–2.5 g should be administered over 6 weeks IV
amphotericin B (*Fungizone*) topical	Candidiasis	3% cream, lotion, or ointment BID–QID for 1–3 weeks
butenafine (*Mentax*)	Athlete's foot only	1% cream once a day for 4 weeks
butaxonazole (*FemStat 3*)	Vulvovaginal moniliasis	2% cream 1 applicator (5 g) intra-vaginally at bedtime for 3–6 days
ciclopiroxolamine (*Loprox*)	Superficial dermatophytic infection, *Candidia* moniliaisis	1% cream or lotion applied BID up to 4 weeks
clioquinol (*Vioform***)		3% ointment,cream applied topically 2–3 times a day; do not exceed 1 week
clotrimazole (*FemCare,** Gyne-Lotrimin,** Lotrimin-AF, Mycelex-G, Mycelex,** Mycelex-OTC***)	Candidiasis Athlete's foot and dermatophytic infections	1% cream, lotion, solution applied topically BID up to 4 weeks; 1 tablet (100 mg) intravaginally inserted for 7days *or* 1 tablet (500 mg) inserted at bedtime
econazole (*Spectazole*)	Dermatophytic infections Superficial fungal infections	1% cream applied BID up to 4 weeks
fluconazole (*Diflucan*)	Candidiasis oroesophageal	200 or 400 mg initially PO followed by 100 mg daily for 2–3 weeks including 2 weeks after resolution
	Candidiasis UTI	50–200 mg PO daily for 2–3 weeks
	Vaginal candidiasis	150 mg single dose
	Candidiasis in bone marrow transplant	400 mg PO daily for several days before and after transplant
	Cryptococcal meningitis	400 mg initially followed by 200 mg PO once a day for 10–12 weeks
flucytosine 5-fluorocytosine (*Ancobon*)	Serious infections *Candidia, Cryptococcus*	50–150 mg/kg in divided doses every 6 hours PO
gentian violet	Candidiasis	1 and 2% solution apply BID
griseofulvin*** (*Fulvicin-U/F, Grifulvin V, Grisactin-250, 500* Griseofulvin (*Gris-PEG*)	Ringworm, *T. corporis, T. crucis, T. capis, T. pedis*	500 mg/day PO microsize (330–375 mg/day ultramicrosize) 0.75–1 g microsize PO (660–750 mg ultrasize) treatment is 4–8 weeks; treatment for fingernails and toes may be 4–6 months
haloprogin (*Halotex*)**	Superficial dermatophytic infections	1% cream or solution applied liberally topically BID up to 4 weeks
itraconazole (*Sporanox*)	Pulmonary and extrapulmonary infections (blastomycosis, histoplasmosis, aspergilosis)	200–400 mg daily PO in divided doses up to several months
	Onychomycosis	200 mg PO daily for 12 weeks

Drugs Effective in the Treatment of Fungal Infections, *continued*

DRUG (TRADE NAME)	USE*	ADULT DOSE
ketoconazole (*Nizoral*)	Blastomycosis, *Candidiasis* Systemic mycosis	200–400 mg PO for 1–2 weeks Can be treated up to 6 months
miconazole* IV	*Candida* in urinary bladder	200 diluted (600–1800 mg/day) IV infused over several hours for 1–20 weeks
	Cryptococcus	1200–2400 mg IV/day for 3–12 weeks
	Coccidioidomycosis	1800–3600 mg/day IV for 3–20 weeks
miconazole (*Micatin*,* *Monistat-Derm*)	Cutaneous candidiasis, dermatophytic infection	2% cream, powder, or spray BID up to 2 weeks; shampoo twice a week for 4 weeks
naftifine (*Naftin*)	Superficial dermatophytic infections	1% cream apply once a day, 1% gel apply BID up to 4 weeks
nystatin (*Mycostatin*, *Nilstat, Nystex*)	Candidiasis intestinal, vulvovaginitis	500,000–1,000,000 units PO BID, including 48 hr after resolution of condition; 1 tablet (100,000 units) intravaginally nightly for 2 weeks
oxiconizole (*Oxistat*)	Dermatophytic infection	1% cream or lotion apply BID up to 2 months
sulconazole (*Exelderm*)	Dermatophytic infection	1% cream or solution apply BID up to 4 weeks
terbinafine (*Lamisil*)	Dermatophytic infections, onychomycosis	1% cream apply BID up to 4 weeks; 250 mg daily for 6 weeks (fingernails) to 12 weeks (toenails)
terconazole (*Terazol-3, Terazol-7*)	Candidiasis, vulvovaginal, moniliasis	1 suppository (2.5 g) intravaginally at bedtime for 3 days; 0.4%, 0.8% cream 1 applicatorful (5 g) at bedtime for 3 or 7 days
tioconazole (*Vagistat-1*)	Candidiasis, vulvovaginal moniliasis	6.5% vaginal ointment; 1 applicator applied at bedtime
tolnaftate** (*Aftate*,** *NP-27*,** *Tinactin*,** *Ting***)	Dermatophytic infections, ringworm, athlete's foot	1% cream, powder, liquid spray gel, or solution applied topically BID up to 6 weeks
triacetin (*Fungoid, Ony-Clear Nail*)	Superficial nail infections	Solution, cream, spray, tincture apply TID up to 4 weeks; tincture may be applied on nails up to 4 months
undecylenic acid (*Breeze Mist Aerosol*,** *Cruex*,** *Desenex***)*	Athlete's foot, diaper rash	Topical powder or ointment, apply liberally

Abbreviations: UTI, urinary tract infection.
*Not an inclusive list of uses.
**These preparations can be obtained over the counter.
***Doses stated are for microsize formulations; these products are also available as ultramicrosize formulations.
Note: Itraconazole is contraindicated for use concurrently with cisapride (antiulcer), astemizole, and terfenadine (antihistamine H_1-antagonists) because serious cardiovascular conduction and rhythm disorders leading to death have occurred.
Note: The FDA has approved the first combination product in the treatment of HIV. *Combivir* is a single tablet containing zidovudine (AZT) and 3TC (lamivudine).

Invasive infections clinically manifest as septicemia, endocarditis, and pulmonary and urinary tract infections. Immunocompromised patients may have infections in any organ or cavity that are particularly difficult to eliminate. Agents that are used in the treatment of serious urinary infections, such as miconazole IV, may require adjunct therapy to achieve a clinical cure.

Topical and/or intravaginal application of antifungal drugs are indicated for use in superficial fungal infections of the scalp, skin, nails, and mucous membranes. Although effective, drugs such as amphotericin B are not recommended for use in conditions where topical application is sufficient. The risk of adverse effects does not warrant the use of such agents in significant but less serious fungal infections.

Mechanism of Action

Drugs useful in the treatment of systemic mycotic infections and candidiasis are usually **fungicidal** (capable of killing fungi). The agents (amphotericin B, ketoconazole, miconazole, itraconazole, and nystatin) bind to fungal membranes and produce a change in cell permeability. The "azole" drugs are believed to impair the synthesis of ergosterol, which is an essential substance for fungal cell membrane integrity. As a result, essential nutrients and inorganic substances (ions) leak out of the cell, causing cell destruction. A drug such as flucytosine, which is 5-fluorocytosine, is thought to prevent fungal multiplication by impairing DNA synthesis in fungal cells; however, the mechanism of action is not absolutely known.

Dermatophytic infections are usually associated with the protein keratin. A drug such as griseofulvin binds to the keratin and prevents the fungi from invading the tissue. Griseofulvin binds to the keratin for months. As the fungus-infected keratin is shed, it is replaced by new normal, uninfected tissue. Griseofulvin also binds to lipid constituents of the actively growing fungi and inhibits cell mitosis. However, the direct effect of griseofulvin on fungal cells is still not understood. Although griseofulvin is fungi*static,* most of the other drugs used in dermatophytic infections are fungicidal.

Pharmacokinetics

Oral Administration

Nystatin exhibits little or no absorption following oral administration. The unmetabolized drug is excreted into the feces. Limiting the effective site of action is advantageous in two ways: (1) for the treatment of intestinal candidiasis, and (2) in the treatment of pregnant women because the drug cannot affect developing fetal tissues. Among the imidazole and triazole derivates used in the treatment of serious infections, ketoconazole absorption depends on the acidity of the stomach for tablet dissolution. Anything that raises gastric pH, such as food or antacids, will impair the absorption of ketoconazole. Once absorbed, it is highly bound (99 percent) to plasma protein, is metabolized in the liver, and excreted in the urine. This drug has proven useful in patients with renal impairment because special dose adjustment is not necessary.

On the other hand, drug administration with food increases the absorption of griseofulvin. This is directly related to the fat content of the meal, as griseofulvin is more fat than water soluble. Since absorption patterns can be quite variable, the available formulations of griseofulvin have been designed to improve the efficiency of surface contact and absorption from the stomach. Ultramicrosize allows more particles to be in contact with the absorptive surface than the conventional microsize formulation. Although this means less ultramicrosize drug may be taken on each dose compared to the microsized formulation, there is no difference in the clinical benefits derived from either formulation.

Flucytosine is well absorbed following oral administration, is not bound to plasma proteins, and is excreted unmetabolized into the urine. Because of free availability, this drug can enter the cerebrospinal fluid (CSF), which may offer an advantage in patient treatment. Among the "azole" drugs, ketoconazole and iatroconazole are highly bound to plasma proteins (98 percent) and metabolized by the liver. These drugs are not distributed within the central nervous system; however, significant concentrations are achieved in fatty tissues. Fluconazole exhibits excellent absorption and enters a variety of tissues including the CSF. It is excreted by the kidney mostly unmetabolized.

Parenteral Administration

Amphotericin B, although bound to plasma proteins (95 percent), does penetrate inflamed tissues to affect fungal colonization. Ultimately it is excreted unchanged in the urine. Amphotericin B is available in a special parenteral liposomal delivery system. This formulation prolongs drug retention through the fat-soluble characteristics of the liposomal vehicle and may distribute differently within fatty tissues. It produces the same spectrum of antifungal activity as other formulations prior to its excretion, and it can be detected in the urine weeks after treatment has stopped. Presumably, this confers an advantage of continuing coverage for some period of time. Miconazole is also highly bound to plasma proteins, metabolized by the liver, and excreted in the urine. Although it penetrates some tissues, it does not cross into the CSF. When needed in the CSF, miconazole can be administered intrathecally. This drug can be used without dose adjustment in patients with renal dysfunction. Duration of treatment usually depends on the response of the patient, underlying conditions, and the chronic nature of the infection. It is not uncommon for these drugs to be continued for a few weeks to several months.

Topical Administration

Topical administration includes application of creams, lotions, ointments, tinctures, sprays, and powders to the surface of the skin and mucous membranes. Less than 10 percent of active drug is absorbed with topical administration. For most of these antifungal drugs, absorption is less than 1 to 5 percent. This permits safe use in pregnant women and may be recommended for use during the second and third trimesters. As a rule, topical antifungal drugs are used to treat less serious fungal infections that occur in the general population. Whether for *Tinea pedis* or diaper rash, these drugs are for external use only. Virtually all of the topical drugs are available over the counter (OTC). A few are available by prescription and OTC (clotrimazole, butaxonazole, miconazole) while nystatin and oxiconizole are prescription only. Many of these agents are broad-spectrum antifungals, and a few such as clioquinol are antibacterial as well. These products may have a single antifungal agent or may contain multiple active drugs. Ingredients may include alcohol, emollients, and talc as vehicles or drying agents. Combination products may also contain benzocaine, phenol, coal tar, camphor, chloroxylenol, and salicylic acid. These provide increased absorption, antiseptic activity, or reduced itching when applied liberally to the infected surface. Except for onychomycoses (nail infections), the intended length of use of topical antifungal drugs is usually less than 4 weeks. If symptoms do not resolve within this time frame, the patient should be reevaluated for complicating conditions as well as a more appropriate antifungal drug.

Adverse Effects

Nystatin is a particularly safe (nontoxic) relative to other drugs used for severe fungal infections. In large doses, oral nystatin has occasionally been associated with diarrhea, nausea, and vomiting. The other antifungal drugs may produce headache, dry mouth, nausea, constipation, gastritis, pruritus, burning, and erythema in addition to their therapeutic effects. Because nystatin and miconazole have proven to be effective and safe with repeated administration, these products have also become available as OTC preparations. Griseofulvin has been reported to produce increased protein in the urine (albuminuria), peripheral neuritis, and photosensitization. Griseofulvin is contraindicated in patients with acute intermittent **porphyria** and hepatic failure, and should not be administered during pregnancy.

Itroconazole and terbinafine may affect the liver, bone marrow, and renal systems during treatment, causing elevations of liver enzymes, creatinine, or blood urea nitrogen (BUN), or changes in the total blood cell count and differential. Similarly, flucytosine must be used with caution in patients with renal disease and bone marrow depression.

Patients are usually hospitalized to receive intravenous antifungal therapy. Antifungal drugs used to treat systemic infections are associated with serious side effects. Amphotericin B, flucytosine, and ketoconazole have been reported to produce adverse effects that include decreased renal function (hypokalemia and acidosis), hepatic failure, elevation in serum creatinine and BUN, ataxia, and thrombophlebitis. Patients receiving these drugs must be monitored for hematologic and hepatic changes. More often, however, the adverse reactions to the systemic antifungals include nausea, diarrhea, abdominal cramps, fever, and allergic dermatitis.

Contraindications

Drug hypersensitivity is the only absolute contraindication for all the antifungal drugs regardless of route of administration. In addition, a few drugs have been associated with specific serious adverse effects mitigating against their use in pregnancy or in combination with particular drugs. Such is the case with itraconazole and flucytosine. These drugs have produced changes in embryos and/or fetuses after administration to animals, which preclude their use during pregnancy. Sexually active women who are taking itraconazole should be using effective contraceptive therapy even up to 2 months after

Patient Administration and Monitoring

Patient Instructions

Serious Fungal Infections

The treatment of serious fungal infections warrants close monitoring of the patient's vital signs, including an electrocardiogram (ECG) for potential evolving cardiac conduction problems. The patient's temperature should be taken frequently during the first 24 hours of treatment. Periodic serum chemistry and hematology tests are warranted to monitor potential elevations in serum creatine (>3 mg/dl) and BUN (>40 mg/dl), indicating changes in renal and liver function that might obligate antifungal dose adjustment or discontinuation of therapy. To minimize the occurrence of thrombophlebitis, indwelling catheters may be rotated to other sites, and heparin may be administered.

Nonserious Fungal Infections

Treatment of less serious though significant fungal infections is dependent upon patient compliance and good hygiene to effect a cure and minimize reinfection. Whether oral or topical formulations are being used, patients must be instructed to complete the entire course of therapy even when signs (cracked skin, redness) and symptoms (itching, burning) have improved. This is particularly true for those infections requiring continuation of medication for 2 weeks after clinical resolution.

Topical Formulations

Creams, ointments, gels, and lotions adhere to skin, providing optimum contact with the infected area. Prior to applying the medication, the skin should always be cleaned with soap and water and dried thoroughly. Hands should always be washed thoroughly after applying medication because of the danger of accidentally touching the eyes or mouth where medication could be deposited. Topical antifungals are for external use only. Application to mucous membranes of the eyes causes intense irritation, burning, and itching. Removal of the offending medication is impossible because of the oily nature of the emollients.

Infected areas that are predisposed to moist conditions, such as the feet, groin, and underarm, may require powder formulations rather than creams or lotions. Powders usually contain talc or cornstarch, which absorbs moisture, so that the medication can perform its action. The advantage of a drier environment has to be balanced against the need to reapply the drug more frequently because the powder does not stay in place. For athlete's foot and jock itch, the cleansed areas should be covered with clean, natural fiber fabric that allows air and moisture to move away from the skin. This means educating patients to the use of cotton socks, preferably white or light colors, whenever wearing shoes. No sockless sneakers or loafers, or polyester briefs, please! Such conditions, usually popular among young adults, are excellent breeding areas for fungi. Patients must be encouraged to change socks, sometimes more than once a day. Occlusive dressings should not be used in lieu of socks.

Discoloration

Certain products may stain clothing, linens, and other fabrics during use. Amphotericin B and clioquinol discolor fabrics and skin but will wash out with soap. Gentian violet, although a lovely color, is a permanent fabric dye. Even when applied to debrided or ulcerative areas, it produces a pattern referred to as "tattooing." This cosmetic effect has caused gentian violet to be replaced by other topical medications even though it is effective.

Drug Interactions

Current medications should be reviewed thoroughly to ascertain whether the patient is taking antacids, cimetidine, or other antiulcer products that could reduce the absorption of oral ketoconazole, fluconazole, or itraconazole. The patient should be instructed to take such medications 2 hours after the antifungal dose.

Adverse Effects

Patients who are using ketoconazole should be alerted that this drug may produce headache, drowsiness, and dizziness that could impair the coordination and concentration required to drive, operate machinery, or perform tasks requiring manual dexterity.

Oral medications such as the imidazole/triazole drugs or flucytosine may cause nausea or gastrointestinal irritation after dosing. Patients may be encouraged to take these medications with meals, or spread the number of tablets or capsules ingested over 15 to 30 minutes.

Intravaginal Use

Intravaginal application of medication may obligate the patient to refrain from sexual intercourse in order to maintain sufficient drug contact with the infected surface. Depending upon the nature of the infection, abstinence may be warranted throughout the course of treatment (up to 4 weeks).

Intravaginal applicators can be designed for reuse. Product information accompanying the drug will specify whether to dispose of the applicator or reuse it. Patients must be orally instructed to wash reusable applicators with soap and water between uses. Oral instruction, whenever possible, is worth the effort because some patients cannot read the print in package inserts. This may be due to poor vision, confusion, inability to read English well, or inability to read at all.

Notifying the Physician

Patients should be instructed to notify the physician if symptoms of rash, itching, blistering, or swelling occur because this may signal the development of hypersensitivity to antifungal drugs. If such symptoms characterize the infection under treatment and persist for more than 2 to 3 weeks during treatment, the physician should be notified. Change of drug, dose, or identification of confounding conditions may be warranted.

The physician should be notified immediately if severe abdominal pain, yellowing of the skin or eyes, dark urine, or diarrhea occurs while taking ketoconazole as this may signal the development of jaundice.

Use in Pregnancy

In general, these drugs are designated Food and Drug Administration (FDA) Pregnancy Category B or C because they have not been adequately studied in pregnant women. Among the systemic drugs, safe use in pregnancy has not been established in humans. Nevertheless, there are situations where their use is clearly indicated, and may be used with caution and close patient monitoring. When amphotericin B has been used in pregnant women, harm to the fetus did not occur. Even with topical administration where absorption is extremely low, these drugs are primarily recommended for use in the second and third trimesters.

Itraconazole and flucytosine have produced changes in animals that indicate these drugs should not be used in pregnant women. Women of childbearing age who are receiving itraconazole must be instructed to use effective contraception during antifungal treatment. Effective contraception must be clearly described to the patient and may include oral contraceptives or barrier methods. Women who become pregnant while on itraconazole or flucytosine treatment should notify their physician immediately for further evaluation and discontinuation of antifungal therapy.

Nystatin is designated FDA Pregnancy Category A because there has been no evidence of risk to the fetus associated with maternal use in the first, second, or third trimester.

antifungal treatment has been discontinued. In the treatment of onychomycoses, terbinafine is not recommended to be given during pregnancy. The rationale is that these infections often require months of continuous treatment to achieve a cure and the nature of the infection allows it to be postponed until pregnancy has ended.

Itraconazole and fluconazole have been associated with serious ventricular arrhythmias, blockade, or prolongation of conduction resulting in cardiac arrest and death in patients concurrently receiving astemizole, terfinadine, or cisapride.

Itraconazole is specifically contraindicated for concurrent use with these drugs.

VIRAL DISEASES AND ANTIVIRAL DRUGS

Influenza

Flu viruses (e.g., Asian influenza) primarily affect the upper (nasal passages and pharynx) and lower (lungs) respiratory tracts. The virus is spread in the aerosolized droplets from the sneeze or cough of an infected person. The inoculated droplets are inhaled directly or transmitted by contact with the uninfected person who inadvertently delivers the virus into the mouth or respiratory tract (e.g., sucking on contaminated pencils, pens, and fingers).

Influenza is a family of viruses categorized as types A, B, and C. Influenza A and B infect humans, although the alternate host for type A is often birds, such as chickens, or pigs prior to human inoculation. Influenza outbreaks occur every year in the Northern Hemisphere between November and April (and May to October in the Southern Hemisphere) coincident with the winter season. A localized wave of infection confirmed as a high incidence (20 percent) in the general population is considered an epidemic. Influenza A epidemics typically begin suddenly, last for several months as the wave of infection spreads throughout the population, and end as abruptly as they began. In contrast, influenza B is less severe and more localized, often occurring in schools and nursing homes. When an outbreak of influenza occurs worldwide, it is considered to be "pandemic." Pandemics, like the influenza outbreak of 1918, which killed 675,000 Americans alone (more than in all the wars of the twentieth century), are facilitated by global travel but, fortunately, occur over a greater cycle of 15 to 20 years. (Go to the Internet at **www.pbs.org/wgbh/ amex/influenza/maps** for a fantastic presentation on the epidemiology of the influenza pandemic.)

Clinical Profile

In the general population (relatively healthy individuals), flu viruses usually produce headache, fever, intense fatigue, dry cough, muscle ache and sensitivity of the eyes to light. The reaction to viral infection is usually mild or moderate with symptom onset within 24 to 72 hours of incubation and resolution after a short period of infection of 7 to 14 days. Flu and its accompanying symptoms are not the same as the constellation of symptoms that occur from "cold" viruses (rhinoviruses). The clinical profile of the common cold differs from flu in that a cold develops gradually, over days, characterized by nasal secretion (rhinorrhea), congestion, and sneezing. Fever (>100.5 °F), muscle and joint aches are usually not associated with a cold.

The problem with flu, especially in children and elderly patients, is that secondary complications may occur, such as bacterial infections, otitis media or bronchitis that prolong the duration of illness in spite of treatment. Moreover, in the elderly and chronically ill, the same flu viruses may produce a more difficult or more intense infection such as pneumonia. Because the immune systems of these patients are often less competent to fight the infection, severe reactions, such as dehydration, convulsions, and death may occur.

Virus Exposure and Immunity

Many viral diseases such as chicken pox, measles, and mumps occur during childhood. Usually, these diseases occur only once because antibodies are produced that protect individuals from reinfection. This protection is referred to as **acquired immunity. Immunity** also can be acquired without experiencing the disease through vaccination. For example, with viruses such as smallpox and polio, vaccination exposes individuals to a weakened (attenuated) virus, which stimulates antibody production without producing the symptoms of disease.

Influenza Vaccine

A vaccine is available for influenza. The influenza vaccine is formulated each year to contain strains of the virus that are expected to produce flu within the population for the following winter. The viruses are grown in highly purified chicken eggs. Usually three strains of virus are included in the vaccine—two type A and one type B. To be optimally effective, vaccinations are given in the United States between October and mid-November. Following a single-dose intramuscular injection, antibody production is initiated and continues over a 2-week period, just in time for the onset of the flu season. The immunity conferred by the antibody response is only effective for the strains contained in the vaccine. Occasionally, despite vaccination, the population succumbs to the wave of influenza or suffers a more severe course than expected. This may occur because a strain of virus (in the wild) changed its antigentic nature during the year when the vaccine was in production. As a result, the antibodies produced from the vaccination no longer recognize the wild virus upon infection.

Despite the variability in effectiveness, vaccination is recommended by the Center for Disease Control for persons over 6 months of age who are at high risk for complications from the flu or who are in a position to transmit the virus to high-risk patients (e.g., health care providers or household members). High-risk persons include persons over 65 years of age, frail elderly, residents of nursing homes or long-term care facilities, and adults and children who have chronic pulmonary (asthma, COPD) or cardiovascular disorders, or those who are immunosuppressed, have HIV, and/or require hospitalization. Other high-risk groups include women who are in their second or third trimester of pregnancy during the flu season and children who require long-term aspirin (salicylates) therapy (i.e., at risk for **Reye's syndrome).**

Vaccination in healthy young adults is up to 90 percent effective in preventing or minimizing the clinical symptoms of flu. Vaccination is recommended for healthy individuals to minimize the incidence of febrile upper respiratory tract illness, and to reduce the economic burden from days of lost work and wages, lost productivity, and visits to health care providers.

The most common adverse reaction to vaccination is soreness at the injection site; however, mild fever and myalgia may also occur. While hypersensitivity reactions such as hives or systemic anaphylaxis are rare, the influenza vaccine should never be given to persons with a history of allergy to eggs.

Herpes

The family of *Herpes* viruses includes *Herpes simplex* (types 1 and 2) and *Herpes (varicella) zoster. Herpes simplex* type 1 is responsible for producing innocuous, though unpleasant, skin lesions known as fever blisters, yet the same virus can produce encephalitis and severe changes in the eye that can lead to blindness (keratitis and corneal scarring). *Herpes simplex* type 2 is associated with adult genital infections and neonatal (generalized) infections while *Herpes zoster* causes inflammation of nerve roots resulting in severe pain. In adults, *Herpes zoster* (the same virus that causes chicken pox) produces lesions on the skin surface known as "shingles."

All of these viral diseases are characterized by their high incidence of recurrence either through seasonal exposure (flu) or because the virus remains within human tissue for years (*Herpes zoster*). Although elderly and immunocompromised patients may die from complications associated with the flu, most people who have been exposed to flu or *Herpes* viruses survive seasonal attacks because the clinical symptoms are usually self-limiting. However, *this is not the case with HIV.*

Acquired Immunodeficiency Syndrome (AIDS)

Incidence of Infection

Today, one of the most notorious virus-induced diseases is **acquired immune deficiency syndrome (AIDS).** Acquired immunodefiency syndrome is caused by the human immunodeficiency virus **(HIV).** The spread of this disease is still escalating worldwide and more than 50,000 new infections occur in the United States each year. Human immunodeficiency virus/acquired immunodeficiency syndrome (HIV/AIDS) is the leading cause of death among young adults in the United States and the virus is reaching younger people each year. More than 80 percent of all people who developed AIDS within 10 years of diagnosis have died. As of 1995, one in four new infections occurs in someone under 21 years of age. The incidence among men has declined slightly since HIV was first identified in 1981; however, the incidence in women continues to escalate. The virus is transmitted through sexual contact, perinatally from an infected mother to the neonate, through infected blood during transfusion, or injection into the blood through IV drug use. Among all AIDS cases in women in the United States, almost half are due to nonmedical IV drug use. Fortunately, measures to protect against blood bank contamination have succeeded in virtually eliminating this route of infection. While the route of transmission varies among communities, more than 95 percent of HIV infection today occurs through sexual contact and/or needle-borne infection.

Clinical Profile

After exposure to the virus, a person may test HIV positive. This only indicates that the person was infected by the virus at some time. It does not give any indication of what the virus is currently doing. The typical course of infection is characterized by an acute clinical illness that varies in severity followed by a prolonged period of clinical latency. Hence, the infected individual may go for years (3 to 10 years) without signs or symptoms associated with active infection. During the clinical latency period, the virus is active within the host—preparing conditions for the onset of AIDS. Finally, patients develop opportunistic infections or cancers that manifest a constellation of clinical symptoms announcing the progression to AIDS. Only 5 to 10 percent of HIV-infected people remain asymptomatic 10 years after the initial infection. Although still used in discussions, the terms *AIDS-related complex (ARC)* and *AIDS* do not accurately reflect the stage of infection. The Centers for Disease Control and Prevention (CDC) in Atlanta have revised the classification of HIV infection to include AIDS-defining illnesses and presentation of critical T-lymphocyte categories (see Table 42:3). Even during the quiet asymptomatic clinical period, HIV is very busy replicating and inducing CD4 T-lymphocyte death. The most significant clinical defect that characterizes AIDS is the profound depletion of T-lymphocytes. Patients are

---

TABLE 42:3   Centers for Disease Control (CDC) Classification of HIV Infections and AIDS-Defining Illnesses

CATEGORIES	DEFINITION
CD4 T-Lymphocytes	
Category 1	> 500 cells/mm^3
Category 2	200–499 cells/mm^3
Category 3	< 200 cells/mm^3
Clinical HIV Infection	
Category A Presence of one or more	Asymptomatic HIV infection Persistent generalized lymphadenopathy Acute (primary) HIV infection
Category B Symptomatic conditions in an HIV-infected adult or adolescent	Meet at least one of the following: 1—Conditions are attributed to HIV or are indicative of a defect in cell-mediated immunity 2—Conditions are considered by the physician to have a clinical course or require management complicated by HIV infection such as* candidiasis, oropharyngeal (thrush), cervical dysplasia Fever or diarrhea > 1 month Idiopathic thrombocytopenic purpura Pelvic inflammatory disease Peripheral neuropathy
Category C AIDS/AIDS-defining illnesses	Includes the clinical conditions: Candidiasis of bronchi, trachea, lungs Candidiasis, esophageal Cervical cancer, invasive CD4 lymphocyte < 14% Crytococcosis, disseminated, or extrapulmonary Cryptosporidiosis, chronic intestinal Cytomegalovirus disease (other than liver, spleen, or nodes) Cytomegalovirus retinitis (loss of vision) Encephalopathy, HIV-related *Herpes simplex:* chronic ulcer(s) Histoplasmosis, disseminated Isosoriasis, chronic intestinal Kaposi's sarcoma Lymphoma, Burkitt's or immunoblastic Lymphoma, primary or brain *Mycobacterium avium* complex *Mycobacterium tuberculosis* *Pneumocystis carinii* pneumonia Pneumonia, recurrent Progressive multifocal leukoencapalopathy *Salmonella* septicemia, recurrent Toxoplasmosis of brain Wasting syndrome due to HIV

*Not an inclusive list of conditions.

monitored for total CD4 cell counts because these numbers reflect the T-lymphocytes available to combat other infections. Some evidence suggests CD4 cells may be a way to quantify viral activity (viral load) in the near future. Signs and symptoms that appear in patients with HIV infection even before the full expression of AIDS-defining illnesses are presented in Table 42:4.

HIV and Immune System Competence

HIV (human immunodeficiency virus) has made a significant negative impact on the health of young adults because there is no acquired immunity or vaccine that can prevent or interrupt the devastating effects of the chronic infection. HIV is significantly different from other viruses already mentioned. Protection from reinfection is conferred by the final outcome of the disease process—death. HIV attacks the heart of the cell-mediated immune system (lymphocytes) so that the human host is progressively **immunosuppressed** and cannot fight disease. As a result, patients become susceptible to multiple infections such as candidiasis, pneumonia, tuberculosis, and toxoplasmosis. Because these patients are incapable of efficiently fighting infection, they are always susceptible to **opportunistic organisms.** The incompetent immune system, specifically a deterioration of cell-mediated immunity, permits patients to develop secondary cancers, such as Kaposi's sarcoma, non-Hodgkin's lymphoma, or primary lymphoma of the brain. Various HIV vaccines, effective in animal models but not yet demonstrated to be effective in humans, are under development. Although AIDS patients take a tremendous variety of drugs during the progression of disease(s), virtually all of the drugs are directed at eradicating pathogenic organisms (antibiotics) or alleviating the symptoms of the AIDS-defining illnesses.

Propagation of Viruses

Unlike other microorganisms, viruses are totally dependent upon the metabolic system of the host's cells. In order to multiply, viruses must enter the cell nucleus. Viruses initially attach to the outer cell membrane and eventually gain access to the nucleus. Viruses have surface proteins (e.g., hemagglutinins) that enable them to attach to the host-cell membrane by binding to specialized structures called receptors. After attaching to the cells, the viruses inject their nucleoprotein (deoxyribonucleic acid [DNA] or ribonucleic acid [RNA]) into the cells. The viral nucleoproteins direct the production of more virus particles by using the substances (host DNA, amino acids, enzymes, bases, and ions) in the cells; therefore, the cells become efficient factories that produce new viruses. Periodically, the cells are triggered to rupture, and new viruses are expelled into the circulation and more host cells become infected.

Attempts have been made to synthesize drugs that arrest the infection after the symptoms have developed. The goal of drug therapy is to destroy the organisms and reduce the severity and length of infection. Since viruses are so closely involved with cells, it is difficult to find a drug that will kill the virus without destroying the host cells. Despite the lethal nature of HIV, you might be surprised that outside of a living cell, HIV is considered a "fragile" virus. When left outside living tissue, household bleach is sufficient to kill

---

TABLE 42:4

Signs and Symptoms in Patients with HIV Infection

Altered mental status

Adenopathy

Cough

Difficulty in swallowing

Diarrhea

Fever

Fatigue

Headache

Numbness

Oral lesions

Retinal lesions

Shortness of breath

Skin lesions

Sweating

Weight loss

Vision changes

Weakness

the HIV virus. This is the recommended disinfectant when cleaning or wiping a surface that has been exposed to fluids containing HIV (for example, infected blood spilled on a countertop).

ANTIVIRAL DRUGS

Mechanisms of Action

Theoretically, viral activity could be interrupted by inhibiting the initial attachment of the virus to the human host cells, injection of viral contents into the host cell, enzymes that transcribe or synthesize viral proteins, and the virus shedding into the circulation to reinfect other cells. Two of these routes (virus attachment and interference with viral protein transcription or synthesis) have proven profitable in the development of antiviral drugs.

The discussion of mechanism and site of antiviral drug action that follows may seem confusing because there are no simple terms for the nucleoproteins and the current cadre of drugs all sound alike. Don't be discouraged! Remember, for the viruses under discussion (HSV, HIV, cytomegalovirus [CMV]), antiviral drugs are effective because they block virus attachment to human cells or they mess up the viral proteins at transcription or synthesis.

Inhibition of Cell Penetration

Amantadine (*Symmetrel*) prevents the Asian (A2) virus that causes influenza from penetrating human cells and releasing viral DNA into the cell. When given prophylactically (within 20 hours after exposure to the flu), amantadine reduces the severity of the infection. It has no effect on other viral infections, including other strains of flu. Therefore, this drug is usually recommended for only high-risk patients (chronically ill, infants, and elderly) who would suffer most from an influenza attack.

In contrast, the neuraminidase inhibitors, the newest group of antiinfluenza drugs, are expected to have a wide range of therapeutic antiviral effectiveness. Drugs in this class include oseltamivir (*Tamiflu*) and zanamivir (*Relenza*). Neuraminidase and hemagglutinin are present on the surface of *all* influenza viruses. Hemagglutinin is responsible for docking the virus onto host cell membranes by bonding to sialic acid molecules (components of glycoproteins and mucoproteins) and inducing cell penetration. After replication, the viral clones are coated with sialic acid as they emerge from the ruptured cells. During the exodus, neuraminidase on the surface of the viral clones releases the sialic acid connections. This critical step directly affects (increases) viral pathogenicity because it frees the hemagglutinin for docking with new sialic acid molecules on the next host cells to be invaded (and not with the sialic acid-coated viruses).

Neuraminidase inhibitors are designed as sialic acid analogs so that the drug preferentially attaches to the virus surface protein but cannot be released by the enzymatic action of neuraminidase. As a result, the bound sialic acid drug causes the viruses to aggregate and clump together, attaching to each other—sialic acid drug to new virus hemagglutinin. In the end, host cell penetration is inhibited and infection (pathogenicity) is reduced because the "virus-clot" cannot be released from the cell and is unable to connect with host cell receptors. Since the sialic acid-binding site is the same for all influenza virus strains, neuraminidase inhibitors are expected to offer a greater therapeutic advantage in the treatment of influenza.

Transcription of Viral Proteins

Other antiviral drugs interfere with one or more sites of viral enzyme activity. For example, HIV infection is initiated when the virus binds to a select group of white blood cells known as T-lymphocytes, helper T-cells, or CD4-positive lymphocytes. Human immunodeficiency virus preferentially attaches to a glycoprotein, known as CD4, present on the membranes of lymphocytes and some macrophages. It is believed that after this fusion of the outside viral coat (lipid envelope), the internal contents of the virus enter the human lymphocyte cytoplasm. Human immunodeficiency virus is a retrovirus, which means it uses its single strand of RNA to manipulate the host cell's DNA into making more retroviruses. To accomplish this, a specific enzyme known as reverse transcriptase (RT) is required. Eventually, the newly produced viral-coded DNA enters the human nuclei so that production of new viruses can begin. As the new viruses are shed into the cytoplasm and meet other helper T-cells, reinfection occurs.

Although cells other than the T-lymphocytes may be the target of the virus—for example, *Herpes* (nervous tissue), cytomegalovirus (CMV; retina, liver, lung), or influenza viruses (respiratory tract), the route of access to host cell nuclei and propagation of viruses is similar. This is simplistically illustrated in Figure 42:1.

Propagation of HIV and Sites of Drug Action

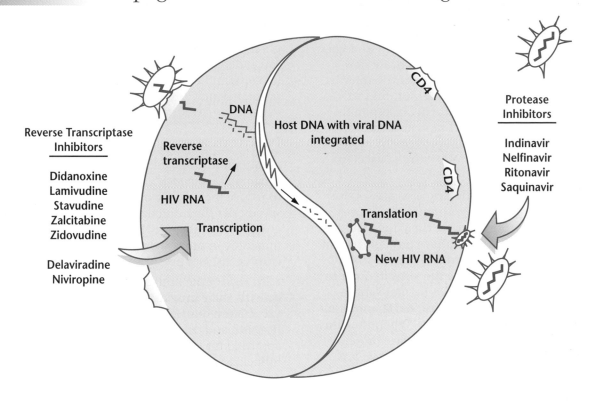

Transcription and/or Synthesis Inhibitors HIV, CMV, HSV

Nucleosides are molecules that contain purine or pyrimidine bases in combination with sugar. Nucleosides are the fundamental building blocks of RNA and DNA. Antiviral drugs such as acyclovir (*Zovirax*), idoxuridine (*Herplex*), vidarabine (*Vira-A*), and trifluridine (*Viroptic*) are purine and pyrimidine analogs that become incorporated into the viral DNA and impair viral protein synthesis. As a result, the newly formed viruses cannot function properly. Virus replication is decreased and the infection is reduced.

Nucleoside analogs such as cidofovir (*Vistide*), didanosine (*ddi, Videx*), lamivudine (*3TC, Epivir*), ganciclovir (*Cytovene*), stavudine (*d4T, Zerit*), zalcitabine (*ddc, Hivid*), and zidovudine (*Retrovir*) are recognized during the synthetic process and incorporated into the new viral-directed DNA. However, because the analog is a "false base" (not the "correct match" that would permit synthesis to continue), the viral DNA chain is terminated at the point where the drug was incorporated. These drugs effectively inhibit viral DNA synthesis and, in HIV, RT is inhibited.

Reverse transcriptase can also be inhibited by drugs that are not nucleosides (nonnucleosides) such as delavirdine (*Rescriptor*) and nevirapine

(*Viramune*). The nonnucleoside reverse transcriptase inhibitors (NNRTI) directly bind to the enzyme RT and block DNA synthesis without harming human DNA activity.

The newest anti-HIV drugs, indinavir (*Crixivan*), nelfinavir (*Viracept*), ritonavir (*Norvir*), and saquinavir (*Invirase*), inhibit HIV protease. This is an enzyme essential for production of other viral proteins that make new viruses infectious. The advantage of these drugs is that new viruses cannot infect more lymphocytes. The site and mechanism of action are removed from RT activity so that combination treatment effectively reduces the number of viruses in circulation (viremia).

Resistance to Antiviral Therapy

Although all of these mechanisms halt viral replication, these drugs do not cure viral diseases. Especially in AIDS/HIV, the course of the disease is delayed but not reversed. The primary reason that drug therapy does not yet result in a cure is that HIV rapidly mutates into a drug-resistant organism. Human immunodeficiency syndrome replicates so frequently and in such large numbers (viral load) that mutations occur in viral proteins that are clinically significant. Mutations are mistakes that occur accidentally during replication of viral genetic material. When this mistake occurs in the code for HIV enzymes such as protease or RT, the drugs that inhibit these enzymes cannot recognize the mutant enzyme. Therefore, the virus with the mutated genetic material is unaffected by drug treatment and goes on to infect more host cells and replicate new HIV with resistant properties. (Go to the Internet activity at the end of this chapter for links to antiviral resistance and treatments.) Despite the inability to cure the disease, each new class of drugs provides substantial improvement in the management of herpes or AIDS until a vaccine becomes available.

Resistance (vaccine ineffectiveness) also occurs with influenza, primarily with influenza type A. During the replication process, the virus is able to make subtle changes in its surface proteins so that antibodies specific to its former biochemistry cannot completely recognize the virus in order to make it inactive. Small changes in viral surface proteins are known as **antigenic drift** and result in decreased vaccine effectiveness. When the virus undergoes a major change in its surface proteins such as hemagglutinin and neuraminidase, it is considered an **antigenic shift.** This could obliterate antibody recognition and has been shown to reduce antiviral drug effectiveness of the neuroaminidase inhibitors in laboratory experiments.

Clinical Indications

Herpes Simplex Virus (HSV)

Drugs available in the United States have selective antiviral activity, which means the drug is effective against one specific virus. Occasionally, these drugs may have activity against two viruses. Idoxuridine (*Herplex*), vidarabine (*Ara-A, Vira-A*), and trifluridine (*Viroptic*) are used in the treatment of *Herpes simplex* infections of the eye, keratoconjuntivitis, and epithelial keratitis. These compounds can be administered topically (ocular instillation) for treatment of acute viral infections of the cornea and conjunctiva. Acyclovir (*Zovirax*) is approved for the treatment of cutaneous and genital *Herpes* infections. Acyclovir is also used to treat infections of *Herpes* and CMV that occur after bone marrow or renal transplant. Valacyclovir (*Valtrex*) is an analog of acylovir that is rapidly converted to acyclovir in the tissues.

Cytomegalovirus (CMV)

Cidofovir (*Vistide*), foscarnet (*Foscavir*), and ganciclovir (*Cytovene*) are approved for use in the treatment of CMV retinitis in patients with AIDS, CMV disease in transplant recipients, and acyclovir-resistant HSV infections in immunocompromised patients. Cytomegalovirus is a member of the *Herpes* group of viruses. In susceptible patients of any age, CMV may cause hepatitis and encephalitis. Exposure during pregnancy may result in abortion or severe brain damage in newborns.

Influenza

Amantadine (*Symadine, Symmetrel*) and rimantadine (*Flumadine*) are used prophylactically to reduce the severity of influenza attacks, specifically the influenza A virus, in susceptible groups. These include the elderly, and immunocompromised patients, and patients with chronic diseases predisposing to infection.

Because of the limited spectrum of antiviral activity, these drugs are often given in addition to vaccination during the flu season. Zanamivir (*Relenza*) and oseltamivir (*Tamiflu*) are FDA-approved for the treatment of uncomplicated influenza (any influenza strain type A or B) in adults who have been symptomatic for less than 3 days. These drugs are not substitutes for annual vaccination and are compatible adjunct therapy in addition to vaccination.

Respiratory Syncytial Virus (RSV)

This virus causes severe bronchitis and pneumonia in infants and children, often leading to death. Although the virus resembles influenza, it responds to treatment as a unique microorganism. Ribavirin (*Virazole*) is used in the treatment of RSV-induced severe lower respiratory infections in hospitalized children. While ribavirin has also been used to treat influenza A and B, it is not approved for this use in adults.

Human Immunodeficiency Virus (HIV)

A significant number of drugs have been recently approved for use alone or in combination for the management of HIV infection. These drugs are indicated for treatment of advanced infection and are not approved for prophylaxis. The frequency of virus mutation results in drug resistance and poor clinical response. Except for the newest agents, monotherapy is not recommended. Among the drugs used against HIV are didanosine (*Videx*), indinavir (*Crixivan*), nelfinavir (*Viracept*), saquinavir (*Invirase*), zalcitabine (*Hivid*), and zidovudine (*Retrovir*). A display of currently available HIV drugs is presented in Table 42:5.

Drugs Effective in the Treatment of Viral Infections

DRUG (TRADE NAME)	PYRIMIDINE OR PURINE BASE	OUTCOME	USE	ADULT DOSE
amantadine (*Symmetrel*)	—	Inhibits release of viral DNA into host cells	Influenza A respiratory tract illness	200 mg PO daily as single dose or 100 mg BID* for at least 10 days
rimantadine (*Flumadine*)	—	Inhibits early viral replication by uncoating the virus	Influenza A respiratory tract illness	100 mg BID* PO for 7 days
cidofovir (*Vistide*)	—	Inhibits viral DNA synthesis	CMV retinitis	5 mg/kg IV every 12 hr for 14–21 days
foscarnet (*Foscavir*)	—	Inhibits viral replication	CMV retinitis	90 mg/kg controlled IV* infusion (1–2 hr) every 12 hr, or 60 mg/kg infused IV over 1 hr every 8 hr for 2–3 weeks
ganciclovir (*Cytovene*)	2'-deoxyguanosine	Inhibits viral DNA synthesis	CMV retinitis CMV disease	5 mg/kg IV infusion* over 1 hr every 12 hr for 14–21 days or 1000 mg PO TID with food or 500 mg PO six times a day
ribavirin (*Virazole*)	—	Mechanism unknown	Severe lower respiratory tract infections in infants and young children, RSV syncytial virus	20 mg/ml aerosolized for 12–18 hr a day for 3–7 days
acyclovir** (*Zovirax*)	Acycloguanosine	Inhibits viral DNA replication	Genital herpes, initial Genital herpes, chronic *Herpes zoster* Chicken pox	200 mg PO* every 4 hr for 10 days 400 mg PO* BID for up to 12 months 800 mg PO every 4 hr for 7–10 days 20 mg/kg QID* for 5 days
famciclovir (*Famvir*)	Penciclovir	Inhibits viral DNA replication	Genital herpes, recurrent *Herpes zoster*	125 mg PO BID for 5 days 500 mg PO every 8 hr for 7 days
idoxuridine (*Herplex*)	5'-iodo-2'-deoxyuridine	Inhibits viral DNA synthesis by blocking incorporation of thymidine	*Herpes simplex* keratitis	1 drop into each infected eye every hour during the day and every 2 hours at night
trifluridine (*Viroptic*)	Trifluorothymidine	Interferes with viral DNA synthesis	*Herpes simplex* 1 and 2, keratoconjuctivitis, keratitis	1 drop into each infected eye every 2 hr not to exceed 9 drops/day up to 7 days
valacyclovir (*Valtrex*)	Acyclovir analog	Inhibits viral DNA replication	Genital herpes, recurrent *Herpes zoster*	500 mg PO BID* for 5 days 1 g PO TID* for 7 days
vidarabine (*Vira-A*)	Acycloguanosine	Inhibits viral DNA enzyme (DNA polymerase)	*Herpes simplex* keratoconjuctivitis, keratitis	0.5 inch of ointment into each infected eye every 3 hr not to exceed 5 applications per day up to 7 days

Drugs Effective in the Treatment of Viral Infections, *continued*

DRUG (TRADE NAME)	PYRIMIDINE OR PURINE BASE	OUTCOME	USE	ADULT DOSE
didanosine (*ddI, Videx*)	Dideoxyinosine	Inhibits viral DNA replication by interfering with viral reverse transcriptase	Advanced HIV infection	200 mg BID PO tablet (250 mg powder) > 60 kg BW*
delavirdine (*Rescriptor*)	—	Inhibits viral DNA replication by interfering with viral reverse transcriptase	Advanced HIV infection	400 mg TID PO in combination with nucleoside analogs
indinavir (*Crixivan*)	—	Inhibits HIV protease	HIV infection	800 mg PO every 8 hr
lamivudine (*3TC, Epivir*)	2'-deoxy-3'-thiacytidine	Inhibits viral DNA replication by interfering with viral reverse transcriptase	HIV infection	150 mg BID PO* in combination with zidovudine
nelfinavir (*Viracept*)	—	Inhibits HIV protease	HIV infection	750 mg TID PO in combination with nucleoside analogs up to 24 weeks
nevirapine (*Viramune*)	—	Inhibits viral DNA replication by infection		200 mg BID PO in combination with nucleoside analogs
ritonavir (*Norvir*)	—	Inhibits HIV protease	HIV infection	600 mg PO BID
saquinavir (*Invirase*)	—	Inhibits HIV protease	Advanced HIV infection	200 mg PO TID in combination with nucleoside analogs
stavudine (*d4T, Zerit*)	2',3'-didehydro-3'–deoxythymidine	Inhibits viral DNA replication by interfering with viral reverse transcriptase	Advanced HIV infection	40 mg BID PO (< 60 kg BW, 30 mg)*
zalcitabine (*ddC, Hivid*)	2',3'-dideoxycytidine	Inhibits viral DNA replication by interfering with viral reverse transcriptase	Advanced HIV infection	0.75 mg PO* every 8 hr
zidovudine** (*Retrovir*)	Azidothymidine (AZT)	Inhibits viral DNA replication by interfering with viral reverse transcriptase	HIV infection in patients with evidence of impaired immunity	100 mg PO every 4 hr up to 600 mg daily

*Doses are adjusted for body weight and/or creatinine clearance.
**Formulations for injection are also available.

Administration and Pharmacokinetics

All of the antiviral drugs presented in this chapter except for those used against CMV and ophthalmic herpes are available as oral formulations. This facilitates patient adherence to therapy, particularly since the treatment of recurrent genital herpes and HIV may be several months to lifelong. In general, these drugs are well absorbed after oral administration, attaining peak blood drug levels within 1 to 2 hours, are metabolized to some extent, and excreted in the urine. Zanamivir (*Relenza*) is a dry powder administered through a breath-actuated diskhaler. Drug is distributed to the pharynx and lower tracheobronchial tree for an immediate onset of action.

Absorption

Most of the drugs presented in this chapter are absorbed as the active antiviral agent. A few, however, must be converted to the active moiety. Oseltamivir (*Tamiflu*), which has no antiviral activity, is readily absorbed following oral administration and is converted in the liver to the active neuraminidase inhibitor. Similarly, famciclovir (*Famvir*) and valacyclovir (*Valtrex*) are metabolized to the active antiherpes component penciclovir and acyclovir, respectively. A few other antiviral drugs exhibit specific problems that must be circumvented in order to achieve therapeutic concentrations in the tissues.

Human immunodeficiency virus inhibitors indinavir (*Crixivan*), ganciclovir (*Cytovene*), nelfinavir (*Viracept*), ritonavir (*Norvir*), saquinavir (*Invirase*), and didanosine (*Videx*) are affected by the presence of food or changes in gastric pH with oral dosing. Food decreases the absorption and bioavailability of indinovir. Acquired immunodeficiency syndrome patients experience a general body wasting at some point in the disease process. It is not unusual for these patients to be on nutritional supplements to boost body weight. However, high-caloric, high-protein, and high-fat meals will decrease indinovir absorption. Didanosine is destroyed in an acidic environment so that the formulation is prepared with special buffering agents to permit maximum absorption. Anything that stimulates acid secretion (such as food) will overcome the buffering effect and degrade the active drug. In contrast, oral absorption is enhanced when the doses are accompanied by food with ganciclovir (*Cytovene*), nefinavir (*Viracept*), saquinavir (*Invirase*), and ritonovir (*Norvir*). This is a desirable interaction with these drugs. All of these actions are the basis of recommendations for drug administration (see Patient Administration and Monitoring) that must be communicated to patients.

Among the other oral antiviral drugs for *Herpes* (acyclovir [*Zovirax*], famciclovir [*Famvir*], valacyclovir [*Valtrex*], or influenza [*Oseltamivir*]) oral absorption is good and unaffected by food or meal content. Famciclovir and valacyclovir are metabolized to the active antiviral components penciclovir and acyclovir, respectively.

Hepatic Microsomal Metabolism (P4503A)

The HIV protease inhibitors inhibit the P450 system to varying degrees, such that metabolism of other concomitant medications going through these enzymes might accumulate in the circulation. Saquinavir (*Invirase*), nelfinavir (*Viracept*), indinavir (*Crixivan*), and delavirdine (*Rescriptor*) are expected to affect drugs such as calcium channel blockers, midazolam, triazolam, clindamycin, dapsone, warfarin, and quinidine. Of particular importance is the concomitant administration of these antivirals with astemizole. Increased concentrations of these antihistamines have been associated with life-threatening cardiac arrhythmias. This hepatic system can also be induced. Concomitant medications that induce P450 would likely eliminate the circulating antiviral through increased metabolism. Nevirapine induces P450 within a few weeks of treatment, increasing its own clearance. While these potential drug interactions have not been frequently observed at this time, the quantity and types of concomitant medications required by patients with advanced AIDS or herpes make this caution noteworthy. The neuraminidase inhibitors do not affect the hepatic microsomal system.

Renal Excretion

Inhibition of glomerular filtration and tubular secretion by any means (drugs, renal impairment) will cause certain antiviral drugs to accumulate. Almost all of the active moieties or their metabolites are excreted via urine. All of the drugs used in the treatment of herpes, CMV, as well as amantidine, stavudine, and zalcitabine, must be dose adjusted in the presence of renal impairment. Anything that decreases renal clearance as evidenced by a creatinine clearance less than 50 ml/min will obligate a reduction in the antiviral dose. Both oral and intravenous doses are reduced.

Amantadine and rimantadine are also dose adjusted for patients over 65 years of age in whom renal clearance is decreased with age. This is to avoid precipitation of central nervous system (CNS) adverse effects including seizures.

Cidofovir must be administered in conjunction with oral probenecid in order to maintain adequate blood levels. Cidofovir is excreted by renal tubular secretion that is actively inhibited by probenecid. Probenecid is administered before (2 hours) and after (2 and 8 hours) cidofovir infusion.

Adverse Effects

Antiviral drugs are used in seriously ill patients or in special populations of elderly patients or young children. Often underlying conditions (flu, diabetes, hypertension, arthritis, liver, or kidney dysfunction) make it difficult to distinguish the onset of adverse effects from those symptoms associated with the progressing disease. This is particularly true in the treatment of AIDS. In this regard, all antiviral drugs may be associated with nausea, gastritis, GI pain, vomiting, diarrhea, headache, confusion, dizziness, insomnia, arthralgia, myalgia, allergic reactions, hypertension, edema and rash. With a few drugs, more unusual adverse effects may occur. Patients taking acyclovir may develop blurred vision or tinnitus. Patients on ritonavir (*Norvir*) who experience dysgeusia (unpleasant taste) often take the medication with chocolate milk or Ensure to improve the taste so that the medication regimen can be completed. Whether given intravenously or orally, serious adverse effects do occur. These include nephrotoxicity, inhibition of hepatic microsomal metabolism, and various anemias that can jeopardize the patient's ability to fight infection, including neutropenia and granulocytopenia.

Influenza

The incidence of adverse effects associated with amantadine is relatively low. The most common adverse effects include slurred speech, ataxia, lethargy, dizziness, nausea, and irritability. Hypotension and congestive heart failure have also been reported. Since amantadine produces anticholinergic effects within the CNS, this drug should be used with caution in the presence of other anticholinergic medication (potentiation). Amantadine (*Symmeterel*) is not indicated for patients who have impaired liver or renal function, epilepsy, or psychosis, and it is not recommended for administration during pregnancy. Rimantidine (*Flumadine*) has a similar profile, and with both drugs elderly patients appear to experience adverse effects more frequently. This does not preclude the use of these drugs in the elderly.

The neuraminidase inhibitors are generally well tolerated. The incidence of adverse effects (nausea, vomiting, diarrhea, abdominal pain, and headache) reported during oseltamivir (*Tamiflu*) treatment is very low and indistinguishable from the clinical course of flu. In addition to the type of adverse effects seen with oseltamivir, zanamivir (*Relenza*) has induced bronchospasm when administered to individuals with mild to moderate asthma. The drug should be discontinued in any patient who develops bronchospasm or reduced pulmonary function.

Herpes

The adverse effects reported to occur in patients include transient elevations of serum BUN and creatinine. When given concurrently with drugs known to decrease renal clearance, nephrotoxicity will develop. The incidence of nephrotoxicity with famciclovir is dose related. Downward dose adjustment is recommended when creatinine clearance is less than 60 ml/min. Acyclovir (*Zovirax*) may cause injection site irritation, mainly due to the alkaline pH. Otherwise, the adverse effects usually reported are headache, nausea, vomiting, and fatigue. Blurred vision, when it occurs, can impair the patient's ability to operate machinery or perform tasks requiring dexterity.

Idoxuridine (*Herplex*), trifluridine (*Viroptic*), and vidarabine (*Vira-A*) may produce local irritation on instillation, edema of the eyelids and cornea, and small defects (clouding) in the corneal tissue. Although some drug is absorbed into ocular tissues, systemic absorption is extremely small.

Idoxuridine produces sensitivity to bright light that can be ameliorated by the use of sunglasses. The effect usually resolves within 7 to 14 days.

Human Immunodeficiency Syndrome (HIV), Cytomegalovirus (CMV)

Even with significant zidovudine overdose (50 times the therapeutic dose), the outcome was not fatal and the effects observed were nausea and vomiting. In the treatment of HIV-infected patients, it is important to have a complete blood count performed frequently to monitor lymphocytes (CD4 level), anemia, or granulocytopenia, so that transfusion or dose adjustment can be made as early as possible. The frequency of testing increases with advanced disease. Ganciclovir (*Cytovene*) is also noted to cause a decrease in platelets (thrombocytopenia), chills, fever, and malaise. Intravenous ganciclovir (*Cytovene*) is associated with fewer adverse effects than via oral administration.

Peripheral neuropathy that is dose dependent occurs with stavudine (*Zerit*), didanosine (*Videx*), and zalcitabine (*Hivid*). The symptoms range from tingling to burning sensations in the hands and feet. This is the primary reason for dose interruption with zalcitabine. When the drug is stopped, the effect may resolve, although slowly with zalcitabine. After the effect subsides, the drug may be restarted at a lower dose. Evidence suggests that this adverse effect occurs more frequently in those patients with a history of neuropathy as well as those patients with low CD4 counts (<200 to 300 cells/mm^3).

There are two areas affected by these drugs that are always serious and can be life-threatening: nephrotoxicity and neutropenia. Zidovudine (*Retrovir*), lamivudine (*Epivir*), and cifodovir (*Vistide*) produce neutropenia. Frequent blood counts are the principal means of following the onset and severity of this effect. These drugs should be used with caution in patients already compromised by bone marrow suppression showing a granulocyte count <1000 cells/mm^3 or hemoglobin, 9.5 mg/dl. Transfusion and/or dose adjustment may be required. Almost all of these drugs produce some degree of interference with renal function in addition to being affected by a decrease in renal clearance. Foscarnet (*Foscavir*) produces nephrotoxicity evidenced by elevated serum creatinine and BUN in most patients, while cifodovir (*Vistide*) may damage the proximal renal tubule. The onset and severity of the renal damage obligates dose adjustment for didanosine (*Videx*), famciclovir (*Famvir*), ganciclovir (*Cytovene*), nevirapine (*Viramune*), stavudine (*Zerit*), and zalcitabine (*Hivid*) when creatinine clearance is less than 50 ml/min, and/or when urine protein is high, for cidofovir. Hydration (1 liter 0.9 percent saline or 5 percent dextrose IV) is recommended with dosing of acyclovir (*Zovirax*), cidofovir (*Vistide*), indinavir (*Crixivan*), and foscarnet (*Foscavir*) to minimize the damage to renal tissue, and to keep the urine flowing and maintain excretion. Renal damage with cidofovir may not return to normal after the drug is discontinued. Lamivudine (*Epivir*) and valacyclovir (*Valtrex*), while not causing renal damage initially, may accumulate in the presence of end organ impairment. Lamivudine and stavudine have special warnings in their directions for use because of their ability to produce lactic acidosis—severe hepatomegaly with elevated liver enzymes. Therefore, these drugs must be used with caution in patients with renal dysfunction and the initial dose reduced.

Miscellaneous Adverse Effects

Foscarnet (*Foscavir*) removes ionized calcium from the blood, causing neuromuscular instability. Since foscarnet is a chelating agent, it ties up metal ions. This is a dose-related effect on calcium, as well as several other electrolytes (potassium, phosphates, magnesium). Patients may experience tetany, muscle pain, spasm, or convulsions. Decreasing the infusion rate may delay the occurrence of these effects. Nevirapine (*Viramune*) has caused life-threatening skin reactions; that is, Stevens-Johnson syndrome, while zalcitabine (*Hivid*) and zidovudine (*Retrovir*) induce a state of acidosis with a decrease in serum bicarbonate levels that can be fatal. Zidovudine produces a myopathy that is sometimes indistinguishable from the progression of the AIDS-defining illnesses.

Special Considerations and Contraindications

Except for the drugs used in the prophylaxis of influenza and treatment of *Herpes zoster,* there is little experience in the use of the antiviral drugs in elderly patients. Specifically for HIV, CMV, and genital herpes, the patient population has been primarily young adults. With the success of the newer treatment strategies and remarkable protease inhibitors, patients may be surviving longer before the onset of AIDS and this will contribute critical information on long-term safety. The newest HIV antiviral drugs are indicated for use in combination with other RT inhibitors such as zidovudine. Experience has shown that monotherapy quickly results in resistance to treatment through viral mutation. Lamivudine (*Epivir*), nevirapine (*Viramune*), delavirdine (*Rescriptor*), and zalcitabine (*Hivid*) are not used as monotherapy for this reason. The combined mechanisms of action reduce the virulent viral load in circulation. However, the incidence and severity of adverse effects such as neutropenia, granulocytopenia, thrombocytopenia, and nephrotoxicity may be potentiated. Therefore, routine chemistry and hematology are performed before all dosing with IV drugs and periodically as determined by the treating physician for oral medication. Absolute contraindication to the use of any of these drugs is hypersensitivity. Otherwise the drugs are used with caution in patients with significant concurrent disease and organ failure.

DRUG INTERACTIONS

The drugs discussed in this chapter are primarily used in patients who are seriously ill and usually have more than one chronic condition. By the nature of this population, patients can easily be exposed to 5 to 15 or more medications daily. This provides ample opportunity for drug interactions to occur, especially with OTC products. Antacids, tetracyclines, and/or H₂-receptor antagonists reduce the absorption of fluconazole, itraconazole, and didanosine when taken concurrently. Specific antihistamines—astemizole, and terfenadine—have been associated with serious cardiac arrhythmias when taken with itraconazole, prompting contraindication of concurrent use and strong warning (not absolute contraindication) to avoid use with indinavir (*Crixivan*) (possibly with other protease inhibitors).

Another significant concern is those interactions that predispose patients to decreased renal clearance of drugs and active metabolites or nephrotoxicity. Since these drugs are indicated for combination treatment, either as antivirals plus antivirals or antifungals plus antivirals, there is a significant opportunity to develop nephrotoxicity. Contributors to renal damage are zidovudine (*Retrovir*), cidofovir (*Vistide*), and foscarnet (*Foscavir*), especially taken concurrently with notoriously nephrotoxic drugs such as amphotericin B, aminoglycoside antibiotics, and IV pentamidine. Interactions associated with decreased renal clearance of other active agents include terfinafine and fluconazole and ganciclovir (*Cytovene*). Probenecid-induced inhibition of tubular secretion is beneficial when given to boost cidofovir blood levels; however, probenecid also affects famciclovir (*Famvir*) and ganciclovir (*Cytovene*) in which increased blood levels may precipitate adverse effects.

The potential for elevating drug blood levels of drugs metabolized through the hepatic microsomal system with chronic protease inhibitors therapy is significant although the clinical implications have not been fully explored. The advantages of drug interaction certainly include the probenecid and cidofovir combination as well as fluconazole, and itraconazole elevation in concomitant cyclosporine blood levels. This interaction has permitted cyclosporine doses to be reduced without jeopardizing clinical effectiveness. A broad presentation of drug interactions with the antifungal or antiviral drugs is provided in Table 42:6.

Patient Administration and Monitoring

The treatment of HIV, especially advanced stages or with opportunistic infections, warrants close monitoring of the patient's vital signs, body temperature, and frequent evaluation of serum chemistry and hematology profiles. Serum analyses forecast changes in electrolytes, liver (ALAT, alanine aminotransferase [AST]), or renal function (serum creatinine, creatine clearance, urine protein) and blood cell production (complete blood count [CBC] with differential, total neutrophil count, hematocrit, hemoglobin, and platelets). The hematology, chemistries, and urine protein should be reviewed prior to each dosing. Patients should be asked frequently about symptoms (tingling, burning sensations) that signal the onset of neuropathy so that dose adjustment or discontinuation of medication can be initiated. Changes in serum bicarbonate (decrease) with or without tachypnea may be an indication of developing acidosis.

Transplant Recipients

Transplant recipients receiving ganciclovir *(Cytovene)* must be evaluated for elevations in serum creatine and BUN, indicating changes in renal function that might obligate dose adjustment or discontinuation of therapy.

Serious Hematologic Changes

The frequency of granulocytopenia and thrombocytopenia obligates frequent complete blood count (CBC) and platelet evaluations. Patients receiving ganciclovir (*Cytovene*) and zidovudine are predisposed to develop severe granulocytopenia.

Medication Review

Current medications should be reviewed thoroughly to ascertain whether the patient is taking (see Table 42:6) products that could potentiate the onset of peripheral neuropathy, hepatitis, or pancreatitis. The prescribing physician may need to adjust or interrupt certain treatments to minimize the potential for serious outcome.

Patient Instruction for Chronic Viral Infections

Treatment of any viral infection, especially HIV, does not produce a cure. Patients with HSV, HIV, or CMV must receive clear instruction that underlying conditions will progress, although more slowly, and opportunistic infections may occur. Medications must be completed as directed whether oral or intravenous. Conversations with patients should present a clear picture of the frequency of clinical evaluation required during treatment and scope of adverse effects so the patient can make a commitment to stay the course of therapy. Pharmacological treatment of HIV or *Herpes is not a substitute for altering lifestyle patterns* that promote the transmission of the virus.

Patients under treatment for genital herpes should receive instructions to avoid sexual intercourse when lesions are visible.

Drug Administration

Patients receiving ganciclovir (*Cytovene*), nelfinavir, ritonavir, or saquinavir must be reminded to take the dose with meals to maximize absorption and bioavailability.

Patients receiving didanosine (*Videx*) and indinavir (*Crixivan*) must be reminded to take the dose on an empty stomach or 2 hours after a meal.

Delavirdine (*Rescriptor*) must be taken 1 hour before antacids to avoid a drug interaction and decreased absorption of delavirdine.

Patients may take ritonavir (*Norvir*) with chocolate milk or Ensure to improve the taste of the medication.

Adverse Effects

Amantadine (*Symmetrel*) may decrease alertness and cause blurred vision that may interfere with driving or performing tasks requiring concentration.

Saquinavir (*Invirase*) may cause photosensitivity so that patients should avoid unnecessary exposure to sunlight until tolerance is evident.

Idoxuridine (*Herplex*) sensitivity to bright light, which should resolve within 7 to 14 days, may be ameliorated by the use of sunglasses.

Notifying the Physician

With any of these drugs, including those for the prophylaxis of cold and flu, patients should receive clear instructions that swelling, edema, shortness of breath, and dizziness should be reported to the prescribing physician.

The physician must be notified immediately if rash, fever, blistering, joint aches, or symptoms of liver dysfunction occur.

Tingling, burning, and pain or numbness in hands or feet may signal the onset of peripheral neuropathy, especially for stavudine (*Zerit*).

With IV adminstration of foscarnet (*Foscavir*), the physician must be notified immediately if the patient reports feeling numbness or tingling, which may indicate changes in serum calcium and other electrolytes.

Use in Pregnancy

In general, antiviral drugs are designated FDA Pregnancy Category B or C because they have not been adequately studied in pregnant women. Among the systemic drugs, safe use in pregnancy has not been established in humans. Nevertheless, there are situations where their use is clearly indicated and may be used with caution and close patient monitoring. There are registry centers that encourage physicians to provide information on antiviral (HIV, herpes) use during pregnancy in order to accumulate information on maternal-fetal outcome. These centers are supported by the specific drug manufacturers.

Ganciclovir (*Cytovene*) should not be administered during pregnancy because of its carcinogenic potential.

Drug Interaction and Pregnancy

Nelfinavir (*Viracept*) counteracts oral contraceptive action by decreasing the blood levels of estrogen and progestins. Patients must be advised to use alternate or additional contraceptives to avoid failure and pregnancy.

Drug Interactions Associated With the Use of Antifungal and Antiviral Drugs

DRUG (TRADE NAME)	ADMINISTERED IN CONJUNCTION WITH	RESULT OF THE INTERACTION
Antifungal Drugs:		
amphotericin B	Antineoplastics	Increase renal toxicity
cyclosporine		Increase serum creatinine levels
digitalis glycoside, corticosteroids, thiazides		Induce potassium loss, hypokalemia; potentiate cardiac arrhythmias and digitalis toxicity
flucytosine		Increase the therapeutic and toxic effects of flucytosine; act synergistically in antifungal effect
miconazole		Decrease the therapeutic effects of miconazole
zidovudine		Increase the nephrotoxicity and myelotoxicity of zidovudine
fluconazole	Antacids, H$_2$-antagonists	Decrease absorption of fluconazole
Anticoagulants		Increase anticoagulant action
cyclosporine		Increase cyclosporine blood levels, dose adjustment may be required
hydrochlorothiazide		Decrease renal clearance of fluconazole
rifampin		Decrease drug blood levels of both drugs
Sulfonylureas		Increase hypoglycemic action of sulfonylureas
theophylline		Decrease clearance of theophylline, increase blood levels, predispose to adverse effects
zidovudine		Increase blood levels of zidovudine, predispose to adverse effects
griseofulvin	Anticoagulants	Decrease warfarin activity
cyclosporine		Decrease cyclosporine blood levels and effectiveness
Oral contraceptives		Decrease contraceptive effectiveness
itraconazole	Antacids, H$_2$-antagonists	Decrease absorption of itraconazole
Anticoagulants, oral		Increase anticoagulant response
Antihistamines, astemizole, terfenadine		Increase serum levels of antihistamine, predispose to serious cardiac arrhythmias
Calcium channel blockers		Edema has occurred
cyclosporine		Increase cyclosporine blood levels, dose adjustment may be required
Digitalis glycosides, thiazides		Induce potassium loss, hypokalemia; potentiate digitalis toxicity
midazolam, triazolam		Decrease blood levels of the antianxiety drugs

(continued)

Drug Interactions Associated With the Use of Antifungal and Antiviral Drugs, *continued*

DRUG (TRADE NAME)	ADMINISTERED IN CONJUNCTION WITH	RESULT OF THE INTERACTION
quinidine	Antacids, H$_2$-antagonists	Cause tinnitus and decreased hearing
rifampin		Decrease drug blood levels of both drugs
Sulfonylureas		Increase hypoglycemic response
ketoconazole		Decrease ketoconazole absorption due to decreased gastric acidity
ketoconazole	Anticoagulants	Enhance the action of the oral anticoagulants
Antihistamines: astemizole, terfenadine		Increase serum levels of antihistamine, predispose to serious cardiac conduction block
Corticosteroids		Decrease steroid clearance, increase blood levels
cyclosporine		Increase cyclosporine blood levels, dose adjustment may be required
isoniazide	cimetidine, terfenadine	Decrease the bioavailability of ketoconazole
rifampin		Decrease serum concentration of both drugs
theophylline		Decrease theophylline serum levels
terbinafine		Decrease clearance of terbinafine, increase potential for adverse effects
cyclosporine		Increase cyclosporine clearance, decrease effectiveness
rifampin		Increase terbinafine clearance, decrease blood level
Antiviral Drugs:		
acyclovir (*Zovirax*)	probenecid	Probenecid decreases renal clearance of acyclovir because probenecid inhibits renal tubular secretion
zidovudine	Nephrotoxic drugs Antacids	Produce severe drowsiness and lethargy
cidofovir (*Vistide*)		Potentiate nephrotoxicity of cidofovir
delaviridine (*Rescriptor*)		Decrease delaviridine blood levels
indinavir (*Crixivan*), saquinavir		Increase indinavir and saquinavir blood levels
didanosine (*Videx*)		Decrease blood level of both drugs
didanosine (*Videx*)	Tetracyclines	Decrease absorption of didanosine
famciclovir (*Famvir*)	probenecid	Decrease renal clearance of penciclovir
foscarnet (*Foscavir*)	Aminoglycosides, amphotericin B, pentamidine IV	Potentiate nephrotoxicity
ganciclovir (*Cytovene*)		Cyclosporine amphotericin B
Cytotoxic drugs		Potentiate or cause additive toxicity on bone marrow
imipenemcilastatin		Generalized seizures occur

(continued)

Drug Interactions Associated With the Use of Antifungal and Antiviral Drugs, *continued*

DRUG (TRADE NAME)	ADMINISTERED IN CONJUNCTION WITH	RESULT OF THE INTERACTION
Potentiate nephrotoxicity	probenecid	Decrease renal clearance of ganciclovir
indinavir (*Crixivan*)		Astemizole, cisapride, midazole, terfenadine, triazolam
		Inhibition of hepatic metabolism may predispose to cardiac toxicity and prolonged sedation
clarithromycin		Increase blood levels of both drugs
didanosine (*Videx*)		Buffering of didanosine may inhibit absorption of indinavir
fluconazole		Decrease in indinavir blood level
ketoconazole		
quinidine		Increase in indinavir blood level
rifampin		Potential induction of liver metabolism, reduce indinavir blood levels
isoniazid		Increase isoniazide blood level
lamivudine (*Epivir*)		Decrease lamivudine blood level
Oral contraceptives		Increase hormone blood levels
rifabutin, stavudine, zidovudine		Increase rifabutin, stavudine, zidovudine blood levels
lamivudine (*Epivir*)	trimethoprim/ sulfamethoxazole	Increase lamivudine blood levels, decrease renal clearance
zidovudine		Increase zidovudine blood levels
Nelfinavir (*Viracept*)	indinavir	Increase both drug blood levels, increase potential toxicity
rifabutin		Decrease nelfinavir blood level but increase rifabutin blood level
rifampin		Decrease nelfinavir blood level
ritonavir, Terfenadine		Increase terfenadine blood levels, predispose to cardiotoxicity
nevirapine (*Viramune*)	rifabutin, rifampin	Decrease trough blood levels of nevirapine
Protease inhibitors, oral contraceptives	acetaminophen, aspirin	Decrease blood levels of protease inhibitors and hormones
rimantidine		Reduce the peak concentration of rimantidine
cimentidine		Rimantidine clearance is decreased, increase blood concentration
ritonavir (*Norvir*)	saquinavir	Inhibit liver metabolism, increase saquinavir blood level

(continued)

Drug Interactions Associated With the Use of Antifungal and Antiviral Drugs, *continued*

DRUG (TRADE NAME)	ADMINISTERED IN CONJUNCTION WITH	RESULT OF THE INTERACTION
didanosine		
sulfamethoxazole	ketaconazole	
theophylline		
zidovudine (*Retrovir*)		Decrease blood levels of these drugs
clarithromycin		
trimethoprim		Increase blood levels of these drugs
disulfiram		
metronidazole		Disulfiram reaction from the alcohol contained within ritonavir formulations
ethinyl estradiol	ketaconazole	Decrease in circulating hormone
fluconazole		
fluoxetine		Increase ritonavir blood level
rifampin		Decrease ritonavir blood level
saquinavir (*Invirase*)		Increase saquinavir blood levels significantly
rifamycins		Decrease saquinavir blood levels
zalcitabine (*Hivid*)	cimetidine, probenecid	Decrease zalcitabine excretion by blocking renal tubular reabsorption
chloramphenicol, cisplatin, dapsone, didansoine, disulfiram, glutethimide, gold, hydralazine, iodoquinol, isoniazid, metronidazole, nitrofurantoin, phenytoin, ribavirin, vincristine		Synergistic potential to produce peripheral neuropathy Synergistic potential to produce pancreatitis Produce severe drowsiness and lethargy Potential to produce renal damage synergistically, decrease RBCs and WBCs
	acyclovir	Increase the risk of hematologic toxicity Potential for increasing hematologic toxicity
pentamidine	ganciclovir (*Cytovene*)	Decrease zidovudine clearance
zidovudine	interferon alpha, nucleoside analog antiviral drugs	Patients have developed flu-like symptoms including fever and rash
adriamycin	phenytoin	
amphotericin B	probenecid	
dapsone		
flucytosine		
pentamidine		
vinblastine		
vincristine		

Abbreviations: RBC, red blood cells; WBC, white blood cells.

Chapter Review

Understanding Terminology

Match the definition or description in the left column with the appropriate term in the right column.

___ **1.** A condition that causes individuals to resist acquiring or developing a disease or infection.

___ **2.** A microorganism capable of causing disease only when the resistance of the host is impaired.

___ **3.** The virus that causes AIDS.

___ **4.** A drug that kills fungi.

___ **5.** Infection of the skin, hair, or nails caused by a fungus.

___ **6.** An incurable disease caused by a virus and characterized by multiple opportunistic infections.

a. AIDS

b. dermatophytic

c. fungicidal

d. HIV

e. immunity

f. opportunistic organism

Acquiring Knowledge

Answer the following questions in the spaces provided.

1. What sites are commonly involved in fungal infections? _____

_____

_____

2. What organism is usually associated with common vaginal fungal infections? _____

_____

_____

3. What is the mechanism of action of amphotericin B? _____

_____

_____

4. Why is griseofulvin useful in the treatment of ringworm? _____

_____

_____

5. How do some viruses protect the host they infect? _____

_____

_____

6. Are vaccines available to treat any virus infection? _____

_____

_____

7. Do patients exposed to HIV always test HIV positive? _____

_____

_____

8. Why are viral infections difficult to treat with drugs? _____

_____

_____

9. How do amantadine and idoxuridine affect viruses without damaging the human cells? _____
_____
_____

10. How do the drugs currently available for the treatment of HIV infection work? _____
_____
_____

Applying Knowledge—On the Job

Use your critical thinking skills to answer the following questions in the spaces provided.

1. Mr. Garcia is admitted to the hospital for treatment of a deep vein thrombosis (blood clot) in his calf. His admitting orders state "Continue meds from home." Upon questioning, Mr. Garcia says he is taking ketoconazole. Warfarin, an oral anticoagulant, is also prescribed. Is there any potential for an adverse reaction? _____
_____
_____

2. Can both drugs (in Question 1) be continued safely? _____
_____
_____

3. How does food affect the absorption of the following medications and how should they be taken with regard to food?
   a. ganciclovir _____
   b. famciclovir _____
   c. indinovir _____
   d. valacyclovir _____
   e. didanosine _____
   f. saquinavir _____

4. A 19-year-old female has been prescribed itraconazole. What should she be told regarding sexual activity during therapy? _____
_____
_____

5. A female patient has been diagnosed with a vaginal yeast infection. Her physician has prescribed *Mycostatin* vaginal tablets - 1 pv qhs × 15d. What should this patient be told regarding proper use and handling? _____
_____
_____

Internet Connection

There are a tremendous number of government, private, and public organizations that maintain web pages specifically to educate and inform the public about virally transmitted diseases. The topics cover cold viruses, guidelines to minimize seasonal symptoms of flu, AIDS databases with computer response to posted questions, daily summary of AIDS news, and coping with herpes through management of herpes during pregnancy. The format of these presentations includes tutorials, color pictures of lesions, interactive chat rooms, and sometimes an accompanying audio narrative. Access to information is as easy as entering *AIDS* or *Herpes* at the search prompt or using search engines such as Yahoo or Altavista to reach preset health and medicine categories. Try any of the following paths as instructed and expand your knowledge of the viruses covered in this chapter. All of the information in these exercises can be printed using on-screen prompts.

1. Flu Viruses

   a. Enter www.yahoo.com. At the home page, type *Influenza* into the search box. Physicians from the University of Florida have provided instructions for surviving the flu with a Patient Information Sheet at http://cme.ufl.edu/media/flu/fluinfo.html. Patient education information is provided by the Institute of Allergy and Infectious Disease on colds versus the symptoms of influenza at www.healthynj.org/dis-con/flu/educat.htm.

   b. At www.yahoo.com, enter *Influenza Virus Replication.* Several excellent sites will appear such as http://www-micro.msb.le.ac.uk/Tutorials/balti/balti.htm. Pick which kind of virus you want to be, from the influenza virus (orthomyxovirus) to human immunodeficiency virus (HIV) (retrovirus).

   c. The Human Genome Project provides a map of how the virus attacks cells and reproduces at http://www.accessexcellence.org/AB/GG/influenza.html.

2. Herpes Viruses

   a. Enter www.yahoo.com then enter *Herpes* into the search box or scroll down the preset list of health topics to the *Herpes* category. This will bring a list of relevant web pages that can be accessed by double-clicking on the topic of interest. Information on transmissions, symptoms, diagnosis, and treatment of *Herpes is* maintained by the National Institutes of Health at http://www.niaid.nih.gov/factsheets/stdherp.htm or through the American Herpes Foundation, a nonprofit foundation seeking to improve infection management through publications, educational symposia, research awards, grants, and the Internet at http://www.**herpes**-foundation.org.

   b. The original **Herpes Home Page** was founded in 1995 for the purpose of providing anonymous information on awareness, treatment, research, and support relating to this disease at http://www.racoon.com/**herpes.**

   c. Another site, formerly the **Herpes Zone,** but now www.valtrex.com, provides information of treatment of *Herpes* infections, including *Shingles.*

3. HIV/AIDS Viruses

   a. Enter www.AIDS.com to enter *NetHealth* (also accessible through www.nethealth.com). This service has more than 500 websites specifically dedicated to sorting and identifying information on AIDS, depression, and Alzheimer's disease.

   The national reference, referral, and distribution service for information on HIV/AIDS, STDs, and TB is sponsored by the Centers for Disease Control and Prevention (**CDC**) at www.cdcnpin.org and for **HIV/AIDS** prevention at www.cdc.gov/hiv/dhap.htm.

Additional Reading

1995. Drugs for AIDS and associated infections. *The Medical Letter* 37: Oct. 13.

Bartlett, J., and Finkbeiner, A. *The Guide to Living with HIV Infections.* Johns Hopkins University Press, Baltimore, MD, 1996.

Danner, S. A. 1995. A short-term study of the safety, pharmacokinetics and efficacy of ritonavir, an inhibitor of HIV-1 protease. *New England Journal of Medicine* 333 (23):1528.

Graybill, J. R. 1996. The future of antifungal therapy. *Clinical Infection Disease* 22 (Suppl. 2): S166.

Petrow, S. (ed.). *The HIV Drug Book.* Project Information, Pocket Books, New York, 1998.

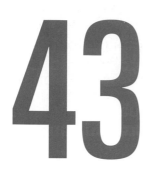

43

ANTIPROTOZOAL AND ANTHELMINTIC DRUGS

This chapter describes the three most common nonbacterial, or protozoal, infections affecting humans: malaria, dysentery, and trichomoniasis. It discusses the drugs used to prevent or reduce the symptoms associated with these infections and explains how these drugs work.

CHAPTER OBJECTIVES

After studying this chapter, you should be able to

- identify three nonbacterial organisms that produce common infections.

- describe the stages of malaria and the site of protozoal activity in each.

- describe the mechanism by which drugs eradicate protozoal organisms.

- differentiate between the symptoms and infecting organisms of dysentery and malaria.

- describe the side effects produced by each class of protozoal drugs.

- describe how parasitic worms gain access to the human host to develop an infestation.

- describe two drugs that are effective against parasitic worm infestation.

DRUG CLASS AT A GLANCE

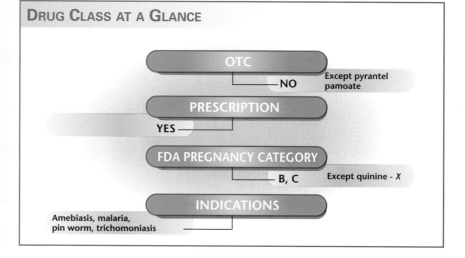

OTC — NO — Except pyrantel pamoate

PRESCRIPTION — YES

FDA PREGNANCY CATEGORY — B, C — Except quinine - *X*

INDICATIONS — Amebiasis, malaria, pin worm, trichomoniasis

Key Terms

asymptomatic: condition in which there is no outward evidence (symptom) that an infection is present.

cinchonism: pattern of characteristic symptoms (central nervous system [CNS] stimulation and headache) associated with the use of cinchona alkaloids (chemicals extracted from the bark of the cinchona tree).

disulfiram reaction: reaction to alcohol ingestion characterized by intense nausea as a result of drug-induced accumulation of acetaldehyde, such as that produced by disulfiram.

dysentery: condition characterized by frequent watery stools (usually containing blood and mucus), tenesmus, fever, and dehydration.

electrolyte: ion in solution, such as sodium, potassium, or chloride, that is capable of mediating conduction (passing impulses in the tissues).

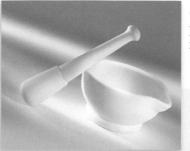

endemic: present continually in a particular geographic region, often in spite of control measures.

gametocyte: organism in an immature stage of development.

malaria: protozoal infection characterized by attacks of chills, fever, and sweating.

prophylaxis: procedure or medication to prevent a disease, rather than to treat an existing disease.

protozoan: single-celled organism belonging to the genus *Protozoa.*

radical cure: arresting of malaria, in which protozoal parasites are eliminated from all tissues.

tenesmus: a painful spasm of the anal sphincter, causing an urgent desire to defecate although little or no material is passed.

trichomoniasis: infection caused by the *Trichomonas* organism; a sexually transmitted disease.

INTRODUCTION

Many microorganisms in addition to bacteria produce infectious disease in humans. Single-cell microorganisms known as **protozoa** produce infection in the circulatory, gastrointestinal (GI), and urogenital systems. The most common diseases associated with protozoal infection in these tissues are malaria, dysentery, and trichomoniasis. Protozoa are frequently introduced into the GI tract through contaminated food and water. However, protozoa can also be transmitted to humans through vectors (mosquitos) or coitus (sexual intercourse).

PROTOZOAL INFECTIONS

Dysentery and trichomoniasis are usually not debilitating diseases. These infections produce symptoms that are primarily more annoying than dangerous (for example, diarrhea and itching). In a compromised patient such as a diabetic, elderly or cancer patient, or children, dysentery can be life-threatening due to loss of fluid (dehydration) and electrolytes. Malaria produces serious alterations in physiological function at any stage of infection. Malaria is characterized by recurrent chills, high fever, sweating, and jaundice. Although malaria is not endemic to the United States, it is a major medical problem throughout some other areas of the world (the South Pacific and Asia). Americans are exposed to malaria as a result of travel or military duty in endemic areas. Fortunately, all of these protozoal infections, especially malaria, readily respond to drug therapy.

The antimicrobial drugs that are presented in this chapter are approved for use in the treatment of acute malaria produced by *Plasmodium falciparum, P. vivax, P. ovale,* or *P. malariae.* This includes treatment of resistant strains as well as pretreatment to prevent infection. Certain agents are also used in the treatment of acute and chronic amebic infections, trichomoniasis, and toxoplasmosis.

MALARIA

Malaria is a protozoal infection of the circulation system and liver. The infectious parasite is a protozoan known as *Plasmodium.* Although four species of *Plasmodia* infect humans, each species produces the same physiological responses. These parasites differ in the severity of the symptoms produced. *Plasmodia* are transmitted to humans by the *Anopheles* mosquito. Normally, the protozoal parasite inhabits the salivary glands of this mosquito. When the mosquito bites an individual, the parasite is injected directly into the human bloodstream (see Figure 43:1).

Initially, the microorganisms invade the liver, where they mature. During this period, no symptoms are produced to suggest the presence of disease. Some of the mature protozoa eventually leave the hepatic tissue and enter the red blood cells (RBCs). In the RBCs, the protozoa rapidly multiply, often causing the cells to rupture. When the cells rupture, chills and high fever are produced, and many protozoa are released to reinfect more red blood cells. In addition, other mosquitos may suck the infected blood and transmit the microorganisms to the next human.

Stages of Malaria Development: Relationship Between *Anopheles* Mosquito and Human Host

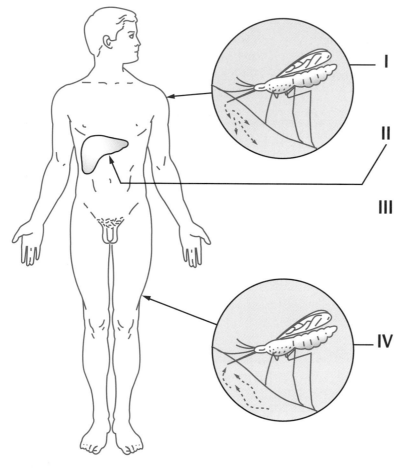

Stages of Malaria

I   Entry of *Plasmodium* through the saliva of the mosquito

II   Maturation of the organisms within the liver

III   Multiplication of the organisms within the red blood cells (RBCs) —rapid multiplication may cause the RBCs to rupture (hemolysis)

IV   Circulating organisms can reinfect more mosquitos when they feed on the contaminated blood

Antimalarial Drugs

The pharmacological treatment of malaria is directed toward preventing the disease **(prophylaxis)** or eradicating the existing parasites from the body. Antimalarial drugs that are administered before and during exposure to malaria to prevent the development of disease are known as prophylactics (see Table 43:1). Most of the antimalarial drugs used today act prophylacticly by destroying the microorganisms as they enter the circulation, thereby preventing the development of hepatic infection.

Certain antimalarial drugs are also useful when administered during an acute malarial reaction (chills and fever). These drugs (chloroquine, mefloquine, and quinine) have a selective action against the parasites that invade the RBCs. Thus, multiplication of the organisms is inhibited, and the disease is arrested. **Radical cure** of malaria is produced when the antimalarial drug eliminates the protozoal parasites from all tissues, especially the liver and RBCs. Primaquine

is an example of an antimalarial agent used to produce radical cure.

Mechanism of Action

All of the available antimalarial agents are protozoacidal drugs. These pharmacological agents destroy *Plasmodia* by interfering with the microorganisms' metabolism or inhibiting normal replication of the protozoa. Pyrimethamine inhibits the conversion of the folic acid to folinic acid in the microorganisms, whereas sulfadoxine inhibits *para*-aminobenzoic acid, another enzyme essential in the folic acid pathway. Since the microorganisms are prevented from producing folinic acid, nucleic acid synthesis is blocked. (See Chapter 30 for an illustration of folic acid synthesis.) As a result, the protozoa cannot produce deoxyribonucleic acid (DNA) and ribonucleic acid (RNA), which are necessary for protein synthesis to sustain life.

Other antimalarial drugs, such as primaquine, act directly on the preformed nucleic acid DNA in the

TABLE 43:1 — Drugs Used in the Treatment of Malaria

DRUG (TRADE NAME)	USE	ADULT ORAL DOSE
chloroquine* (Aralen phosphate)	Acute malarial attacks and causal prophylaxis	300 mg weekly 2 weeks prior to exposure and up to 4 weeks after leaving an endemic area
doxycycline	Causal prophylaxis	100 mg daily 1–2 days before, continuously during, and 4 weeks after travel
hydroxychloroquine (Plaquenil)	Acute attacks and causal prophylaxis	600 mg initially, then 300 mg weekly 2 weeks prior to exposure and up to 4 weeks after leaving an endemic area
mefloquine (Lariam)**	Acute attacks and causal prophylaxis	5 tablets as a single dose with 8 ounces water 250 mg once a week, then every other week before, during, and up to 4 weeks after leaving an endemic area
primaquine	Causal prophylaxis and radical cure	15 mg for 14 days
pyrimethamine (Daraprim)	Prophylaxis	25 mg once a week up to 10 weeks
quinine	Acute malarial attacks alone or in combination with sulfonamide or tetracyclines	260–650 mg every 8 hr for 6–12 days
sulfadoxine (500 mg) and pyrimethamine (25 mg) (Fansidar)	Acute attacks for chloroquine-resistant patients	2–3 tablets daily
	Prophylaxis	1 tablet weekly for up to 6 weeks after leaving an endemic area

*Chloroquine hydrochloride is parenterally given IM, 4–5 ml (160–200 mg), repeated in 6 hours for 3 days.
**Mefloquine increases the potential for convulsions and cardiac arrest when given concurrently with other cardiac depressants such as quinine, quinidine, or beta-blocking drugs. Mefloquine should be given at least 12 hours after the last dose of quinine to minimize the cardiotoxic effect.

microorganisms. These drugs accumulate in the parasites and bind to the components of the DNA molecules. In this manner, the drugs prevent DNA from directing the synthesis of normal protozoal proteins that are essential for the organism. The advantage of this mechanism of action is that parasites at various stages of development (**gametocytes**—immature or mature) or in different locations (RBC or tissue) are equally affected, so that relapse is less likely to occur.

Occasionally, patients are intolerant to one of the antimalarial drugs or, more frequently, the organism *P. falciparum* is resistant to the effects of chloroquine. In these situations, quinine, tetracycline, and/or folic acid antagonist therapy may be initiated alone or in combination.

Drug Administration

Antimalarial drugs include derivatives of quinolone—4-amino quinolone, chloroquine and hydroxychloroquine, 8-amino quinolone, primaquine, mefloquine, quinine, and pyrimethamine. Table 43:1 identifies which agents are used for acute attacks and which are better suited to prophylaxis. Drugs for the treatment of acute malaria exacerbations are usually administered orally for relatively short periods (2 days to 2 weeks). Patients are often given chloroquine to destroy the parasites within the RBCs quickly and end the cycle of chills and fever. This initial course of treatment may be followed by primaquine to eradicate the parasites completely. If the oral route is not available, chloroquine hydrochlorine injection is available for parenteral administration.

Prophylaxis requires a longer duration of treatment. Persons planning to enter an area where malaria is **endemic** should begin treatment 1 to 2 weeks prior to their arrival. Treatment should continue throughout the stay and for up to

6 weeks after leaving the area. Short-term travelers (1 to 2 weeks) may be advised to begin a course of daily tetracycline (*Doxycycline*) that continues up to 4 weeks following their return home.

Pharmacokinetics

These drugs are well absorbed following oral administration. They are highly bound to plasma proteins and are primarily metabolized in the liver. Because these drugs are bases, anything that alkalinizes the urine will enable these drugs to be reabsorbed rather than excreted. Conversely, acidification of the urine will promote excretion.

Miscellaneous Therapeutic Actions

Among the antimalarial drugs, tetracycline and chloroquine have value in the treatment of infection caused by other microorganisms, such as amebic dysentery. Quinine is readily available over the counter (OTC) as tablets, capsules, and a beverage ingredient (for example, in tonic water). At doses of 260 to 300 mg taken once or twice before bedtime, quinine relieves nocturnal leg cramps. Because it exerts a direct action on skeletal muscle to affect calcium ions, muscle excitability is decreased resulting in muscle relaxation. Quinine, which is related to quinidine, has the ability to depress cardioconduction as well. In uterine muscle, quinine acts as an oxytocic; that is, it stimulates labor contractions. Although not medically used for this purpose, it is not uncommon to encounter patients who have unsuccessfully used quinine to induce miscarriage. Such attempts end by treating the patient for toxicity because the doses selected tend to be exorbitant.

Chloroquine, like its close relative quinine, induces antiinflammatory responses that make it medically useful in the treatment of chronic immuno/inflammatory diseases. Chloroquine is used in the management of rheumatoid arthritis, systemic lupus erythematosus, scleroderma, and polymyositis (degenerative disease of connective tissue and muscle).

Adverse Effects

The adverse effects associated with the use of these drugs are seldom serious, but the intensity of the effects increases with the dose of the drug and the length of treatment. The most common side effects include nausea, diarrhea, headache, blurred vision, vertigo, and rash. Quinine may produce cinchonism in sensitive individuals. **Cinchonism,** a symptom complex characterized by central nervous system (CNS) stimulation, ringing in the ears, and headache, is derived from cinchona, the South American tree from which quinine is obtained.

Primaquine produces hemolytic anemia in individuals who are genetically deficient in the enzyme glucose-6-phosphate dehydrogenase (G6PD). This condition, which occurs primarily in Caucasians, is genetically transmitted through the X-chromosome. It is characterized by hemolysis of RBCs. In their metabolism, drugs such as primaquine, salicylates, and sulfonamides produce peroxide, which oxidizes hemoglobin and RBC membranes. The severity of the anemia will vary with the genetic sensitivity of the patient—that is, the degree of G6PD deficiency. Large doses of primaquine and chloroquine have also been associated with methemoglobinemia and leukopenia. Therefore, the recommended doses should not be exceeded. The folic acid antagonists have been associated with Stevens-Johnson syndrome. This is a severe inflammatory reaction where lesions on the skin and mucous membranes cause the patient's eyes to be swollen and pruritic, and the patient may not be able to swallow. Since this can be a fatal condition, the offending agent is discontinued immediately and supportive treatment provided. If a rash appears, or if the RBC count is reduced significantly or an active fungal infection occurs, these drugs should be stopped immediately.

Mefloquine increases the potential for cardiotoxicity when given concurrently with quinine or beta-blocking drugs. Increases in PR and QT intervals, indicative of conduction blockage, are evident on the electrocardiogram (ECG). Mefloquine is a myocardial depressant. Since it is likely to be given in conjunction with other antimalarials in severe cases, mefloquine should be given at least 12 hours after the last dose of quinine. Mefloquine also produces Stevens-Johnson syndrome.

Overdose

There is no antidote for overdose of the antimalarial drugs. Treatment is supportive according to the evolving symptoms. Children are particularly sensitive to the 4-aminoquinolines, with death resulting from exposure to even small doses. The symptoms range from headache, drowsiness, nausea, vomiting, cardiovascular collapse, and convulsions. Death is usually a result of respiratory and cardiac arrest.

Contraindications

Antimalarial drugs are contraindicated in patients who are hypersensitive to the drug or known to be hypersensitive to a related compound. Quinine is the only antimalarial that is contraindicated in pregnancy due to its spectrum of muscle depressant actions. Quinine is designated Food and Drug Administration (FDA) Pregnancy Category X: risk to the fetus from administration to a pregnant woman outweighs any possible benefit to the mother.

DYSENTERY

Two protozoal organisms, *Entamoeba histolytica* and *Giardia lamblia*, are frequently responsible for producing **dysentery** in humans. These organisms gain access to the human GI tract through contaminated food and water and irritate the intestinal muscles, causing the inflammation, pain, **tenesmus**, and diarrhea characteristic of dysentery. The severity of the symptoms depends on the organism producing the response. For example, when the infection is limited to the intestinal tract, diarrhea is the primary symptom. Diarrhea may result in loss of body water and

electrolytes, which leaves patients feeling fatigued and dehydrated. *Entamoeba histolytica* can cause additional damage because it invades hepatic tissue and produces hepatic amebiasis (amebic hepatitis). In the stages of amebic hepatitis, the organisms burrow into the wall of the liver and create an inflammatory reaction; this usually results in the formation and accumulation of pus (liver abscess) even though no overt symptoms may be present.

Antidysenteric Drugs

Several drugs are useful for the treatment of dysentery. The choice is often based on the site of protozoal infection (see Table 43:2). Acute intestinal amebiasis is currently treated with a combination of drugs.

Mechanism of Action

Paromomycin and tetracyclines are antibiotics that reduce protozoal infections in the intestines by inhibiting the availability of nutrients to the microorganisms. Since the normal intestinal flora

TABLE 43:2	Drugs Effective in the Treatment of Protozoal Infections	
SITE OF INFECTION	**DRUG (TRADE NAME)**	**ADULT ORAL DOSE**
Entamoeba histolytica:		
Intestine	iodoquinol *(Yodoxin)*	650 mg TID for 20 days
	metronidazole *(Flagyl, Metizol, Protostat)*	500–750 mg TID for 5–10 days
	paromomycin sulfate *(Humatin)*	25–35 mg/kg in three divided doses for 5–10 days
	tetracyclines *(Doxycycline)*	100 mg once daily as an adjunct to amebicide treatment
Liver and intestinal wall	chloroquine* *(Aralen phosphate)*	1000 mg/day for 2 days then 500 mg/day up to 3 weeks
	metronidazole *(Flagyl, Protostat)*	500–750 mg TID for 5–10 days
Giardia lamblia:		
Intestine	metronidazole *(Flagyl, Protostat)*	250 mg TID for 7 days
Trichomonas vaginalis:		
Genitourinary tract	metronidazole *(Flagyl, Protostat)*	2 g in 1 day for women; 500 mg BID for 7 days for men

*Chloroquine hydrochloride is the parenteral formulation given IM 4 to 5 mg (200–250 mg) for 10–12 days.

(bacteria) provide nutrients that are necessary for the survival of the infectious protozoa, antibiotics such as paromomycin and tetracyclines destroy the intestinal flora and thereby affect the survival of the protozoa. Elimination of intestinal bacteria "starves" the protozoa and decreases the multiplication of the parasites. Paromomycin also has a direct amebicidal action against *Entamoeba histolytica*. Metronidazole represents a great advance in the treatment of dysentery because it is a systemic drug active against various anaerobic bacteria and protozoa. Metronidazole is distributed very well to many tissues, including bone, bile, intestines, and abscesses within the liver. Therefore, metronidazole has amebicidal activity in all stages of amebiasis (intestinal and hepatic).

Most of the other agents in this class are useful only in the intestinal protozoal infections. At present, metronidazole is considered a drug of choice in the treatment of acute intestinal dysentery. In moderate to severe cases of amebiasis, iodoquinol and chloroquine are used. Chloroquine is of primary value in the treatment of amebic hepatitis. These drugs probably damage the protozoal DNA so that the organism cannot replicate properly. As a result, these two drugs are direct-acting amebicides.

Pharmacokinetics

Metronidazole and chloroquine are readily absorbed following oral administration. Chloroquine is very slowly redistributed among tissue, metabolized slightly (30 percent), and excreted into the urine mostly unchanged (70 percent). Metronidazole is metabolized in the liver to active trichomonicidal conjugates. Therefore, the drug may accumulate in patients with severe liver disease. These patients must be monitored more closely; however, the drug can be given. The major route of metronidazole elimination is the urine. Paromomycin is not absorbed or metabolized within the GI tract. This feature facilitates its contact with the microorganisms within the intestine. Then it is excreted unchanged (100 percent) in the feces.

Metronidazole does cross the placenta and is distributed within fetal tissues. Although it has not been associated with human abnormalities, metronidazole has produced mutagenic activity *in vitro* (test tube analyses). For this reason metronidazole is not recommended to be used in the first trimester of pregnancy when active cell division and development occur. It is given for trichomoniasis during the second and third trimesters.

Adverse Effects

Most of the amebicides produce side effects such as nausea, vomiting, abdominal cramps, and diarrhea. The diarrhea usually subsides once the drug is discontinued and the infectious microorganisms are eradicated. The usual side effects of metronidazole include nausea, diarrhea, vaginal and urethral burning, and headache. Individuals taking metronidazole should not drink alcoholic beverages, since metronidazole produces a **disulfiram reaction** with alcohol that can be very unpleasant.

The quinoline derivatives are probably the most toxic agents in this class. These drugs have been associated with the production of CNS stimulation, amnesia, peripheral neuropathy, and optic atrophy, which can be permanent. The amebicidal drugs are contraindicated in patients who have liver or renal damage, visual dysfunction, or known hypersensitivity to the drugs.

Paromomycin is an aminoglycoside antibiotic produced by the mold, *Streptomyces rimosus*. Like its cousins, neomycin and kanamycin, paromomycin develops cross-resistance bactericidal effects. Since it is not absorbed, it is unlikely to produce the same renal toxicity and impaired hearing produced by the other aminoglycosides. Nevertheless, with protracted use in severe infection, the potential for producing adverse effects should be kept in mind.

OTHER PROTOZOAL INFECTIONS

Giardia lamblia

Giardia lamblia is a flagellated protozoa that resides in the intestine. It gains access through unsanitary conditions such as sewage entering the local water supply. Travelers and children are among the largest groups affected. The organism attaches to the membranes of the intestine. As it multiplies it spreads into the feces, is excreted into the water, or transmitted to sex partners through intercourse. The waterborne infestation can exist in chlorinated water that is not adequately filtered. Treatment of choice is metronidazole, 250 mg daily for 7 days.

Toxoplasma

Toxoplasmosis is caused by another protozoa, *Toxoplasma gondii*, which uses any mammal as a host. Most commonly *Toxoplasma* has been identified in the fecal material of domestic cats. Presumably the animals eat raw or undercooked meat containing the protozoan cysts, which then attach to the intestinal tissue and multiply. The asymptomatic host sheds the oocysts in the stool and provides an opportunity for children and adults to become exposed to the oocysts. Humans access contaminated fecal matter by routinely cleaning pet cat litterboxes and distributing the material into the air, which is then inhaled, or on hands that are not adequately washed after the task. Children may also be exposed to the same contact in play areas where cats have defecated. Women are cautioned not to clean pet litterboxes during pregnancy in order to minimize the opportunity for exposure to potential infection. This has also been termed "cat scratch disease" because of the potential for an infected animal to transmit cysts to a human host by scratching the skin or mucous membranes around the eyes, either in play or aggressive behavior, bringing blood in contact with the organism.

If the patient is infected very early in pregnancy, *Toxoplasma* will induce abortion, viewed in the patient as a miscarriage of the first trimester. Miscarriage, in general, is not uncommon during this period, and in the absence of significant symptomatology toxoplasmosis goes undetected. Pregnant women who contract the infection during the second and third trimesters can pass the organism onto the newborn. Symptoms can range from mild malaise, muscle pain, and low-grade fever that is self-limiting to an acute fulminating infection. The more severe manifestations usually occur in patients who are compromised, such as those with acquired immunodeficiency syndrome (AIDS). In the United States, toxoplasmosis is most commonly encountered as encephalitis.

Pharmacotherapy

Drugs that are effective in the treatment of toxoplasmosis include pyrimethamine, 25 to 50 mg/day PO for 4 weeks, in conjunction with sulfonamide treatment. Congenitally infected infants may be given pyrimethamine every 2 or 3 days for up to 1 year. Similarly, the relapse rate in AIDS patients warrants indefinite drug administration. Because pyrimethamine affects folic acid metabolism, 10 mg of folinic acid is taken daily for the duration of treatment.

Trichomonas

Trichomonas vaginalis is a protozoan that infects the male urogenital (bladder and urethra) tract. Since this organism is frequently transmitted to females through sexual intercourse, **trichomoniasis** is considered a sexually

transmitted disease (STD). Sexual intercourse with an infected male may result in a vaginal trichomonal infection in the female partner. Trichomoniasis is associated with the use of nonbarrier methods of contraception. Usually, the female is made aware of the infection because a pungent vaginal discharge is produced, accompanied by intermenstrual spotting and itching. However, many women harbor the organism without experiencing discomfort (are **asymptomatic).** Proper treatment of this protozoal infection should include treatment of both partners. If the infected individuals are not treated simultaneously, the infection will rapidly recur in either person.

The drug of choice used to eradicate *Trichomonas vaginalis* is metronidazole. It is an effective trichomonacide when administered orally (either 2 g as a single or divided dose in 1 day, or 250 mg TID for 7 consecutive days) to both men and women. Occasionally, metronidazole is used in conjunction with vinegar douches.

The usual side effects of metronidazole include nausea, diarrhea, vaginal and urethral burning, and headache. Metronidazole produces a disulfiram reaction with alcohol so that patients should be cautioned to avoid alcohol consumption during treatment (this includes OTC products with 10 to 20 percent alcohol content). Metronidazole has been suspected of being potentially carcinogenic in animals, so metronidazole should not be used indiscriminately in the treatment of trichomoniasis. But for short-term use, metronidazole is a relatively safe drug valuable in the treatment of trichomoniasis. Although metronidazole has been used during pregnancy with no adverse results, as a precaution metronidazole should not be administered during the first trimester of pregnancy. When given in the second or third trimester, the 7-day schedule should be used rather than the single 2-g dose.

ANTHELMINTIC DRUGS

Parasitic worm infestations are a major cause of disease throughout the world. However, in the United States, the most frequently encountered parasitic infestations are limited to pinworms, roundworms, and tapeworms, as shown in Table 43:3. These parasites gain access to the human GI tract when food or soil contaminated with worm eggs is ingested. The worms then mature and multiply in the intestines. Frequently, worms can be seen in the stools when there is a heavy infestation. Occasionally, certain worms also gain access to muscle tissue and burrow into the tissue. Usually parasitic worm infestations produce symptoms such as diarrhea, nausea, loss of appetite, intense itching, and abdominal cramping. Hookworms and tapeworms are especially dangerous because these parasites can perforate the intestinal membranes, resulting in loss of blood, anemia, and hemorrhage. When diagnosed early, most parasitic worm infestations are confined to the intestinal tract. Oral administration of anthelmintic drugs brings the drugs into direct contact with the parasites throughout the GI tract (see Table 43:4).

Mechanism of Action

Most anthelmintic drugs are not well absorbed and, therefore, remain in close contact with the parasites. In general, these drugs produce muscle paralysis in the worms and decrease their motility. They also may inhibit the metabolic functions of the parasites. After the parasites are immobilized, the peristaltic action of the intestine can carry worms and eggs out of the body. Usually, a laxative is administered to increase intestinal activity and facilitate bowel flushing, so that worms and eggs are excreted into the feces. Encysted forms of parasites (in the muscle) may require more intensive drug therapy to remove them.

Two drugs in this class, pyrantel *(Antiminth)* and piperazine *(Antepar),* directly affect muscle contraction in the worms through different mechanisms. Piperazine blocks the worms' responses to acetylcholine (ACH), causing flaccid paralysis (receptor inactivation) whereas pyrantel inhibits cholinesterases (elevating ACH), leading to depolarizing neuromuscular blockade. These two drugs should not be coadministered to treat roundworms because their mechanisms of action will counteract the therapeutic effect when given together. Drug interactions reported to occur with anthelmintics, antivirals, and antifungal drugs are presented in Table 43:5.

Adverse Effects

Many anthelmintic drugs are derivatives of antimony, which is usually well tolerated by human hosts. The common adverse effects include nausea, fever, headache, cramps, and diarrhea. Tinnitus, hypotension, and paresthesia have also been reported. These drugs must be used with caution in patients who have severe renal, cardiac, or liver disease. Pregnant women and young children may be especially sensitive to the adverse effects of these drugs.

TABLE 43:3	Parasitic Worms That Infect Humans
SCIENTIFIC NAME	**COMMON NAME**
Ascarsis lumbricoides	Roundworm
Enterobius vermicularis	Pinworm
Hymenolepis nana	Tapeworm
Taenia saginata	Beef tapeworm
Taenia solium	Pork tapeworm
Necator americanus	Hookworm
Trichinella spiralis	Trichinae

TABLE 43:4	Drugs Effective in the Treatment of Parasitic Worm Infestations	
DRUG (TRADE NAME)	**USE**	**ORAL ADULT DOSE**
mebendazole *(Vermox)*	Pinworms	100 mg one time
	Roundworms and hookworms	100 mg BID for 3 days
praziquantel *(Biltricide)*	Tapeworm	20 mg/kg TID for 1 day
pyrantel pamoate *(Antiminth, Pin-Rid, Pin-X)*	Roundworms and pinworms	11 mg/kg of body weight up to maximum dose of 1 g
thiabendazole *(Mintezol)*	Roundworm	22 mg/kg/dose < 70 kg; 1.5 g/dose > 70 kg at 2 doses daily for 2–3 days

Special Considerations

In the treatment of parasitic worm infestations, all family members must be counseled to wash their hands and fingernails before eating meals and after bowel movements. To avoid reinfection, the family must be reminded to wash the perianal area daily. Usually, all family members receive treatment until there is no evidence that the worms are still present. For some infestations (pinworms), medication is taken as an initial dosage and then repeated 3 weeks later if the worms persist in stool samples. In the treatment of tapeworm, patients are not considered cured until the stools are negative for worms for 3 months.

Drug Interactions

The most critical adverse effects involve precipitation of convulsions or cardiac arrhythmias. Halofantrine, chloroquine, and valproic acid must be used with caution if given concomitantly with mefloquine because of the significant risk of producing convulsions. Beta-blocking drugs and cardiac depressants such as quinine administered with mefloquine are apt to induce conduction disorders leading to arrhythmias and potential arrest.

Drugs that decrease the clearance of antiprotozoal drugs, such as cimetidine, increase the blood levels and predispose the patient to possible adverse effects. Cimetidine treatment may be interrupted until the protozal infection is stabilized. Conversely, antibiotics such as rifampin may induce hepatic metabolism of the quinolines and quinine and therefore reduce their effectiveness.

Antacids containing aluminum can bind these drugs within the intestinal tract when given concurrently reducing absorption and effectiveness. Specific drug interactions are presented in Table 43:5.

TABLE 43:5 Drug Interactions Associated with the Use of Antiprotozoal Drugs

DRUG	ADMINISTERED IN CONJUNCTION WITH	RESULT OF THE INTERACTION
chloroquine	Cimetidine kaolin or magnesium trisilicate	Decrease absorption of chloroquine Decrease clearance of chloroquine
mefloquine	Beta-adrenergic blockers	Cardiac arrest has occurred
	Chloroquine	Increased risk of convulsions
	Halofantrine	Increased risk of prolonged cardiac conduction blockade
	Valproic acid	Decrease seizure control of valproic acid
pyrimethamine	Methotrexate, sulfonamides	Synergistic folic acid deficiency, increase the risk for bone marrow suppression
	Lorazepam	Mild hepatotoxicity has occurred
quinine	Antacids with aluminum	Decrease quinine absorption
	Antibiotics rifabutin, rifampin	Induce hepatic microsomal metabolism of quinine
	Cimetidine	Decrease quinine clearance
	Neuromuscular blockers	Quinine may potentiate the neuromuscular blockade causing respiratory difficulty
	Oral anticoagulants	Quinine may depress the hepatic synthesis of vitamin K clotting factors
	Urinary alkalinizers acetazolamide, sodium bicarbonate	Increase renal reabsorption leading to toxic levels of quinine

Patient Administration and Monitoring

Routine CBC and platelet count should be periodically performed during prolonged therapy. A drop in hematocrit and hemoglobin may indicate the onset of anemia. Quinine and amino-quinolines in particular may induce hemolysis resulting in hemolytic anemia in susceptible patients. Prior to beginning treatment with the quinolines, the patient interview should interrogate the possibility of G-6PD deficiency in the family or personal history. Susceptible individuals should have the drug schedule changed to weekly administration.

Vital signs and ECG should be performed before and during therapy to identify potential changes in cardiac conduction. Especially with mefloquine and quinine, prolongation in conduction may precipitate escape foci leading to arrhythmias, fibrillation, and arrest.

General Instructions to Patients

Patients should be instructed to use caution when driving, operating equipment, or performing tasks requiring coordination and dexterity because quinine and mefloquine may cause blurred vision, dizziness, and confusion.

Instruct patients to keep any of these drugs out of the reach of children. Overdose is especially dangerous with the quinolines. In the event of overdose, the patient should be taken to the emergency room for proper symptomatic treatment.

Drug Administration

Patients must be told to complete the full course of treatment in order to assure eradication of the microorganisms. In order to assure optimum compliance with the treatment schedule, patients can be instructed to take these drugs with meals. This will minimize any gastric irritation.

Metronidazole may have a metallic taste that is unpleasant and noticeable to some patients. Encourage patients to continue the medication until it has been used up. This drug will darken the urine. Although the effect is not harmful, patients should be alerted to this to avoid unnecessary concern and deviation from the treatment schedule.

Notify the Physician

Patients should be clearly instructed to notify the physician immediately for evaluation and potential discontinuation of the drug if they develop itching, rash, or fever (indicative of allergy), or stomach pain, difficulty breathing, severe diarrhea, vomiting, visual disturbances, or ringing in the ears.

Use in Pregnancy

Quinine should not be given to pregnant women. It is designated FDA Pregnancy Category X: risk to the fetus outweighs any possible benefit to the mother. If the patient becomes pregnant during treatment, the physician should be notified immediately and the drug discontinued.

Metronidazole, although designated FDA Pregnancy Category B, should not be given in the first trimester.

Other antiprotozoal and anthelmintic drugs are designated FDA Pregnancy Category B or C. While safe use in pregnant women has not been established through clinical trials, the drugs can be given if clearly needed.

Chapter Review

Understanding Terminology

Match the definition or description in the left column with the appropriate term in the right column.

___ **1.** Examples include sodium, potassium, and chloride.

___ **2.** A protozoal infection carried by mosquitos.

___ **3.** Procedures or medications to prevent, rather than to treat, an existing disease.

___ **4.** A condition in which there is no outward evidence that an infection is present.

___ **5.** A sexually transmitted disease.

___ **6.** A painful spasm of the anal sphincter.

___ **7.** Present continually in a particular geographic region.

___ **8.** A condition characterized by frequent watery stools, tenesmus, fever, and dehydration.

a. asymptomatic

b. dysentery

c. electrolytes

d. endemic

e. malaria

f. prophylactic

g. tenesmus

h. trichomoniasis

Acquiring Knowledge

Answer the following questions in the spaces provided.

1. Which diseases are commonly produced by protozoa? _____

_____

2. How do these infectious protozoa gain access to the body? _____

_____

3. Describe the cycle of infection produced by *Plasmodium*. _____

_____

4. What is meant by prophylactic treatment of malaria? _____

_____

5. How does prophylaxis differ from radical cure? _____

_____

6. Which organisms produce dysentery in humans? _____

_____

7. Which drugs are effective against protozoally induced dysentery? _____

_____

8. Why is trichomoniasis considered an STD? _____

_____

_____

9. What is the drug of choice in the treatment of trichomoniasis? _____

_____

_____

10. Why should alcoholic beverages be avoided during metronidazole therapy? _____

_____

_____

11. What are the common parasitic worm infestations found in the United States? _____

_____

_____

12. Why are tapeworms and hookworms potentially dangerous? _____

_____

_____

13. How do anthelmintic drugs act? _____

_____

_____

14. Why are laxatives administered as adjunct medication in treating parasitic worm infestations?

_____

_____

Applying Knowledge—On the Job

Use your critical thinking skills to answer the following questions in the spaces provided.

1. Mrs. Bell is leaving her gynecologist's office with prescriptions for herself and her husband for metronidazole because of her diagnosis of trichomoniasis. As she is chatting with you on her way out, she mentions that she and her husband will be going out to a four-star restaurant two nights from now to celebrate their third anniversary. What potential drug interaction should Mrs. Bell be warned of?

_____

_____

2. Mr. Green calls his physician's office complaining of significant foul-smelling diarrhea, abdominal discomfort, and weight loss. He is requesting a prescription for something, such as *Lomotil,* to control the diarrhea. You recall talking to him several weeks ago about his upcoming trip to Yellowstone Park, where he planned backpacking for a couple of weeks. Could Mr. Green's recent vacation be related to his current diarrhea?

_____

_____

3. Which is the only antimalarial that is contraindicated in pregnancy and why?

_____

_____

4. Susan is traveling to Mexico for a 1-week vacation. She has asked for travel medications in case she develops dysentery during her trip. She is 7 months pregnant. Her physician has decided to prescribe paromomycin. Why is this the medication of choice?

_____

_____

5. Becky is 5 months pregnant and has just been diagnosed with trichomoniasis. Her physician has decided to medicate her and her partner with *Flagyl*. This may be administered orally as 2 g as a single or divided dose in 1 day, or 250 mg TID × 7 d. Which dosing schedule should be prescribed for Becky? Why? Can her partner be treated with a different dosing schedule? Why or why not?

Internet Connection

Since we can access the *Worldwide Web* through the Internet, countries that have endemic outbreaks of malaria, giardiasis, and toxoplasmosis provide excellent information about the management and prevention of these diseases and the protozoa that cause them. It is amazing to see the low number of cases of these diseases in the United States compared to other countries. Try the following net connection. Enter www.yahoo.com/science/biology/parasitology. At the web page, enter either *Malaria* or *World of Parasites* in the search box.

a. Malaria is presented as a category that links to other disease websites such as the **Malaria Database.**

b. The website **World of Parasites** contains animated color pictures of the parasites and the associated disease. Click on the world map to any country and an incidence list of parasitic diseases for that area will be provided. Select the United States to see the occurrence of malaria, trichomoniasis, and giardiasis. Then compare the incidence to that of our neighbors in North America. How does Canada compare to the United States? Why does Mexico have a greater number of cases for the parasites listed?

c. Return to the parasitology menu (yahoo.com/science/biology/parasitology). This time enter *Parasitology Images List,* then click on *Protozoa.* This website presents color pictures of the different organisms as found in body fluids—for example, *Trichomonas vaginalis* from a vaginal smear, or *Plasmodium vivax* in blood or liver tissue.

d. Go to www.parasitology-online.com/ for a complete portal to journals and medical information on parasitology and tropical medicine.

The Centers for Disease Control & Prevention National Center for Infectious Diseases Division of Parasitic Diseases, CDC maintains a national user-friendly website on parasites at www.dpd.cdc.gov/dpdx/. This site links to the *Medical Letter,* an online update from the FDA on recent drug alerts and warnings.

Go to www.findarticles.com to locate published articles on any of the topics (giardiasis, malaria, dysentery) covered in this chapter. At the home page enter the word or phrase of interest in the search box.

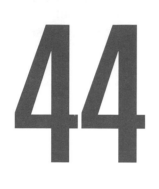

chapter

44

ANTISEPTICS AND DISINFECTANTS

CHAPTER FOCUS

This chapter describes chemicals that reduce the potential for acquiring infection. It explains how antiseptics and disinfectants, which are used to control and prevent infection, are different from antibiotics, which are used to treat infection.

CHAPTER OBJECTIVES

After studying this chapter, you should be able to

- explain the difference between reducing bacterial growth and inhibiting all bacterial growth (eradication).

- describe the mechanisms by which antiseptics reduce bacterial function.

- list four common chemicals that inhibit infectious microorganisms.

- explain why these chemicals are not administered by mouth to treat infection.

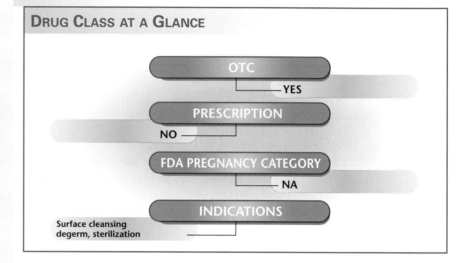

DRUG CLASS AT A GLANCE

OTC — YES

PRESCRIPTION — NO

FDA PREGNANCY CATEGORY — NA

INDICATIONS — Surface cleansing degerm, sterilization

Key Terms

antiseptic: substance that inhibits the growth of microorganisms without totally destroying them; refers to substance used on living tissue.

argyria: permanent black discoloration of skin and mucous membranes caused by prolonged use of silver protein solutions.

-cidal: suffix denoting killing, as of microorganisms.

decubitis ulcer: bedsore.

denaturing: causing destruction of bacterial protein function; also adulteration of alcohol, rendering it unfit for drinking.

disinfectant: substance that inhibits the growth of disease-causing microorganisms; refers to substances used on nonliving surfaces.

eschar: thick crust or scab that develops after skin is burned.

hypersensitivity: exaggerated response, such as rash, edema, or anaphylaxis, that develops following exposure to certain drugs or chemicals.

iodophor: compound containing iodine.

irrigation: washing (lavage) of a wound or cavity with large volumes of fluid.

lyse: to disintegrate or dissolve.

nosocomial: infection acquired as a result of being in a hospital.

-static: suffix denoting the inhibition of, as of microorganisms.

sterilization: process that results in destruction of all microorganisms.

INTRODUCTION

Antiseptics and disinfectants are used to control and prevent infection. These drugs can be distinguished from other antimicrobials in that they are usually chemical solutions (for example, alcohols, aldehydes, or iodophors) that are topically applied to surfaces such as skin, mucous membranes, or inanimate objects (floors, walls, or instruments) where microorganisms may be present. The primary mode of application is via swab, sponge, scrub solution, or, occasionally, as a mouthwash.

Antiseptics and disinfectants destroy microorganisms on contact. The term **antiseptic,** however, is more frequently associated with the eradication or inhibition of microbial growth on living tissue surfaces. **Disinfectants,** on the other hand, reduce the risk of infection by destroying pathogenic microbes on nonliving surfaces. Neither antiseptics nor disinfectants are intended to be swallowed or injected in order to destroy microorganisms.

MECHANISM OF ACTION

Antiseptics and disinfectants destroy bacteria by interfering with cell metabolism or by **denaturing** bacterial protein. In addition, these agents can decrease the surface tension of bacterial cell walls, causing the cells to swell and **lyse** (disintegrate or dissolve). Chemicals that denature protein or decrease surface tension have a more immediate onset of action than do those that exert an antimicrobial action through cell metabolism. Solutions of heavy metals (mercury or silver) and hexachlorophene inhibit cell enzyme systems. Alcohol, formaldehyde, glutaraldehyde, and chlorhexidine directly disrupt cell membrane integrity.

Chemicals that kill microorganisms **(-cidal)** are termed *germicidal, bactericidal, fungicidal,* or *virucidal,* depending on the type of microorganism they affect. Chemicals that reduce or inhibit growth without eradicating the microorganisms are considered **-static** agents, such as *bacteriostatic* or *fungistatic.* Antiseptics and disinfectant solutions differ in their antimicrobial potency (bactericidal versus bacteriostatic), spectrum of activity, and duration of action. Some of these chemicals are nonselective in their antimicrobial action and have broad-spectrum activity. Formaldehyde,

glutaraldehyde, and iodine-containing solutions, which are effective against bacteria, bacterial spores, fungi, viruses, and protozoa, are broad-spectrum agents. More selective chemicals, such as hexachlorophene and benzalkonium chloride, are primarily effective against gram-positive bacteria. Alcohol (40 to 70 percent ethyl alcohol solutions) is bactericidal for vegetative forms of gram-positive and gram-negative bacteria, whereas benzalkonium chloride, cetylpyridinium chloride, and thimerosal may be more bacteriostatic. Examples of commonly used antiseptics and disinfectants are presented in Table 44:1 on page 558.

Sterilization

The complete eradication of all microorganisms may be achieved with disinfectants. It is not practical to steam-sterilize large areas, such as an entire operating room. It is often easier to disinfect the area. Since microorganisms are affected to different degrees by the spectrum of available disinfectants, a sequence of disinfectant solutions usually is applied.

Surfaces, whether walls, fingernails, or open wounds, must be thoroughly cleaned prior to using disinfectants or antiseptics. Organic matter (pus, mucus, or protein exudate), dirt, or other foreign material reduce the activity of the

TABLE 44:1 Examples of Antiseptics and Disinfectants

DRUG (TRADE NAME)	PRIMARY ANTIMICROBIAL ACTIVITY
Alcohols*	
ethanol, ethyl alcohol; isopropanol, isopropyl alcohol	Vegetative bacteria
Aldehydes*	
formaldehyde	Bacteria, spores, fungi, viruses
glutaraldehyde *(Cidex)*	
Biguanides*	
chlorhexidine *(Exidine skin cleanser, Hibiclens liquid)*	Bacteria, spores, fungi, viruses
Halogenated Compounds*	
iodine, tincture of iodine	
sodium hypochlorite *(Dakin's* solution)	Bacteria, spores, fungi, viruses
sodium hypochlorite mixture *(Chlorpactin-XCB, Chlorpactin-WCS-90)*	
Iodophors**	
povidone-iodine *(Betadine, Isodine)*	Vegetative microorganisms and spores
poloxamer-iodine *(Prepodyne, Septodyne)*	
Heavy Metals**	
nitromersol (mercurial) *(Metaphen)*	
thimerosal (mercurial) *(Merthiolate)*	
silver nitrate	Vegetative forms of bacteria and fungi
silver protein *(Argyrol)*	
silver sulfadiazine *(Silvadene)*	
Oxidizing Agents	
peroxide, hydrogen peroxide	Vegetative microorganisms
Phenols**	
hexachlorophene *(pHisoHex, Septisol)*	Vegetative gram-positive bacteria
triclosan/Irgasan *(Septisoft, Septisol)*	Vegetative gram-positive and gram-negative bacteriostatic
Quaternary Ammonium Compounds**	
benzalkonium chloride *(Benz-all, Zephiran)*	Vegetative gram-positive bacteria
cetylpyridinium chloride *(Ceepryn, Cepacol)*	

*Bactericidal   **Bacteriostatic

Note: Antiseptics in general and disinfectants in particular should never be swallowed or injected in order to destroy microorganisms.

disinfectant or antiseptic by complexing the active ingredient (iodine, hexachlorophene, or formaldehyde) or by simply blocking penetration to an area of microbial activity. Dirt and organic matter can be removed first by washing with medicated soap or detergent. Depending on the nature of the surface to be treated, a combination of alcohol, phenols, or iodophors may then be generously washed over the area. Some disinfectant combinations are incompatible; for example, quaternary ammonium compounds are inactivated by contact with soaps or cotton.

Under optimal conditions (that is, application of an appropriate concentration of chemical solutions to a particular surface for a specified length of time), even narrow-spectrum disinfectants may be effective in **sterilizing** a local area. Bacterial spores are particularly difficult to destroy and may be eliminated by increasing the disinfectant-to-surface contact time. Various disinfectant-to-surface exposure times have been recommended, particularly prior to surgical procedures. These periods include a 2-minute wash with soap followed by a 2-minute alcohol wash followed by a 5- to 10-minute iodophor scrub. The particular ritual for surgical disinfection varies among individual institutions. Despite an inherently low or moderate potency, antimicrobial efficiency can be increased by combining the agent with alcohol. It is not unusual to find ethyl or isopropyl alcohol as an active vehicle for clorhexidine, benzalkonium chloride, hexachlorophene, and iodine. The term "active vehicle" means that the solution used to dissolve or dilute the antiseptic is capable of killing microorganisms by itself. Therefore the activity of the active vehicle contributes to the overall germ killing activity.

Main Uses

Microorganisms are ubiquitous and migrate freely on skin, hair, and furniture and in air currents. Given an optimal environment that supports colonization, any microbe can produce an infection. An infectious process that is localized to the skin surface can frequently be treated expeditiously without the use of systemic antibiotics, thus minimizing the risk of further infection.

A serious consequence of any infection, including one originally localized on the skin surface, is migration of the pathogenic microorganisms to the general circulation. At home, simple wounds and skin abrasions provide potential pathogens an access route to the circulation. In hospitals and other health care institutions, the risk of infection is complicated by the type of wound—**decubitis ulcer** (bedsore), trauma, or surgical—as well as the potential for contracting a nosocomial infection. **Nosocomial** infections (hospital-acquired infections) develop while patients are in the hospital and characteristically are virulent and difficult to eradicate. Hospital-acquired infections may result from catheterizations (for example, urinary tract or intravenous therapy), which provide a pathway for microorganisms to enter the body. These infections result from prolonged hospitalization or decreased patient resistance (for example, high-risk, elderly, malnourished, burned, or immunosuppressed patients).

In this era of highly effective systemic antibiotics, antiseptics have limited application in the treatment of infections. Antiseptics and disinfectants are useful for reducing microbial growth and contamination, and thus for reducing the risk of infection (especially wound infection) from exogenous sources. This aspect is particularly important during surgical procedures, in which local infection could significantly delay wound (incision) healing as well as jeopardize the general patient health should a systemic infection develop.

Antiseptics are used to cleanse and **irrigate** wounds, cuts, and abrasions, to prepare (degerm) patients' skin prior to surgery or injection, and to prepare the surgical team prior to surgery. An ideal antiseptic kills bacteria with a persistent duration of action and does not irritate or sensitize the skin. It is impossible to sterilize the skin without damaging tissue. Therefore, the objectives of antiseptic treatment are to decrease the opportunity for bacteria to enter the body and to permit normal defense mechanisms to continue uninterrupted in the healing process. Table 44:2 on pages 560–61 lists examples of antiseptic use.

Iodine is probably superior to all other antiseptics for degerming the skin. Iodine is a rapid-acting, potent germicide effective against bacteria, protozoa, and viruses. Although much more effective than the aqueous solution, iodine tincture is associated with residual staining and local pain. The stinging sensation is principally due to the alcohol vehicle of the tincture (2 percent iodine in 50 percent ethanol). Iodine complexes (**iodophors**) cause less irritation and staining and although they are only bacteriostatic, they are used frequently as surgical preps. In general, preparations containing iodine are for topical use and are not to be taken orally.

Indications for the Use of Antiseptics and Disinfectants

CHEMICAL NAME	CONCENTRATION	DISINFECTANT USE	ANTISEPTIC USE
alcohol, ethyl isopropyl	40–70% solution 70–90% solution	Disinfect instruments, ampules	Prepare skin prior to injection
benzalkonium chloride	0.02–0.5% solutions	Preservation of instruments, ampules, rubber articles; disinfect operating room equipment	Preoperative treatment of denuded skin, mucous membranes; irrigation of deep wounds, vagina; topical treatment of acne; preservative in ophthalmic products
chlorhexidine gluconate	1% solution 4% emulsion	—	Cleanse skin wounds, surgical scrub, hand washing, mouthwash for aphthous ulcers; keep out of ears and eyes
formaldehyde	10–37% solution	Cold sterilization of equipment; tissue fixative, preserve cadavers	Avoid contact with skin or mucous membranes; always dilute 37% solution
glutaraldehyde	2% solution	Cold sterilization of surgical instruments; fumigation (aerosol) of operating rooms	Use only on inanimate objects
hexachlorophene	0.25–3% foam, soaps, lotions	—	Surgical scrub, skin cleanser; use with caution in infants and burn patients where absorption can occur
hydrogen peroxide	1.5–3% solution	—	Wound cleansing, mouthwash for Vincent's infection; excessive oral use causes hairy tongue
iodine	2% solution	—	Topical treatment of skin; germicide; stains skin and linens
nitromersol	0.2% solution 0.5% tincture	Disinfect instruments	Topical treatment of skin abrasions, irrigate mucous membranes
oxychlorosene calcium	0.5% solution	—	Preoperative skin cleanser, local irrigation during surgery, ophthalmic irrigant
poloxamer-iodine	1–5% scrub, swab, solution	—	Preoperative skin preparation, cleanse wounds; less irritating than iodine
povidone-iodine	0.5–10% foam, swab, douche, gel	Disinfect instruments	Preoperative scrub, postoperative antiseptic, often used for bedsores, burns, lacerations; skin preparation prior to injections and hyperalimentation line; whirlpool solution
Silver nitrate	0.1–0.5% solution	—	Treatment of conjunctiva, burned skin

(continued)

Indications for the Use of Antiseptics and Disinfectants, *continued*

CHEMICAL NAME	CONCENTRATION	DISINFECTANT USE	ANTISEPTIC USE
silver protein	5–25% solution	—	Topical treatment of inflammation of the eye, nose, or throat; prolonged use results in permanent discoloration of skin (argyria)
silver sulfadiazine	1% cream	—	Topical treatment of wound sepsis in second- and third-degree burns
sodium hypochlorite	4–6% solution 0.15–0.5% antiseptic	Disinfect walls, floors	Wound irrigation; avoid contact with hair (bleach)
thimerosal	0.1% cream, ointment 0.02% ophthalmic	—	Preoperative skin preparation, antiseptic for eyes, nose, throat, urethral membranes, wounds; contraindicated in patients sensitive to mercury compounds

Ethyl alcohol is an effective antiseptic in concentrations of less than 70 percent, whereas isopropyl alcohol (rubbing alcohol) is bactericidal at all concentrations (50 to 90 percent). Alcohol can be used alone or in combination with other topical agents to degerm the skin prior to surgery or hypodermic injection. Alcohol preparations such as tinctures frequently increase the penetrability of additional antiseptic ingredients, which improves antiseptic efficiency but may lead to increased skin irritation. Most "prep" wipes or swabs contain isopropyl alcohol, which quickly evaporates following topical application. Because isopropyl alcohol causes local vasodilation, increased bleeding at the venipuncture site occasionally occurs.

Hexachlorophene is a bacteriostatic preparation that is primarily effective against gram-positive bacteria. Despite its selectivity, hexachlorophene is useful as a skin cleanser and surgical scrub because potential pathogens that reside on the skin surface are frequently gram-positive bacteria. With repeated use, hexachlorophene accumulates in the skin and maintains its bacterial response.

Hydrogen peroxide, an oxidizing agent, has limited usefulness because it does not penetrate well and rapidly breaks down to molecular oxygen and water. The standard medicinal solution is a weak antiseptic that contains 3 percent hydrogen peroxide in water. The effervescence may facilitate mechanical cleansing of debris surrounding a superficial wound. Hydrogen peroxide is recommended as a mouthwash for the treatment of Vincent's infection (trench mouth); however, continued use may produce hypertrophied papillae of the tongue, known as "hairy tongue." This effect subsides when treatment is discontinued. Chlorhexidine, a bactericidal surgical preparation, is also useful as a mouthwash for the treatment of aphathous ulcers and to decrease the amount of plaque deposited on teeth.

Among the heavy metal solutions currently available as antiseptics are organic mercurials and inorganic silver complexes. Silver nitrate is commonly used as an ophthalmic antiseptic in newborns to reduce the risk of gonococcal infection. Gonococcal resistance to silver nitrate is unlikely to occur as it might if systemic antibiotics were used. Silver nitrate has also been used in the treatment of burn patients. However, it has been displaced by silver sulfadiazine, which penetrates the crust of burns better and does not produce residual skin staining. Other silver solutions will produce **argyria,** a permanent black discoloration of the skin and mucous membranes.

The bacteriostatic organic mercurials (nitromersol and thimerosal) are not as effective as are other available antiseptics, despite their popularity as over-the-counter first aid preparations. Some antiseptics, notably benzalkonium chloride, thimerosal, and cetylpyridinium chloride are also found in eye care and contact lens preparations as preservatives to reduce microflora growth.

Disinfectants are used to clean and store surgical instruments, to disinfect operating room walls and floors, and to sterilize (cold sterilization) objects that cannot tolerate the high temperatures associated with routine sterilization procedures. Common disinfectants include formaldehyde, glutaraldehyde, sodium hypochlorite, alcohol, and nitromersol (see Table 44:2). Certain solutions, such as formaldehyde and glutaraldehyde, are irritating to the skin, eyes, and respiratory tract at any concentration and should be used on inanimate surfaces only.

Adverse and Toxic Effects

The most common side effects associated with the topical use of disinfectants and antiseptics in general are dryness, irritation, rash, and **hypersensitivity** at the contacted surface. Formaldehyde cannot be used as an antiseptic because concentrations large enough to be antimicrobial will damage living tissue. Formaldehyde toxicity is usually limited to local irritation or allergic reaction. However, repeated topical exposure may result in eczematoid dermatitis. Similarly, with topical iodine preparations, individuals occasionally may exhibit a hypersensitivity reaction. Iodophors have been reported to penetrate the **eschar** of burn patients, leading to increased absorption of iodine. Iodine toxicity can manifest as erosion of the gastrointestinal (GI) tract or hypothyroidism. In cases of accidental iodine ingestion, sodium thiosulfate is the antidote of choice. It can also be used to remove iodine stains.

Antiseptics and certain disinfectants should not be taken orally. Some agents are toxic when taken internally or absorbed in significant amounts through the skin. Absorption of hexachlorophene via the skin has been reported to cause neurotoxicities, which may manifest as convulsions and can be fatal. Hexachlorophene use should not be prolonged with patients who may be predisposed to absorb the compound through the skin, such as premature infants or burn patients. When taken orally, hexachlorophene can produce anorexia, vomiting, abdominal cramps, convulsions, and death. Although ethanol is a constituent of alcoholic beverages, ingestion of pure ethyl alcohol (99 percent) can be fatal. Ethyl alcohol and isopropyl alcohol antiseptics are not for consumption because these products contain denaturing agents, methylisobutylketone, and color additives that are poisonous.

Sodium hypochlorite used as a wound irrigant may dissolve blood clots and delay further clotting. In concentrations greater than 0.5 percent (modified *Dakin's* solution) sodium hypochlorite may be irritating to the skin.

Chapter Review

Understanding Terminology

Match the definition or description in the left column with the appropriate term in the right column.

___ **1.** Includes responses such as a rash, edema, or anaphylaxis that develop following administration of certain drugs.

___ **2.** Compound that contains iodine.

___ **3.** A permanent darkening of skin and mucous membranes caused by prolonged use of silver protein solutions.

___ **4.** A process that kills all microorganisms.

___ **5.** The destruction of bacterial protein function.

___ **6.** A scab that develops after skin is burned.

a. argyria

b. denaturing

c. eschar

d. hypersensitivity

e. iodophor

f. sterilization

Answer the following questions in the spaces provided.

7. Explain the difference between an *antiseptic* and a *disinfectant*. _____

_____

_____

8. Differentiate between a *-static* solution and a *-cidal* solution. _____

_____

_____

Acquiring Knowledge

Answer the following questions in the spaces provided.

1. How are disinfectants and antiseptics similar in their clinical uses? _____

_____

_____

2. How do antiseptics differ from antibiotics? _____

_____

_____

3. What is cold sterilization? _____

_____

_____

4. What are nosocomial infections? _____

_____

_____

5. What are two objectives of antiseptic treatment? _____

_____

_____

6. Why aren't antiseptics given parenterally or by mouth? _____

_____

_____

7. Why is silver nitrate frequently used for newborns? _____

_____

_____

8. Why is alcohol frequently a vehicle for other antiseptics such as benzalkonium chloride?

_____

_____

Additional Reading

Alfa, M. J. 2001. A new hydrogen peroxide—based medical-device detergent with germicidal properties: comparison with enzymatic cleaners. *American Journal of Infection Control* June 29 (3):168.

Gardiner, A. 1995. Knowledge of disinfection. *Nursing Times* 91 (20):59.

Garland, J. S. 2001. A randomized trial comparing povidone-iodine to a chlorhexidine gluconate-impregnated dressing for prevention of central venous catheter infections in neonates. *Pediatrics* June 107 (6):1431.

Gould, D. 1994. The significance of hand drying in the prevention of infection. *Nursing Times* 90 (47):33.

Kasuda, H. 2002. Skin disinfection before epidural catheterization: Comparative study of povidone-iodine versus chlorhexidine ethanol. *Dermatology* 204 Suppl 1:42.

Webster, J. 2001. Water or antiseptic for periurethral cleaning before urinary catheterization: A randomized controlled trial. *American Journal of Infection Control* December 29 (6):389.

Wicks, J. 1994. Handle with care, aldehyde disinfectants. *Nursing Times* 90 (12):67.

ANTINEOPLASTICS AND DRUGS AFFECTING THE IMMUNE SYSTEM

Chapter 45

Antineoplastic Agents

Types of Cancer
Alkylating Drugs
Antimetabolites
Miscellaneous Antineoplastic Drugs

Chapter 46

Immunopharmacology

Immune System
Immunosuppressive Drugs
Immunostimulant Drugs

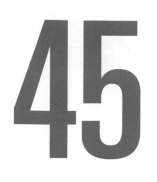

45

ANTINEOPLASTIC AGENTS

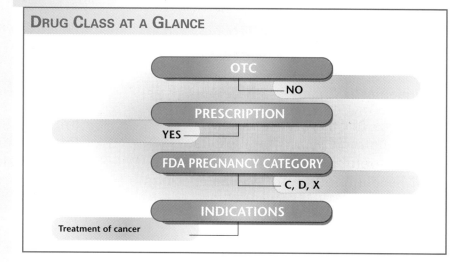

DRUG CLASS AT A GLANCE

OTC — NO

PRESCRIPTION — YES

FDA PREGNANCY CATEGORY — C, D, X

INDICATIONS — Treatment of cancer

Key Terms

alkylation: irreversible chemical bond that some drugs form with nucleic acids and DNA.

antimetabolite: drug whose chemical structure is similar to that of normal body metabolites and that inhibits normal cell function.

antineoplastic: drug that inhibits tumor growth or cell reproduction; used to treat cancer.

cancer: disease that involves the development and reproduction of abnormal cells.

chemotherapy: use of drugs to inhibit the growth of or to destroy infectious organisms or cancer cells.

drug resistance: lack of responsiveness of cancer cells to chemotherapy.

malignant: life-threatening; refers to growth of a tumor that causes the normal cell population to decrease.

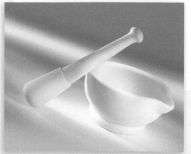

metastasis: spread of cancer cells throughout the body, from primary to secondary sites.

myelosuppression: suppression of bone marrow activity that interferes with the production of all blood cells; causes anemia, increased infections, and bleeding problems.

remission: period when cancer cells are not increasing in number.

teratogenic: causing birth defects or fetal abnormalities.

tumor: group of new cells having no useful function and exhibiting abnormal, uncontrolled growth; also called a neoplasm.

INTRODUCTION

The ability of cells to reproduce (mitosis) is one of the most vital characteristics of living organisms. A frequently stated biological principle is "like produces like," which means that, when a cell reproduces, it forms another cell that is identical to itself. Unfortunately, this is not always true; there is always the possibility for the development of an abnormal cell. **Cancer** is a disease process that involves the development and reproduction of abnormal cells.

There are two consistent findings with cancerous cells. First, regardless of the type of cell (for example, epithelial, muscle), there is structural alteration accompanied by a loss of function. Second, normal cell reproduction is controlled, whereas cancer cell reproduction is uncontrollable. As a result, groups of cells (a **tumor** or neoplasm) that have no useful function are produced. Also, these cells often multiply at a faster rate than many normal body cells. The term **malignant** (life-threatening) tumor, or cancer, is used to describe this situation of abnormal cell growth. As a malignant tumor increases in size, it robs normal body cells of vital nutrients. Therefore, as the tumor increases, the normal body cell population decreases. In the later stages of cancer, there is significant loss of body weight and vitality.

TYPES OF CANCER

The original location of a tumor is referred to as the primary site. As the tumor enlarges, there is an increased likelihood that some of the tumor cells will detach and relocate in other body areas. These new sites of tumor development are referred to as secondary sites. This spread of cancer is referred to as **metastasis.** The route of metastases is usually through the lymphatic system or the circulatory system.

There are many different types of cancer that can affect a variety of body cells. The different forms of cancer can be broadly classified into solid tumors and diffuse tumors. Solid tumors (breast, prostate, and lung) are stationary and can usually be palpated if they are significantly large and accessible. The diffuse tumors (leukemias and Hodgkin's disease)—especially the leukemias that involve cancer of the white blood cells—are not restricted to any one location. The successful treatment of any cancer depends mainly on the type of cancer present and its location.

There are three main approaches to the treatment of cancer: surgery, radiation, and chemotherapy. Surgery is the best method for solid tumors that are surgically accessible. Radiation (X-ray treatments) is used after surgery in an attempt to kill any cancer cells located in the area around where the tumor was located. However, even after surgery and radiation, there is no guarantee that all cancerous cells have been eliminated.

Chemotherapy

Chemotherapy is the use of drugs to kill cancer cells. This form of treatment is the primary therapy for diffuse tumors. In addition, chemotherapy is often used after surgery and irradiation of solid tumors in order to eliminate the possibility of any remaining cancer cells that may have metastasized.

Many drugs are used to treat cancer. The term **antineoplastic** refers to drugs that inhibit tumor growth or cell reproduction. Unfortunately, the antineoplastic drugs cannot differentiate cancer cells from normal cells. Therefore, antineoplastic drugs usually kill some normal cells and are, in general, very toxic drugs. This is the major problem with cancer chemotherapy—there is very little selectivity of action. The goal of chemotherapy is to kill more cancer cells than normal cells and eventually rid the body of all cancer cells.

Cells that have the fastest rates of metabolism and reproduction are most affected by antineoplastic drugs. Consequently, cancer cells are readily affected by cancer chemotherapy. However, normal cells of the bone marrow, gastrointestinal (GI) tract, and skin have growth rates that are equal to those of most cancer cells. During chemotherapy, there is always some degree of drug toxicity to these tissues. One of the major toxicities is **myelosuppression,** or bone marrow suppression. This can reduce the number of red blood cells (anemia), white blood cells (leukopenia, increased infections), and platelets (thrombocytopenia, bleeding problems). Myelosuppression usually requires 1 to 2 weeks to develop. In addition, disturbances and ulcerations of the skin and GI tract are also common. Many of the drugs cause temporary hair loss (alopecia). In order to limit toxicity, the antineoplastic drugs may be administered in a series of treatments, which allows a drug-free period (2 to 6 weeks) between each treatment. The hope is that during the drug-free periods, the normal body cells will multiply and regenerate at a faster rate than the remaining cancer cells.

Remission

One of the early goals of chemotherapy is **remission,** which refers to an inactive period when cancer cells are not actively reproducing and increasing in number. Remission occurs when a drug treatment kills all of the actively dividing cancer cells. Other cancer cells that are dormant (resting) usually become active with time, but during remission the cancer is not growing. Although remission is not a cure, it does offer patients more time and respite from the disease.

Drug Resistance

Drug resistance is a lack of responsiveness of cancer cells to chemotherapy. When this occurs, the cancer cells continue to reproduce even in the presence of the drug. When resistance occurs, alternate drugs must be substituted for those that have lost their effectiveness.

One method used to prevent the development of drug resistance is combination therapy. When two or three different antineoplastic drugs are used in combination, there is usually a significant decrease in the incidence of drug resistance. Drugs with different mechanisms of action are able to attack different areas of the cancer cells and are therefore more efficient in destroying the cells. The antineoplastic drugs are divided into several groups based on chemical structure or mechanism of action. The main features of each group will be presented in the following sections.

ALKYLATING DRUGS

One of the frightening developments of World War I was the introduction of chemical warfare. These compounds were known as the nitrogen mustard gases. The nitrogen mustards were observed to inhibit cell growth, especially of bone marrow. Shortly after the war, these compounds were investigated and shown to inhibit the growth of cancer cells.

Mechanism of Action

Nitrogen mustards inhibit cell reproduction by binding irreversibly with the nucleic acids (deoxyribonucleic acid, DNA). The specific type of chemical bonding involved is **alkylation.** Hence, the nitrogen mustards are also referred to as alkylating drugs. After alkylation, DNA is unable to replicate and therefore can no longer synthesize proteins and other essential cell metabolites. Consequently, cell reproduction is inhibited and the cell eventually dies from the inability to maintain its metabolic functions.

The nitrosoureas are a newer type of alkylating agent. The advantage of the nitrosoureas is that they are very lipid soluble and therefore pass into the brain, where they are particularly useful for treating brain tumors. Another drug, cisplatin, appears to be effective in testicular and ovarian cancers. Cisplatin contains platinum, a heavy metal, and may cause nephrotoxicity, which is common in heavy metal poisoning.

Administration

The routes of administration of the alkylating drugs and their main uses are summarized in Table 45:1. Many of the alkylating drugs can be administered orally. Administered by IV infusion, mechlorethamine requires caution in handling because of its vesicant (blistering) action; splashing on skin or infiltration into soft tissue will cause tissue damage. Dosages of the alkylating drugs must be adjusted to individual requirements.

TABLE 45:1 Alkylating Drugs and Their Main Uses

DRUG (TRADE NAME)	ROUTE	MAIN USES
busulfan (*Myleran*)	PO	Chronic granulocytic leukemia
carboplatin (*Paraplatin*)	IV	Ovarian tumors
chlorambucil (*Leukeran*)	PO	Lymphocytic leukemia, cancer of the breast, ovary, testes
cisplatin (*Platinol*)	IV	Testicular and ovarian tumors
cyclophosphamide (*Cytoxan*)	PO, IV	Hodgkin's disease, lymphomas, acute leukemias
ifosfamide (*Ifex*)	IV	Testicular cancer, sarcomas
mechlorethamine (*Mustargen*)	IV, IP	Hodgkin's disease, lymphomas
melphalan (*Alkeran*)	PO	Multiple myeloma
nitrosoureas		
carmustine (*BiCNU*)	IV	
lomustine (*CeeNU*)	PO	Brain tumors, Hodgkin's disease, lymphomas
semustine (*Methyl-CCNU*)	PO	
thiotepa	IV, IP	Cancer of the breast and ovary, melanoma

Adverse Effects

Nausea and vomiting are characteristic side effects produced by the alkylating agents, especially mechlorethamine. These effects occur shortly after drug administration and usually last for 1 or 2 days. Varying degrees of bone marrow depression occur (anemia, leukopenia, and thrombocytopenia) in all patients. Blood cell counts (red blood cells [RBCs], white blood cells [WBCs], and platelets) are determined periodically to avoid the development of aplastic anemia. In addition, ulceration of the skin and GI tract and hair loss are common. Because of their growth-inhibiting properties, the antineoplastic drugs are **teratogenic** (cause birth defects). These drugs should not be used during pregnancy if at all possible, but especially not during the first trimester.

ANTIMETABOLITES

The **antimetabolites** are a group of drugs whose chemical structures are similar to those of certain normal body metabolites. The antimetabolite competes with the normal substance for use by the body cells. However, the antimetabolite is a fraud. When the antimetabolite is used, inhibition or blockade of some cell function or chemical reaction that is vital to cell growth and reproduction occurs. The antimetabolites are classified according to the substances they interfere with.

Folic Acid Antagonists

Folic acid is a vitamin that is essential to the synthesis of the nucleic acids. Deficiency of folic acid decreases the production and replication of DNA. The symptoms of folic acid deficiency usually involve the development of various anemias and GI disturbances. The enzyme folic acid reductase converts folic acid into its active form, tetrahydrofolate.

Methotrexate is an antimetabolite that inhibits folic acid reductase and prevents the formation of tetrahydrofolate. Because of their faster rates of metabolism, cancer cells take up methotrexate more rapidly than do most normal cells. Methotrexate is administered (PO, IV) daily for approximately 5 days. This treatment is usually repeated after 4 weeks. The main use of methotrexate is in the treatment of choriocarcinoma and acute leukemia.

Overdosage of methotrexate is treated by the administration of folinic acid, referred to as leucovorin rescue, which prevents many of the adverse effects caused by methotrexate therapy. The administration of leucovorin after methotrexate provides the bone marrow with activated folic acid so that blood cell production can occur. The adverse effects of methotrexate include nausea, vomiting, diarrhea, bone marrow depression, and GI ulceration. Bone marrow depression may be significant and the development of aplastic anemia is an ever-present danger.

Purine Antagonists

Several substances are essential to the synthesis of DNA. Two of these substances are the purine bases adenine and guanine. Mercaptopurine (*Purinethol*), a purine antagonist, has a chemical structure similar to that of adenine. Mercaptopurine competes with adenine in the formation of the nucleotide adenylic acid. When mercaptopurine is utilized, an abnormal nucleotide is formed that prevents the successful replication of DNA. Consequently, normal cell reproduction does not occur.

Mercaptopurine is administered orally in the treatment of acute and chronic leukemias. The major adverse effects include nausea, vomiting, bone marrow depression, and liver toxicity.

Newer purine antagonists include cladribine (*Leustatin*), which is used in hairy cell leukemia; fludarabine (*Fludara*), which is used in chronic lymphocytic leukemia (CLL); and pentostatin (*Nipent*), which is used in hairy cell leukemia. These drugs are all administered intravenously and produce bone marrow suppression as their major toxicity.

Pyrimidine Antagonists

Three pyrimidine bases are required in the synthesis of deoxyribonucleic acid (DNA) and ribonucleic acid (RNA): cytosine, thymine, and uracil. Two pyrimidine antagonists currently used are fluorouracil (*Adrucil*) and cytarabine (*Cytosar-U*). Fluorouracil competes with uracil, whereas cytarabine competes with cytosine. The pyrimidine antagonists prevent the normal synthesis and replication of DNA. Administered orally or intravenously, fluorouracil is used in the treatment of solid tumors. The major adverse effects include nausea, vomiting, GI ulceration, bone marrow depression, and hair loss. Cytarabine is administered IV in the treatment of certain leukemias. The adverse effects are similar to those for fluorouracil.

MISCELLANEOUS ANTINEOPLASTIC DRUGS

A number of plant extracts, hormones, antibiotics, and radioactive compounds are used to treat cancer. These drugs are usually used in combination with other antineoplastic drugs. Table 45:2 summarizes the miscellaneous antineoplastic drugs and their main uses.

Plant Extracts

The periwinkle plant (*Vinca rosea*) contains several alkaloids that inhibit tumor growth. The two most important alkaloids are vincristine (*Oncovin*) and vinblastine (*Velban*), which appear to inhibit the process of mitosis by binding to the microtubules to cause metaphase arrest. The primary toxicity of vincristine is neurotoxicity (paraesthesias and loss of reflexes); the primary toxicity of vinblastin is leukopenia. Both drugs cause severe pain and local toxicity if there is leakage of drug out of the blood vessels and into the tissues (extravasation). In addition, vinblastin may cause a fatal reaction if administered intrathecally.

Etoposide (*VePesid*) and teniposide (*Vumon*) are two derivatives of the extract from the mandrake or mayapple plant. These drugs inhibit an enzyme necessary for the function of DNA. The main adverse effects of etoposide is alopecia, leukopenia, and nausea and vomiting.

Paclitaxel (*Taxol*) is a drug that was originally isolated from the bark of the yew tree. The drug binds to the microtubules and leads to arrest of mitosis. Bone marrow suppression and peripheral neuropathy are the main adverse effects. The plant-derived drugs and their main uses are listed in Table 45:2.

Hormone Antagonists

Certain tumors—usually those involving the reproductive organs (prostate, uterus, and breast)—are hormone dependent, which means that the hormone must be present in order for the tumor to grow. It was discovered that in certain patients, surgical removal of the testes (prostatic cancer) and ovaries (breast cancer), which eliminates production of the sex hormones, decreased the growth of these cancers. Removal of sex organs is a drastic measure and is done only as a last resort. The current approach involves the uses of drugs that act as hormone antagonist. These drugs bind to hormone receptors to block the actions of the sex hormones, which results in inhibition of tumor growth.

Miscellaneous Antineoplastic Drugs

DRUG (TRADE NAME)	MAIN USES
Plant Extracts:	
vinblastine (*Velban*)	Hodgkin's disease, solid tumors
vincristine (*Oncovin*)	Leukemias, solid tumors
vinorelbine (*Navelbine*)	Non-small-cell lung cancer
etoposide (*VePesid*)	Testicular tumors, lung cancer
teniposide (*Vumon*)	Acute childhood leukemia
paclitaxel (*Taxol*)	Ovarian and breast cancer
Antibiotics:	
bleomycin (*Blenoxane*)	Skin cancer, lymphomas
dactinomycin (*Cosmegen*)	Wilms' tumor, choriocarcinoma
doxorubicin (*Adriamycin*)	Leukemias, solid tumors
idarubicin (*Idamycin*)	Acute adult myeloid leukemias
Radioactive Isotopes:	
gold (^{198}Au)	To reduce peritoneal and pleural effusions caused by metastatic cancer
iodine (^{131}I)	Cancer of thyroid gland
phosphorus (^{32}P)	Polycythemia vera
Other Drugs:	
asparaginase (*Elspar*)	Acute leukemia
pegaspargase (*Oncaspar*)	Acute leukemia in patients allergic to asparaginase
procarbazine (*Matulane*)	Hodgkin's disease

Tamoxifen (*Nolvadex*)

Tamoxifen is an estrogen antagonist that blocks the estrogen receptor. By blocking the estrogen receptor, tamoxifen prevents the actions of estrogen to stimulate the growth of the hormone-dependent tumor. Tamoxifen is primarily used to treat breast cancer, particularly after surgery to prevent the growth of any cancer cells that may remain. The common side effects of tamoxifen are similar to the postmenopausal syndrome and include nausea, vasomotor hot flashes, rash, and vaginal bleeding.

Leuprolide (*Lupron*)

Leuprolide is an analog of gonadotropin-releasing hormone (GnRH). Gonadotropin-releasing hormone normally stimulates the release of follicle-stimulating hormone (FSH) and luteinizing hormone (LH) from the pituitary gland (see Chapters 35 and 37). Leuprolide therapy leads to inhibition of FSH and LH release. Subsequently, the actions of FSH and LH to stimulate sex hormone production (estrogen or testosterone) are blocked. Leuprolide is primarily used in the treatment of prostate cancer and other hormonal conditions (in both males and females) where inhibition of hormone production is desired. Common side effects include headache, vasomotor hot flashes, and impotence in males.

Goserelin (*Zoladex*)

Goserelin is a drug similar to leuprolide in mechanism and therapeutic use. The drug is designed for subcutaneous injection with continuous release over a 28-day period.

Antibiotics

Certain antibiotics, such as dactinomycin, doxorubicin, bleomycin, and idarubicin interfere with the synthesis of DNA and therefore inhibit cell reproduction. These antibiotics are generally too toxic to use in the treatment of bacterial infections. Bone marrow suppression is the most common toxicity produced by these drugs. These antibiotics and their main uses are listed in Table 45:2.

Radioactive Isotopes

Radioactive compounds emit radiation, which is damaging to the cell nucleus. These compounds have rather limited use.

Cautions and Contraindications

Pregnancy

The majority of antineoplastic drugs are designated either Food and Drug Administration (FDA) Pregnancy Category D or X, indicating that they have been shown to cause harmful fetal effects. These drugs should not be used during pregnancy, and women of childbearing age should use contraceptive methods if there is any possibility of pregnancy while taking these drugs. Only in circumstances where the benefits of treatment far outweigh the risks of harm to the fetus should these drugs be considered.

Patient Administration and Monitoring

Monitor vital signs during and after administration of drugs.

During parenteral drug administration, especially prolonged infusions, check the IV site frequently for extravasation of drug. If extravasation occurs, stop the infusion and notify the physician immediately.

Since most cancer chemotherapy causes nausea and vomiting, be prepared to assist the patient.

Observe for and instruct patient to report fever, chills, sore throat, swollen glands, and other signs of infection.

Explain to patient the common side effects of the drugs administered.

Instruct patients to report any significant symptoms such as difficulty with breathing, central nervous system (CNS) effects, sores on the skin or in the mouth, or any other symptoms that suggest drug toxicity.

Chapter Review

Understanding Terminology

Match the definition or description in the left column with the appropriate term in the right column.

___ **1.** The spread of cancer cells.

___ **2.** A period, usually after chemotherapy, when cancer cells are not increasing in number.

___ **3.** The use of drugs to inhibit the growth of cancer cells.

___ **4.** A disease that involves the development of abnormal cells.

___ **5.** A drug used to treat cancer by inhibiting tumor growth or cancer cell reproduction.

___ **6.** Lack of responsiveness of cancer cells to chemotherapy.

___ **7.** Also called a neoplasm; a group of new cells with no useful function.

___ **8.** Life-threatening; refers to tumor whose growth can cause normal cell population to decrease.

___ **9.** Refers to a drug that can cause birth defects.

a. antineoplastic

b. cancer

c. chemotherapy

d. drug resistance

e. malignant

f. metastasis

g. remission

h. teratogenic

i. tumor

Acquiring Knowledge

Answer the following questions in the spaces provided.

1. What are two cell changes caused by cancer? _____

_____

_____

2. What process occurs with the development of secondary cancer sites? _____

_____

_____

3. List three main approaches to the treatment of cancer. _____

_____

_____

4. What are the main disadvantages of chemotherapy? _____

_____

_____

5. What is the mechanism of action of the alkylating drugs? _____

_____

_____

6. What is the function of folic acid? How does methotrexate interfere with folic acid utilization?

_____

_____

7. What is leucovorin rescue, and when is it used? _____

_____

_____

Antineoplastic Agents   573

8. Give an example of a purine antagonist and a pyrimidine antagonist. What is the mechanism of action of these drugs? _____

_____

_____

9. Briefly describe the mechanism of action of the plant extracts, hormone antagonists, and antibiotics in the treatment of cancer. _____

_____

_____

Applying Knowledge—On the Job

Use your critical thinking skills to answer the following questions in the spaces provided.

1. Cancer drugs are often administered in various combinations and at specific time intervals that allow time periods (usually several weeks) that are drug free. What is the logic behind these two practices? _____

_____

_____

2. Mr. White presented at his physician's office with enlarged lymph glands, hepato-splenomegaly, anemia, fever, chills, night sweats, loss of appetite, and loss of weight. The diagnosis was Hodgkin's disease. Mr. White was administered a combination of drugs referred to as MOPP (mechlorethamine, *Oncovin*, procarbazine, prednisone), which included mechlorethamine (M) and vincristine (*Oncovin*).

   a. What is the major precaution to be observed in the handling and administration of mechlorethamine and vincristine? _____

   _____

   _____

   b. Mr. White asks you to explain how these drugs are going to get rid of his cancer. What will you tell him? _____

   _____

   _____

   c. Mr. White complains about feelings of numbness in his hands and feet. Which drug might be causing this? _____

   _____

   _____

   d. What are the most common immediate adverse effects of mechlorethamine? What is the most serious delayed adverse effect of mechlorethamine? _____

   _____

   _____

3. Following the diagnosis of breast cancer and bilateral mastectomy, Mrs. Smith was prescribed tamoxifen and told she would be taking the drug for the next 2 years.

   a. What is this drug and why was it prescribed after the breast tumors were removed?

   _____

   _____

   b. Explain to Mrs. Smith the expected adverse effects and why these particular effects occur.

   _____

   _____

4. High doses of methotrexate were administered to a young patient for the treatment of acute lymphocytic leukemia (ALL).

    a. How does this drug work to kill these cancer cells? _____

_____

_____

    b. What is the most serious adverse effect that can occur after methotrexate therapy?

_____

_____

    c. Eight days after drug treatment, the patient became extremely debilitated with fever, breathing difficulties, blood in the urine, and there was evidence of bacterial infection. What do you suppose is happening? _____

_____

_____

    d. What would be the immediate treatment for the patient's condition? What is this treatment called? _____

_____

_____

Use the appropriate reference books to answer the following questions.

5. Many chemotherapeutic agents are prepared prior to administration. Because many of these medications are not stable once reconstituted or diluted, strict storage guidelines must be followed. How far in advance can *Mustargen* be prepared? _____

_____

_____

6. All patients receiving *Taxol* therapy must be premedicated prior to *Taxol* treatment. What does the premedication consist of and what is the dosing schedule? _____

_____

_____

7. Both *Oncovin* and *Velban* are contraindicated for intrathecal use. Why? _____

_____

_____

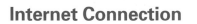

Internet Connection

Visit the MedicineNet web site (http://www.medicinenet.com) and click on the *Diseases and Conditions Index* heading. Highlight the letter "C" for cancer and click on the various topics: *Cancer Causes, Cancer Detection, Cancer of the Lung,* etc. to acquire additional information and background on cancer and its treatment. Students could select a topic and give a presentation to the class.

Additional Reading

Held, J. L. 1995. Caring for a patient with lung cancer. *Nursing* 25 (10):34.

MaCarron, E. G. 1995. Supporting the families of cancer patients. *Nursing* 25 (6):48.

Machia, J. 2001. Breast cancer: Risk, prevention, and tamoxifen. *American Journal of Nursing* 101(4):26.

Meissner, J. E. 1996. Caring for patients with liver cancer. *Nursing* 26 (1):52.

O'Brien, J. F. 1996. The oncologic crisis Part 1: Septic, hematologic, and metabolic emergencies. *Emergency Medicine* 28 (6):24.

O'Brien, J. F. 1996. Assessing and managing oncologic emergencies Part 2: Cardiorespiratory and neurologic complications. *Emergency Medicine* 28 (7):20.

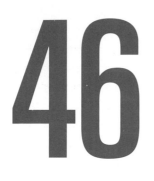

chapter

46

IMMUNOPHARMACOLOGY

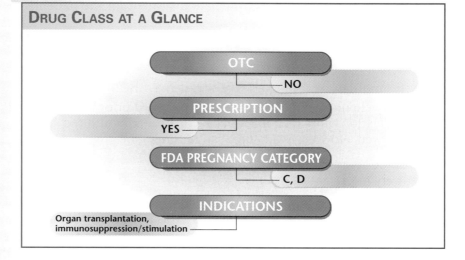

DRUG CLASS AT A GLANCE

OTC — NO

PRESCRIPTION — YES

FDA PREGNANCY CATEGORY — C, D

INDICATIONS — Organ transplantation, immunosuppression/stimulation

Key Terms

antibody: protein that attacks and helps destroy infectious organisms.

carcinogenic: causing cancer.

immunopharmacology: study of drugs with immunosuppressive and immunostimulant effects.

immunostimulation: ability to stimulate and increase immune function.

immunosuppression: ability to reduce the activity of immune function.

interferon: chemical mediator produced by immune cells that increases immune function.

interleukin: chemical mediator produced by immune cells that helps regulate and increase immune function.

lymphopenia: decrease in the number of circulating lymphocytes.

mutagenic: having the ability to cause mutations.

teratogenic: capable of causing abnormal development.

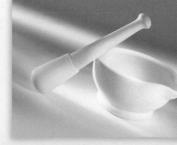

INTRODUCTION

Immunology is the study of how normal body defenses resist and overcome invasion from infectious organisms (bacteria, viruses) and other foreign substances. Recent advances in this field have identified various drugs that affect the activity of the immune system. **Immunosuppression** refers to decreasing immune activity. It is used after organ transplantation and in the treatment of severe allergic conditions when the immune system is hyperactive and causing harmful effects. **Immunostimulation** refers to stimulating or increasing the activity of the immune system. Immunostimulating drugs are desirable in the treatment of cancer and acquired immunodeficiency syndrome (AIDS), which are characterized by deficiencies of the immune system. **Immunopharmacology** is the study of drugs that affect the immune system. To understand how drugs act to affect immunity, it is necessary to have a basic understanding of the immune system.

IMMUNE SYSTEM

The immune system is made up of different lymphoid tissues (tonsils, lymph nodes, spleen) and cells (macrophages, lymphocytes) that are found in the blood and most body organs. There are two very important kinds of lymphocytes: T-cells, which mature in the thymus gland, and B-cells, which originate in the bone marrow. When the immune system is activated, these cells multiply and help protect the body. Lymphocytes also produce chemical mediators that help regulate the activity of the immune system. Two important classes of mediators are the **interleukins** and the **interferons.**

Cells Involved in the Immune Response

Many different types of cells are involved in the immune response; however, macrophages and lymphocytes are the most important.

Macrophages

Macrophages are scavenger white blood cells that phagocytize (eat the cells of) infectious organisms and foreign substances. Macrophages are usually the first cells that come in contact with foreign invaders and are responsible for initiating the immune response.

Helper T-cells

These T-cell lymphocytes play a key role in regulating the activity of the immune system.

Helper T-cells stimulate other T-cells—killer T-cells and B-cells—to become active, to multiply, and to increase the activity of the immune response.

Killer T-cells

Killer T-cells have the ability to attack the cell walls of infectious organisms, leading to destruction of these foreign invaders.

B-cells

B-cells, also known as plasma cells, produce **antibodies.** Antibodies are proteins that attack and help destroy infectious organisms and foreign cells.

Suppressor T-cells

Suppressor T-cells turn off the immune system after the immune system response is no longer needed.

Memory Cells

Some B-cells remain in the body for many years and can quickly become reactivated to produce antibodies against an organism that previously infected the body. These cells provide long-term immunity against reinfection from many childhood diseases (for example, measles, chicken pox). The purpose of vaccination is to produce memory cells and antibodies against a specific organism in order to produce long-term immunity and protection against infection. Figure 46:1 on page 578 summarizes the actions of these immune cells during a typical immune response to an infectious organism.

Response of Immune Cells to Viral Infection

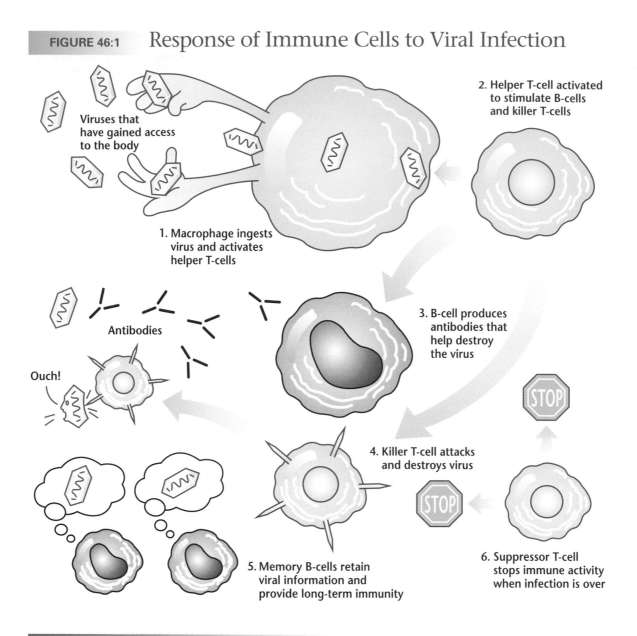

1. Macrophage ingests virus and activates helper T-cells

Viruses that have gained access to the body

2. Helper T-cell activated to stimulate B-cells and killer T-cells

3. B-cell produces antibodies that help destroy the virus

Antibodies

Ouch!

4. Killer T-cell attacks and destroys virus

STOP

STOP

5. Memory B-cells retain viral information and provide long-term immunity

6. Suppressor T-cell stops immune activity when infection is over

IMMUNOSUPPRESSIVE DRUGS

Drugs that have the ability to suppress the immune response are useful in the treatment of severe allergic reactions and immune-based diseases such as multiple sclerosis, myasthenia gravis, and systemic lupus erythematosus. These drugs are also essential in preventing organ rejection following organ transplantation. In these conditions, inappropriate activation of the immune system causes inflammatory reactions that lead to destruction of body tissue and rejection of transplanted organs.

Corticosteroid Drugs

The corticosteroids produce potent anti-inflammatory and antiallergic effects (see Chapter 36). Corticosteroids also have the ability to suppress the immune response. Prednisone (*Deltasone*) and prednisolone (*Delta-Cortef*) are the two most widely used corticosteroid drugs.

Mechanism of Action

The main immunosuppressive effect of the corticosteroids is to cause lymphocytes in the blood to be redistributed into the bone marrow. This immunosuppressive effect **(lymphopenia)** occurs 4 to 6 hours following drug administration and significantly reduces the number of circulating lymphocytes in the blood. Lymphopenia decreases the ability of lymphocytes to initiate and participate in an immune response. Continued therapy maintains this drug action and effectively reduces the number of T-cells and B-cells and the activity of the immune system.

Clinical Indications

Corticosteroids are usually used in combination with other immunosuppressive drugs. Initially, a large dose is administered parenterally, followed by smaller oral doses on a daily schedule to maintain the effect. Corticosteroids are used to prevent rejection of transplanted organs, to treat severe allergic reactions, and to control inflammatory responses in other immune-based diseases.

Adverse Effects

Chronic administration of corticosteroids is associated with many serious adverse effects (see Chapter 36).

Azathioprine (*Imuran*)

Azathioprine is a derivative of the antineoplastic drug mercaptopurine. Following absorption, azathioprine is rapidly converted in the body to mercaptopurine and exerts a similar cytotoxic effect. Azathioprine inhibits the synthesis of purine nucleotides (adenine, guanine) that are required for the synthesis of deoxyribonucleic acid (DNA) and for cell growth and reproduction. Inhibition of vital cell processes leads to the death of many existing lymphocytes and suppresses the formation of new B-cells and, in particular, T-cells.

Clinical Indications

Azathioprine is widely used in organ transplantation to prevent rejection. It is usually administered along with corticosteroids. In addition, it is used to control many immune-based diseases, such as lupus erythematosus and rheumatoid arthritis.

Adverse Effects

Adverse effects are similar to those observed with methotrexate. Gastrointestinal disturbances include nausea, vomiting, diarrhea, and ulceration. Excessive reductions in blood cells and depression of bone marrow function may occur, which, along with the immunosuppressive effect, can increase susceptibility to serious infection. Azathioprine is **mutagenic, carcinogenic,** and **teratogenic;** therefore, the benefits and risks of treatment must be carefully evaluated.

Cyclophosphamide (*Cytoxan*)

Cyclophosphamide is an alkylating drug used in the treatment of certain cancers. Like azathioprine, it is a cytotoxic drug that kills and suppresses the function of lymphocytes. The major immunosuppressive effect of cyclophosphamide is to reduce the number of B-cells that produce antibodies. Reduction of antibody formation is useful in the treatment and control of various immune-based diseases that involve abnormal antibody activity, especially severe rheumatoid arthritis.

Adverse Effects

Similar to other alkylating drugs used to treat cancer, cyclophosphamide causes nausea, vomiting, alopecia (hair loss), and bone marrow depression. During the metabolism of cyclophosphamide, a toxic metabolite is formed, which during urinary excretion may cause hemorrhagic cystitis along with hematuria and bladder dysfunction. Increased fluid intake can minimize the incidence of these adverse effects.

Cyclosporine (*Sandimmune*)

Cyclosporine is a polypeptide metabolite produced by a particular fungus. It is a potent immunosuppressive drug and, unlike azathioprine and cyclophosphamide, is not cytotoxic.

Cyclosporine suppresses T-cell function, especially the activity of helper T-cells. Since helper T-cells play a key role in regulating the activation of other immune cells (killer T-cells and B-cells), the immune response is significantly depressed. Cyclosporine inhibits the production of interleukin-2 (IL-2), a chemical mediator necessary for the growth and multiplication of T-cells. Upon cessation of drug treatment, normal T-cell function resumes.

Clinical Indications

The major use of cyclosporine is to prevent organ rejection after transplantation. The selective action is to suppress T-cell function. The low toxicity compared to that of the cytotoxic drugs has made cyclosporine the drug of choice for this indication. Cyclosporine is usually administered along with corticosteroid drugs.

Adverse Effects

The major concern is the development of nephrotoxicity, characterized by renal tubule damage. This effect occurs in about one-fourth of individuals treated. Reduction of the dosage usually eliminates tubular damage. Liver toxicity and central nervous system (CNS) disturbances such as paresthesias and seizures occur less frequently.

Tacrolimus (*Prograf*)

Tacrolimus is a macrolide antibiotic that has a similar mechanism of action as cyclosporine—to inhibit T-cell lymphocyte activity. This drug is more potent than cyclosporine and is primarily used in organ transplantation to prevent rejection. The adverse effects of tacrolimus are similar to those of cyclosporine.

Mycophenolate Mofetil (*CellCept*)

Mycophenolate mofetil is a cytotoxic drug that inhibits the activity of both T-cells and B-cells. The primary use of this drug is in renal organ transplantation to prevent rejection. Adverse effects include diarrhea, vomiting, leukopenia, and increased susceptibility to infection.

Leflunomide (*Arava*)

Leflunomide is a new immunosuppressant drug currently used in the treatment of rheumatoid arthritis. The drug is converted to a long-acting metabolite that inhibits the synthesis of pyrimidines and DNA. This action inhibits the

Patient Administration and Monitoring

Patients receiving immunosuppressive drugs usually have disease conditions that require hospitalization or they have recently undergone organ transplantation, which also requires prolonged hospitalization. Consequently, these patients receive intensive care treatment and close clinical observation. Of greatest importance is the detection of any signs that indicate infection or organ rejection. Blood counts are taken periodically to ensure that blood cells do not fall below acceptable levels. It is extremely important to observe all the precautions for infection control.

Monitor vital signs and body temperature during and after drug administration; fever is often the first indication of infection.

Explain to patient the common side effects of the administered drugs.

Instruct patient to report fever, chills, swollen glands, sore throat, tiredness, and malaise or any other symptoms that suggest infection or possible organ rejection, especially after hospitalization.

Instruct other family members on the importance of cleanliness and infection control.

proliferation of both T-cells and B-cells involved in rheumatoid arthritis. Leflunomide is taken orally and has a half-life (on average) of 15 days. Adverse drug effects include diarrhea and other GI disturbances, liver and renal impairment, and the potential to cause birth defects.

Muromonab-CD3 (*Orthoclone OKT3*)

New discoveries in molecular biology have led to the development of commercially prepared monoclonal antibodies designed to attack specific aspects of the immune system. The first of these antibodies has been approved and is marketed as muromonab-CD3. The immunosuppressive effect occurs when the CD3 antibody (administered IV) binds specifically to T-cells. This binding quickly decreases the activity of the T-cells. Since T-cells play a major role in regulating immune activity, the overall activity of the immune system is reduced. The major use of CD3 is to prevent organ rejection after renal transplantation. Nausea, vomiting, fever, shortness of breath, and chest pain are associated adverse effects.

Daclizumab (*Zenapax*)

Daclizumab is a monoclonal antibody that binds to and blocks the interleukin-2 receptor. This action inhibits the activation of lymphocytes and the immune reaction that occurs during the rejection of transplanted organs. The main indication for daclizumab is for the prevention of renal allograft rejection. Common adverse drug reactions include weakness, chills, muscle and joint ache, GI disturbances, and renal impairment.

Infliximab (*Remicade*)

Infliximab is a monoclonal antibody that binds to and inhibits the activity of tumor necrosis factor (TNF-alpha). TNF-alpha is a mediator of inflammation and immune activation. The main indication for infliximab is in the treatment of Crohn's disease, which is an inflammatory condition of the intestinal tract. Administration of infliximab is associated with an infusion reaction that may occur following IV injection. The reaction can include fever, chills, hives, hypotension, and chest pain. There is also an increased incidence of bacterial infection that occurs in infliximab-treated patients. Other adverse effects include headache, nausea, and GI disturbances.

TABLE 46:1 Newer Immunopotentiating Drugs

IMMUNOPOTENTIATORS	MECHANISM OF ACTION
Colony Stimulating Factors (CSFs)	
Filgrastim (granulocyte-CSF, G-CSF)	Increases formation of granulocytes and immune activity
Sargramostim (macrophage-CSF, GM-CSF)	Increases formation of macrophages and immune activity
Beta-interferon (β-IFN)	Antiviral activity, activation of macrophages
Gamma-interferon (γ-IFN)	Antiviral activity, activation of macrophages
Levamisole (*Ergamisol*)	Immunomodulator used with fluorouracil in the treatment of colon cancer

IMMUNOSTIMULANT DRUGS

Drugs that increase the activity of the immune system are desirable in the treatment of cancer, AIDS, and other conditions where immunological deficiencies exist. At present, there are a limited number of drugs available. Many of these immunostimulant drugs are commercial preparations of growth factors and mediators that are normally produced by body cells.

Alpha-Interferon

Alpha-interferon (α-IFN) is one kind of interferon produced in the body in response to viral infection. In addition to its antiviral effect, α-IFN appears to stimulate immune function, and it has been effective in the treatment of some cancers. Leukemia and certain cancer tumors have regressed after α-IFN treatment. Further research is needed to evaluate the effectiveness and use of α-IFN. Nausea, diarrhea, headache, fever, and flu-like symptoms are common adverse effects.

Interleukin-2 (*Proleukin*)

Interleukin-2 (IL-2) is one of the chemical mediators known as a lymphokine. It is produced by lymphocytes and other cells. Interleukin-2 is especially important for the activity of helper T-cells. It functions to stimulate B-cell production of antibodies and killer T-cell activity. These actions increase the function and response of the immune system. Killer T-cells, in particular, attack and destroy infectious organisms. Consequently, there is a great interest in developing interleukins for the treatment of cancer and AIDS. Fever, flu-like symptoms, and fluid retention are common adverse effects.

Newer immunopotentiating drugs have recently become available; they are still being evaluated to determine their most appropriate clinical uses. These agents are presented in Table 46:1.

Chapter Review

Understanding Terminology

Match the definition or description in the left column with the appropriate term in the right column.

___ **1.** The study of drugs with immunosuppressive or immunopotentiating effects.

___ **2.** Proteins that attack and help destroy infectious organisms.

___ **3.** The ability to stimulate and increase immune function.

___ **4.** Having the capability of causing cancer.

___ **5.** Capable of causing abnormal development (birth defects).

___ **6.** A decrease in the number of circulating lymphocytes.

___ **7.** Capable of causing mutations.

___ **8.** A chemical mediator produced by immune cells that helps regulate and increase immune function.

___ **9.** A chemical mediator produced by immune cells that increases immune function.

___ **10.** The ability to suppress or decrease immune function.

a. antibodies

b. carcinogenic

c. immunopharmacology

d. immunostimulation

e. immunosuppression

f. interferon

g. interleukin

h. lymphopenia

i. mutagenic

j. teratogenic

Acquiring Knowledge

Answer the following questions in the spaces provided.

1. In what diseases or conditions is it useful to suppress immune function? _____
_____
_____

2. When is it desirable to stimulate immune function? _____
_____
_____

3. Briefly describe the function of macrophages, helper T-cells, B-cells, and killer T-cells. _____
_____
_____

4. What is the function of suppressor T-cells and memory cells? _____
_____
_____

5. Describe the main immunosuppressive effect of corticosteroid drugs. _____
_____
_____

6. Compare the actions of azathioprine and cyclophosphamide with that of cyclosporine. Is there any advantage with cyclosporine? _____
_____
_____

7. What adverse effects are associated with cyclosporine? _____

_____

_____

8. What is the mechanism of action of muromonab-CD3? _____

_____

_____

9. Explain the immunopotentiating actions of α-interferon and interleukin-2. _____

_____

_____

Applying Knowledge—On the Job

Use your critical thinking skills to answer the following questions in the spaces provided.

1. As a nurse, you often get to know your patients personally as well as medically. Mary Peters is one of your patients. You know she feels lucky that a heart was found for her transplant surgery and glad just to be alive, but she still has to deal with organ rejection.

   a. What is the immunosuppressive drug of choice that Mary should be prescribed?

_____

_____

   b. Why is this the drug of choice?

_____

_____

   c. What adverse effects should Mary be monitored for while being administered this drug?

_____

_____

   d. What can be done to reduce the drug's adverse effects?

_____

_____

2. Assume you assist a family practice physician in a small town. Mr. Clark presents at the physician's office with hives, itching, a rash, and edema in his face, particularly around his eyes. The physician diagnoses it as an allergic reaction, cause unknown, and prescribes prednisone. Use the *Physicians' Desk Reference (PDR)* to help Mr. Clark use the drug safely.

   a. What would you ask Mr. Clark to see if he has contraindications to prednisone?

_____

_____

   b. Why should you warn Mr. Clark to avoid stress and infections while taking prednisone?

_____

_____

   c. For what adverse reactions should you monitor Mr. Clark?

_____

_____

   d. How should the prednisone be administered to Mr. Clark?

_____

_____

3. All patients taking immunosuppressants should be cautioned to watch for and report any signs of infections. Why is this important?

_____

_____

4. Patients receiving *Imuran* should be warned of the common adverse effects, GI disturbances, etc. What additional adverse effects should they be warned of?

_____

_____

5. Patients using alpha interferon should be warned of the common adverse reactions. Which adverse reactions are most likely to occur?

_____

_____

Internet Connection

Visit the MedicineNet website (http://www.medicinenet.com) and click on the *Diseases and Conditions Index* heading, highlight the letter "I" for immunotherapy, also referred to as biological therapy, and read about the role of immunotherapy in the treatment of various conditions.

Additional Reading

Graham, R. M. 1994. Cyclosporine: Mechanism of action and toxicity. *Cleveland Clinic Journal Medicine* 61:308.

Jaret, P. 1986. Our immune system: The war within. *National Geographic* June:706.

Life, death, and the immune system. 1993. *Scientific American* 269 (9):Special issue.

Overmyer, R. H., and Frohlick, E. D. 1991. Cyclosporine targets diabetic, arthritic, dermatologic, and other conditions. *Modern Medicine* 59:136.

Stephenson, K. S. 2002. Immunization update 2002. *Physician Assistant* 26 (5):44.

INDEX

Page numbers followed by f indicate figures;
those followed by t indicate tables.

Abortifacients, 370, 380
Abortions, therapeutic, 486–487
Absence seizure, 166, 167, 170
Absorption, drug, 14, 15, 16f, 17–19, 24–25,
    31, 33t, 529
Acarbose (Precose), 474t, 475, 476t, 477
ACE (angiotensin-converting enzyme)
    inhibitors, 242, 242t, 279, 281,
    284, 284t
Acebutolol (Sectral), 64t
Acetaminophen (Datril, Tylenol), 202t, 214,
    215t, 220–222, 220t, 224, 225, 226t,
    249t, 354t, 536t
Acetate, 464, 469
Acetazolamide (Diamox, Dazamide), 269t,
    270–271, 270t, 551t
Acetohexamide (Dymelor), 473, 474t
Acetylcholine (ACH), endogenous, 51, 54,
    71–76, 71f, 88, 98, 175, 176, 179
Acetylcholine (ACH) (Miochol-E), 74t
Acetylcholinesterase, 70, 71, 71f, 74
Acetylcysteine (Mucosil), 221, 364
Acid drugs, 19
Acid rebound, 370, 386
Acidification, 265, 268
Acidosis, 265, 268, 305, 316
Acne, 310
Acquired immunity, 511, 520
Acquired immunodeficiency syndrome
    (AIDS), 511, 521–523, 522t
Action potential, cardiac, 247f
Activated partial thromboplastin time
    (APTT), 296, 298
Acyclovir (Zovirax), 525–526, 527t, 529–531,
    535t, 537t
Addiction, 122, 193, 197, 204, 438
Addison's disease, 416, 417, 423
Additive effects, 25t
Adenosine (Adenocard), 253
Adenosine triphosphate (ATP), 238, 239
ADH (antidiuretic hormone), 125, 193, 203,
    268, 409, 484, 485, 487
Adipose tissue, 183, 187, 464, 465
Adrenal cortex, 416t
Adrenal steroids, 415–424
Adrenergic nerve endings, 58, 58f
Adrenergic neuronal blockers, 57, 60, 65–66,
    65f, 66f, 84t
Adrenergic receptors, 51, 54, 58–60,
    59t, 66f
Adrenocorticotropic hormone, (ACTH,
    Acthar, Corticotropin), 410t, 421t
Adriamycin, 537t
Adsorbents, 397, 399, 400t
Adverse effect, 2, 4, 7–8. See also
    specific drugs
Advice for the Patient, 8

Afferent nerve, 51, 52
Age, drug effects and, 22, 31–39
Agonist, 2, 5, 5f, 193, 199
Agranulocytosis, 288, 294, 450, 455
AIDS (acquired immunodeficiency
    syndrome), 511, 521–523, 522t
Akathisia, 131, 133
Albumin, 19, 32, 33
Albuterol (Proventil, Ventolin), 61t, 362t
Alcohol, 26, 125–127, 557, 558t, 559, 560t,
    561, 562
Alcoholic preparations, 15
Aldehydes, 558t
Aldosterone, 267, 273, 279, 281, 420–421
Alendronate (Fosamax), 457t, 458, 460
Alfentanil (Alfenta), 197t, 198t
Alkalosis, 265, 305, 316
Alkylating drugs, 568–569, 569t
Alkylation, 566, 568
Allopurinol (Zyloprim), 223–224, 223t,
    226t, 336
Alopecia, 288, 291
Alpha-adrenergic blockers, 57, 59, 62, 63t, 66f
Alpha-adrenergic drugs, 60, 60t, 66f, 122
Alpha-adrenergic receptors, 57, 58–59, 59t
Alpha-glucosidase inhibitors, 474t,
    475–477, 477f
Alpha-interferon (α-IFN), 581
Alprazolam (Xanax), 137t
Alteplase (Activase), 299–300
Alternate-day therapy, 420
Aluminum hydroxide, 384t, 385t, 386
Alzheimer's disease, 76
Amantadine (Symmetrel, Symadine), 177t,
    178–179, 524, 526, 527t, 529, 530, 533
Ambenonium (Mytelase), 74, 74t, 75
Amenorrhea, 427, 438
Amide local anesthetic, 98, 100, 101t
Amikacin (Amikin), 46, 189, 501t
Amiloride (Midamor), 269t, 273, 274t
Amino acid solutions
    (Aminosyn, Travasol), 315t
Amino acids, essential, 305, 306, 306t
Aminocaproic acid (Amicar), 301
Aminoglycosides, 501–502, 501t
Aminophylline, 362
Amiodarone (Cordarone), 252
Amitriptyline (Elavil), 146t
Amlodipine (Norvasc), 259, 283
Ammonium chloride, 201, 202t
Amobarbital, 121t, 122
Amoxapine (Asendin), 146t
Amoxicillin (Amoxil), 373, 375t,
    497–498, 498t
Amoxicillin-clavulanic acid (Augmentin), 499
Amphetamines, 148, 148t, 157–158,
    157f, 354t
Amphotericin B (Fungizone, Abelcet,
    Amphotec), 423, 512, 513, 513t, 514t,
    516, 517, 532, 534t, 537t

Ampicillin (Omnipen), 497–498, 498t
Ampicillin-sulbactam (Unasyn), 499
Amyl nitrite, 258t
Anabolism, 427, 441
Analgesia, 183, 184, 193, 196, 211
Analgesics
    adjunct to general anesthesia, 188, 189t
    for gout, 223, 223t
    nonopioid, 213–222, 215t–216t, 220t,
    224–226
    opioid (narcotic), 193–207
    patient-controlled, 206
Anandamide, 161
Anaphylaxis, 8, 61, 211, 217, 221
Androgens, 24t, 427, 441–444, 442t
Anemia, 211, 217, 332, 333
    causes of, 333, 334t
    cyanocobalamin deficiency, 336–338
    erythropoietin for, 340
    folic acid deficiency, 338–340
    iron deficiency, 217, 334–336
Anesthesia
    complete, 185
    epidural, 98, 102
    general, 183–190
    local, 98–105
Angina pectoris, 232, 235, 256, 257, 294
    antianginal drugs, 63, 256–260
    types, 256, 257
Angiotensin, 279, 281
Angiotensin receptor blocking drugs, 285
Angiotensin-converting enzyme (ACE)
    inhibitors, 242, 242t, 279, 281,
    284, 284t
Anion, 305, 315, 450
Anisindione (Miradon), 293t
Anistreplase (Eminase), 299
Anovulation, 437
ANS. See Autonomic nervous system
Antacids, 370, 372f, 376–378, 377t, 384–386,
    384t, 385t, 386t, 391–392, 551, 551t
Antagonism, 2, 5, 5f, 25t, 193, 196
Anthelmintic drugs, 549–552, 550t
Antiallergic agents, 346–350, 349f
Antianemics, 332–341
Antianginal drugs, 256–260
    beta-adrenergic blocking drugs, 259–260
    calcium antagonists, 259
    clinical indications, 260
    nitrites and nitrates, 257–259, 258t
    patient administration and
    monitoring, 260
Antianxiety drugs, 123–124, 131, 136–139,
    137t, 188, 189t
Antiarrhythmic drugs, 245, 247–253
    adjunct to general anesthesia, 188, 189t
    Class 1, 248–251
    Class 2, 251–252
    Class 3, 252
    Class 4, 252–253

Antiarrhythmic drugs—*Cont.*
 patient administration and
  monitoring, 253
 special considerations of use, 253
 uses, table of, 248t
Antibacterial drugs. *See also specific drugs*
 aminoglycosides, 501–502, 501t
 cephalosporins, 499–501, 500t
 chemoprophylaxis, 507
 chloramphenicol, 505–506
 clindamycin, 506
 fluoroquinolones, 505, 505t
 macrolides, 504–505
 penicillins, 497–499, 498t
 resistance, 497, 499, 506
 spectrum, 496–497
 sulfonamides, 503–504, 503t
 tetracyclines, 502–503, 502t
 for tuberculosis, 506–507
 vancomycin, 506
Antibacterial spectrum, 494, 496–497
Antibiotic susceptibility, 494, 495–496
Antibiotics, 188, 189t, 373, 494, 496, 572.
  See also Antibacterial drugs;
  specific drugs
Antibodies, 577, 578f
Antibody, 576
Anticholinergic drugs, 70, 76–78, 77t
 adjunct to general anesthesia, 188, 189t
 adverse and toxic effects, 78
 antidotes to poisoning, 76
 as antiemetics, 390t
 for asthma, 362–363
 clinical indications, 76–77, 77t
 for gastrointestinal disorders, 372f,
  382–384, 383t, 400, 400t, 401
 interaction with ganglionic blocking
  agents, 84t
 for Parkinson's disease, 179, 179t
 patient administration and monitoring, 78
Anticholinesterase drugs, 73–76
Anticoagulant effects, of salicylates, 218
Anticoagulants, 288–298, 534t, 535t, 551t
 antiplatelet drugs, 289–290, 290t,
  294–295
 antithrombins, 290t, 292
 chelators, 290t, 295
 clinical indications, 295
 comparison of, 293t
 contraindications, 293–294
 coumarin derivatives, 290, 292–293
 drug interactions, 295–296, 297t–298t
 heparins, 290–292, 290t, 293t, 294
 indandiones, 294
 mechanism of action, 289–290, 290t
 patient administration and monitoring,
  296, 298
 peripherally acting, 291
 special considerations, 296
 vitamin K derivatives, 294
Anticonvulsant drugs, 166, 168, 171
Antidepressant drugs, 144–148
 monamine oxidase inhibitors, 144–145,
  145t, 149
 patient administration and
  monitoring, 149
 selective serotonin reuptake inhibitors,
  147–148, 147t, 149
 tricyclic, 145–147, 146t, 147t, 149
Antidiarrheals, 398–401, 399t, 400t
Antidiuretic hormone (ADH), 125, 193, 203,
  268, 409, 484, 485, 487

Antiemetics, 77, 188, 388–389 390t, 392
Antiepileptic drugs, 166–171
Antifungal drugs, 512–519
 adverse effects, 517
 clinical indications, 513, 516
 contraindications, 517, 519
 doses, table of, 514t–515t
 mechanism of action, 516
 patient administration and
  monitoring, 518
 pharmacokinetics, 516–517
Antigenic drift, 511, 526
Antigenic shift, 511, 526
Antigens, 346, 347
Antigout drugs, 222–224, 226t
Antihistaminic agents, 346, 347, 350–355,
  534t, 535t
 adverse reactions, 352–353
 as antiemetics, 388
 cautions and contraindications, 353
 clinical indications, 352
 cold and allergy preparations, 352t
 dosages, table of, 351t
 drug interactions, 353–354, 354t
 H_2-receptor antagonists, 372f, 374t,
  376–380, 377t
 for Parkinson's disease, 179
 patient administration and
  monitoring, 355
 site of action, 349f
Antihypertensive drugs
 angiotensin receptor blocking drugs, 285
 angiotensin-converting enzyme (ACE)
  inhibitors, 284, 284t
 beta-adrenergic blockers, 283
 calcium antagonists, 283–284, 284t
 diuretic agents, 281–282, 322t
 for hypertensive crisis, 285
 patient administration and
  monitoring, 285
 sympathetic blocking drugs, 282–283, 283t
 vasodilators, 283
Antiinflammatory action, 211, 418
Antiinflammatory drugs, 212. *See also*
  Nonsteroidal antiinflammatory drugs
  (NSAIDs)
 for asthma, 363–364, 363t
 for pain relief, 195f, 196
Antimalarial drugs, 544–547, 545t
Antimanic drugs, 149–150
Antimetabolites, 566, 569–570
Antimicrobial drugs, 494, 496
Antineoplastic agents, 566–572
 alkylating drugs, 568–569, 569t
 antimetabolites, 569–570
 drug resistance, 568
 patient administration and
  monitoring, 572
 use in pregnancy, 572
Antiparkinson drugs, 175–180
Antiplatelet drugs, 289–290, 290t, 294–295
Antipsychotic drugs, 131, 132–136, 134t, 188
Antipyresis, 211, 212
Antisecretory drugs, 370, 376–384, 379t
 anticholinergics, 382–384
 antispasmodics, 382–384
 gastrointestinal stimulants, 381–382
 H_2-receptor antagonists, 376–380
 prostaglandins, 380
 proton pump inhibitors, 380–381
Antiseptics
 definition, 556

 mechanism of action, 557
 uses, 559, 560t–561t, 561–562
Antiserotonin drugs, 382, 383t
Antispasmodic drugs, 76, 383–384, 383t
Antithrombins, 290t, 292
Antitussives, 193, 196, 200–201, 201t, 202t
Antiviral drugs
 absorption, 529
 adverse effects, 530–531
 clinical indications, 526
 contraindications, 531
 drug interactions, 532, 534t–537t
 hepatic microsomal metabolism, 529
 mechanisms of action, 524–525
 patient administration and monitoring,
  532–533
 renal excretion, 529–530
 resistance, 525–526
 table of, 527t–528t
Anuria, 193, 203, 265, 268
Anxiety, drugs to control, 123–124, 131,
  136–139, 137t, 188, 189t
Aplastic anemia, 332, 339
Apothecaries' system, of measurement, 43
APTT (activated partial thromboplastin
  time), 296, 298
Aqueous humor, 265, 271
Aqueous preparations, 15
Ardeparin (*Normiflo*), 290–291, 293t, 295
Argatroban, 292
Argyria, 556, 561
Arrhythmia, 98, 102, 245, 246–247, 246t
Arteriosclerosis, 232, 235
Arthralgia, 211, 212
Arthritis, 211, 212
 nonopioid analgesics for, 214, 215t–216t
Articaine (*Septocaine*), 101t
Asparaginase (*Elspar*), 571t
Aspirin (*Anacin, Bayer, Bufferin, Empirin*), 5,
  19, 214, 215t, 217–220, 220t, 223t,
  225, 226t, 249t, 290, 294–295, 536t
Assisted reproductive technologies (ART), 437
Astemizole (*Hismanal*), 353–354, 532,
  534t, 535t
Asthma, 347, 358–359
 autonomic nervous system, role of,
  360–361
 treatment
  antiallergic agents, 364
  anticholinergic drugs, 362–363
  antiinflammatory drugs, 363–364, 415f
  bronchodilators, 361–362, 413f
  mucolytics, 364
Asymptomatic, 542, 549
Atenolol (*Tenormin*), 63, 64t
Atherosclerosis, 232, 235, 289, 322–323
Atorvastatin (*Lipitor*), 325, 325t
Atracurium besylate (*Tracrium*), 90t
Atrioventricular (AV) node, 234, 246,
  249, 252
Atropine, 75, 76–77, 77t, 179, 189, 354t,
  382, 383t
Attapulgite (*Rheaban Maximum, Kaopectate
  Maximum Strength*), 400t
Autoimmune disease, 450, 454
Automatism, 118, 122
Autonomic ganglia, drugs affecting, 82–84
Autonomic nervous system (ANS), 51–54
 parasympathetic nervous system, 51,
  52–54, 53f, 54f, 54t
 physiology and pharmacology, 52
 role in asthma, 360–361

sympathetic nervous system, 51, 52–54, 53f, 54f, 54t
Autorhythmicity, 234
Azapirones, 139
Azatadine (Optimine), 350
Azathioprine (Imuran), 579
Azithromycin (Zithromax), 354t, 504
Aztreonam (Azactam), 499

B vitamins, 313–314
Baclofen (Lioresal), 89f, 92, 93, 93t, 94
Bacteria, 494, 495–496, 496t
Bacterial resistance, 494, 497
Bactericidal drugs, 494, 496
Bacteriostatic drugs, 494, 496
Barbiturates, 20, 26, 118, 120–123, 168–169, 186–189, 382
Basal ganglia, 111, 113, 133, 175–177, 179
Basal metabolic rate (BMR), 451
Basic drugs, 19
B-cells, 577–581
Beclomethasone (Beclovent, Vanceril), 363t
Belladonna (Bellafoline), 383t
Belladonna alkaloids, 382, 383t, 384, 400t
Benazepril (Lotensin), 284t
Bendroflumethiazide (Naturetin), 269t, 272t, 322t
Benzalkonium chloride (Benz-all, Zephiran), 557, 558t, 559, 560t, 561
Benzocaine (Boil-ease, Dermoplast, Lanacane, Solarcaine), 101t
Benzodiazepines, 32, 118, 123–124, 136–139, 137t, 170
Benzthiazide (Exna), 269t, 272t, 322t
Benztropine (Cogentin), 179, 179t
Bepridil (Vascor), 259
Beta-adrenergic blockers, 63–65, 64t, 66f, 251–252, 259, 283, 551t
Beta-adrenergic drugs, 60–61, 61t, 66f, 72t, 361, 362t
Beta-adrenergic receptor, 57, 59, 59t
Beta-carotene, 309
Beta-interferon (β-IFN), 581t
Beta-lactamase, 497
Beta-lactamase inhibitors, 499
Betamethasone (Celestone, Cel-U-Ject, Selestoject), 418t, 421t
Bethanechol (Urecholine), 73, 74t, 377t
Biguanides, 558t
Bile acid sequestrants, 324–325, 325t, 327–328, 329t
Bioavailability, 14, 21
Biperiden (Akineton), 179t
Biphasic, 427, 430
Bisacodyl, 403t, 404
Bismuth subsalicylate (Pepto-Bismol, Bismatrol, Pepto-Bismol Maximum Strength), 375t, 400t
Bisoprolol (Zebeta), 64t
Bisphosphonates, 435, 459, 460
Bitolterol, 362t
Bivalirudin, 292
Bleomycin (Blenoxane), 571t
Blood drug levels, 21
Blood flow
    drug distribution and, 19
    through the heart, 233f
Blood pressure
    antihypertensive drugs, 281–285
    definition, 279, 280
    physiological factors controlling, 280–281
Blood-brain barrier, 20

BMR (basal metabolic rate), 451
Body fat, percent, 22, 32
Body water, 314
Bowel function, 398
Brain, 112–115, 113f
Brainstem, 113
Bran, 403t
Breast milk, drugs in, 23, 24t
Bretylium (Bretylol), 252
Broad-spectrum drugs, 495, 497
Bromocriptine (Parlodel), 177t, 178
Bromodiphenhydramine, 201t
Brompheniramine (Brovex), 351t, 352, 354t
Bronchitis, 34t
Bronchodilators, 58, 59, 61, 90, 358, 361–362, 362t
Buccal absorption, 427, 443
Buccal, administration, 18t
Budesonide (Entocort E. C., Pulmicort, Rhinocort), 363t, 421t
Bumetanide (Bumex), 269t, 273, 274t, 282
Bupivacaine (Marcaine), 101t, 102
Buprenorphine (Buprenex), 198t
Bupropion (Wellbutrin), 148
Buspirone (BuSpar), 139
Busulfan (Myleran), 569t
Butabarbital (Butisol), 121t
Butalbital, 220t
Betaconazole (FemStat 3), 514t, 517
Butenafine (Mentax), 514t
Butorphanol (Stadol), 198t, 199
Butorphanol nasal spray (Stadol NS), 198t
Butyrophenones, 134–135, 134t

Caffeine, 220t, 269t, 274, 361
Calcifediol (Calderol), 311
Calcitonin, 456, 459
Calcitonin, salmon (Calcimar, Miacalcin), 457t, 458
Calcitriol (Rocaltrol, Calcijex), 311
Calcium, 316
    homeostasis, 456
    hypercalcemia, 456, 457–458
    hypocalcemia, 456
    for osteoporosis, 435
    patient administration and monitoring, 317
Calcium antagonists, 283–284, 284t
    adverse effects, 260
    for angina, 259–260
    mechanism of action, 259
Calcium carbonate, 384t, 385t, 386
Calcium channel blockers, 534t
Calcium chloride, 457t
Calcium gluconate, 457t
Calcium lactate, 457t
Calcium pantothenate, 313
Cancer, 566
    antineoplastic drugs, 567–572, 569t, 571t
    sex hormones and, 438, 439–440
    types, 567
Candesartan (Atacand), 285
Candidiasis, 511, 512–513, 513t, 514t
Cannabinoids, 154, 161
Capsules, 16
Captopril (Capoten), 242t, 284
Caramiphen edisylate, 201t
Carbachol (Miostat), 74t
Carbamazepine (Tegretol), 168t, 169, 171
Carbamazine, 24t
Carbenicillin indanyl (Geocillin), 498, 498t
Carbidopa (Lodosyn), 177, 177t

Carbohydrate solution (Emetrol), 390t
Carbonic anhydrase inhibitors, 269t, 270–271, 270t
Carboplatin (Paraplatin), 569t
Carboprost tromethamine (Hemabate), 486–487, 488t
Carboxymethylcellulose, 403t
Carcinogenic drugs, 576, 579
Cardiac arrhythmia, 98, 102, 245, 246–247, 246t
Cardiac glycosides, 239–241, 240t
    adverse and toxic effects, 240–241
    clinical indications, 241
    drug interactions, 241
    patient administration and monitoring, 241
    pharmacokinetics, 240
    pharmacological effects, 239–240
    serum electrolyte levels and, 240
Cardiac output (CO), 279, 280, 320
Cardiovascular disease
    hormone replacement therapy effect, 435
    thyroid hormones effect on, 453–454
Cardiovascular effects of drugs
    anticholinergics, 76
    general anesthetics, 186
    histamine, 348
    local anesthetics, 102
    opioids, 203
    salicylates, 218
    skeletal muscle relaxants, 90
Carisoprodol (Rela, Soma), 89f, 93t
Carmustine (BiCNU), 569t
Carvedilol (Coreg), 64t
Castor oil, 403t
Cat scratch disease, 549
Catabolism, 415, 417
Catecholamines, 57, 58
Catechol-O-methyltransferase (COMT) inhibitors, 178
Cathartics, 397, 401
Cation, 305, 315
Caudal anesthesia, 98, 102
Cefaclor (Ceclor), 500t
Cefadroxil (Duricef), 500t
Cefazolin (Kefzol), 499, 500t
Cefepime (Maxipime), 500, 500t
Cefixime (Suprax), 500t
Cefonicid (Monocid), 500t
Cefoperazone (Cefobid), 500t
Cefotaxime (Claforan), 500t
Cefotetan (Cefotan), 500t
Cefoxitin (Mefoxin), 499, 500t
Ceftazidime (Fortaz), 500t
Ceftriaxone (Rocephin), 500t
Ceiling effect, 6
Celecoxib (Celebrex), 214, 216t, 217
Cellulose, oxidized, 301
Central nervous system (CNS), 52, 111–115
    alcohol effects on, 125
    anticholinergic drug effect on, 77
    depression, 119–126, 120f
    general anesthetic, 185–186, 185f
    local anesthetic effects on, 103
    opioid effects on, 199–200, 200f
Centrally acting skeletal muscle relaxant, 87, 88, 92–93, 93t
Centrally acting sympatholytic drugs, 282–283
Cephalexin (Keflex), 500t
Cephalosporinases, 495, 497
Cephalosporins, 499–501, 500t

Cephradine (*Velosef*), 500t
Cerebellum, 111, 114
Cerebral cortex, 111, 112–113, 120
Cerebral medulla, 111, 113
Cerebrum, 111, 130
Cerivastatin (*Baycol*), 325, 326
Cetirizine (*Zyrtec*), 350, 351t
Cetylpyridinium chloride (*Ceepryn, Cepacol*), 557, 558t, 561
Chelate, definition of, 332, 336
Chelators, 295
Chemical mediators, 358, 360
Chemical name, 2, 8
Chemoprophylaxis, 495, 507
Chemoreceptor trigger zone (CTZ), 200f, 387, 388f, 389
Chemotherapy, 495, 566, 567–568. *See also* Antineoplastic agents
Chicken pox, 219
Chloral hydrate (*Noctec, SK-Chloral*), 121t, 124
Chlorambucil (*Leukeran*), 569t
Chloramphenicol (*Chloromycetin*), 505–506
Chlordiazepoxide (*Librium*), 92, 93, 93t, 136, 137t, 382
Chlorhexidine (*Exidine skin cleanser, Hibiclens liquid*), 557, 558t, 559, 561
Chlorhexidine gluconate, 560t
Chloroform, 187t
Chloroprocaine (*Nesacaine*), 101t
Chloroquine (*Aralen phosphate*), 544–546, 545t, 547t, 548, 551, 551t
Chlorothiazide (*Diuril, Diurigen*), 269t, 271, 272t, 275–276, 322t
Chlorotrianisene (*TACE*), 431t
Chlorpheniramine (*Allerchlor, Chlor-Trimeton*), 201, 202t, 350, 351t, 353, 354t
Chlorpromazine (*Thorazine*), 133, 134t, 159, 189, 352, 389, 390t, 453
Chlorpropamide (*Diabinese*), 473, 474t, 475
Chlortetracycline (*Aureomycin*), 502
Chlorthalidone (*Hygroton*), 269t, 271, 272t, 282, 322t
Chlorzoxazone (*Parafon Forte DSC*), 93t
Cholecalciferol (D_3) (*Delta-D, Vitamin D_3*), 311
Cholesterol, 321, 322–329, 324f, 435, 439
Cholesterol absorption inhibitors, 326
Cholestyramine (*Questran*), 241, 324–325, 325t, 327–328, 329t, 453
Choline salicylate (*Arthropan*), 223t
Cholinergic crisis, 75
Cholinergic, definition of, 70, 71
Cholinergic drugs, 73–75, 74t
    adjunct to general anesthesia, 188, 189t
    adverse and toxic effects, 75
    clinical indications, 73, 75–76
    direct-acting, 73, 74t
    indirect-acting, 73–74, 74t
    interaction with ganglionic blocking agents, 84t
    patient administration and monitoring, 75
Cholinergic nerve endings, 71, 71f
Cholinergic receptors, 51, 54, 72–73, 72f
-chromic, definition of, 332, 333
Chronic bronchitis, 358, 359
Chronic, definition of, 332
Chronic illnesses, 333
Chronic obstructive pulmonary disease (COPD), 358, 359
Chylomicrons, 322
Ciclopiroxolamine (*Loprox*), 512, 514t
-cidal, definition of, 556, 557

Cidofovir (*Vistide*), 525, 527t, 530–532, 535t
Cimetidine (*Tagamet*), 124, 139, 171, 336, 354t, 374t, 377–379, 377t, 379t, 391, 535t, 536t, 537t, 551, 551t
Cinchonism, 245, 249, 542, 546
Ciprofloxacin (*Cipro*), 505, 505t
Cisapride, 381, 392
Cisatracurium besylate (*Nimbex*), 90t
Cisplatin (*Platinol*), 568, 569t
Citalopram (*Celexa*), 147t
Cladribine (*Leustatin*), 570
Clarithromycin (*Biaxin*), 354t, 373, 375t, 504, 536t, 537t
Clavulanic acid, 499
Clemastine (*Tavist*), 350, 351t
Clindamycin (*Cleocin*), 506
Clioquinol (*Vioform*), 514t
Clofibrate, 329
Clomiphene (*Clomid, Milophene, Serophene*), 437
Clonazepam (*Klonopin*), 137t, 138, 168t, 170
Clonic, 166, 167
Clonidine (*Catapres*), 16, 282–283, 283t
Clopidogrel (*Plavix*), 290, 293t, 294
Clorazepate (*Tranxene*), 137t
Clotrimazole (*FemCare, Gyne-Lotrimin, Lotrimin-AF, Mycelex-G, Mycelex, Mycelex-OTC*), 512, 514t, 517
Cloxacillin sodium (*Tegopen*), 498t
Clozapine (*Clozaril*), 134t, 135
CMV (cytomegalovirus), 524, 526, 530–531
CNS. *See* Central nervous system
Coagulants, 300–301
Coagulation, 288, 289
    monitoring, 296, 298
Cocaine, 101t, 102, 157, 158–160
Codeine, 196, 197t, 198t, 200–201, 201t, 202t, 207, 220t
Colchicine, 223, 223t
Colesevelam (*Welchol*), 324, 325t
Colestipol (*Colestid*), 324–325, 325t
Colony stimulating factors, 581t
Compliance, 23
COMT (catechol-O-methyltransferase) inhibitors, 178
Conduction system, heart, 232, 233–234, 234f
Congestive heart failure (CHF), 34t, 235, 238, 239
    cardiac glycoside therapy, 239–241
    diuretic therapy, 241–242
    vasodilator therapy, 241–242, 242t
Conjugated estrogens (*Premarin*), 431t
Constipation, 207, 401–402
Contraception, 427, 430
Contraindications, 2, 4. *See also specific drugs*
Controlled substance, 2, 9, 9t
Conversions, measurement, 43–44
Convoluted, 265
COPD (chronic obstructive pulmonary disease), 358, 359
Coronary artery, 256, 257
Coronary artery disease (CAD), 235, 323
Coronary heart disease (CHD), 323
Corticosteroids, 354t, 534t, 535t
    adverse effects, 363
    aerosol inhalation, 363, 363t
    for asthma, 363–364, 363t
    for immunosuppression, 578–579
Corticotropin (adrenocorticotropic hormone, ACTH), 416–419, 421t
Cortisol, 416–417

Cortisone (*Cortisone acetate, Cortone*), 214, 418t, 421t
Cosyntropin (*Cortrosyn*), 417, 421t
Coumarin derivatives, 290, 292–293, 354t
Creatinine, 30, 32
Creatinine clearance, 30, 32
Cretinism, 408, 409, 450, 451, 455
Crohn's disease, 580
Cromolyn sodium (*Gastrocrom, Intal, Nasalcrom, Spinhaler*), 348–350, 350t, 364
Cross-tolerance, 154, 156
CTZ (chemoreceptor trigger zone), 200f, 387, 388f, 389
Curare, 88–91, 89f, 90t
Cushing's disease, 420
Cyanocobalamin (vitamin B_{12}), 313
    deficiency, 336–338
    preparations, 337, 338t
Cyclic adenosine monophosphate (cyclic AMP), 361
Cyclic guanosine monophosphate (cyclic GMP), 361
Cyclizine (*Marezine*), 389, 390t
Cyclobenzaprine (*Flexeril*), 93t
Cyclooxygenase (COX), 211, 213–214, 294
Cyclophosphamide (*Cytoxan*), 569t, 579
Cycloplegia, 77, 83
Cyclosporine (*Sandimmune*), 532, 534t, 535t, 579
Cyproheptadine (*Periactin*), 350, 351t, 353
Cytarabine (*Cytosar-U*), 570
    cytic, definition of, 332, 333
Cytokines, 360
Cytomegalovirus (CMV), 524, 526, 530, 531

Daclizumab (*Zenapax*), 580
Dactinomycin (*Cosmegen*), 571t
Dalteparin (*Fragmin*), 290–291, 293t, 295
Dantrolene (*Dantrium*), 89f, 90t, 91–92, 94
Dapsone, 537t
Decimal, 39, 41–42
Decubitus ulcer, 556, 559
Deep vein thrombosis (DVT), 295
Defecation, 397, 398, 401, 402
Dehydration, 275
Dehydroepiandrosterone (DHEA), 443, 445
Delavirdine (*Rescriptor*), 525, 528t, 529, 531, 533, 535t
Delayed-release products, 16
Delta receptor, 199
Demecarium (*Humorsol*), 74t
Demeclocycline (*Declomycin*), 502t
Denaturing, 556, 557
Denominator, 39, 40
Dental anesthesia, 105
Dependency, 14, 26, 154, 155
    amphetamine, 158
    antianxiety drugs, 139
    barbiturate, 122
    cocaine, 159
    LSD, 156
    marijuana, 162
    opioid, 196, 203–204
    PCP, 160
Depolarizing blocker, 87, 89
Depression, 34t, 143
    antidepressant drugs for, 144–148, 149
    endogenous, 143, 144
    exogenous (reactive), 143, 144
    from quinidine, 249

Depression, CNS, 119–126, 120f
 in general anesthesia, 184–190, 185f
Dermatitis, 346, 352
Dermatophytic infections, 511, 512–513,
  513t, 516
DES (diethylstilbestrol), 24t, 430, 438, 440
Designer drug, 154, 157, 160
Desipramine (Pertofrane), 146t
Desloratadine (Clarinex), 351t
Desmopressin acetate (DDAVP), 486,
  487, 488t
Desogestrel, 432t, 436
Dexamethasone (Dalone LA, Decadron,
  Decadron-LA, Decaject LA, Dexone,
  Dexameth, Hexadrol), 418t, 419t, 421t
Dexamethasone with lidocaine (Decadron
  with Xylocaine), 422t
Dexchlorpheniramine, 351t
Dexmethylphenidate (Focalin), 148t
Dextran, 315t
Dextroamphetamine (Dexedrine), 148t, 157
Dextromethorphan, 196, 197, 199, 200–201,
  202t, 207, 354t
Dextrose, 315t
Dextrothyroxine, 327, 328
Dezocine (Dalgan), 198t
DHEA (dehydroepiandrosterone), 443, 445
Diabetes insipidus, 484, 485–486, 488t
Diabetes mellitus, 34t
  causes, 465
  complications, 466
  symptoms, 466, 466t
  thyroid hormone effect on, 453, 454
  treatment, 466–480
    biguanides, 477–479
    glucose absorption inhibitors, 474t,
      475–477, 477f, 479
    insulin sensitizers, 474t, 479–480
    insulin therapy, 467–471, 468t, 472t
    oral hypoglycemic secretagogues,
      471–475, 474t, 476t
    patient administration and
      monitoring, 478–479
Diarrhea, 398–401, 399t, 400t
Diazepam (Valium), 32, 89f, 92, 93, 93t, 103,
  136, 137t, 138, 158, 159, 168t, 170,
  171, 188, 378
Diazoxide (Hyperstat), 275, 285
Dibucaine (Nupercaine, Nupercainal),
  101t, 102
Dichlorphenamide (Daranide), 269t, 270t
Diclofenac (Cataflam, Voltaren), 215t
Dicloxacillin sodium (Dynapen), 498t
Dicumarol, 292, 293t
Dicyclomine (Bentyl, Dyspas), 77t, 383t, 384
Didanosine (ddI, Videx), 525, 526, 528t, 529,
  531–533, 535t, 536t, 537t
Diet. See also Nutrition
  dietary recommendations, 307–308
  disease and, 306–307
  food guide pyramid, 308–309, 308f
  recommended daily food
    consumption, 308t
  recommended dietary allowances (RDA),
    307, 307t
  vitamins, 307t, 309–314, 317
Diethylstilbestrol (DES), 24t, 430, 438, 440
Difenoxin and atropine (Motofen), 400t, 401
Diflunisal (Dolobid), 215t, 226t
Digestion, 371, 372f, 373
Digitalis, 3, 423, 534t

Digitalization, 238, 240
Digitoxin (Purodigin), 240, 240t
Digoxin (Lanoxin, Lanoxicaps), 46, 240, 240t
Digoxin Immune Fab (Digibind), 241
Dihydrotachysterol (DHT, Hytakerol),
  311, 457t
Diltiazem (Cardizem), 241, 253, 259, 283, 284t
Dimenhydrinate (Dramamine), 350, 351t, 390t
2,5-dimethoxy-4-methylamphetamine
  (DOM), 156–157
Dimethyltryptamine, 156
Dinoprostone (Prostin E₂), 487, 488t
Diphenhydramine (Benadryl), 179, 350, 351t,
  354t, 389, 390t
Diphenidol (Vontrol), 389
Diphenoxylate, 401
Diphenoxylate and atropine (Logen, Lomotil,
  Lonox), 400t, 401
Diplopia, 427, 439
Dipyridamole (Persantine, Aggrenox), 290, 294
Dirithromycin (Dynabac), 504–505
Disease presence, drug response and, 22,
  33, 34t
Disinfectants, 556–562
  adverse and toxic effects, 562
  definition, 556
  mechanism of action, 557
  sterilization with, 557, 559
  uses, 559, 560t–561t, 561–562
Disopyramide (Norpace), 248t, 250, 253
Dissociative anesthesia, 183, 188
Distal convoluted tubule (DCT), 265, 266, 267f
Distribution, drug, 14, 15, 16f, 19, 25,
  31–32, 33t
Disulfiram (Antabuse), 127, 537t
Disulfiram reaction, 475, 479, 542, 548, 549
Diuresis, 265, 268
Diuretics
  adverse effects, 282
  as antihypertensive drug, 281–282
  carbonic anhydrase inhibitors, 269t,
    270–271, 270t
  classes of, 269t
  clinical indications, 269
  for congestive heart failure, 241–242
  drug interactions and incompatibilities,
    275–276
  mechanism, 281–282
  organic acid, 269t, 273, 274t
  osmotic, 269–270, 269t, 270t
  overdose, 276
  patient administration and
    monitoring, 276
  potassium-sparing, 269t, 273–274, 274t
  refractory, 271
  thiazide, 269t, 271–273, 272t
  xanthine derivatives, 269t, 274
DMMS (drug microsomal metabolizing
  system), 14, 20, 121
Dobutamine (Dobutrex), 62
Docusate calcium, 403t
Docusate sodium, 403t, 404
Donepezil (Aricept), 74t, 76
Dopamine (Intropin), 62
Dopamine agonists, 178
Dopamine, endogenous, 133, 157, 175, 176
Dosage
  adjustment, 25
  calculations, 42, 44–46
  pediatric, 45–46
Dose, 2, 6

Dose-response curve, 6, 6f
Doxacurium (Nuromax), 90t
Doxazosin (Cardura), 63t
Doxepin (Sinequan), 146t
Doxorubicin (Adriamycin), 571t
Doxycycline (Vibramycin), 502, 502t, 545t, 546
Doxylamine, 202t, 352, 354t
Dronabinol (C-III Marinol), 180, 389, 390t
Drug, 2
  absorption, 14, 15, 16f, 17–19, 24–25,
    31, 33t, 529
Drug abuse, 26
Drug addiction, 14, 26, 122, 193, 197,
  204, 438
Drug allergy, 8
Drug compliance, 30, 34–35
Drug dependence, 14, 26. See also
  Dependency
Drug distribution, 14, 15, 16f, 19, 25,
  31–32, 33t
Drug Enforcement Agency (DEA), 197
Drug excretion, 20–21, 25, 32, 33t
Drug forms, 15–16
Drug formulation, 19
Drug indications, 2, 4
Drug Information - American Hospital
  Formulary Service, 8
Drug Information for the Health Care
  Professional, 8
Drug interactions, 25, 25t. See also
  specific drugs
  anticoagulants, 295–296, 297t–298t
  antipsychotic drugs, 136
  antiviral drugs, 532, 534t–537t
  benzodiazepines, 139
  beta-blockers, 64
  cardiac glycosides, 241
  with disease in the elderly, 33, 34t
  hypolipidemic drugs, 327–328, 329t
  local anesthesia, 103–104
  nonopioid analgesics, 224, 226t
  nonsteroidal antiinflammatory drugs
    (NSAIDs), 224, 226t
  opioid analgesics, 206–207
  tricyclic antidepressants, 147t
Drug ionization, 19
Drug metabolism, 20, 25, 32, 33t
Drug microsomal metabolizing system
  (DMMS), 14, 20, 121
Drug nomenclature, 8, 8f
Drug references, 8
Drug resistance, 525–526, 566, 568
Drug response, in geriatric patients, 33–34, 34t
Drug safety, 7–8
Drug sources, 3–4
Drug tolerance. See Tolerance
Drugs of abuse, 4, 11t, 154–162
Dwarfism, 408, 409
Dynorphin, 199
Dysentery, 542
Dyskinesia, 175, 177
Dysmenorrhea, 211, 214, 215t–216t, 427, 438
Dysphoria, 193, 199
Dystonia, 177
Dystonic reaction, 131, 133

ECF-A (eosinophilic chemotactic factor of
  anaphylaxis), 360
Echothiophate (Phospholine), 74
Econazole (Spectazole), 514t
Ectopic beat, 238, 240

Ectopic focus, 245, 246, 247f
Eczematoid dermatitis, 346, 353
ED50, 2, 6
Edema, 268, 271, 273, 275
Edrophonium (Tensilon), 74, 74t, 90
EDTA (ethylenediamine tetraacetic acid), 457
Efferent nerve, 51, 52
Elderly. See Geriatrics
Electrocardiogram (ECG), 232, 234, 234f, 518
    indications of the toxic effects of
        quinidine, 249f
    monitoring of arrhythmias, 246t,
        247, 247f
Electroencephalogram (EEG), 111, 113, 167
Electrolytes, 305, 315–316, 315t, 397, 398,
    542, 547
Electrophysiology of the heart, 247, 248t
Emesis, 194, 200, 387–389, 388f, 390t
    antiemetics, 77, 188, 388–389 390t, 392
    emetics, 387–388
EMLA (lidocaine, prilocaine), 101t, 102
Emollients, 397, 402
Emphysema, 34t, 358, 359
Enalapril (Vasotec), 242t, 284t
Endemic, 542, 545
Endocrine system, 408–412. See also
        Hormones; specific hormones
Endogenous, 194, 484, 485
Endogenous depression, 143, 144
Endometrium, 427, 429
Endorphins, 194, 199
Enemas, 402
Enflurane (Ethrane), 186, 187t
Enkephalin, 199
Enoxacin (Penetrex), 505t
Enoxaparin (Lovenox), 290–291, 293t, 295
Entacapone (Comtan), 178
Entamoeba histolytica, 547–548, 547t
Enteric-coated products, 16, 332, 336
Enterohepatic cycling, 30, 32
Enuresis, 77
Enzyme induction, 14, 20
Enzyme inhibition, 14, 20
Eosinophilic chemotactic factor of
        anaphylaxis (ECF-A), 360
Ephedrine, 60t, 201
Epidural anesthesia, 98, 102
Epilepsy, 166, 167, 271
    antiepileptic drugs, 168–171, 168t
    types, 167–168
Epinephrine, 51, 54, 58–61, 59t, 61t,
    102, 362t
Eprosartan (Teveten), 285
Equipotent, 428, 430
Ergocalciferol (D₂) (Calciferol Drops, Drisdol
        Drops, Vitamin D, Deltalin Gelseals),
        311, 457t
Ergonovine (Ergotrate), 486, 488t
Erythema, 211, 213, 346, 347
Erythromycin (Erythrocin, E-Mycin), 189,
        354t, 504
Erythropoiesis, 428, 441
Erythropoietin (Epogen, Procrit), 340
Eschar, 556, 562
Escitalopram (Lexapro), 147t
Esmolol (Brevibloc), 64, 64t, 251–252
Esomeprazole (Nexium), 375t, 377t, 380
Esophageal sphincter, 374, 376t
Essential amino acids, 305, 306, 306t
Essential fatty acids, 305, 306, 306t
Essential hypertension, 279, 280
Estazolam (ProSom), 121t

Ester local anesthetic, 98, 99–100, 101t
Estradiol (Estrace), 431t
Estradiol cypionate (Depogen,
        depGynogen), 431t
Estradiol valerate (Delestrogen, Duragen, Estra-
        L-40, Gynogen), 431t
Estrogens, 16, 24t, 428–430, 429f, 431t,
        432t, 433–441, 445, 453, 460
Estrone (Aquest, Theelin), 431t
Ethacrynic acid (Edecrin), 269t, 273, 274t, 275
Ethambutol (Myambutol), 507
Ethanol, 558t, 560t, 561, 562. See also Alcohol
Ether, 187t
Ethinyl estradiol (Estinyl, Feminone), 430,
        431t, 432t, 436, 537t
Ethosuximide (Zarontin), 168t, 170
Ethotoin (Peganone), 169
Ethyl alcohol. See Alcohol; Ethanol
Ethyl chloride, 101t
Ethylenediamine tetraacetic acid (EDTA), 457
Ethynodiol diacetate, 432t
Etidocaine (Duranest), 101t
Etidronate (Didronel), 457t, 458, 460
Etodolac (Lodine), 215t
Etomidate (Amidate), 186–188, 187t
Etoposide (VePesid), 570, 571t
Euphoria, 183, 184
Evacuation, 397, 398
Excretion, drug, 20–21, 25, 32, 33t
Exertional angina, 256, 257
Exogenous, 484, 485
Exogenous depression, 143, 144
Expectorants, 194, 201, 364
Extracellular, 265, 266–267
Extracellular fluid (ECF), 314
Eyes, opioid effects on, 203
Ezetimibe (Zetia), 325t, 326

False transmitter, 57, 65
Famciclovir (Famvir), 527t, 529, 531, 532, 535t
Famotidine (Pepcid), 374t, 377–378, 377t
Fasciculation, 87, 89
Fat emulsions (Intralipid, Liposyn), 315t
Fatty acids, essential, 305, 306, 306t
Felbamate (Felbatol), 168t, 170
Felodipine (Plendil), 259, 283
Fenofibrate (Tricor), 325t, 327, 329t
Fenoprofen (Nalfon), 215t
Fenoterol (Berotec), 61t
Fentanyl (Sublimaze), 198t, 199
Fentanyl citrate-droperidol (Innovar), 185,
        186, 187, 187t, 189
Fentanyl transdermal (Duragesic), 198t
Fentanyl transmucosal (Actiq), 198t
Fertility drugs, 428, 437–438, 439
Fexofenadine (Allegra), 350, 351t
Fibric acid derivatives, 327
Fibrocystic breast disease, 428, 443
Fight or flight reaction, 51, 53
Filgrastim (granulocyte-CSF), 581t
Filtration, renal, 266
First-pass metabolism, 14, 20
Flashback, 154, 156
Flecainide (Tambocor), 251
Fluconazole (Diflucan), 354t, 513, 513t, 514t,
        519, 532, 534t, 536t, 537t
Flucytosine (Ancobon), 513, 513t, 514t, 516,
        517, 519, 534t, 537t
Fludarabine (Fludara), 570
Fludrocortisone (Florinef), 421
Fludrocortisone acetate (Florinef acetate), 421t
Fluid balance, 314

Fluid retention, 417
Flumazenil (Romazicon), 93, 139
Flunisolide (Aerobid), 363t
Fluori-methane, 101t
Fluoroquinolone antimicrobials, 505, 505t
Fluorouracil (Adrucil), 570
Fluoxetine (Prozac), 147, 147t, 537t
Fluoxymesterone (Halotestin), 442t
Flurazepam (Dalmane), 121t, 123, 137t
Flurbiprofen (Ansaid), 215t
Fluroethylchloride, 101t
Fluticasone (Flonase), 363t, 422t
Fluvastatin (Lescol), 325, 325t
Fluvoxamine (Luvox), 147t
Folic acid, 171, 313
    antagonists, 569–570
    deficiency, 338–340, 386f
Follicle-stimulating hormone (FSH), 410t,
        429–430, 433, 436, 437
Food guide pyramid, 308–309, 309f
Formaldehyde, 557, 558t, 559, 560t, 562
Foscarnet (Foscavir), 527t, 531, 532, 533, 535t
Fosinopril (Monopril), 284t
Fosphenytoin (Cerebyx), 169
Fraction, 39, 40–41, 40f
FSH (follicle-stimulating hormone), 410t,
        429–430, 433, 436, 437
Fungicidal, 511, 516
Furosemide (Lasix), 47, 241, 269t, 273, 274t,
        275, 282

Gabapentin (Neurontin), 168t, 170
Galantamine (Reminyl), 74t
Gallamine (Flaxedil), 88–90, 89f, 90t
Gametocytes, 543, 545
Gamma-aminobutyric acid (GABA), 118,
        120, 123, 137, 169
Gamma-interferon (γ-IFN), 581t
Ganciclovir (Cytovene), 525, 527t, 529, 531,
        532, 533, 535t, 537t
Ganglionic blocker, 82, 83–84, 84t
Ganglionic stimulant, 82, 83
Gastric lavage, 221, 332, 336
Gastritis, 125
Gastroesophageal reflux disease (GERD),
        373–374, 376, 377t
Gastrointestinal disorders, therapy of, 370–392
Gastrointestinal effects of drugs
    alcohol, 125
    anticholinergics, 76
    general anesthetics, 186
    opioids, 200, 200f, 207
    salicylates, 218
Gastrointestinal excretion of drugs, 20
Gastrointestinal stimulants, 375t, 377t,
        381–382
Gelatin capsules, 16
Gelatin film (Gelfilm), 301
Gelatin sponge (Gelfoam), 301
Gemfibrozil (Lopid), 325t, 327, 328, 329t, 475
General anesthesia, 98, 99
    adjuncts to, 188, 189t
    cautions and drug interactions, 188–190
    defined, 183, 184
    induction and maintenance, 184, 185
    inhalation anesthetics, 186, 187t
    injectable anesthetics, 186–188, 187t
    patient administration and
        monitoring, 190
    physiologic effects, 185–186
    route of administration, 185
    signs and stages of, 184–185, 185f

Generalized seizure, 166, 167
Generic name, 2, 8
Genetic variation, drug effects and, 22
Genitourinary system, anticholinergic drug
    effect on, 76–77
Gentamicin (Garamycin), 501t
Gentian violet, 512, 514t
GERD (gastroesophageal reflux disease), 370,
    373–374, 376, 377t
Geriatrics, 30–35
    anticholinergic drug use in, 78
    drug compliance, 34–35
    drug response, 33–34, 34t
    pharmacokinetics, 31–32, 33t
Giardia lamblia, 548
Gigantism, 408, 411
Glaucoma, 73, 188, 271
Glimepiride (Amaryl), 473, 474t
Glipizide (Glucotrol), 473, 474t
Glucagon, 465
Glucocorticoids, 415, 416–420, 418t, 419t,
    421t, 422t, 423t
Gluconeogenesis, 417, 420t, 464, 465
Glucose absorption inhibitors, 474t,
    475–477, 477f, 479
Glucose-6-phosphate dehydrogenase
    (G6PD), 546
Glutaraldehyde (Cidex), 557, 558t,
    560t, 562
Glyburide (DiaBeta, Glynase, Micronase),
    473, 474t
Glycerin (Osmoglyn), 269t, 270, 270t
Glycopyrrolate (Robinul, Robinul Forte), 77t,
    382, 383t
Glycosuria, 464, 466
Goiter, 450, 452, 455
Gold (^{198}Au), 571t
Gonadal hormones
    female sex hormones, 428–441
    male sex hormones, 441–444
Goserelin (Zoladex), 571
Gout, 222–224, 226t
Gram negative, 495
Gram positive, 495
Gram stain, 495
Grand mal seizure, 166, 167
Granisetron (Kytril), 389, 390t
Grepafloxacin (Raxar), 505t
Griseofulvin (Fulvicin-U/F, Grifulvin V,
    Grisactin-250, 500, Gris-PEG), 513t,
    514t, 516, 517, 534t
Growth hormone (somatotropin), 409, 411
Growth-stimulating hormone, 410t
Guaifenesin, 201, 202t
Guanabenz (Wytensin), 282
Guanadrel (Hylorel), 66
Guanethidine (Ismelin), 66, 283t
Guanfacine (Tenex), 282
Gynecomastia, 273

Halazepam (Paxipam), 137t
Half-life, drug, 14, 21
Hallucinogenic drug, 154, 155–157
Halofantrine, 551, 551t
Halogenated compounds, 183, 186, 558t
Haloperidol (Haldol), 134, 134t, 159
Haloprogin (Halotex), 513, 513t, 514t
Halothane (Fluothane), 186, 187t
Hashish, 154, 161
HDL. See High-density lipoprotein
HDN (hemorrhagic disease of the
    newborn), 292

Heart
    antiarrhythmic drugs, 247–253
    arrhythmias, 245–247, 246t
    blow flow through, 233f
    conduction system, 233–234
    diseases of, 234–235
    electrophysiology of, 247, 248t
    function, 233–234
    nerve supply, 234
Heart rate, 279, 280
Heavy metals, 557, 558t
Helicobacter pylori, 373, 392
Helper T-cells, 577, 578f, 581
Hemagglutinin, 524
Hematinics, 332, 335–336, 382t
Hematuria, 288, 292
Hemoglobin, 333
Hemorrhage, 288, 291
Hemorrhagic disease of the newborn
    (HDN), 292
Hemorrhoids, 402
Hemostatics, 300–301
Heparins, 290–292, 290t, 293t, 295,
    296, 299
Hepatic microsomal metabolism, 370,
    377, 529
Hernia, 397, 401
Heroin, 197, 197t, 198t
Herpes, 521, 526, 530
Herpes Zoster neuralgia, 103
Hexachlorophene (pHisoHex, Septisol), 557,
    558t, 559, 560t, 561, 562
Hexamethonium, 83
High-density lipoprotein (HDL), 322–323,
    324f, 325–328, 435, 439
Hirsutism, 428, 443
Histamine, 103–104, 346, 347–348, 348t,
    349f, 360
HIV. See Human immunodeficiency virus
HMG-CoA reductase inhibitors, 325–326,
    325t, 328–329, 329t
Homatropine, 77t
Homeostasis, 51, 52
Hormone antagonists, 570
Hormone replacement therapy (HRT), 430,
    431t, 433–434, 439–440
Hormones, 408, 409
    anterior pituitary, 409–412, 410f, 410t
    regulation of secretion, 411
    uses of, 409
Household system, of measurement, 43
H_2-receptor antagonists, 372f, 374t,
    376–380, 377t, 391
Human chorionic gonadotropin (HCG)
    (A.P.L., Chorex-5, Gonic, Pregnyl),
    437–438
Human immunodeficiency virus (HIV), 511,
    521–524, 522t, 523t
    antiviral drugs for, 524–526, 525f, 528t,
    529–533
    clinical profile, 521–523, 522t
Hydantoins, 169
Hydralazine (Apresoline), 242t, 283
Hydrochlorothiazide (Esidrix, Ezide,
    HydroDIURIL, Oretic), 269t, 272t,
    322t, 534t
Hydrocodone (Dicodid), 196, 197t, 200–201,
    201t, 220t
Hydrocortisone (Cortef, Cortisol,
    Hydrocortone), 418t, 419, 422t
Hydrocortisone acetate (Hydrocortone
    acetate), 419t, 422t

Hydrocortisone sodium phosphate
    (Hydrocortone phosphate), 422t
Hydrocortisone sodium succinate
    (A-hydroCort, Solu-Cortef), 422t
Hydroflumethiazide (Diucardin, Saluron),
    269t, 271, 272t
Hydrogen (H^+), 316
Hydrogen peroxide, 558t, 560t, 561
Hydromorphone (Dilaudid), 197t, 198t,
    200–201
Hydroxychloroquine (Plaquenil), 545, 545t
Hydroxycyanocobalamin (alpha-Redisol,
    Hydrobexan), 337
Hydroxyzine (Atarax, Vistaril), 351t, 352, 382
Hyoscyamine (Levsin), 77t, 382
Hyperacidity, 370, 373
Hyperalgesia, 194, 196
Hypercalcemia, 238, 240, 371, 385, 450, 456,
    457–458
Hyperchlorhydria, 371, 373
Hyperglycemia, 245, 251, 273, 464, 465
Hyperkalemia, 238, 240
Hyperkinesis, 148
Hyperlipidemia, 321, 323–324
Hypermotility, 371, 382
Hyperphosphatemia, 371, 386
Hypersensitivity, 98, 103, 104, 105, 556, 562
Hypertension, 34t
    antihypertensive therapy, 62–66, 84,
    281–285
    classification of, 281t
    definitions, 279–280
    essential, 279, 280
    malignant, 279, 285
    patient administration and
    monitoring, 285
    patient education, 285
    role of kidneys in, 281
    secondary, 280
Hyperthermia, 91, 189, 190
Hyperuricemia, 222, 271, 273
Hypervitaminosis, 305, 310, 311, 312, 313
Hypnotic drug, 118, 119
Hypochloremia, 265
Hypochloremic alkalosis, 272
Hypochromic, 333
Hypoglycemia, 465
Hypokalemia, 34t, 238, 240, 265, 271, 272,
    275, 397, 402, 423
Hypolipidemic drugs, 321–329
    adverse effects, 328
    bile acid sequestrants, 324–325, 325t,
    327–328, 329t
    cholesterol absorption inhibitors, 326
    clinical indications, 327
    contraindications, 327
    doses, table of, 325t
    drug interactions, 327–328, 329t
    fibric acid derivatives, 327
    HMG-CoA reductase inhibitors, 325–326,
    325t, 328, 329t
    nicotinic acid, 326–327
    patient administration and
    monitoring, 328
    use in pregnancy, 328–329
Hyponatremia, 397, 402
Hypoparathyroidism, 456
Hypophosphatemia, 385
Hypotension, 103, 122, 203
    orthostatic, 93, 272, 275, 276
Hypothalamus, 5, 111, 114, 183, 184, 409
Hypoxia, 183, 186, 190

IBS (irritable bowel syndrome), 76, 382, 384
Ibuprofen (Advil, Motrin, Nuprin), 215t, 220t, 296
ICSH (interstitial cell-stimulating hormone), 441
Idarubicin (Idamycin), 571t
Idoxuridine (Herplex), 525, 526, 527t, 530, 533
Ifosfamide (Ifex), 569t
Imipenem (Primaxin), 499, 535t
Imipramine (Tofranil), 146t, 354t, 453
Immunity, 511, 520
Immunopharmacology, 576, 577
Immunostimulant drugs, 581, 581t
Immunostimulation, 576, 577
Immunosuppression, 512, 523, 576, 577
Immunosuppressive drugs, 578–580
Impotence, 444
Improper fraction, 39, 40
Incompatibility, drug, 25t, 87, 91
Indandiones (anisindione), 294
Indapamide (Lozol), 269t, 272t, 322t
Indinavir (Crixivan), 525, 526, 528t, 529, 531–533, 535t, 536t
Individual variation, 14, 15, 22–23
Indomethacin (Indocin), 214, 215t, 223t, 226t, 460
Induction of general anesthesia, 184, 185
Infarction, 288
Infiltration anesthesia, 98, 102
Inflammation, 212–213, 213f
Infliximab (Remicade), 580
Influenza, 519–521, 526, 530
Inhalation administration, 17, 18t
Inhalation anesthetics, 186, 187t
Injectable anesthetics, 186–188, 187t
INR (international normalized ratio), 296, 298
Insomnia, 124
Insulin, 45
    secretion, 465
    therapy, 467–471, 468t, 472t
Interferons, 576, 577
Interleukin-2 (Proleukin), 581
Interleukins, 576, 577
International normalized ratio (INR), 296, 298
Interstitial cell-stimulating hormone (ICSH), 441
Intestinal motility, drugs affecting, 397–404
Intestinal stasis, 75–76
Intoxication, 212, 219
Intraarterial, administration, 18t
Intracellular fluid (ICF), 314
Intradermal anesthesia, 99, 102
Intramuscular (IM) injection, 14, 17, 18t
Intrathecal, administration, 18t
Intravenous (IV) fluid therapy, 314, 315t, 316
Intravenous (IV) infusion rates, monitoring, 46–47
Intravenous (IV) injection, 14, 17, 18t
Intrinsic factor, 333, 336
Iodine, 459, 558t, 559, 560t, 562
Iodine (^{131}I), 454–455, 455t, 459, 571t
Iodophors, 558t, 559, 562
Iodoquinol (Yodoxin), 547t, 548
Ipecac, 387–388
Ipratropium bromide (Atrovent), 362–363
Irbesartan (Avapro), 285
Iron deficiency anemia, 334–336
Iron preparations, 335–336, 335t
Irrigation, 557, 559
Irritable bowel syndrome (IBS), 76, 382, 384
Ischemia, 212, 214
Isocarboxazid (Marplan), 145t

Isoetharine (Bronkometer), 61t, 362t
Isoflurane (Forane), 186, 187t
Isoniazid (INH), 506–507, 535t, 536t
Isopropamide, 382
Isopropyl alcohol, 558t, 559, 561, 562
Isoproterenol (Isuprel, Medihaler-Iso, Mistometer), 61, 61t, 362t
Isosorbide (Ismotic, Isordil), 258t, 269t, 270, 270t
Isotonic, 305, 315
Isotretinoin (Accutane, Retin-A), 310
Isradipine (DynaCirc), 259, 283
Itraconazole (Sporanox), 328, 354t, 475, 513, 513t, 514t, 516, 517, 519, 532, 534t

Kanamycin (Kantrex), 189, 501t
Kaolin/pectin (Kaopectate), 241
Kappa receptor, 199
Keratinized tissues, 512
Ketamine (Ketalar), 186, 187t, 188–190
Ketoconazole (Nizoral), 354t, 513, 513t, 515t, 516, 517, 519, 535t, 536t, 537t
Ketoprofen (Orudis, Actron, Orudis-KT), 214, 215t, 296
Ketorolac tromethamine (Toradol), 215t
Ketosis, 464, 466, 467
Kidneys. See also Renal system
    conditions associated with dysfunction, 268–269
    renal physiology, 266–268
    role in hypertension, 281
Killer T-cells, 577, 578f, 581
Korsakoff's psychosis, 126

Labetalol (Normodyne), 64t
Labor induction, 486
Lactated Ringer's solution, 315t
Lactation, 428, 429
    drug exposure during, 23, 24t
Lactulose, 402, 403t
Lamivudine (3TC, Epivir), 525, 528t, 531, 536t
Lamotrigine (Lamictal), 170
Lansoprazole (Prevacid), 375t, 377t, 379t, 380–381
Laryngospasm, 190
Lavage, 212, 221
Laxatives, 401–402, 403t, 404
LD50, 2, 7
LDL. See Low-density lipoprotein
Lecithin (Phoschol), 76
Leflunomide (Arava), 580
Lepirudin, 292
LET (lidocaine, epinephrine, tetracaine), 101t, 102
Leukopenia, 212, 224
Leukotriene inhibitor drugs, 363
Leukotrienes, 360
Leuprolide (Lupron), 571
Levamisole (Ergamisol), 581t
Levetiracetam (Keppra), 170
Levodopa (Dopar, Larodopa), 176–178, 177t, 336
Levodopa/Carbidopa (Sinemet), 177, 177t
Levofloxacin (Levaquin), 505t
Levomethadyl (Orlaam), 204, 205t
Levonorgestrel (Norplant System), 432t, 436
Levorphanol (Levo-Dromoran), 197t, 198t, 207
Levothyroxine sodium (Levothroid, Synthroid), 452t
LH (luteinizing hormone), 410t, 429–430, 436, 437, 441
L-hyoscyamine (Levsin), 383t

Lidocaine (Xylocaine, Solarcaine, Aloe Extra, Lidoderm), 101t, 102, 103, 189, 248t, 250
Limbic system, 111, 114–115, 137
Linezolid (Zyvox), 506
Liothyronine sodium (Cytomel), 452t
Lipid solubility, 18–19
Lipodystrophy, 464, 470
Lipolysis, 291
Lipoprotein, 321, 322–328. See also High-density lipoprotein (HDL); Low-density lipoprotein (LDL)
Lipoprotein lipase, 290
Lisinopril (Prinivil, Zestril), 242t, 284t
Lithium (Eskalith, Lithobid), 24t, 143, 144, 149–150, 275, 453, 454
Liver
    general anesthetic effect on, 186
    metabolism, 322
Loading dose, 14, 21
Local anesthesia, 98–105
    adverse effects, 102–103
    characteristics of commonly employed, 101t
    clinical applications, 103
    drug interactions, 103–104
    mechanism of action, 99, 100f, 100t
    patient administration and monitoring, 105
    pharmacology, 99–100
    route of administration, 100, 102
    site of action, 195f
Lomefloxacin (Maxaquin), 505t
Lomustine (CeeNU), 569t
Loop diuretics. See Organic acid diuretics
Loop of Henle, 267f, 268
Loperamide, 401
Loratadine (Claritin, Alavert), 350, 351t, 352
Lorazepam (Ativan), 137t, 138, 170, 551t
Losartan (Cozaar), 285
Lovastatin (Mevacor), 325–326, 325t, 327, 328
Low-density lipoprotein (LDL), 322–328, 324f, 435, 439
Loxapine (Loxitane), 134t, 135
Lozenges, 16
LSD (lysergic acid diethylamide), 155–156
Luteinizing hormone (LH), 410t, 429–430, 436, 437, 441
Lymphocytes, 577–581
Lymphopenia, 576, 578
Lypressin (Diapid), 485–486, 488t
Lyse, 557
Lysergic acid diethylamide (LSD), 155–156
Lysosomes, 415, 418

Macrolide antibiotics, 504–505
Macrophages, 577, 578f
Mafenide (Sulfamylon), 503t
Magnesium citrate, 403t, 404
Magnesium hydroxide, 384t, 385t, 386, 403t
Maintenance dose, 14, 21, 238, 240
Maintenance of general anesthesia, 184, 185
Malabsorption, 333, 335
Malaria, 543
    antimalarial drugs, 544–547, 545t
    stages of, 544f
Male sex hormones, 441–444, 442t
Malignant, 566, 567
Malignant hypertension, 279, 285
Malignant hyperthermia, 87, 91, 92, 189, 190
Mania, 143, 149

Mannitol (Osmitrol), 269, 269t, 270t,
275–276
MAO inhibitors. See Monoamine oxidase
(MAO) inhibitors
Maprotiline (Ludiomil), 146t
Marijuana, 160–162
Mast cells, 349f, 378
Measurement, systems of, 42–44
Mebendazole (Vermox), 550t
Mecamylamine (Inversine), 84, 283t
Mechanism of action, 2, 5
Mechlorethamine (Mustargen),
568–569, 569t
Meclizine (Antivert, Bonine), 351t, 389, 390t
Meclofenamate (Meclomen), 214, 215t
Meclofenamic acid (Ponstel), 214, 215t
Medroxyprogesterone (Amen, Curretab,
Cycrin, Depo-Provera, Provera), 431t,
436, 438
Medulla oblongata, 111, 114
Medullary depression, 184
Medullary paralysis, 184
Mefloquine (Lariam), 544–546, 545t, 551,
551t, 552
Mega-, definition of, 333
Megaloblastic anemia, 212, 217, 339
Megaloblasts, 333
Megestrol (Megace), 438
Meloxicam (Mobic), 215t
Melphalan (Alkeran), 569t
Memory cells, 577, 578f
Menarche, 428
Menopause, 428, 433–434, 445–446
Menotropins (Pergonal, Humegon), 437–438
Menstrual bleeding disorders, 438
Menstruation, 428, 429
Mental illness, 132
Meperidine (Demerol), 45, 197t, 198t, 203,
206–207
Mephenytoin, 169
Mepivacaine (Carbocaine), 101t, 102
Meprobamate, 220t, 382
Mercaptopurine (Purinethol), 570
Mescaline, 156
Mestranol, 432t
Metabolic acidosis, 268, 316
Metabolic alkalosis, 316
Metabolic waste products, 266, 268
Metaproterenol (Alupent), 61t, 362t
Metaraminol (Aramine), 60t
Metastasis, 567
Metaxalone (Skelaxin), 93t
Metformin (Glucophage, Glucophage XR),
474t, 477–479
Methacholine, 73
Methadone (Dolophine, Intensol, Methadone),
197t, 198t, 199, 204, 205t, 234
Methamphetamine (Desoxyn), 148t, 157
Methaqualone, 124
Methazolamide (Neptazane), 269t, 270t
Methdilazine (Tacaryl), 351t
Methicillin (Staphcillin), 189, 498t
Methimazole (Tapazole), 455, 455t
Methocarbamol (Robaxin), 89f, 93t
Methohexital (Methohexital), 186–187,
187t, 189
Methotrexate, 551t, 569–570
Methoxamine (Vasoxyl), 60t
Methoxyflurane (Penthrane), 186, 187t
Methscopolamine (Pamine), 77t
Methyclothiazide (Aquatensen, Enduron),
269t, 272t

Methyl salicylate (oil of wintergreen,
Ben-Gay, Deep-Heat), 217
Methyldopa (Aldomet), 65, 189, 282,
283t, 336
Methylenedioxyamphetamine (MDA), 160
Methylenedioxyethamphetamine (MDEA),
160
Methylenedioxymethamphetamine
(MDMA), 160
Methylergonovine (Methergine), 486, 488t
Methylphenidate (Ritalin), 148t
Methylprednisolone acetate (A-Methapred,
depMedalone 40, Depo-Medrol,
Depoject, D-Med 80, Medrol,
Solu-Medrol), 418t, 419t, 422t
Methyltestosterone (Oreton Methyl, Android-
25, Testred, Virilon), 442t
Methylthiouracil, 455
Metoclopramide (Reglan, Maxolon, Clopra,
Octamide, Reclomide), 375t, 377t,
379t, 381–382, 389, 390t
Metolazone (Zaroxolyn), 269t, 271, 272t
Metoprolol (Lopressor), 64t, 283t, 378
Metric system, of measurement, 42–43
Metronidazole (Flagyl, Metizol, Protostat),
373, 392, 537t, 547t, 548, 549, 552
Mexiletine (Mexitil), 251
Mezlocillin sodium (Mezlin), 498t
Miconazole (Micatin, Monistat-Derm), 354t,
512, 513, 513t, 515t, 516, 517, 534t
Micro-, definition of, 333
Midazolam (Versed), 93, 139, 186, 187t, 188,
190, 534t
Miglitol (Glyset), 474t, 475
Mineral oil, 403t, 404
Mineralocorticoids, 415, 420–421, 420t, 421t
Minerals, 314–315
deficiency, 307t
recommended dietary allowance, 307t
Minocycline (Minocin), 502, 502t
Minoxidil (Loniten), 283
Miosis, 203
Misoprostol (Cytotec), 374t, 380, 392
Mivacurium (Mivacron), 90t
Mixed number, 39, 40
Mixed-function oxidase system, 30, 32
Molindone (Moban), 134t, 135
Mometasone (Nasonex), 422t
Monoamine oxidase (MAO), 58, 58f, 143, 144
Monoamine oxidase (MAO) inhibitors,
144–145, 145t, 149, 207
Monoamine Theory of Mental Depression,
143, 144, 149
Monophasic, 428, 430
Montelukast (Singulair), 364
Moricizine (Ethmozine), 251
Morning sickness, 389, 390t
Morphine, 5, 19, 45, 189, 197, 197t, 198t,
199, 202, 207, 400–401
Morphology, 333
Motion sickness, 352, 387
Mountain sickness, 271
Moxifloxacin (Avelox), 505t
Mucolytics, 358, 364
Mucopolysaccharide, 288, 290
Multiple sclerosis, 92, 93
Muromonab-CD3 (Orthoclone OKT3), 580
Muscarinic receptors, 70, 72–73, 72f
Mutagenic drugs, 576, 579
Myalgia, 212
Myasthenia gravis, 74, 75, 89, 91

Mycophenolate mofetil (CellCept), 580
Mycosis, 512
Mydriasis, 77, 78, 83, 203
Myelosuppression, 567, 568
Myocardial infarction, 232, 235
Myocardium, 232, 233
Myoclonic seizures, 167
Myxedema, 450, 452

Nabumetone (Relafen), 215t
Nadolol (Corgard), 63, 64t
Nafcillin sodium (Unipen), 498t
Naftifine (Naftin), 515t
Nalbuphine (Nubain), 198t, 199
Nalmefene (Revex), 204, 205t
Naloxone (Narcan), 5, 199, 204–205, 205t
Naltrexone (ReVia), 205t
Nandrolone (Durabolin), 442t
Nandrolone decanoate (Deca-Durabolin), 442t
Naproxen (Aleve, Anaprox, Naprosyn), 215t,
223t, 296
Narcolepsy, 148
Narcotic analgesics. See Opioid analgesics
Narcotic (opioid) antagonists, 194, 204–205,
205t
Narcotics, 194, 400t, 401
Nateglinide (Starlix), 473, 474t
Nausea, 190, 387, 388
Nedocromil (Tilade), 364
Nefazodone (Serzone), 148
Nelfinavir (Viracept), 525, 526, 528t,
529, 533, 536t
Neomycin (Neobiotic), 501t
Neostigmine (Prostigmin), 74, 74t, 76, 90
Nephritis, 266, 268
Nephrotoxicity, 531, 532
Nerve conduction, 99, 100f
Nerve depression, 99, 100t
Nerve supply, cardiac, 234
Neural tube defects, 171
Neuraminidase inhibitors, 524, 530
Neuroleptanalgesia, 184, 188
Neuroleptanesthesia, 184, 188
Neuroleptic, 131, 132
Neuroleptic malignant syndrome, 133–134
Neuromuscular blocking drugs, 188, 551t
Neuromuscular junction, 87, 88, 89f
Neurons, 112, 113f
Neuropathic pain, 194, 195
Neuropathy, 464, 466
Neurosis, 131, 132
Neurotransmitter, 51, 53–54, 112, 113f, 176
Neutropenia, 531
Nevirapine (Viramune), 525, 528t, 531, 536t
Niacin (Niacor), 325t, 326–327
Niacin, dietary, 313, 317
Niacin and lovastatin (Advicor), 325t, 326
Nicardipine (Cardene), 259, 283, 284t
Nicotine (Nicorette, Nicoderm, Habitrol), 82, 83
Nicotinic acid (Niacor), 325t, 326–327
Nicotinic acid, dietary, 313, 317
Nicotinic-II (NII) receptors, 88, 89, 91
Nicotinic-muscle (Nm) receptor, 70, 73
Nicotinic-neural (Nn) receptor, 70, 73, 82, 83
Nifedipine (Procardia), 259, 283, 284t
Nitric oxide (NO), 257
Nitrites and nitrates
adverse effects, 258
for angina, 257–259, 258t
clinical use of nitroglycerin, 257–258
mechanism of action, 257
patient education, 258–259

Nitrogen mustards, 568
Nitroglycerin *(Nitro-bid, Nitrostat, Nitrogard, Transderm-Nitro)*, 16, 242t, 257–259, 258t
Nitromersol *(Metaphen)*, 558t, 560t, 561, 562
Nitrosoureas, 568, 569t
Nitrous oxide, 185, 186, 187t, 188
Nizatidine *(Axid)*, 374t, 377–378, 377t, 379t
NNRTI (nonnucleoside reverse transcriptase inhibitors), 525
NO (nitric oxide), 257
Nociceptin, 199
Nociceptive pain, 195
Nociceptor, 194, 195
Nocistatin, 199
Nonbarbiturate drug, 118, 119
Nondepolarizing blockers, 87, 88–89
Nonnucleoside reverse transcriptase inhibitors (NNRTI), 525
Nonopioid analgesics, 194, 196, 213–222, 224–226. *See also* Nonsteroidal antiinflammatory drugs (NSAIDs)
    acetaminophen, 220–222, 249t
    doses, recommended adult, 215t–216t
    drug interactions, 224, 226t
    drug mixtures containing, 220t
    patient administration and monitoring, 225
    salicylates, 217–220
Nonprescription drug, 2, 8
Nonselective beta-adrenergic blocker, 57, 59, 66f
Nonsteroidal antiinflammatory drugs (NSAIDs), 196
    absorption and metabolism, 216
    acetaminophen, 220–222, 249t
    adverse effects, 216–217
    clinical indications, 214, 216
    doses, recommended adult, 215t–216t
    drug interactions, 224, 226t
    mechanism of action, 213, 214
    patient administration and monitoring, 225
    salicylates, 217–220
    special considerations, 217
Norepinephrine *(Levophed)*, 60t
Norepinephrine, endogenous, 51, 54, 58–60, 58f, 59t, 63, 65–66, 65f, 157, 157f, 429f
Norethindrone *(Norlutin)*, 431t, 432t
Norethynodrel and mestranol *(Enovid)*, 431t
Norfloxacin *(Noroxin)*, 505t
Norgestrel, 432t
Normocytic anemia, 333, 339
Nortriptyline *(Aventyl)*, 146t
Noscapine, 200
Nosocomial infections, 557, 559
NREM (nonrapid eye movement) sleep, 118, 119, 124
NSAIDs. *See* Nonsteroidal antiinflammatory drugs
Nucleoside analogs, 525
Nucleosides, 512, 525
Numerator, 39, 40
Nursing, drug exposure during, 23, 24t
Nutrition, 305–317
    alcohol effect on, 126
    body water and, 314
    diet and disease, 306–307
    dietary recommendations, 307–308
    electrolytes, 315–316

food guide pyramid, 308–309, 308f
    minerals, 314–315
    patient administration and monitoring, 317
    recommended dietary allowances (RDA), 307, 307t
    vitamins, 307t, 309–314, 317
Nutritional status, drug response and, 33
Nystagmus, 245, 251
Nystatin *(Mycostatin, Nilstat, Nystex)*, 512, 513t, 515t, 516, 517, 519

Obsessive-compulsive disorders (OCD), 147
Ocular effects, of anticholinergic drugs, 77
Ofloxacin *(Floxin)*, 505t
Ointments, 16
Olanzapine *(Zyprexa)*, 134t, 135
Oligospermia, 428, 443
Oliguria, 194, 203, 266, 268
Omeprazole *(Prilosec)*, 375t, 377t, 379t, 380–381
Ondansetron *(Zofran)*, 389, 390t
Opiates, 194, 197, 400, 400t
Opioid analgesics, 193–207
    absorption and metabolism, 203
    acute poisoning, 204
    adverse effects, 203–204
    antagonists to, 204–205, 205t
    antitussives, 200–201, 201t, 202t
    cardiovascular effects, 203
    cautions and contraindications, 204–205
    clinical indications, 205
    CNS effects, 199–200, 200f
    doses, table of, 198t
    drug interactions, 206–207
    eye effects, 203
    gastrointestinal effects, 200, 200f, 207
    patient administration and monitoring, 206–207
    pharmacologic effects, 197t, 199–203
    respiratory depression from, 200, 204, 205t
    schedule classification, 197, 201t
    site and mechanism of action, 195f, 199
    smooth muscle effects, 202–203
    tolerance and physical dependence, 196, 203–204
    withdrawal (abstinence syndrome), 204
Opioid antagonists, 204–205, 205t
Opium *(Opium Tincture)*, 198t, 400, 400t, 401
Opportunistic organisms, 512, 523
Oral administration, 15, 17, 18t
Oral contraceptives, 392, 424, 430, 432t, 433, 435–438, 440–441, 445, 534t, 536t
Oral hypoglycemic drugs, 471–475, 474t, 476t
Organic acid diuretics, 269t, 273, 274t
Orphenadrine, 89f
Orthostatic hypotension, 203, 272, 275, 276
Oseltamivir *(Tamiflu)*, 524, 526, 529, 530
Osmosis, 398, 402
Osmotic diuretics, 122, 269–270, 269t, 270t
Osmotic pressure, 19
Osteoporosis, 428, 434–435, 451, 458, 460
Ototoxic drugs, 502
Over-the-counter (OTC) drug, 2, 8
Ovulation, 428, 429
Ovulation stimulants, 437–438
Oxacillin sodium *(Prostaphlin)*, 498t
Oxandrolone *(Oxandrin)*, 442t
Oxaprozin *(DayPro)*, 215t
Oxazepam *(Serax)*, 137t

Oxazolidinediones, 170
Oxiconazole *(Oxistat)*, 515t, 517
Oxidized cellulose *(Oxycel, Surgicel, Hemo-Pak)*, 301
Oxidizing agents, 558t
Oxybutynin *(Ditropan, Ditropan XL)*, 77t
Oxychlorosene calcium, 560t
Oxycodone *(Roxicodone)*, 197t, 198t, 199, 220t
Oxymetholone *(Anadrol 50)*, 442t
Oxymorphone *(Numorphan)*, 197t, 198t, 199
Oxyntic cells, 376
Oxyphenbutazone, 257f
Oxyphencyclimine *(Daricon)*, 383t, 384
Oxytetracycline *(Terramycin)*, 502t
Oxytocics, 486–487, 488t
Oxytocin *(Pitocin, Syntocinon)*, 409, 484–486, 488t

Paclitaxel *(Taxol)*, 4, 570, 571t
Paget's disease, 451, 458, 460
Pain, 195–196, 195f
Pamabrom, 269t, 274
Pamidronate *(Aredia)*, 457t, 458
Pancuronium *(Pavulon)*, 88–90, 89f, 90t
Pantopon, 198t
Pantoprazole *(Protonix)*, 375t, 377t, 380–381
Paramethadione *(Paradione)*, 170
Parasitic worm infestations, 549–552
Parasympathetic nervous system, 51, 52–54, 53f, 54f, 54t
    drugs affecting, 70–78
Parasympatholytic, 70, 76
Parasympathomimetic, 70, 73, 74
Parathyroid hormones, 456
Paregoric *(Paregoric)*, 198t, 400, 400t
Parenteral administration, 15, 17, 18t
Parietal (oxyntic) cells, 371, 376
Parkinsonism, 131, 133, 175, 176
Parkinson's disease, 77, 175, 176
    drugs used to treat, 175–180
Paromomycin *(Humatin)*, 547–548, 547t
Paroxetine *(Paxil)*, 147t
Partial seizure, 166, 167–168, 170
Partial thromboplastin time (PTT), 296, 298
Pathogenic, 495
Patient-controlled-analgesia, 206
PCP (phencyclidine), 160
Pediatrics
    dosage calculations, 45–46
    drug considerations, 23–25, 28t
Pegaspargase *(Oncaspar)*, 571t
PEG-ES (polyethylene glycol-electrolyte solution), 402, 403t
Penicillamine, 336
Penicillin G, 189, 497, 498t
Penicillin G benzathine *(Bicillin)*, 498t
Penicillin G procaine *(Wycillin)*, 498t
Penicillin V, 497
Penicillin V potassium K *(Pen-Vee K, V-Cillin K)*, 498t
Penicillinase, 495, 497, 499
Penicillins, 497–499, 498t
Pentamidine, 532, 537t
Pentazocine *(Talwin)*, 197t, 198t, 207
Pentobarbital *(Nembutal)*, 121t, 122
Pentolinium, 83
Pentostatin *(Nipent)*, 570
Percent, 39, 42
Percent composition, 306, 315
Perforation, 371, 373
Pergolide *(Permax)*, 178

Perimenopause, 428, 433
Peripheral nerve, 194, 195
Peripheral neuropathy, from antivirals, 531
Peripheral resistance, 280
Peripheral skeletal muscle relaxant,
    88–91, 106f
Peristalsis, 398
Pernicious anemia, 336–337
Pernicious, definition of, 333
Peroxide, 558t
Perphenazine (Trilafon), 352, 389, 390t
Petechia, 212, 218
Petit mal. See Absence seizure
Phagocyte, 212, 222–223, 224f
Pharmacodynamics, 4t, 33–34
Pharmacokinetics, 4t, 31–32, 33t
Pharmacology, 2, 3, 3t
Pharmacotherapeutics, 4t
Phenacetin, 221
Phencyclidine (PCP), 160
Phenelzine (Nardil), 145t
Phenethylamine derivatives, 156–157
Phenindamine (Nolahist), 351t
Phenobarbital (Luminal, Solfoton), 8f, 121,
    121t, 168t, 169, 171, 424
Phenolphthalein, 402
Phenols, 558t, 559
Phenothiazines, 133–134, 134t
Phentolamine (Regitine), 63t
Phenylbutazone, 257f
Phenylephrine, 60t, 201
Phenylpropanolamine, 201, 201t, 202t
Phenytoin (Dilantin), 24t, 168t, 169, 171,
    251, 253, 424, 537t
Pheochromocytoma, 62
Phlegm, 194, 201
Phosphate, 464, 467
Phosphodiesterases (PDE), 444
Phosphorated carbohydrate solution
    (Emetrol, Nausetrol), 389, 392
Phosphorus (^{32}P), 571t
Phthalylsulfathiazole, 503t
Physical dependence, 194, 196, 203–204. See
    also Dependency
Physician's Desk Reference (PDR), 8
Physostigmine (Antilirium, Eserine), 74, 74t,
    76, 78
Phytoestrogens, 435
Pilocarpine (Pilocar, Ocusert-Pilo), 73, 74t
Pimozide (Orap), 134t, 135
Pindolol (Visken), 64t
Pinworms, 549, 550t, 551
Pioglitazone (Actos), 474t, 480
Pipecuronium (Arduan), 90t
Piperacillin (Pipracil), 498t
Piperacillin-tazobactam (Zosyn), 499
Piperazine (Antepar), 550
Pirbuterol (Maxair), 362t
Piroxicam (Feldene), 214, 215t
Pituitary gland, 114, 409–412, 410f, 470f
Placebo effect, 22
Plant extracts, as antineoplastics, 570, 571t
Plasma protein binding, 19, 25, 32
Poloxamer-iodine (Prepodyne, Septodyne),
    558t, 560t
Polycarbophil, 403t
Polydipsia, 464, 466
Polyethylene glycol-electrolyte solution
    (PEG-ES), 402, 403t
Polypeptide, 451, 458, 484, 485
Polyphagia, 464, 466

Polypharmacy, 30, 34
Polythiazide (Renese), 269t, 272t, 322t
Polyuria, 466
Pons, 111, 114
Porphyria, 512, 517
Posology, 4t
Posterior pituitary powder, 485
Postpartum, 484, 486
Potassium (K$^+$), 316
Potassium bitartrate, 403t
Potassium iodide and iodine (Lugol's solution,
    Thyro-Block), 454, 455t
Potassium-sparing diuretics, 269t,
    273–274, 274t
Potency, 2, 6
Potentiation, of effect, 88, 91
Povidone-iodine (Betadine, Isodine), 558t, 560t
Powders, 15
Pralidoxime (Protopam), 74
Pramipexole (Mirapex), 177t, 178
Pravastatin (Pravachol), 325, 325t, 327
Prazepam (Centrax), 137t
Praziquantel (Biltricide), 550t
Prazosin (Minipress), 63t, 242t, 283t
Prednisolone (Delta-Cortef, Hydeltra-TBA,
    Predcor 25, Predcor 50, Prelone), 418t,
    422t, 578
Prednisolone acetate (Key-Pred, Predcor,
    Articulose, Predaject-50), 419t, 422t
Prednisolone tebutate (Hydeltra-TBA,
    Predalone-TBA), 419t
Prednisone (Deltasone, Meticortone, Orasone,
    Panasol), 363, 418t, 422t, 578
Pregnancy, drug use in, 23, 23t
    adrenal steroids, 425
    alcohol, 126–127
    aminoglycoside, 501
    anticoagulants, 300
    antidiarrheals and laxatives, 404
    antiepileptic drugs, 171
    antifungals, 519
    antihistamines, 355
    antineoplastic drugs, 572
    antipsychotics, 136
    antivirals, 533
    barbiturates, 142
    benzodiazepines, 124, 139
    diuretics, 276
    estrogens, 440
    gastrointestinal drugs, 392
    hypolipidemic drugs, 328–329
    lithium, 150
    local anesthetics, 105
    metronidazole, 549, 552
    nicotine, 83
    nonopioid analgesics, 225
    opioids, 205, 207
    quinine, 552
    sex hormones, 446
    skeletal muscle relaxants, 94
    tetracyclines, 502–503
    thyroid hormones, 454, 459
    vitamin A, 310
    vitamin supplements, 317
Premature atrial contraction, 245, 246, 246t
Premature rupture of obstetrical membranes
    (PROM), 488
Premature ventricular contraction (PVC),
    240, 245, 246, 246t, 247f
Prescription drug, 2, 8
Pressor, 484

Prez-Pak, 101t
Prilocaine (Citanest), 101t, 102
Primaquine, 545, 545t, 546
Primidone (Mysoline), 169
Probenecid, 223t, 224, 226t, 530, 532, 535t,
    536t, 537t
Procainamide (Procanbid), 248t, 250, 253
Procaine (Novocain), 101t, 102, 104, 105
Procarbazine (Matulane), 571t
Prochlorperazine (Compazine), 134t, 189,
    352, 389, 390t
Procyclidine (Kemadrin), 179t
Progesterone, 429–430, 429f, 431t, 436,
    438–440
Progestogen drugs, 431t
Prolactin, 410t
Promazine, 189
Promethazine (Phenergan), 134t, 189, 201t,
    350, 351t, 352, 353, 389, 390t
Propafenone (Rythmol), 251
Propantheline (Pro-Banthine), 77t, 382, 383t
Proper fraction, 39, 40
Prophylactic, definition of, 347
Prophylactic drugs, 348
Prophylaxis, 212, 223, 543, 544
Propofol (Diprivan), 186–188, 187t
Proportion, 39, 42
Propoxyphene (Darvon, Dolene), 197t,
    198t, 220t
Propranolol (Inderal), 63, 64t, 160, 248t, 251,
    253, 259, 283, 283t
Propylthiouracil, 455, 455t
Prostacyclin, 294
Prostaglandins, 212–213, 213f, 218, 221,
    359, 360, 372f, 374t, 380
    for therapeutic abortion, 486–487
Prostatic cancer, 431t
Prostatic hypertrophy, 34t
Protamine sulfate, 291
Protein catabolism, 417, 420t
Proteolytic, 371
Prothrombin time (PT), 296, 298
Proton pump inhibitors, 372f, 375t, 377t,
    380–381
Protozoal infections, 543–549, 547t, 551t
Protozoan, 543
Protriptyline (Vivactil), 146t
Proximal convoluted tubule (PCT),
    266, 267f
Pseudoephedrine, 60t, 201, 201t, 202t, 354t
Pseudomembranous colitis, 506
Psilocybin, 156
Psychomotor stimulants, 143, 148, 148t,
    157–160
Psychosis, 131, 132, 158, 159
Psychotomimetic drugs, 154–162
Psyllium hydrophilic, 403t
PT (prothrombin time), 296, 298
PTT (partial thromboplastin time),
    296, 298
Puberty, 428
Purine antagonists, 570
PVC (premature ventricular contraction),
    240, 245, 246, 246t, 247f
Pyrantel pamoate (Antiminth, Pin-Rid, Pin-X),
    550, 550t
Pyrazinamide, 507
Pyriamine/pheniramine/phentoloxamine
    (Poly-Histine Elixir), 351t
Pyridostigmine (Mestinon), 74t, 75
Pyridoxine, 313

Pyrilamine, 201
Pyrimethamine *(Daraprim)*, 544, 545, 545t, 549, 551t

Quantal dose-response curves, 6
Quaternary ammonium compounds, 558t, 559
Quazepam *(Doral)*, 121t
Quetiapine *(Seroquel)*, 134t
Quinestrol *(Estrovis)*, 431t, 436
Quinethazone *(Hydromox)*, 269t, 272t, 282, 322t
Quinidine *(Cardioquin, Quinaglute, Quinidex)*, 241, 248–250, 248t, 253, 535t, 536t
Quinine, 3–4, 544–548, 545t, 551, 551t, 552
Quinolones, 336
Quinupristin-dalfopristin *(Synercid)*, 506

Rabeprazole *(Aciphex)*, 375t, 377t, 380–381
Radical cure, 543, 544
Radioactive iodide (^{131}I), 454–455, 455t, 459, 571t
Radioactive isotopes, 571t, 572
Raloxifene *(Evista)*, 434
Ramipril *(Altace)*, 284t
Ranitidine *(Zantac)*, 374t, 377–379, 379t, 391, 460
Ranitidine bismuth citrate *(Tritec)*, 375t
Rapacuronium *(Raplon)*, 90t
Ratio, 39, 42
Raynaud's disease, 62
Reactive depression, 143, 144
Receptor, 3, 5
Recommended Dietary Allowance (RDA), 307, 307t
Rectal, administration, 18t
Red blood cell (RBC), 333
Referred pain, 194, 196
Reflexes, 114
Refractory, definition of, 266
Refractory diuretic, 271
REM (rapid eye movement) sleep, 118, 120, 124
Remifentanil *(Ultima)*, 198t
Remission, 567, 568
Renal system
    alcohol effects on, 125–126
    dysfunction, 34t, 268–269
    excretion, of drugs, 20, 529–530
    filtration, 266
    physiology, 266–268
    tubular reabsorption, 266–268
    tubular secretion, 268
Renin, 280, 281
Repaglinide *(Prandin)*, 473, 474t, 475
Replacement therapy, 415, 416, 417–418
Repository preparation, 415, 419
Reproductive cycle, female, 428–430, 429f
Reserpine, 65–66
Resistance, to drugs, 525–526, 566, 568
Respiratory acidosis, 316
Respiratory alkalosis, 316
Respiratory excretion, of drugs, 21
Respiratory syncytial virus (RSV), 526
Respiratory system
    anticholinergic drug effect on, 76
    disease, 34t, 359–360
    skeletal muscle relaxant effect on, 90
Reteplase *(Retavase)*, 299
Reticular formation, 111, 114, 120, 137–138
Retinoic acids, 24t, 310

Retinol, 309
Reye's syndrome, 219, 512, 521
Rhabdomyolysis, 326
Rheumatic fever, 212, 218
Ribavirin *(Virazole)*, 526, 527t
Riboflavin, 313–314, 317
Rifabutin, 536t, 551t
Rifampin *(Rifadin)*, 424, 475, 507, 534t, 535t, 536t, 537t, 551, 551t
Rimantadine *(Flumadine)*, 526, 527t, 530, 536t
Ringer's solution, 315t
Risedronate *(Actonel)*, 457t, 458
Risperidone *(Risperdal)*, 134t, 135
Ritodrine *(Yutopar)*, 487–488, 488t
Ritonavir *(Norvir)*, 525, 528t, 529, 530, 533, 536t
Rofecoxib *(Vioxx)*, 214, 216t
Rocuronium *(Zemuron)*, 90t
Ropinirole *(Requip)*, 177t, 178
Ropivacaine *(Naropin)*, 101t
Rosiglitazone *(Avandia)*, 474t, 480
Roundworms, 549–550, 550t
Routes of administration, 17, 20t
RSV (respiratory syncytial virus), 526

SA (sinoatrial) node, 234
Salicylamide, 217
Salicylates, 215t, 217–220, 225, 226t
Salicylic acid *(Amigesic, Disalcid, Arthra-G)*, 215t
Salicylism, 212, 219
Salivary and bronchial secretions, general anesthetic effect on, 186
Salmeterol *(Serevent)*, 61t, 362t
Saquinavir *(Invirase)*, 525, 526, 528t, 529, 533, 535t, 536t, 537t
Sargramostim (macrophage-CSF), 581t
Schilling test, 337
Schizophrenia, 131, 132
Scopolamine *(Transderm-Scop)*, 76–77, 77t, 179, 189, 382, 383t, 390t, 391
Secobarbital *(Seconal)*, 45, 121t, 122
Secondary hypertension, 280
Secretagogues, 471–475, 474t, 476t
Sedative, 118, 119
Sedative-hypnotic drugs, 118–127, 121t
    as adjunct to general anesthesia, 188, 189t
Seizures, 166, 167
    absence, 167
    drugs for control of, 168–171, 168t
    generalized, 167
    myoclonic, 167
    partial, 167–168
    tonic-clonic, 167
Selective beta-1 adrenergic blocker, 57, 59
Selective beta-2 adrenergic blocker, 58, 59, 66f
Selective COX-2 inhibitors, 212, 214, 216t, 227
Selective estrogen receptor modulators (SERMs), 434
Selective serotonin reuptake inhibitors (SSRIs), 147–148, 147t, 149
Selegiline *(Eldepryl)*, 177t, 178
Semisolid preparations, 15
Semustine *(Methyl-CCNU)*, 569t
Senna preparations, 403t
Sensitize, 347
SERMs (selective estrogen receptor modulators), 434
Serotonin, 133, 139

Serotonin (5-HT) antagonists, 388, 390t
Sertraline *(Zoloft)*, 147t
Sex hormones
    female, 428–430, 429f, 433–441
    male, 441–444, 442t
Side effect, 3, 4
Sildenafil *(Viagra)*, 444
Silver nitrate, 558t, 560t, 561
Silver protein *(Argyrol)*, 558t, 561t
Silver sulfadiazine *(Silvadene)*, 503t, 558t, 561, 561t
Simvastatin *(Zocor)*, 325, 325t, 327
Sinoatrial (SA) node, 249, 252
Site of action, 3, 5, 15
Skeletal muscle, general anesthetic effect on, 186
Skeletal muscle relaxants, 87–94
    adjunct to general anesthesia, 188, 189t
    antidotes to, 76
    centrally-acting, 87, 88, 92–93, 93t
    direct-acting, 91–92
    patient administration and monitoring, 94
    peripherally-acting, 88–91, 106f
Sleep cycle, 119–120, 124, 417
Smoking, 26
Smooth muscle
    histamine effects on, 348
    opioid effects on, 202–203
Sodium (Na$^+$), 315
    reabsorption along the nephron, 266–268, 267f
    retention, 421
Sodium bicarbonate, 219, 220t, 384–386, 385t, 403t, 551t
Sodium biphosphate, 403t
Sodium chloride, 315t
Sodium hypochlorite *(Dakin's solution)*, 558t, 561t, 562
Sodium hypochlorite mixture *(Chlorpactin-XCB, Chlorpactin-WCS-90)*, 558t
Sodium nitroprusside *(Nipride)*, 242t, 285
Sodium phosphate, 403t
Sodium thiosalicylate *(Rexolate)*, 223t
Solid preparations, 15
Solute, 39, 44
Solution, 39, 44
Solution incompatibilities, 189–190
Solvent, 39, 44
Somatic motor neurons, 89f
Somatic nerves, 52
Somatotropin *(Humatrope)*, 408, 411
Somatrem *(Protropin)*, 411
Sotalol *(Betapace)*, 252
Sparfloxacin *(Zagam)*, 505t
Spasmogenic activity, 194, 202–203
Spinal anesthesia, 99, 102
Spinal cord, 114
Spironolactone *(Aldactone)*, 269t, 273–274, 274t
Spironolactone and hydrochlorothiazide *(Aldactazide)*, 274t
Sponges, hemostatic, 301
SRS-A (slow-reacting substance of anaphylaxis), 359, 360
SSRIs (selective serotonin reuptake inhibitors), 147–148, 147t, 149
Stanozolol *(Winstrol)*, 442t
-static, definition of, 557
Statins, 325–326
Status asthmaticus, 187

Status epilepticus, 167, 171
Stavudine (d4T, Zerit), 525, 528t, 529, 531, 533, 536t
Sterilization, 557, 559
Steroids, 416
    adrenal, 415–424
Stevens-Johnson syndrome, 504, 546
Streptokinase (Streptase), 299–300
Streptomycin, 19, 189, 501t
Stress, 417
Stroke volume (SV), 280
Subcutaneous (SC), administration, 18t
Sublingual, administration, 18t
Succinimides, 170
Succinylcholine (Anectine, Quelicin, Sucostrin), 88–91, 89f, 90t, 188, 189
Sucralfate (Carafate), 372f, 376, 386–387, 391
Sufentanil (Sufenta), 197t, 198t
Sulbactam, 499
Sulconazole (Exelderm), 515t
Sulfacetamide (Sulamyd), 503t
Sulfadoxine, 544
Sulfadoxine-pyrimethamine (Fansidar), 545t
Sulfameter (Sulla), 503t
Sulfamethizole (Thiosulfil), 503t
Sulfamethoxazole (Gantanol), 503t, 537t
Sulfanilamide, 503
Sulfasalazine (Azulfidine), 503t
Sulfinpyrazone (Anturane), 223t, 224, 226t
Sulfisoxazole (Gantrisin), 503t
Sulfonamides, 503–504, 503t, 549, 551t
Sulfonylureas, 534t, 535t
Sulindac (Clinoril), 214, 215t, 223t
Summation, 25t
Suppositories, 16, 402
Suppressor T-cells, 577, 578f
Supraventricular arrhythmia, 245, 246
Suspension, 468
Sympathetic blocking drugs, 282–283, 283t
Sympathetic nervous system, 51, 52–54, 53f, 54f, 54t, 57–66, 132
Sympatholytic, 58, 59
Sympathomimetic, 58, 59, 122
Synergism, 25t, 184, 188
Synesthesia, 154, 155
Synthetic drugs, 194, 196
Systemic, definition of, 371
Systemic mastocystis, 378

Tablets, 16
TAC (tetracaine, adrenaline, cocaine), 100, 101t
Tacrine (Cognex), 74t, 876
Tacrolimus (Prograf), 579–580
Tamoxifen (Nolvadex), 571
Tamsulosin (Flomax), 63t
Tapeworms, 549–550, 550t
Tardive dyskinesia, 132, 133
Target organ, 408, 409
Tazobactam, 499
TBG (thyroxine-binding globulin), 452
TCAs (tricyclic antidepressants), 145–147, 146t, 147t, 149, 160
T-cells, 577–581
Tegaserod (Zelmac), 382, 383, 383t
Telmisartan (Micardis), 285
Temazepam (Restoril), 121t, 123, 137t
Tenesmus, 543, 547
Teniposide (Vumon), 570, 571t
Teratogenicity, 23, 24t, 567, 569, 576, 579
Terazosin (Hytrin), 63t

Terbinafine (Lamisil), 515t, 517, 535t
Terbutaline (Brethine), 61t, 362t, 487, 488t
Terconazole (Terazol-3, Terazol-7), 515t
Terfenadine (Seldane), 353, 532, 534t, 535t, 536t
Terminology, related to drug effects, 4
Terpin hydrate, 201
Testosterone, 441–444, 442t, 445
Testosterone (Andro-LA 200, Delatestryl, Depo-Testosterone, Depotest 100, 200, Duratest-100, 200, Everone 200, Testosterone Enanthate), 442t
Testosterone (Histerone 100, Tesamone Testosterone Aqueous), 442t
Testosterone (Testosterone propionate), 442t
Testosterone transdermal system (Transderm, Androderm), 442t
Tetanus antitoxin, 45
Tetany, 456, 485, 486
Tetracaine (Protocaine), 101t, 105
Tetracycline(s) (Doxycycline, Sumycin), 189, 336, 373, 392, 502–503, 502t, 546–548, 547t
Tetrahydrocannabinol (THC), 154, 160, 161
Tetrahydrozoline (Tyzine, Visine), 60t
Thalamus, 111, 113–114
Thalidomide, 24t
Theobromine, 269t, 274, 361
Theophylline, 269t, 274, 361–362, 534t, 535t, 537t
Therapeutic drug range, 21f
Therapeutic effect, 4, 5
Therapeutic index (TI), 3, 7
Thiabendazole (Mintezol), 550t
Thiamin (Thiamilate, Biamine), 313
Thiamylal (Surital), 186, 187t
Thiazide diuretics, 269t, 271–273, 272t
Thiethylperazine (Torecan), 390t
Thimerosal (Merthiolate), 557, 558t, 561, 561t
Thiopental (Pentothal), 185, 186, 187, 187t, 189
Thioridazine (Mellaril), 134t
Thiotepa, 569t
Thiothixene (Navane), 134t
Thioxanthenes, 134t, 135
Thrombin (Thrombogen, Thrombostat), 301
Thrombocyte, 288
Thrombocytopenia, 291–292, 295
Thromboembolism, 288, 289
Thrombolytic enzymes, 299–300
Thrombophlebitis, 289, 290, 438, 440
Thromboplastin, 289
Thromboxane, 294
Thrombus, 289, 301
Thrush, 512
Thyrocalcitonin, 451
Thyroid (desiccated thyroid) (Armour Thyroid, S-P-T, Thyrar), 452t
Thyroid gland
    antithyroid drugs, 454–456, 455t
    function, 451, 451f
    hormonal control of, 411–412, 411f
    hormone replacement, 452–454, 452t
    hypersecretion of hormones, 454
    hyposecretion of hormones, 451–452
Thyroid-stimulating hormone (TSH), 410t, 411–412, 451–455, 451f, 452t
Thyrotoxic crisis, 451, 455
Thyrotropic-releasing hormone (TRH), 412
Thyroxine, 411–412, 451–455, 451f, 452t
Thyroxine-binding globulin (TBG), 452

Tiagabine (Gabitril), 170–171
Ticarcillin disodium (Ticar), 498, 498t
Ticlopidine (Ticlid), 290, 293t, 294
Tiludronate (Skelid), 457t, 458, 460
Time-response curve, 6–7, 6f
Timolol (Blocadren), 64t
Tinea, 512, 513t, 517
Tioconazole (Vagistat-1), 515t
Tissue plasminogen activator (tPA), 289, 299
Tizanidine (Zanaflex), 92, 93, 93t
Tobramycin (Nebcin), 501t
Tocainide (Tonocard), 251
Tocolytics, 487–488, 488t
Tolazamide (Tolinase), 473, 474t
Tolbutamide (Orinase), 473, 474t, 475
Tolcapone (Tasmar), 178
Tolerance, 14, 25–26, 154, 155, 194
    amphetamine, 158
    barbiturate, 122
    cocaine, 159
    LSD, 156
    marijuana, 162
    opioid, 196, 203
    PCP, 160
Tolmetin (Tolectin), 214, 215t
Tolnaftate (Aftate, NP-27, Tinactin, Ting), 513, 513t, 515t
Tolterodine (Detrol, Detrol-LA), 77t
Tonic, definition of, 167
Tonic-clonic seizures, 167
Topical administration, 17, 18t, 99, 100, 102
Topical antifungals, 517, 518
Torsemide (Demadex), 269t, 273, 274t
Total parenteral nutrition (TPN), 306, 316
Tourette's disorder, 135
Toxic effect, 3, 4, 7
Toxicology, 4t
Toxoplasma gondii, 548–549
Trade name, 8, 44
Tramadol (Ultram), 198t
Trandolapril (MAVIK), 284t
Tranquilization, 132
Tranquilizers, 188, 189t
Transdermal absorption, 428, 430
Transdermal administration, 18t
Transdermal products, 16
Tranylcypromine (Parnate), 145t, 354t
Trazodone (Desyrel), 148
Tretinoin (Accutane, Retin-A), 310
TRH (thyrotropic-releasing hormone), 412
Triacetin (Fungoid, Ony-Clear Nail), 515t
Triamcinolone (Aristocort, Atolone, Azmacort, Aristospan, Kenacort, Kenalog-40), 363t, 418t, 422t
Triamterene (Dyrenium), 269t, 273, 276
Triazolam (Halcion), 121t, 123–124, 137t, 534t
Trichlormethiazide (Diurese, Metahydrin, Naqua), 269t, 272t
Trichomoniasis, 543, 549
Triclosan/irgasan (Septisoft, Septisol), 558t
Tricyclic antidepressants (TCAs), 145–147, 146t, 147t, 149, 160
Trifluoperazine (Stelazine), 134t
Triflupromazine (Vesprin), 134t, 352, 389
Trifluridine (Viroptic), 525, 526, 527t, 530
Triglycerides, 321, 322–323, 324f, 325, 327, 329
Trihexyphenidyl (Artane), 179, 179t
Triiodothyronine, 451–455, 451f
Trimethadione (Tridione), 168t, 170, 171
Trimethaphan, 83

Trimethobenzamide *(Tigan)*, 390t
Trimethoprim, 537t
Trimethoprim-sulfamethoxazole *(Septra, Bactrim)*, 401, 504
Trimipramine *(Surmontil)*, 146t
Triphasic, 428, 430
Triprolidine *(Zymine)*, 351t
Triprolidine/pseudoephedrine *(Actagen, Actifed)*, 351t
Troches, 16
Troglitazone *(Rezulin)*, 479–480
Troleandomycin, 354t
Tropic, definition of, 416
Tropic hormones, 416
Tryptamine derivatives, 156
TSH (thyroid-stimulating hormone), 410t, 411–412, 451–455, 451f, 452t
Tuberculosis, 506–507
Tubocurarine, 90t, 188
Tubular reabsorption, 266–268
Tubular secretion, 266, 268
Tumor, 567
Tumor necrosis factor (TNF-alpha), 580

Ulcerogenic drugs, 371, 373
Ulcers, 371
    management of, 373, 374t–375t, 391
    production of, 371, 373
    sites of, 372f
Undecylenic acid *(Breeze Mist Aerosol, Cruex, Desenex)*, 513, 515t
United States Pharmacopeia/National Formulary (USP/NF), 8
Urea *(Ureaphil)*, 269t, 270, 270t
Uremia, 266, 268
Uric acid, 222–224, 222f, 224f
Urinary retention, 75–76
Urofollitropin *(Metrodin)*, 437–438
Urokinase *(Abbokinase)*, 299–300
U.S.-Recommended Daily Allowance (U.S.-RDA), 307
Uterine muscle, drugs affecting
    oxytocics, 486–487, 488t
    tocolytics, 487–488, 488t

Vaccine, influenza, 520–521
Vaginal, administration, 18t
Vagolytic, 88, 90
Valacyclovir *(Valtrex)*, 527t, 529, 531
Valdecoxib *(Bextra)*, 214, 216t
Valproic acid *(Depakene)*, 168t, 169, 171, 551, 551t
Valsartan *(Diovan)*, 285
Vancomycin *(Vancocin)*, 506
Vascular effects of drugs. *See also* Cardiovascular effects of drugs
    alcohol, 125
    local anesthetics, 102

Vasoconstriction, 99, 102
Vasodilation, 99, 102
Vasodilators, 88, 90
    for congestive heart failure, 241–242, 242t
    for hypertension, 283
    interaction with ganglionic blocking agents, 84t
Vasopressin, 485–486
Vasopressin injection *(Pitressin)*, 485, 488t
Vasospastic angina, 256, 257
Vecuronium *(Norcuron)*, 90t
Venlafaxine *(Effexor)*, 148
Ventricular fibrillation, 245, 246t, 247
Verapamil *(Calan, Isoptin)*, 241, 248t, 252–253, 259, 283, 284t
Very-low-density lipoprotein (VLDL), 322, 325–327
Vidarabine *(Ara-A, Vira-A)*, 525, 526, 527t, 530
Vinblastine *(Velban)*, 537t, 570, 571t
Vincent's infection, 561
Vincristine *(Oncovin)*, 537t, 570, 571t
Vinorelbine *(Navelbine)*, 571t
Viral infections
    antiviral drugs, 524–533, 525f, 527t–528t, 535t–537t
    herpes, 521, 526, 530
    human immunodeficiency virus (HIV), 521–524, 522t, 523t
    influenza, 519–521, 526, 530
    propagation of virus, 523
Virilization, 428, 443
Visceral nerves, 52
Vitamin A
    clinical indications, 309–310
    contraindications, 310
    deficiency, 310
    function in body, 309
    overdose, 310
    patient administration and monitoring, 317
    products, 310
    source, 309
Vitamin B_{12} (cyanocobalamin), 313, 336–338, 338t
Vitamin C (ascorbic acid), 314, 317
Vitamin D (cholecalciferol), 456–457
    clinical indications, 310–311
    deficiency, 311
    drug interactions, 311
    function in the body, 310–311
    overdose, 311
    patient administration and monitoring, 317
    products, 311
    source, 310

Vitamin E
    clinical indications, 312
    deficiency, 312
    drug interactions, 312
    function in the body, 311
    overdose, 312
    products, 312
    source, 311
Vitamin K_1 (phytonadione), 292, 293, 294, 312
Vitamin K_3 (menadione), 294
Vitamin K_4 (menadiol), 294
Vitamins, 309–314. *See also specific vitamins*
    B vitamins, 313–314
    deficiency, 307t
    fat-soluble, 309–312
    recommended dietary allowance, 307t
    water-soluble, 312–314
VLDL (very-low-density lipoprotein), 322, 325–327
Volume in volume (V/V), 44
Volumes, conversion table of, 43
Vomiting, 387, 388f, 390t. *See also* Emesis
Vomiting center, 200, 200f, 387, 389 388f

Warfarin, 24t, 292, 293t
Weight, body, 22, 46
Weight in volume (W/V), 44
Weight in weight (W/W), 44
Weights, conversion table of, 43
Wernicke's encephalopathy, 126
Withdrawal
    amphetamine, 158
    barbiturate, 122
    cocaine, 159
    LSD, 156
    marijuana, 162
    opioids, 204
    PCP, 160

Xanthine derivatives, 269t, 274
Xerostomia, 347, 352

Yohimbine *(Aphrodyne)*, 63t

Zafirlukast *(Accolate)*, 364
Zalcitabine *(ddC, Hivid)*, 525, 526, 528t, 529, 531, 537t
Zaleplon *(Sonata)*, 121t, 125
Zanamivir *(Relenza)*, 524, 526, 529, 530
Zidovudine *(Retrovir)*, 340, 525, 526, 528t, 531, 532, 534t, 535t, 536t, 537t
Zileuton *(Zyflo)*, 364
Zinc undecylenate, 513t
Zollinger-Ellison syndrome, 378–379
Zolpidem *(Ambien)*, 121t, 124–125